Immunization

CHILDHOOD AND TRAVEL HEALTH

This fourth edition edition
is dedicated to my wife Karen
and our children Juliana,
Nicholas and Alexis
for their love and unfailing support.

Immunization

CHILDHOOD AND TRAVEL HEALTH

GEORGE C. KASSIANOS
General Medical Practitioner

FOREWORD BY
PROFESSOR MIKE PRINGLE CBE

Blackwell
Science

© 1990, 1994, 1998, 2001 by
Blackwell Science Ltd
Editorial Offices:
Osney Mead, Oxford OX2 0EL
25 John Street, London WC1N 2BS
23 Ainslie Place, Edinburgh EH3 6AJ
350 Main Street, Malden
  MA 02148-5018, USA
54 University Street, Carlton
  Victoria 3053, Australia
10, rue Casimir Delavigne
  75006 Paris, France

Other Editorial Offices:
Blackwell Wissenschafts-Verlag
GmbH
Kurfürstendamm 57
10707 Berlin, Germany

Blackwell Science KK
MG Kodenmacho Building
7–10 Kodenmacho Nihombashi
Chuo-ku, Tokyo 104, Japan

Iowa State University Press
A Blackwell Science Company
2121 S. State Avenue
Ames, Iowa 50014-8300, USA

First published 1990
Fourth edition 2001

Set by BookEns Ltd, Royston, Herts
Printed and bound in Great Britain
by The Alden Press, Oxford and
Northampton.

The Blackwell Science logo is a
trade mark of Blackwell Science Ltd,
registered at the United Kingdom
Trade Marks Registry

A catalogue record for this title
is available from the British Library

ISBN 0-632-05581-2

Library of Congress
Cataloging-in-publication Data

Kassianos, George C.
  Immunization: childhood and
travel health
  / G.C. Kassianos; foreword by Mike
Pringle.–4th ed.
    p.; cm.
  Includes bibliographical references
and index.
  ISBN 0-632-05581-2
  1. Immunization of children–
Handbooks, manuals, etc. 2. Travel–
Health aspects–Handbooks, manuals, etc.
3. Immunization–Handbooks, manuals,
etc. 4. Vaccination–Handbooks,
manuals, etc.
I. Title. [DNLM: 1. Immunization–
Child–Handbooks.
2. Communicable Disease Control–
Handbooks.
3. Disease Outbreaks–Handbooks.
4. Travel–Handbooks. 5. Vaccines–
Handbooks. QW 39 K19i 2000]
RJ20 .K37 2000
614.4'7–dc21   00-051941

DISTRIBUTORS
Marston Book Services Ltd
PO Box 269
Abingdon, Oxon OX14 4YN
(*Orders*: Tel: 01235 465500
       Fax: 01235 465555)

USA
Blackwell Science, Inc.
Commerce Place
350 Main Street
Malden, MA 02148-5018
(*Orders*: Tel: 800 759 6102
              781 388 8250
       Fax: 781 388 8255)

Canada
Login Brothers Book Company
324 Saulteaux Crescent
Winnipeg, Manitoba R3J 3T2
(*Orders*: Tel: 204 837 2987)

Australia
Blackwell Science Pty Ltd
54 University Street
Carlton, Victoria 3053
(*Orders*: Tel: 3 9347 0300
           Fax: 3 9347 5001)

For further information on
Blackwell Science, visit our website:
www.blackwell-science.com

Contents

Part 5
Travel Health

Part 6
Immunization and Travel Information Resources

Foreword

It is a pleasure to write a foreword to the fourth edition of this remarkable book. In it George Kassianos offers even more advice and information and has updated the previous edition. Even more so than before, this is now the indispensable bible of the control of infectious disease, especially for primary healthcare.

When I was a medical student, the emphasis on infectious diseases was low. Tuberculosis was 'beaten'. Smallpox was being eradicated. Diphtheria, rheumatic fever and tetanus were becoming increasingly rare. For other bacterial diseases, antibiotics gave a sense of complacency. In a large part these successes were a result of improved living conditions and sanitation in the UK. However, they were also the result of an alliance between general practice and public health medicine in applying the new sciences of immunization, vaccination and disease control.

Those optimistic days are long past. While successes such as smallpox and diphtheria are still with us, the re-emergence of infections such as tuberculosis, the advent of antibiotic resistance, and the emergence of new types of meningitis and hepatitis and the spread of HIV have all dramatically raised the profile of infectious disease.

General practice has a key part to play. For prevention to be effective, immunizations and vaccines must be available and made acceptable. This means overcoming some understandable fears, counselling patients and parents, and ensuring that all are educated in the availability and benefits of such procedures. And this book is an essential part of that enterprise. Only with accurate and consistent messages can we persuade the public to join with us in the prevention of these major causes of morbidity and mortality.

But the contents of this book go much wider. Many infectious diseases are more common abroad and foreign travel advice is an important facet of modern general practice. Every practice needs to take this responsibility seriously and needs access to authoritative advice, as given here.

I recommend this valuable book to general practitioners, practice nurses and all those concerned with the reduction in infectious diseases in the UK.

Professor Mike Pringle, CBE
Council Chairman
Royal College of General Practitioners

Preface

It is now generally accepted that no other measure taken by man, apart from the provision of clean water, has ever saved more lives than immunization against infectious disease. Vaccines are among the safest and most successful public health tools available for preventing infectious diseases and their complications. Immunization is one of the areas at the forefront of family care in general practice. Effective and safe immunization, providing lasting immunity against infectious diseases, has made a major contribution to human welfare. Smallpox has been eradicated and, in countries with successful immunization programmes, we are witnessing virtual elimination of tetanus, diphtheria, poliomyelitis, pertussis, measles, mumps and rubella. The better the immunization programme, the greater the reduction in the morbidity and mortality of both bacterial and viral infectious diseases. *Failure to control infectious disease is primarily not because of vaccine failure but vaccination failure.*

Vaccines have provided us with the means of living without infectious disease. By using the vaccine to immunize, we aim to prevent infectious disease in the individual and the community. The ultimate goal of immunization is to eradicate infectious disease.

In 1974, when the Expanded Programme on Immunization (EPI) was launched by the WHO, less than 5% of the world's children were immunized against the six target diseases—diphtheria, tetanus, whooping cough, poliomyelitis, measles and tuberculosis—during their first years of life. By 1994, almost 80% of children under one, throughout the world, were immunized against these target diseases.

None the less, vaccine-preventable diseases kill 3 million children every year [Gwatkin D.R. & Guillot M. (1999) *The burden of disease among the global poor*. World Bank, Washington DC]. Millions more die from diseases, such as malaria and AIDS, that should be preventable by vaccines if they have been successfully developed. AIDS, tuberculosis, measles, malaria, diarrhoeal diseases such as dysentery and cholera, and acute respiratory infections such as pneumonia were responsible for 90% of all deaths due to infectious diseases around the world in 1998.

Unfortunately, existing vaccines are not reaching these millions of children because of failure in delivery systems, lack of resources, and high price of some newer vaccines. Moreover, new vaccines may not be developed because private companies cannot foresee a good return. The same has already happened with drugs. Of 1223 drugs developed between 1975 and 1997 only 11 were for tropical conditions [Trouiller P.T. & Olliaro P.I. (1999) Drug development output from 1975 to 1996: what proportions for tropical diseases? *Int. J. Infect. Dis.* 3, 61–3].

Infectious disease kills 17 million people worldwide every year. The WHO is aiming to stop neonatal tetanus and congenital rubella, as well as eliminate poliomyelitis from the world by the year 2000 (realistically this has been put back to year 2002 and after). It had a policy for universal hepatitis B immunization by the year 1997 but not all countries (including the UK) have taken up the challenge.

A new third world vaccination programme was launched in the year 2000, courtesy of Bill Gates' charitable foundation. The Global Fund for Children's Vaccines, which received $750 million from Gates, has made initial grants of $150 million to fund hepatitis B immunization programmes in 13 countries, including Cambodia, Mozambique and Rwanda. Around 30 million children do not have complete protection against vaccine-preventable diseases, and 3 million die every year.

Dramatic advances in molecular biology and the use of genetic engineering techniques are ensuring that over the next few years we will witness the introduction of a new generation of vaccines that will save the lives of millions of children every year. They include improved existing vaccines as well as vaccines for diseases for which no vaccines currently exist. We are going to see a range of combination vaccines as well as new delivery systems (oral, nasal).

In most circumstances immunization, particularly of young children, is an elective procedure. The vaccines used to immunize children against infectious diseases are among the safest medicines available to health professionals. It is, therefore, important to ascertain that no contraindications exist before any vaccination is carried out. *To deny a child vaccination can be to deny that child health.*

The aim of immunization is to protect the individual from suffering from serious infections, prevent local outbreaks, achieve high levels of immunization uptake thus creating 'herd immunity', prevent epidemics and eradicate infectious disease. Despite, or perhaps because of, the success of the UK immunization programme some parents have come to doubt the need to have their children immunized, particularly with the measles, mumps and rubella combined vaccine. This (in)action not only places their own children at risk, but also the population as a whole.

Part of the GP's and nurse's work is confidently to promote the benefits of immunization. This has to be done in the face of sporadic media scares and not only some hostility but also apathy among a minority of our patients.

Immunization is the most cost-effective public health intervention. The benefits of immunization are greatly under-recognized by a number of people. Vaccines have safely and effectively prevented more disease and death than any other medical intervention or treatment, including antibiotics. Improvement in living conditions, sanitation and the provision of clean water along with vaccines are contributing to the reduction in the loss of life all over the world.

In England and Wales we have seen a dramatic reduction of cases of infectious disease notified, thanks to the dedication of the healthcare workers, the Department of Health, the vaccine manufacturers and the availability of vaccines. Table 1 below shows the maximum number of cases notified in England and Wales in one year compared to the number notified in 1998. Soon we shall see the replacement of infectious disease by heart disease as the biggest killer in the world. Table 2 below shows the ten top causes of death in 1990 and those projected in year 2020 as estimated by the Harvard School of Public Health.

Table 1

	Number of cases reported	Maximum (year)	In 1998
Diphtheria	46,281	(1940)	23
Tetanus	24	(1976)	7
Pertussis	>100,000	(1975)	1,577
Poliomyelitis	4,000	(1955)	1
*Haemoph.infl.*b	1,259	(1989)	29
Measles	800,000	(1968)	3,728
Mumps	20,713	(1989)	1,587
Rubella	24,570	(1989)	3,208
Tuberculosis	50,000	(1950)	6,087

Members of the primary care team involved in immunization should speak with one voice and give similar and consistent advice and information to parents. This book is intended to help the GP, practice nurse and health visitor to present a united front in the fight for the total elimination of infectious diseases.

This fourth edition has been greatly revised and extended to include comprehensive advice on all immunizations performed in general practice. The previous style of starting with the contraindications to the vaccine and side-effects has been

Table 2

	1990	2020
1	Respiratory infections	Heart disease
2	Diarrhoeal disease	Severe depression
3	Complications of birth	Traffic accidents
4	Severe depression	Stroke
5	Heart disease	Chronic pulmonary disease
6	Stroke	Respiratory infections
7	Tuberculosis	Tuberculosis
8	Measles	War injuries
9	Traffic accidents	Diarrhoeal disease
10	Congenital anomalies	HIV/AIDS

retained, as this is the most commonly sought information in busy clinics.

I am very grateful to all those who have helped in the production of this book at Blackwell Science. Also to Ursula Shine and Jeannette Martin for their useful comments, and the Medical Information and Vaccines Departments of Aventis Pasteur MSD and SmithKline Beecham for their assistance. Special thanks to Usha Gungabissoon, information officer at the London Public Health Laboratory Service, Communicable Disease Surveillance Centre, Immunization Division.

Finally, I would welcome and value any reader feedback. Please contact me on authors@blacksci.co.uk.

George C. Kassianos

List of abbreviations

AAFB	Acid and alcohol-fast bacilli
ABPI	Association of British Pharmaceutical Industry
ACIP	Advisory Committee on Immunization Practices (USA)
Ads	Adsorbed
AIDS	Acquired immune deficiency syndrome
Anti-HBc	Antibody to hepatitis B core antigen
Anti-HBe	Antibody to hepatitis B e antigen
Anti-HBs	Antibody to hepatitis B surface antigen
APV	Acellular pertussis vaccine
BCG	Bacillus Calmette–Guérin vaccine
BMA	British Medical Association
BNF	British National Formulary
BP	British Pharmacopoeia
BW	Body weight
CABG	Coronary artery by-pass graft
CDC	Centers for Disease Control and Prevention (USA)
CDSC	Communicable Disease Surveillance Centre
CMO	Chief Medical Officer
COCP	Combined oral contraceptive pill
COPD	Chronic obstructive pulmonary disease
CRS	Congenital rubella syndrome
CSM	Committee on Safety of Medicines
d	Low-dose diphtheria vaccine for adults
DHF	Dengue haemorrhagic fever
DNA	Deoxyribonucleic acid
DoH	Department of Health
DOTS	Directly observed treatment short course
DT	Diphtheria/tetanus combined vaccine
DTaP	Diphtheria/tetanus/acellular pertussis combined vaccine
DTP, DTwP	Diphtheria/tetanus whole-cell pertussis combined vaccine
EEA	European Economic Area
eIPV	Enhanced potency inactivated polio myelitis vaccine
ELISA	Enzyme-linked immunosorbent assay
EPI	Expanded Programme on Immunization
ERVL	Enteric and Respiratory Virus Laboratory
ETEC	Enterotoxinogenic *Escherichia coli*
EU	European Union
FP10	General Practitioner's prescription
GMC	General Medical Council
GP	General Practitioner (family doctor)
h	Hour
HAV	Hepatitis A virus
HB	Hepatitis B
HBeAg	Hepatitis B e antigen
HBIG	Hepatitis B immunoglobulin
HBsAg	Hepatitis B surface antigen
HBV	Hepatitis B virus
HCV	Hepatitis C virus
HDCV	Human diploid cells virus
HEV	Hepatitis E virus
Hib	*Haemophilus influenzae* b
HIV	Human immunodeficiency virus
HNIG	Human normal immunoglobulin
HVZIG	Human varicella-zoster immunoglobulin
ID	Intradermal
Ig	Immunoglobulin
IHPS	Infantile hypertrophic pyloric stenosis
IM	Intramuscular
IOS	Item of service
IPV	Inactivated poliomyelitis vaccine

IU	International unit	PCR	Polymerase chain reaction
IV	Intravenous	PCT	Primary Care Trust
kg	kilogram	PHLS	Public Health Laboratory Services
L	litre	POEC	Progesterone-only emergency
LMWH	Low molecular weight heparin		contraception
m	Months	POM	Prescription-only medicine
Map	*Mycobacterium avium*	POP	Progesterone-only pill
	paratuberculosis	PPA	Prescription Pricing Authority
MASTA	Medical Advisory Service for	RIBA	Recombinant immunoblot assay
	Travellers Abroad	RNA	Ribonucleic acid
MCA	Medicines Control Agency	RVA	Rabies vaccine adsorbed
MDR	Multiple drug resistance	s	seconds
MenC	Meningococcal C conjugate vaccine	SC	Subcutaneous
min	Minutes	SFA	Statement of Fees and Allowances
MMR	Measles/mumps/rubella combined	SIDS	Sudden Infant Death Syndrome
	vaccine	SSPE	Subacute sclerosing panencephalitis
NOIDS	Notifications of Infectious Diseases	Td	Tetanus and low-dose diphtheria
OMP	Outer membrane protein		vaccine for adults and adolescents
ONS	Office for National Statistics	UK	United Kingdom
OP	Original pack	UKCC	United Kingdom Central Council
OPCS	Office of Population Censuses and		for Nursing, Midwifery and
	Surveys		Health Visiting
OPV	Oral poliomyelitis vaccine	US/USA	United States of America
OTC	Over the counter medicine	VAPP	Vaccine-associated paralytic
PA	Per annum		poliomyelitis
PCG	Primary Care Group	VZV	Varicella-zoster virus
PCEC	Prurified chicken embryo cell	WHO	World Health Organization
PCO	Primary Care Organisation		

Part 1

Introduction to
Immunization and Vaccines

Chapter 1

History of immunization

There is no doubt that immunizations have had a profound impact upon the incidence and prevalence of infectious diseases in the whole world. The vaccines have been used mainly in two ways: on an individual basis to protect specific persons at risk, and on a population basis to provide 'herd immunity', which is so important in combating infectious disease.

The origins of modern immunology are a matter of controversy. Some researches attribute fundamental notions about contagion and resistance to ancient Greek medicine, particularly to the Hippocratic notion of a constitution

The observation that recovery from smallpox prevented subsequent attacks of the disease was made in both ancient Greece and China. The concept of the protective effect of 'immunity' was established. About 1000 years ago the Chinese developed the technique of obtaining dried crusts from the pustules of smallpox patients, grinding them up and making them into powder, which was blown into the nose of the person being protected. Their aim was to induce immunity after a mild illness. This was perhaps the first attempt to induce immunity artificially by the process of immunization. This method of protection was not taken up to any significant extent outside the Far East at the time.

At the beginning of the eighteenth century it was becoming known that in the Middle East 'variolation' was being practiced. This involved the introduction of material from smallpox crusts into scarified areas of the skin, usually on the arm. The recipient would develop a mild form of the disease and then be afforded some protection against it. Variolation was introduced into Britain in 1721 by **Lady Mary Wortley Montagu** (1679–1762) who volunteered her daughter to be variolated. Lady Mary had observed the technique while she was in Constantinople, where her husband was the British ambassador to Turkey. During the same year this new technique was also introduced in America.

In the years 1720 and 1721, London was in the grip of a smallpox epidemic. Caroline, Princess of Wales, had seen one of her daughters nearly die from smallpox and sought to protect her other children by the new method introduced to England by Lady Montagu. Before going ahead with the treatment, Caroline requested that it be tried out on condemned prisoners. In 1721, an experiment was performed on six 'volunteers' from Newgate prison. Following variolation five developed mild smallpox but survived. The sixth had already had smallpox therefore no reaction was seen. They were duly pardoned. In order to test the technique, one of the five was later employed to work in an area with a high incidence of smallpox. When a local boy developed smallpox, she was ordered 'to lie every night in the same bed with this boy, and to attend him constantly from the first beginning of the distemper to the very end'. The experiment was thought to be successful as, in spite of this close contact, she did not develop smallpox.

In the eighteenth century in Britain, it was observed that dairymaids and cowmen did not seem to catch smallpox, although they were prone to develop cowpox. This observation led a Hampshire farmer, **Benjamin Jesty**, to believe he could protect his family against smallpox by 'inoculating' (the term was introduced around this time by the physician Emmanuel Timoni) them with cowpox material. Similar propositions were put forward by Jon Fauster, an apothecary, in 1765.

Twenty-two years later, on 14 May 1796, the first scientific attempt at immunization was made by **Edward Jenner** (1749–1823) in a hut in the garden of

18th century	Smallpox 1796
19th century	Anthrax 1881, rabies 1885, diphtheria antitoxin 1891, plague 1897, cholera 1896, typhoid 1898
Early 20th century	BCG 1921, diphtheria toxoid 1923, pertussis 1926, tetanus 1927, yellow fever 1935, influenza 1945
Post World War II	Poliomyelitis (injectable 1955, oral 1962) measles (1960), mumps (1967), rubella (1962), pneumococcal, meningococcal, *Haemophilus influenzae* b, hepatitis A (1992), hepatitis B (1981)

Table 1.1 The development of human vaccination.

his house in Berkeley, Gloucestershire. Jenner took some material from a cowpox pustule on the arm of Sarah Nelmes, a milkmaid, and scratched this into the arm of a young local boy named James Phipps. Young James developed a pustule and a mild fever following the experiment. He remained healthy when three months later Edward Jenner inoculated him with smallpox. This was the beginning of 'vaccination' (see Table 1.1 for the development of human vaccination).

Edward Jenner published his work in 1798 under the title *An inquiry into the causes and effects of the variolae vaccinae*. The word 'vaccinae' means 'of the cow'. The original meaning of the word 'vaccination' means 'protection against smallpox'. In the 50 years following Jenner's first inoculation, the number of deaths from smallpox in England fell from about 23 000 to 5000 a year. In 1853 smallpox vaccination of infants within 4 months of birth became compulsory in England. By 1980, smallpox had been eradicated from the world.

After Edward Jenner, the world had to wait for about a century for the next major advance which came from the work of **Louis Pasteur** (1822–1895), a brilliant chemist, physicist and microbiologist (he was not a medical practitioner). His earliest work on microbes, a term he coined from the Greek, was carried out when studying ways of preventing wine, beer and vinegar from spoiling. His discovery of the tiny creatures that spoiled these products, and his invention of a method of destroying them by heating the product, such as wine, to 60° C for a few moments, now known as 'pasteurization', has led to innumerable benefits for both industry and public health.

His aim was always prevention of disease. His

words reflect exactly this: 'When meditating over a disease, I never think of finding a remedy for it, but instead a means of preventing it.' He worked tirelessly and with passion in his laboratory observing and experimenting. 'Nothing great has ever been accomplished without passion' was one of his comments. Speaking at his installation as professor and dean of the Faculty of Science, University of Lille, on 7 December 1854, he said: 'In the field of observation, chance only favours prepared minds.'

His work on the fatal illness of sheep called anthrax ('splenic fever') led to the discovery of the basic principles of immunity. Pasteur treated cultures of the anthrax bacillus in various ways until he found that microbes grown at a particular temperature range became harmless without losing their capability to provoke resistance in injected animals.

He demonstrated his new discovery in 1881 in front of the public and many scientists. Virulent cultures of the anthrax bacillus were injected into healthy sheep and an equal number of sheep previously inoculated with attenuated, harmless cultures. Within a few days all the unprotected sheep died and all the prepared sheep remained well. Pasteur had by now established the principal of immunity that attenuated cultures of an organism could afford protection against the disease caused by that organism. Jenner had obtained the same protection from smallpox by producing another illness, vaccinia or cowpox. Pasteur paid tribute to Jenner's work by calling his own method 'vaccination'.

Louis Pasteur's greatest achievement, however, was the discovery of a rabies vaccine. This followed earlier work he had undertaken on anthrax which had shown him, as mentioned above, that old, and therefore weakened, bacilli could be injected into an animal, producing a mild form of the disease and giving lasting immunity. Partly paralysed by a stroke, Pasteur would work long hours in his laboratories with his assistants, **Pierre Roux** and **Charles Chamberland**, trying to identify the rabies organism, which he called virus from the Latin word for poison. All attempts to grow it *in vitro* failed. However, he succeeded in growing the rabies virus in the brain and spinal cord. He went on to discover a way of reducing its strength so that, when injected into an animal, it would give immunity without causing the disease.

On 6 July 1885, nine-year-old Joseph Meister from Alsace was bitten by a rabid dog. The family doctor believed he must risk vaccination or face a certain death. Pasteur injected young Joseph with the first of 14 daily doses of rabbit spinal cord suspensions containing progressively inactivated rabies virus. The vaccination was completely successful and Joseph Meister went on to become concierge at the Pasteur Institute in Paris. In 1940, he killed himself rather than admit the invading Nazis to the crypt where Pasteur is buried. Pasteur's method was so successful that it was rapidly adopted throughout the world.

Robert Koch (1843–1910) described the anthrax bacillus. In 1882 he isolated the tubercle bacillus and in 1883 the cholera bacillus. By 1884 he was able to define the four conditions that should be satisfied if the cause of a particular disease was to be ascribed to an organism:

- the organism must be present in every case of the disease;
- the organism must be isolated and grown as a pure culture;
- the culture should produce the disease when inoculated into a susceptible animal;
- the organism must be recovered from an infected animal and grown again as a pure culture.

Addressing a scientific meeting in Berlin, on 28 November 1902, Robert Koch advanced the idea of a healthy carrier of infection and applied it to the epidemiology of typhoid fever.

Two former assistants of Robert Koch first provided a treatment for the horrifying disease of diphtheria. **Emil von Behring** (1854–1917) and **Shibasaburo Kitasato** (1852–1931) were first to observe the formation of an antibody to a toxin—

in this case, the toxin produced by the diphtheria bacillus. Von Behring showed that the body had a natural defence mechanism against toxins and that an animal injected with a sublethal dose of diphtheria bacilli would form antibodies, or antitoxins, which would enable it to fight off a later attack of the disease. On Christmas Eve 1891, a little Berlin girl suffering from diphtheria was treated with antitoxin prepared in a sheep and recovered. The concept of 'passive immunization' was now established. The work of von Behring and Kitasato led to the production of diphtheria (Ramon, 1923) and tetanus (Ramon and Zoeller, 1927) toxoids. The diphtheria antitoxin was first isolated by Paul Ehrlich (1854–1915).

In the meantime, the world saw the production of a plague vaccine by **Yersin** in 1897, typhoid vaccine by **Almroth Wright** in 1898, BCG (Bacillus Calmette–Guérin) vaccine by **Calmette** and **Guérin** in 1921, and typhus vaccine by **Weigl** in 1933.

A major landmark was the preparation of a highly successful yellow fever vaccine using chick embryo cells. It was introduced by **Theiler** in 1935. In 1941 experiments started with an influenza vaccine and in 1945 an influenza vaccine was developed by **Salk**. **John Huxham** (1692–1768), from Devon, was the first physician to use the term 'influenza' in 1750 in *An Essay on Fevers*.

The wall paintings of ancient Egypt showed children suffering from a mysterious illness, which wasted and crippled the limbs. Priests believed the disease was a mark of God's displeasure. In the nineteenth century poliomyelitis outbreaks became more common, with the worst one hitting the USA in 1916. Franklin D. Roosevelt lost the use of both legs when he contracted the disease in 1921 immediately after his defeat as a vice-presidential candidate. Roosevelt was later instrumental in promoting research, which made the USA the world leader in conquering the disease.

The three poliomyelitis viruses were first identified by an American team led by **John Enders** in 1949. The discovery that polio viruses could be grown in tissue culture enabled **Jonas Salk** of the University of Pittsburgh to produce an inactivated polio vaccine in 1954, and **Albert Sabin**—a Polish-born US microbiologist—an oral, attenuated form in 1957. John Enders and his coworkers, **John**

Franklin and **Thomas Weller**, were awarded the Nobel Prize for Medicine in 1954.

Soon thereafter, many viral vaccines were introduced. In 1954, Enders and **Peebles** isolated the virus causing measles from the blood and secretions of patients, which allowed Enders to develop the measles vaccine in 1960. In 1962, Weller developed the rubella vaccine. By 1967, the Jeryl Lynn strain of live attenuated mumps virus vaccine was introduced, **Maurice Hillman** having isolated the virus from specimens he obtained from his daughter Jeryl Lynn. In the 1970s, the work of **Krugman** paved the way for the successful development of a vaccine against hepatitis B, while the hepatitis A vaccine was developed in the early 1990s.

In the 1990s, we witnessed biotechnology open entirely new, highly scientific approaches to vaccine development. Examples are the rational and precise attenuation of bacteria and viruses to serve as live vaccines, the direct inoculation with plasmid DNA encoding protective antigens, and the microencapsulation of antigens to enhance immunogenicity and modulate the kinetics and type of immune response. The result is vastly improved vaccines (e.g. acellular pertussis vaccine) as well as vaccines, which are still being developed, against other diseases (e.g. malaria and Lyme disease).

The smallpox chapter of the history of immunization was closed when the World Health Organization (WHO) declared the disease officially eradicated in 1980. The eradication of measles in the Americas and the global eradication of poliomyelitis are the targets of WHO for the year 2000. Already, poliomyelitis has been eradicated in the Americas.

If a disease is eradicated, is then humanity safe? Well, it appears not. Take the case of smallpox. The WHO has now to rethink its policy to abandon and for ever destroy the last of the smallpox vaccine. One of the problems is monkeypox, a relative of smallpox and cowpox. The infection is spread from chimpanzees, other species of monkeys and squirrels, who are probably the most important reservoir of the virus. Monkeypox causes a syndrome clinically similar to smallpox and carries a high mortality—over 1 in 10 people who catch the disease in the rainforests of central and western Africa. Until recently, transmission was mainly from animal to human. During the 1996–97 outbreak of monkeypox in former Zaire, the main mode of transmission was person-to-person. Smallpox vaccination protects against monkeypox. Are we to reintroduce smallpox vaccination in any form or should we destroy the last remaining laboratory stocks of the smallpox virus?

It appears that clinical considerations are not enough. Smallpox virus is a most dangerous organism that might be used by bioterrorists. The international black market trade in weapons of mass destruction is probably the only means of acquiring the deadly virus. Officially, the smallpox virus now exists in two government-run laboratories in the USA and the Russian Federation; at the Centre for Disease Control and Prevention in Alabama, and at the Russian State Centre for Research on Virology and Biotechnology in Siberia. Many scientists believe that samples are also being held in secret elsewhere.

The last recorded cases of smallpox were in Somalia in 1978, and also in Birmingham, UK, during the same year, when the virus escaped from a laboratory, killing one person and driving the scientist in charge of the laboratory to suicide. Smallpox samples in laboratories around the world were progressively destroyed throughout the 1980s. It is possible that not all laboratories complied fully. The possible use of smallpox virus as a weapon by terrorists has stimulated growing international concern and led to a review by WHO of the global availability of smallpox vaccine. This review (1999) found approximately 60 million doses worldwide. It is estimated that the USA alone will need to stockpile at least 40 million doses of the vaccine for emergency use, including in case of a terrorist release of smallpox virus.

In 1996, the World Health Assembly agreed the destruction, by 30 June 1999, of the two known stocks in the USA and the Russian Federation mentioned above. The new decision is 'the temporary retention, up to but not later than 2002, of the existing stocks of variola virus'. The final elimination of all variola virus remains the goal of WHO.

Furthermore, an international group of scientific and public health experts who met at WHO, Geneva, Switzerland, in December 1999, has recommended that more research should be undertaken on the smallpox virus before the end of 2002 when the two remaining collections of the virus would have been destroyed. The experts said that the DNA of the virus should be sequenced more completely, tests should be devised to detect human smallpox infection, and drugs should be developed to treat smallpox infections.

Bioterrorism fears have prompted the USA to set up a study on the safety and effectiveness of Dryvax. This smallpox vaccine is no longer produced but part of the limited supply still available in the USA will be used for a study in which 60 people will be given a full, one-tenth or one-hundredth dose of the vaccine. Information can be obtained from the Saint Louis University website: www.slu.edu. Readers can obtain further information on the subject of smallpox via the internet on the WHO home page: www.who.int.

About 200 million children are born worldwide each year, of whom 140 million are born in less developed countries. Despite all the efforts of the world community, 2 million children still die every year from immunization-preventable diseases. Yet, immunization coverage is levelling off in many countries and falling in others. The world community is responding; an International Vaccine Institute has opened in Seoul, Korea (www.ivi.org): new or expanded cooperative research efforts include the Multilateral Initiative on Malaria (http://www. malaria.org/MIM.html), and the international AIDS Vaccine Initiative (http://www.iavi.org).

Fighting infectious diseases in the developing world is a priority for all nations if we are to control and eventually eliminate them. An important element in this is the Millennium Vaccine Initiative (MVI) announced in February 2000. UNICEF, WHO and various other organizations are creating a new Global Alliance for Vaccines and Immunization (GAVI) http://www.who.int/gpr-aboutus/gavi. It aims to help lower the toll of infectious diseases, which accounts for a quarter of all deaths worldwide. In addition to the extra $150 million in the US budget for the year 2001 to fight human immunodeficiency virus (HIV)/acquired immune deficiency syndrome (AIDS) and other infectious diseases, the US President proposed a new tax credit to speed development of new vaccines. The Bill and Melinda Gates Foundation has pledged $750 million over 5 years for the GAVI (http://www.gatesfoundation.org). Merck has pledged 5 million doses of its hepatitis B vaccine over 5 years. American Home Products have pledged 10 million doses of its *Haemophilus influenzae* b vaccine. SmithKline Beecham announced it would undertake paediatric trials of its malaria vaccine in Africa and renewed a pledge made in 1998 to work with WHO to donate 5 billion doses of albendazole over the next 20 years to eradicate lymphatic filariasis; Aventis Pharma has pledged 50 million doses of its polio vaccine for 'war-torn nations of Africa'.

The twentieth century witnessed a revolution in immunology and saw the introduction of vaccines that led to the reduction or elimination of 21 infectious diseases. Can the twenty-first century do better? It should!

Chapter 2

Timescale of vaccine introduction in the UK

1938	Smallpox vaccination—the only routine immunization
	Tetanus toxoid—for military personnel
1940	Diphtheria toxoid (in some cities it began in 1937)
1946	Trials of pertussis vaccine
1948	Compulsory smallpox vaccination ended
1949	BCG vaccination for health service staff and contacts of tuberculous patients
1953	BCG vaccination in general use
	Pertussis vaccine (usually combined with diphtheria)
1956–61	Tetanus toxoid routinely for children, initially in some areas as monovalent and nationally in 1961 as diphtheria/tetanus/pertussis (DTP)
1961	DTP combined vaccine
1961	Oral polio vaccine (Sabin)
1967	Influenza vaccine
1968	Measles vaccine
1970	Rubella vaccine
1971	Smallpox vaccination discontinued
1975	Human diploid cell rabies vaccine
1979	Pneumococcal (14-valent) vaccine
1982	Hepatitis B plasma-derived vaccine
1987	Hepatitis B recombinant yeast vaccine
1988	Measles/mumps/rubella (MMR) combined vaccine
1989	Meningococcal A and C polysaccharide vaccine
1992	Hepatitis A vaccine
	Haemophilus influenzae b vaccine
	Pneumococcal (23-valent) vaccine
	Oral and Vi antigen typhoid vaccines
1994	Tetanus and low-dose diphtheria vaccine for adults and adolescents (Td)
	Acellular monovalent pertussis vaccine
	Measles/rubella combined vaccine
1997	Combined hepatitis A and B vaccine
	Combined DTP-Hib vaccine
1999	Combined hepatitis A and typhoid vaccine
	Meningococcal C conjugate vaccine
	Diphtheria/tetanus/acellular pertussis vaccine
	Diphtheria/tetanus/acellular pertussis–inactivated polio vaccine
	Diphtheria/tetanus/acellular pertussis–haemophilus influenza b vaccine
2000	Acellular monovalant pertussis vaccine no longer available

Chapter 3

Immunology, immunization and vaccine development

In the Golden Age of immunology and bacteriology (1870–1910) it was discovered that particular microbes were responsible for specific diseases. This eventually led to the development of vaccines, which have controlled several major infectious diseases. Vaccines are probably biomedical science's greatest triumph.

Immunization is the induction of artificial immunity through the administration of a vaccine or immunoglobulin. The term is commonly used interchangeably with *vaccination* (protection against smallpox)—it refers to the process of immunization. Vaccination is the administration of one or more doses of vaccine. As a result of this, and if vaccination is successful, the vaccinee is immunized (acquires immunity) against a specific infectious disease, thus becoming immune to that disease.

Immunity is the development of a relative resistance to an infection. This can be acquired from the mother *in utero* and during breast-feeding, actively from a pathogen able to mount an immunological response (infection, vaccine), or passively through the administration of ready-made anti-bodies in the form of immunoglobulins. Following natural infection, immunity may be lifelong.

Immune response is the recognition of antigens associated with pathogenic organisms by the body's defence system and operates in the form of a collection of tissues, cells and molecules. This response can be *antibody-mediated* (directed against extracellular pathogens) or *cell-mediated* (against intracellular pathogens) and is specific. A *memory* developed from previous experiences of foreign material ensures that a future challenge provokes a faster and more vigorous response.

Passive immunity

Immunity that can be induced by giving preformed antibodies is referred to as passive immunity. This is short-term immunity and can be achieved by giving nonspecific human normal immunoglobulin, collected from pooled human blood donations that contain antibodies to infectious agents prevalent in the community (e.g. for hepatitis A, measles), or specific immunoglobulin, formed from high-titre sera from humans or animals recently vaccinated or who have had the infection (e.g. varicella zoster, hepatitis B, tetanus, rabies). A neonate can acquire passive immunity from the mother's antibodies crossing the placental barrier and/or in breast milk.

Although passive immunization gives rapid protection within 24–48 h of intramuscular administration of the immunoglobulin, it does not last long, up to 6 months depending on dose given.

Active immunity

Active immunity is created by giving an antigen as a vaccine, containing organisms that have been:
- killed (e.g. heat-killed whole-cell typhoid vaccine; no longer available in the UK);
- attenuated—live organism with low virulence (e.g. measles, mumps, rubella, oral polio, BCG);
- inactivated bacterial toxins (e.g. with formaldehyde as in the case of diphtheria and tetanus);
- inactivated organisms (e.g. parenteral polio vaccine, hepatitis A);
- inactivated selected antigens of the organisms (e.g. pneumococcal capsular polysaccharide, influenza);
- genetically engineered (as in the case of hepatitis B vaccine).

Vaccines produce humoral immunity (i.e. most bacterial vaccines) or cell-mediated immunity (i.e.

the live virus vaccines, including the live bacterial BCG vaccine).

Humoral immunity

Activation of B-lymphocytes produced by the bone marrow (so known from the 'bursa of Fabricius', a gut-associated lymphoid organ where chicken lymphocytes were found to require a period of differentiation) by an antigen results in the production of millions of *antibodies*. Their task is to bind to the antigen and neutralize it.

Each B-cell is programmed to encode a surface receptor specific to a particular antigen (the surface antigen of a microorganism, a toxin, etc.). Once B-cells have recognized their specific antigens, they multiply and differentiate into plasma cells capable of producing large amounts of the receptor molecule in a soluble form—the antibody. Antibodies are large glycoproteins (*immunoglobulins, Ig*) and can be found in the blood and tissue fluids. They are virtually identical to the original receptor molecule, therefore they bind to the antigen that initially activated the B-cell.

Early in the humoral immune response IgM antibody is produced (primary response—disappears after a few months), but later large amounts of IgG mature antibodies (longer lasting—secondary response) are released in the blood and body tissues. When IgA antibodies are formed, they are secreted across mucosal surfaces in order to provide protection in the respiratory tract or the gut. An example here is the oral vaccines, which can produce local gut immunity as well as antibodies in the general circulation. These responses are important first-line defences against future infection.

Simultaneously, large numbers of *memory cells* are produced. These are antigen-specific B-cells. Further antigen exposure provokes a fast and vigorous antibody response.

Neutrophils are white cells that migrate to the site of invasion and destroy microorganisms by *phagocytosis* (from the Greek *phago* to ingest and *cytos* the cell). *Macrophages* are mononuclear white cells, able to ingest bacteria that have been coated with complement component (one of the main mediators of the inflammatory response) or antibody.

Following completion of the immunization course, the IgG levels will remain high for some time. When the level falls, a further dose of the vaccine (a booster) will reinforce immunity by increasing the IgG level again. This is not the case after polysaccharide vaccines when a booster dose does not increase the response (does not raise the antibody titre) but just sustains it.

Cell-mediated immunity

The cell-mediated immune response is a system of lymphocyte-mediated immunity that does not depend on major production of antibody. It relies more on a system of antigen recognition and cytokine production among macrophages and T-cells.

T-cells are lymphocytes that require a period of differentiation in the thymus gland and this gives rise to the designation *T-lymphocytes*. Once activated, T-cells produce cytotoxic cells, which destroy in-fected cells, and cytokinins, which prevent microorganisms from replicating within cells.

There are two major types of T-cells: CD4 (T-helper cells) and CD8 (T-suppressor or cytotoxic cells). CD4 T-cells stimulate B-cells to produce antibodies and also produce cytokinins—soluble mediators of immunity. Cytokinins, in turn, activate macrophages to destroy intracellular pathogens.

CD4 lymphocytes can be categorized according to the cytokinins they produce. These subsets have distinct functional characteristics: T-helper 1 (Th1) cells make γ-interferon (activates macrophages and T-cytotoxic cells, has a major role in eradication of viruses) and are associated with cell-mediated immunity, while T-helper 2 (Th2) cells make interleukin-4 and -5, and help B-cells produce antibody.

Within the past five years comparable populations of CD8 lymphocytes have been identified. Their task is to destroy host cells which have become infected by viruses or other intracellular pathogens—this action is called cytotoxicity. T-cells generate their effects by releasing soluble proteins (cytokinins), or by direct cell–cell interactions. The T-cytotoxic 1 (Tc1) lymphocytes make γ-interferon, an efficient killer cell that also inhibits Th2 cells. T-cytotoxic 2 (Tc2) lymphocytes make interleukin-4 and -5, less efficient killer cells that inhibit Th1 cells.

Immunological memory

Immunological memory is the situation where the vaccine-induced immunological 'memory' sustains immunity in the absence of detectable, or the presence of low, antibody. A rapid response in the antibody titres after a booster dose of vaccine is indicative of immunological 'memory'. An example is the case of hepatitis B when the anti-HBs level is below 10 mIU/mL or not detectable. Some lymphocytes become 'memory' cells with capacity for clonal expansion, differentiation and production of antibody upon subsequent stimulation by hepatitis B surface antigen (HBsAg). The principle of immunological memory could apply to other immunizations such as tetanus, hepatitis A, and probably diphtheria and measles.

Acquired immunity

A mother passes her antibodies to infectious diseases (passive immunity), which she has acquired through infection or vaccination, to her newborn child via the placenta and breast milk. Once these maternal antibodies wane, the child becomes susceptible. The child can acquire (active) immunity by vaccination or infection.

For infectious diseases to which a newborn child will be at immediate risk (such as tuberculosis in prevalent areas or hepatitis B where the mother giving birth is infected), the vaccines are given at birth. For a short period after birth (2 or 3 months) infants have some passive immunity from antibodies passed on to them *in utero* for diseases such as diphtheria, tetanus, pertussis, polio, *Haemophilus influenzae* and meningococcal infection. This depends greatly on whether the mother is immune, and whether this immunity is by natural infection or immunization (and how recent vaccination was). Breast milk does not give protection against infections such as diphtheria, tetanus and pertussis.

In deciding when to commence immunizations one has to balance the time an infant will obtain good immunity from immunization against the risk of disease. Pertussis kills very young infants and most of the deaths are seen in those under 2 months old. Pertussis vaccine will take from birth, but maternal antibodies to tetanus persist in the child for several weeks and would 'mop up' the tetanus vaccine. This is why in the UK we commence childhood immunizations at the age of 2 months. The WHO recommends starting the primary course at 6 weeks, so it is safe to start early—for example, if the family is flying abroad. With regard to measles, any persisting passively acquired (*in utero* and breast milk) maternal antibodies can interfere with the ability of the child to respond to the vaccine, if given during the first year of life, hence the postponement of vaccination until the child is over 1 year of age.

The killed organism vaccines are generally given more than once in order to produce sustained immunity, while live vaccines are generally given only once.

Vaccine production

Vaccines are produced in different ways depending on the microorganism and whether viral or bacterial, live or inactivated.

Viruses are parasites that can only grow in living cells, therefore they have to be produced in live cell cultures. The viruses for some viral vaccines are grown in hens' eggs. The process starts with a small 'laboratory' culture that is progressively scaled up to larger and larger culture vessels. This process takes time and cannot be accelerated. Bacterial vaccines are produced in a similar way, with production being scaled up over a period.

Once the microorganism is grown, it is inactivated or split into smaller units. The active component of the vaccine is then highly purified and blended with the other constituents of the vaccine to produce 'the bulk'. This process takes 4–9 months.

The next step is the testing of the bulk in order to ensure that it contains the correct organism; it has not changed during the growth period; it is free of contamination; and it does contain the correct ingredients in the correct amounts. Testing can take a further 1–3 months. If the vaccine is combined (e.g. MMR or DTP), the bulk of all constituents has to be further blended and tested. Once the manufacturer is satisfied that the bulk vaccine meets the stringent criteria set by the product licence, samples of the bulk are released to the authorities so that they can perform their tests. The whole process can take a year or more.

Once quality control is secured, the bulks are then used to fill in the appropriate containers (syringes, ampoules, vials). Before a vaccine is released, further tests are carried out to ensure that it conforms to the product licence. This process takes a further 4–10 weeks. The next step is further testing of the bulk and the finished product by one of several European Official Medicines Control Agencies—for vaccines to be used in Europe. This takes up about 2 months. Once satisfied of the quality of the product, the manufacturer proceeds to packing and distribution. By now, and provided no delays were encountered, an average of 20 months have elapsed since the start of production of the vaccine.

Planning vaccine production is essential for the manufacturer as well as the immunization authority of a country. Despite every effort by the manufacturer to produce enough vaccines, we frequently witness shortages of vaccine worldwide. Among the reasons for these shortages are the following:
- epidemics, and emergency programmes;
- new national immunization campaigns;
- new recommendations being adopted;
- steadily increasing vaccine demand;
- manufacturing capacity limits and manufacturing problems.

Conjugate vaccine technology

A good example of conjugate vaccine technology are the *Haemophilus influenzae* b and meningococcal C vaccines as well as others developed since the early 1970s. Such vaccines contained purified capsular polysaccharides (long-chain sugars forming 'bacterial coats' covering the surface). While effective in adults, they were generally ineffective in children under 18 months of age— the most vulnerable group. In this age group polysaccharide vaccines are unable to induce memory in T-lymphocytes and therefore give them only brief protection.

The aim was to produce vaccines that would be effective in preventing disease in children of all ages as well as adults. This was achieved by new conjugate vaccine technology which permanently links (conjugates) purified polysaccharides to pur-ified proteins (carrier molecules) rendering them immunogenic, thereby improving the vaccine immunogenicity, even in children under the age of 1 year. A nontoxic derivative of diphtheria toxin, group B meningococcal outer membrane protein, diphtheria and tetanus toxoids, among others, have been used to conjugate capsular polysaccharides.

Adjuvant

In order to enhance the antibody response to the antigen and prolong the stimulatory effect, some inactivated vaccines contain adjuvants. These are most commonly derived from minerals, oily materials or derivatives of certain microorganisms. Examples are aluminium phosphate and aluminium hydroxide.

Preservatives, stabilizers, antibiotics

In order to prevent bacterial growth or to stabilize the antigen, trace amounts of chemicals (e.g. mercurials such as thiomersal, antibiotics such as streptomycin, neomycin or penicillin) are frequently needed. Allergic reactions can occur if the vaccinee is allergic to these additives. The vaccine is contraindicated if the person to be vaccinated is expected to exhibit an anaphylactic reaction as a result of contact with these substances.

Thiomersal is 49.6% mercury by weight, and metabolizes to ethylmercury and thiosalicylate. It has been used for over 60 years as an antibacterial preservative in vaccines, and is particularly useful in maintaining bacteriological safety of opened multidose vials. At doses much higher than those used in vaccines, this preservative has been reported to cause neurotoxicity and nephrotoxicity. However, the precise nature of toxicity from low concentrations of exposure to thiomersal remains uncertain.

There are no data on and no evidence of the toxicity of ethylmercury at such low levels as in vaccines, but new guidelines make the (as yet unproven) assumption that it has the same toxicity as methylmercury. The WHO supports the 1999 statement from the American Academy of Paediatrics that it is to be phased out over the next few years, although it is accepted that there is no evidence that thiomersal has caused any harm in the amount contained in vaccines (< 0.05 mg). The USA Public Health Services, the American Academy of Paediatrics and vaccine manufacturers have agreed that thiomersal-containing vaccines should be replaced to avoid any theoretical risk and unnecessary exposure to mercury. This action is not urgent, but will take place as expeditiously as possible.

The UK childhood immunization schedule contains a much smaller number of routine vaccinations than the USA schedule and it is therefore unlikely that the use of thiomersal is a significant problem there.

The WHO has stressed the importance of continuing to use existing children's vaccines in the light of moves to phase out the use of thiomersal. It notes that the risk to unvaccinated children of death and complications from vaccine-preventable diseases is 'real and enormous', while the risk from side-effects of thiomersal is 'theoretical', uncertain and, at most, extremely small. Thiomersal has been in vaccines for many years with no adverse effects being seen. Furthermore, the WHO states that although there are other chemicals which could be used as preservatives, none is as effective as thiomersal. Also, if a new preservative is used in a vaccine, or thiomersal is omitted, the vaccine will have to undergo regulatory approval as a new product, which could be a lengthy process. Already, hepatitis B vaccines are available in the USA that do not contain thiomersal.

Serum albumin

Concern has been raised over the risk of transmission of bovine spongiform encephalopathy (BSE) and Creutzfeld–Jakob disease (CJD) from vaccines resulting from the production process and final constituents of vaccine. This risk remains hypothetical. None the less, no vaccine used in the UK childhood immunization programme since 1994 has contained UK human albumin. All UK vaccines using bovine albumin have been sourced from outside the UK since well before 1994. The rabies vaccine currently issued by the Public Health Laboratory Service (PHLS) is the only vaccine that does contain UK

human albumin. Until further advice is received from the Committee on Safety of Medicines (CSM) it will be issued for pre- and postexposure prophylaxis where there is clear indication for the use of this vaccine.

Testing the vaccine

In the UK no vaccine is licensed until it has been tested for safety, efficacy and acceptability. Before obtaining a licence a vaccine has to undergo testing in three phases.

Phase I

The safety and overall tolerability of the vaccine is tested on a small number of human healthy adult volunteers.

Phase II

Here it must be proved that the vaccine is safe and effective in producing antibodies capable of preventing the disease among the population. The dose, age ranges and vaccination schedules are also worked out.

Phase III

The vaccine is now tried on the population it is meant to protect, e.g. the Hib vaccine in the under 4- and especially under 1-year-olds.

Beyond phase III is continued *postmarketing surveillance* of the vaccine. The Post Licensing Division of the MCA has a responsibility for monitoring the safety of vaccines.

'Named-patient' basis

Some vaccines or immunoglobulins that have not been submitted to the UK authorities for licensing or that have not obtained a licence, can be made available on a 'named-patient' basis. In legal terms, supply of a product under this provision renders ultimate liability for its use with the prescribing clinician.

'Black triangle'

A new vaccine or immunoglobulin may carry the 'black triangle' in the British National Formulary (BNF). In this case we are asked to report *all* suspected reactions, however minor, that could conceivably be attributed to the preparation bearing the black triangle. Reports should be made despite uncertainty about a causal relationship, irrespective of whether the reaction is well recognized, and even if other drugs have been given concurrently.

Definition of terms used in clinical trials of vaccines

To define terms used in clinical trials of vaccines, let us take as an example the hepatitis B recombinant vaccine.

Immunogenicity (*immunogenic efficacy*) refers to the titre of anti-HBs antibody produced in the person receiving the vaccine. It can be assessed by the sero-conversion rate (the percentage of individuals who seroconvert—see below) and the geometric mean titre (GMT) of anti-HBs generated by the vaccines after primary vaccination.

Seroconversion is the creation by vaccination of an anti-HBs titre that is equal or greater than 1 mIU/mL. It means that antibodies have been developed and detected by current laboratory techniques in a person whose blood did not previously contain these antibodies, following the introduction of an antigen into the body. Before seroconversion the subject is said to be *seronegative* while after seroconversion the subject is *seropositive*.

Seroprotection, in the case of hepatitis B vaccine, is where the vaccine produced an anti-HBs titre equal or greater than 10 mIU/mL (minimum required to protect).

Protective efficacy is the prevention by the administration of hepatitis B vaccination of future acute symptomatic hepatitis B and hepatitis B virus (HBV) carriage.

Combined vaccines

If the British child received the vaccines in single antigens, by the time the child was 2 years of age, it would have received three oral doses and 18 injections. At the moment, it receives three oral doses and seven injections thanks to combination vaccines. Future vaccines will predominantly be combined vaccines. This involves combining a number of antigens in one syringe in order to minimize the number of injections required. The US Food and Drug Administration (FDA) requires that a combination vaccine not be inferior in 'purity, potency, immunogenicity, or efficacy' to each agent given separately.

Paediatric vaccines are being developed which will eventually combine the following antigens into one vaccine: diphtheria, tetanus, whole-cell or acellular pertussis, inactivated polio, *Haemophilus influenzae* type b, meningococcal A, B, C, hepatitis B, hepatitis A and yellow fever. Already a combination vaccine has been developed that incorporates DTaP–IPV–HBV–Hib (Infanrix HeXa, Smith Kline Beecham; HEXAVAC, Aventis Pasteur).

In the UK, vaccines that combine various antigens have been licensed:
- diphtheria/tetanus combined vaccine (DT);
- tetanus and low-dose diphtheria vaccine for adults and adolescents (Td);
- diphtheria/tetanus/whole-cell pertussis combined vaccine (DTwP);
- DTwP and Hib;
- DTaP (Infanrix);
- DTaP–IPV (Tetravac)
- MMR;
- meningococcal A + C;
- hepatitis A + B (Twinrix);
- hepatitis A and typhoid (Hepatyrix).

The benefits of combined paediatric vaccines are:
- fewer injections, thus less discomfort for the children;
- less stress for the accompanying parents;
- improved acceptance of existing and newly recommended vaccines;
- increased compliance;
- a more effective immunization programme;
- lower drop-out rates;
- greater convenience for doctor/nurse;
- lower administration cost;
- simpler logistics (transport, storage, records);

- less time to prepare and administer the vaccines;
- lower overall cost of immunization programmes;
- fewer visits to the doctor—fewer inoculations, contacts;
- simpler to protect against more than one infectious disease;
- real chance to eradicate polio if the inactivated form in the combined vaccine is used universally (we still see, rarely, vaccine-associated paralysis with the live oral polio vaccine);
- simplification of immunization schedule;
- enabling of reluctant countries to accept a particular vaccine, as may happen with the UK and childhood hepatitis B immunization.

The future vaccines

The success of existing vaccines depends on their ability to induce production of antibodies, which are the principal agents of immune protection against most viruses and bacteria. There are, however, exceptions, including intracellular organisms such as *Mycobacterium tuberculosis*, the malaria parasite, *Leishmania* and possibly the human immunodeficiency virus (HIV), in which protection depends more on the cell-mediated immunity than on induction of antibodies (humoral immunity). With the exception of vaccines prepared from live attenuated organisms, the others do not bring about cellular immunity. For these reasons, a new approach to vaccination, which involves the injection of a piece of DNA that contains the gene for the antigen, has been developed.

It is my belief that DNA vaccines will have a very important role in the future. We are witnessing an explosion of DNA vaccine research and some exciting results are coming out of many laboratories.

The new DNA vaccines (polynucleotide expression vectors) represent a new generation of vaccines to come. By encoding proteins derived from various pathogens, researchers have demonstrated that this can be an effective way of generating both humoral and cellular immune responses following intramuscular injection (see Fig. 3.1). In a DNA vaccine, the gene for the antigen is cloned into a bacterial plasmid that is engineered to augment the expression of the inserted gene in the mammalian cells. After being injected into the muscle, the plasmid enters a host cell, where it remains in the nucleus as an episome (from Greek meaning additional body); it is not integrated into the cell's DNA. Using the host cell's metabolic machinery, the plasmid DNA in the episome directs the synthesis of the antigen it encodes.

DNA vaccines are generally:
- fundamentally different from other vaccines;
- easier to produce and purify;
- easy to modify;
- relatively inexpensive;
- may not require cold chain;
- are highly immunogenic, especially for CD8 T-lymphocyte cells.

Fig. 3.1 The DNA vaccine.

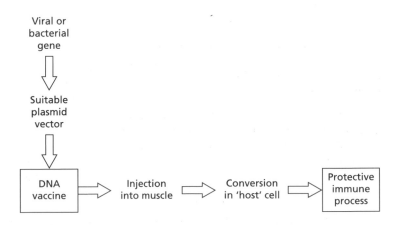

Viral or bacterial gene → Suitable plasmid vector → DNA vaccine → Injection into muscle → Conversion in 'host' cell → Protective immune process

Experimental work with DNA influenza vaccine has demonstrated three very important advantages over existing vaccines:

1 it produces a higher antibody level in monkeys than the inactivated whole-cell or split virion vaccines;

2 it stimulates strongly the cell-mediated immune response (it evokes a strong cytotoxic T-cell response to viral nucleoprotein);

3 it demonstrates the ability to protect from antigenic shifting of the influenza strains (one of the reasons for the yearly vaccination). Mice immunized with DNA encoding the nucleoprotein on an H1N1 1934 strain of influenza were greatly protected from death and morbidity (90% of them survived as opposed to 20% of the controls) following challenge with an H3N2 1968 strain of influenza virus.

Work is now continuing to apply this DNA technology to tuberculosis, genital herpes, influenza, HIV, hepatitis B and C, rabies, malaria, papillomavirus, Japanese b encephalitis, dengue and carcinogen antigens.

Remaining issues for the scientists are the full safety profile of these DNA vaccines, induction of anti-DNA antibodies, autoimmunity, induction of tolerance, their human efficacy and stability.

Vaccines under development

Some of the vaccines currently under development are:

• asthma/pneumonia vaccines (respiratory syncytial virus, house dust mite, cat antigens);

• prostate cancer vaccine;

• gastric cancer (*Helicobacter pylori*);

• cervical cancer (human papillomavirus);

• breast cancer;

• metastatic renal carcinoma—immunotherapy;

• leukaemia;

• melanoma;

• hepatocarcinoma (hepatitis C, complementing existing hepatitis B vaccine);

• malaria;

• dengue fever

• schistosomiasis;

• tuberculosis (adults);

• AIDS;

• diarrhoeal diseases (rotavirus, cholera, *Shigella*, enterotoxigenic *Escherichia coli*);

• meningitis and otitis media (*Streptoccocus pneumoniae*, *Neisseria meningitidis* group B);

• autoimmune diseases (insulin-dependent diabetes mellitus, multiple sclerosis);

• Alzheimer's disease;

• Angiotensin vaccine for hypertension.

Already vaccines for Lyme disease and rotavirus infections exist, and clinical trials are in their final stages for dengue fever vaccines. Phase I and III trials have commenced in the UK with different human papillomavirus vaccines; already trials are being completed in the USA. One early application this vaccine may have in the UK is its use in women who are at high risk of cervical cancer or have mildly abnormal smears. It will have to be shown to be cost-effective to be used on a large scale.

Vaccine strategy for the future

The US Institute of Medicine's 1999 report *Vaccines for the 21st century: tools for decision making*, uses a cost-effectiveness model to develop a priority list of 26 vaccines for infections and chronic diseases in the USA. The model was based on vaccine impact on morbidity and mortality, the cost of health care for the illness, and the costs of the vaccine itself and its development.

The vaccines with the highest priority and feasibility were those for cytomegalovirus, influenza, group B streptococcus, and *S. pneumoniae*. Vaccines with a lower but still favourable rating were those for chlamydia, *Helicobacter pylori*, hepatitis C, herpes simplex virus, human papillomavirus, *Mycobacterium tuberculosis*, gonococcus, and respiratory syncytial virus (RSV).

In high income countries, new vaccine prospects are for rotavirus, conjugate pneumococcal vaccine, live attenuated influenza vaccines and vaccines for RSV and parainfluenza vaccines—all with potential impact on child health.

The reality in poorer countries, where 70% of childhood deaths are caused by infectious diseases, is that about half of these deaths could be prevented by better use of vaccines widely available in the developed world. For example, *Haemophilus influenzae* b and hepatitis B vaccines are not available to most children in poor countries. Every child in the world, no matter where they live, should have access to vaccines that could immunize them against the major causes of death.

In arriving at a decision whether to immunize or not a public health organization measures the severity of the infection, the incidence of the disease, and the efficacy of the vaccine against the risk from the vaccine, and the price of the vaccine and the programme that will implement the vaccination campaign.

Non-parenteral routes and methods of vaccine administration

In most countries and most cultures, oral immunization is more readily accepted than vaccines that require injections. Moreover, the WHO Global Programme for Vaccines and Immunization has 'declared war' on unsafe injections with nonsterile needles and syringes, which in developing countries inadvertently transmit HIV, HBV and HCV from one infant to another. In fact the WHO estimates that worldwide more than one billion injections (not just vaccines) are given each year. Analysis at the WHO suggests that at least 50% of the injections given in some parts of the developing world are unsafe, and that more than 8 million HBV infections and almost 2 million HCV infections occur each year from unsafe injections.

Safer methods of vaccine administration have been developed. These include needleless devices that administer a liquid vaccine through the skin via a high-pressure air jet. A similar device uses high-pressure gas to deliver the vaccine in a powder form.

Another method of vaccine delivery under development involves the injection of a biosphere—a tiny starch ball, into the skin. It takes months to dissolve, thus releasing the vaccine steadily or in sudden bursts. The aim here is to avoid the need for booster injections.

Vaccines that preferably stimulate the mucosal immune response to provide an effective barrier against pathogens are highly desirable because mucosal surfaces are the most common site for pathogen entry, and because over 90% of all infections are acquired via mucosal routes. The mucosal immune system consists of molecules, cells and organized lymphoid structures intended to provide immunity to pathogens that impinge upon mucosal surfaces. Mucosal infection by intracellular pathogens results in the induction of cell-mediated immunity, as manifested by CD4-positive ($CD4^+$) T-helper type 1 cells, as well as $CD8^+$ cytotoxic T-lymphocytes. These responses are normally accompanied by the synthesis of secretory immunoglobulin A (S-IgA) antibodies, which provide an important first line of defence against invasion of deeper tissues by pathogens.

Recent advances in vaccinology have created new vaccines, antigen-delivery systems and adjuvants that can be administered via the mucosal surfaces by the rectal, vaginal, conjunctival, oral or nasal routes. The rectal route is highly efficient at eliciting immune responses but would be unpopular in several cultures, including Britain. The vaginal route excludes half the population. The conjunctival route leads on occasions to inflammation and purulent infection. Therefore, the oral and nasal immunizations are the most practical options. New generation, live, attenuated viral vaccines, such as the cold-adapted, recombinant nasal influenza and oral rotavirus vaccines have already been developed.

We already have three oral vaccines—polio, typhoid and cholera (the latter not yet available in the UK). Many other vaccines have been developed and are undergoing evaluation. A live attenuated influenza vaccine administered intranasally has been found to be safe, and effective when given to children in a USA study [Belshe R. *et al*. (1998) *N. Engl. J. Med.* 338, 1405–12].

The most exciting development in vaccine research has been the recruitment of plant science to the field. Two strategies have been used. One involves the integration into the host plant's chromosome of a microbial gene encoding an antigenic protein. A second approach exploits expression of a desired foreign gene that has been incorporated into the genome of a common plant virus. Once ingested, these bioencapsulated vaccines would release the antigen as food is degraded in the human gastrointestinal tract. Contact of the vaccine with the extensive gastrointestinal-associated lymphoid tissue could induce mucosal immunity followed soon after by humoral mucosal immunity, secondary to the trafficking of lymphoid cells. Successful experiments have been carried out with potatoes and bananas.

Vaccination in utero may reduce vertical transmission of infectious diseases. Canadian scientists have introduced DNA herpes vaccine into the amniotic fluid of fetal lambs and elicited a powerful immune response to it. This approach may eventually reduce the need for Caesarian sections in women at high risk of passing on infections such as herpes and hepatitis to their offspring [*Nature Medicine* (2000) 6, 929–932].

Needle length

With the increased use of prefilled syringes with needles already welded to the syringe, there is a possibility of inappropriate placement of the vaccine, particularly in obese individuals. Already the UK Department of Health (DoH) recommends for deep subcutaneous and intramuscular immunizations the use of a 23G (blue) or 25G (orange) needle for infants, and 23G (blue) for adults.

The US Advisory Committee on Immunization Practices (ACIP) recommends that 'the needle should be long enough to reach the muscle mass and prevent the vaccine from seeping into the subcutaneous tissue' [the ACIP for the Centers for Disease Control and Prevention (USA) (CDC)] publishes statements for each recommended childhood vaccine: http://www.cdc.gov/nip/publications/aciplist.htm). Furthermore, it recommends that 'an individual decision on needle size should be made for each person based on age, volume of drug, size of the muscle and the depth below the muscle surface into which the material is to be injected'. The Australian advisory body recommends the longer needle for all but very small infants so that the vaccine can reach the substance of the muscle.

If the needle is too fine, the vaccine may not dissipate over a wide enough area. If the needle is too short, it may not enter the muscle and especially the bulk of the muscle. Such poor technique or inappropriate needle size may result in sometimes severe local reactions and/or the vaccine may not take. Aluminium-adsorbed vaccines should be given by the intramuscular route because subcutaneous or superficial administration leads to an increased incidence of local reactions.

In a paper published in 1997 [Gregory A. *et al.* (1997) *J. Am. Med. Assoc.* 277, 1709–11] researches surveyed the deltoid fat pad thickness. Using ultrasound measure-ments of the skin and fat thickness overlying the deltoid, the research team confirmed that deltoid penetration to a depth of 5 mm was only possible using:
- 1 inch (25 mm—23G blue) needle in men between 59 and 118 kg;
- 5/8 inch (16 mm—25G orange) needle in women less than 60 kg;
- 1 inch (25 mm—23G blue) needle in women between 60 and 90 kg;
- 1.5 inch (37.5 mm—21G green is 40 mm) needle for women over 90 kg.

By implication, according to data presented in that paper, for children we need to use the 5/8 (16 mm—25G orange) needle length.

Researchers from the Oxford Vaccine Group at the University Department of Paediatrics, John Radcliffe Hospital, studied redness, swelling and tenderness at the injection sites of 119 healthy infants, following their routine 16-week (third) DTP and Hib immunizations. The study was conducted in eight general practices in Buckinghamshire. 61 infants were vaccinated with the shorter, 25G orange hub needles, and 58 with the longer 23G blue hub needles. After six hours, the longer (blue) needle group suffered only two-thirds the rate of redness, and one-third the risk of swelling of those injected with the shorter (orange) needles. Three days later, the rate of redness with the blue needles was only one-seventh of the orange needle group, with the rate of swelling still one third. Rates of tenderness were also lower with the longer needle throughout follow up, but the difference was not statistically significant.

The researchers concluded that the use of the 25G blue needle significantly reduced rates of local reaction to routine infant immunization. On average, for every five infants vaccinated, use of the longer needle instead of the shorter needle would prevent one infant from experiencing any local reaction [Diggle L., Deeks, J. (2000) Effect of needle length on incidence of local reactions to routine immunisation in infants aged 4 months: randomised controlled trial. *BMJ* 321, 931–933].

When a vaccine with a needle welded to the syringe is licensed, it has to demonstrate that the vaccine given with that needle, at the recommended site, is immunogenic. The doctor or nurse should ensure that the vaccine is given to the licensed site (e.g. deltoid or anterolateral thigh). In this case, there are no fears that the vaccine will not 'take', provided that the operator is skilled. If no needle is supplied with the vaccine, a (25 mm) 23G blue needle should be used, but consider a (37.5 mm) 21G green needle for all those over 90 kg. Practically, this means that children and a large number of adults will receive their immunizations using a blue needle. For very small infants a (16 mm) 25G orange needle may be used.

The WHO recommends the 23G blue needle be used for all infant vaccinations. It also recommends the following injection technique in order to ensure the vaccine is delivered to the muscle.

1 The thumb and forefinger should be placed on the anterolateral thigh.
2 The skin should be stretched flat between finger and thumb.
3 The 23G blue needle should be pushed quickly straight down through the skin between the finger and thumb, deep into the muscle.

Topical anaesthesia before injection

The eutectic mixture of local anaesthetic (EMLA) cream, which is applied topically under an occlusive dressing, has been evaluated in multiple placebo-controlled, randomized trials and has been demonstrated to provide pain relief during injection. It required one hour to work adequately but, in my practice, a few minutes will suffice.

Site of vaccine administration—multiple injections

Apart from BCG, all parenteral vaccines are given by intramuscular or deep subcutaneous injection. The preferred site is the anterolateral thigh (high up) in infants. Beyond this age (see below), the deltoid muscle is the preferred site for injections.

The gluteal muscle (buttock) should not be used for the administration of vaccines. There is past evidence of sciatic nerve damage from immunizations given into the buttock. Furthermore, the plentiful adipose tissue at that site (especially in infants that have not as yet walked to develop their gluteal muscle) can reduce the absorption and efficacy of administered vaccines. This is particularly true for rabies, hepatitis A and hepatitis B vaccines. The buttock can be a dirty area with a risk of infection and formation of subcutaneous fibrous nodule. The British Paediatric Association recommends either the anterolateral thigh or deltoid.

When more than one vaccine needs to be injected at the same time, they should be given on contralateral thighs or deltoids—depending on age. Live-virus vaccines must be given simultaneously and on different sites. This way antibody response is not impaired and the rate of adverse events is not increased. Otherwise, they should be separated by a time period of 3 weeks.

Inactivated vaccines can be given either simultaneously or at any time before or after another inactivated or a live-virus vaccine. Ideally, each recommended site should receive one injection. In the event where you have more than two injections to give on one site, the live-virus vaccines should be given on contralateral sites and the inactivated vaccines should be either postponed for later or given about 1 cm away from another vaccine.

With regard to children and intramuscular vaccinations, the following 'rule of thumb' may be applied:
● under 1 year of age the anterolateral thigh is the preferred site;
● between 1 and 6 years of age the anterolateral thigh or the deltoid are suitable;
● over 6 years of age the deltoid is the preferred site.

Interchangeability of vaccines

Similar vaccines made by different manufacturers are considered interchangeable when administered according to their licensed indications. Whenever possible a primary immunization course or booster should be completed with the same vaccine used initially. There may be situations when:

● the brand name of the vaccine used previously is not known;

● the vaccine is not currently available in the Travel Clinic;

● the vaccine is not available due to manufacturing delays or production problems; or

● the vaccine has been withdrawn from the market.

In such cases, it is acceptable to use another manufacturer's similar schedule vaccine, in order to complete the primary course or for a booster dose.

Revaccination after adverse reaction

In an Australian study [Gold M. *et al.* (2000) Re-vaccination of 421 children with a past history of an adverse vaccine reaction in a special immunization service. *Archives of Disease in Childhood* 83, 128–31) 469 children had an adverse event: 63% had a local reaction, fever or irritability, while 37% had a hypotonic hyporesponsive episode, convulsions, rash or anaphylaxis. In 90% the reaction was associated with DTP vaccine, and 10% with acellular pertussis, MMR, Hib, OPV, hepatitis B, combined diphtheria and tetanus.

After review, 90% were re-vaccinated. Acellular pertussis was given if the reaction involved the whole-cell vaccine. Of all the re-vaccinated children, 83% had no adverse reaction, 17% had fever and/ or a local reaction, and only one had a significant episode, but made a full recovery.

Chapter 4

The cold chain and vaccine storage

'Cold chain' is the maintenance of vaccine and immunoglobulin potency by maintaining the manufacturer's recommended temperature (+2–+8 °C) during storage and distribution from the manufacturer to the user. The previous Medeva oral poliomyelitis vaccine (Evans OPV), which required temperatures of 0 to 4 °C, is not available in the UK. All immunoglobulins require temperatures of 2 to 8 °C. Temperatures above or below the above will cause deterioration of the vaccine or even breakage of the glass vials or syringes if they should freeze.

One person (with a deputy) in the practice/clinic should be designated to have overall responsibility for the care of the vaccines.

- Sufficient supplies of vaccines should be ordered, taking care to avoid stockpiling. Expiry dates on existing vaccine stocks should be checked and brought forward to be used first. Date-expired vaccines should be removed.
- On receipt of vaccines, they should be checked, recorded and refrigerated immediately.

The vaccines refrigerator should not be a domestic one but a special pharmacy refrigerator, which is of a higher specification and may incorporate an internal fan, an external thermometer and should have an external lock. Larger practices should consider a large pharmacy refrigerator for vaccine stocks and a small one in the treatment room for everyday vaccinations. Nothing other than vaccines should be stored in the practice pharmacy refrigerator, and in particular no food.

- The vaccines refrigerator should be supplied from a switchless electrical socket. If this is not available, protect the socket with tape or something similar to avoid accidental switching off, and label it clearly.
- Avoid opening the refrigerator door unnecessarily and, once opened, close the door as soon as possible.

Consider locking the refrigerator when it is not in use.

- Defrost the refrigerator regularly if it has no automatic defrost. Keep vaccines in another refrigerator or cool box while doing this.
- Consider an internal maximum/minimum thermostat, even if there is an external thermometer fitted to the refrigerator. Some are able to record the maximum and minimum temperatures achieved.
- Keep a notebook close to the refrigerator and record the daily temperatures as well as the maximum and minimum temperatures reached, if possible. In case of refrigerator failure or electricity interruption, seek advice from the local community services pharmacist or the Drug Information Centre. Failing this, consider contacting the vaccine manufacterer/s.
- Inside the refrigerator, the vaccines should not be stored too tightly. Air should be allowed to circulate around the packages. No vaccines should be stored in such a way that they could come into contact with ice. Avoid shelves or storage compartments on the refrigerator door—this is especially important if, against good clinical practice, a domestic refrigerator is used.
- Reconstituted vaccines must be used within the manufacturer's recommended period—usually 1h but some are viable up to 4h. Unused vaccines and opened multidose vials should be discarded, although the oral polio multidose vaccine may be re-refrigerated and re-used for a short time, usually the same morning or afternoon (manufacturers advice). The DoH advises up to 4 weeks when the OPV is stored at appropriate cold chain conditions and is in date. Unused whole vials that have been left out of the refrigerator for any appreciable length of time, are out of date or frozen, should also be discarded.
- Remove vaccines from the refrigerator just before the beginning of a vaccination session and

return them to the refrigerator as soon as possible, and not later than 3 hours, after. Remove only the required number of vaccines. Unused vaccine that is put back in the refrigerator should be used first at the next immunization session as repeated warming and cooling of vaccines shortens their shelf life.

• Some vaccines need to be protected from light, e.g. OPV, BCG, reconstituted MMR.

• Vaccine in an already opened ampoule can be destroyed by soaking it in hypochlorite solution for 20 min (e.g. Milton). Such treated ampoules can then be discarded into the Sharps bins.

• Partly used vials should be stored in a marked container and returned via the Pharmacy Collection Service for unused medicines.

• Empty vials should be discarded into a Sharps bin.

The supply of vaccines is through an appointed distribution service (e.g. Farillon Ltd), the local pharmacy, a courier service, or by post from the manufacturer. If vaccines are sent by post, check the dispatch date and time. They should not be accepted if posted more than 48 h prior to receipt. If in doubt, do not accept. Where coolboxes or insulated containers are used, the vaccines should not come into contact with frozen ice packs.

In case of disruption of the cold chain (electricity supply interruption, accidental switching off of the refrigerator etc.), and before seeking advice from the local community services pharmacist, the local Drug Information Service or the manufacturer, be prepared to answer questions including:

• How long has the refrigerator been off?

• What are the last minimum/maximum recorded temperatures?

• What is the temperature around the outside of the refrigerator?

• What vaccines are in the refrigerator, including their manufacturers?

• When will the clinic need and which vaccines?

Do not discard any vaccines until expert advice is taken. The thermostability of the vaccines varies. For example, at room temperature (21°C) the potency of the Fluarix (SKB) vaccine is not affected for one week, while that of polio (SKB) vaccine is 2 days.

For advice on supplies of *refrigeration equipment and accessories* telephone the Communicable Disease Branch at the DoH on 020 7972 1430.

Insulated containers for vaccine transport are available from Thermos Ltd (Tel.: 01277 213 404) and Mailbox International Ltd (Tel.: 0161 330 5577).

For active *temperature management system combined with continuous monitoring containers* contact ISOsafe Ltd, Woodlands Business Village, Basingstoke, Hants, RG21 4JX (Tel.: 01256 362 700. Fax: 01256 869 911).

Chapter 5

Transmission of infection

Infection can be transmitted from patients suffering active infection as well as from carriers. Diseases that spread to humans from animals are called zoonoses.

Horizontal spread occurs between people in the same population, and person-to-person is the most common method.

Vertical spread is where infection is passed on from mother to fetus (congenital rubella, hepatitis B).

Infection spreads by one of the methods detailed below.

Inhalation

Infected droplets from the respiratory tract, mouth, throat and nose are expelled during coughing, sneezing and speaking, and these are then inhaled by the new host. Diseases that may spread this way are whooping cough, influenza, pulmonary tuberculosis, diphtheria, mumps, measles, rubella, chickenpox and scarlet fever.

Ingestion

The pathogens present in the faeces, vomit, urine or respiratory secretions contaminate hands, fingers, cooking and eating utensils, clothing, toilets, etc. Diseases that spread this way are typhoid, cholera, hepatitis A and E, salmonellosis, dysentery and poliomyelitis. A common form of transmission is direct contact between faecally contaminated hands and oral mucosa (faecal–oral transmission). Another way is by ingestion of contaminated food, e.g. brucellosis, *Campylobacter* enteritis and salmonellosis. Food-borne transmission is most likely to occur if contaminated food is eaten raw or undercooked. It is important that milk is pasteurized, water is supplied by reputable organizations and a very good sewage system is in place.

Inoculation/direct contact/bites

Pathogens can be inoculated directly into the body through a defect in the skin, can penetrate the mucosal surfaces or are introduced via a bite. Examples are hepatitis B virus (HBV), human immuno-deficiency virus (HIV), malaria, anthrax, tetanus, rabies, leptospirosis (if the urine of infected animals contaminates fresh water or swimming facilities).

Venereal route

The pathogen is transmitted by sexual contact, e.g. HBV, HIV, herpes genitalis, syphilis, gonorrhoea, lymphogranuloma venereum.

Iatrogenic

Infection can be transmitted from contaminated gloves, instruments, transfusions, blood, blood products, nonsterile needles or syringes, e.g. HBV, HCV, HIV, malaria. Iatrogenic is from *iatros*, Greek for doctor.

Vectors

Some living creatures are able to transmit infection from one host to another, and they are called vectors. Important vectors in humans are:
- mosquito—malaria, yellow fever, Japanese B encephalitis, dengue fever, filariasis;
- tick—relapsing fever, encephalitis, typhus, Lyme disease;
- flea—plague, rickettsial infection;
- louse—typhus, relapsing fever;
- sandfly—sandfly fever, leishmaniasis;
- fly—trypanosomiasis, onchocerciasis;
- mite—typhus, scabies;
- cone-nosed bug—Chagas' disease.

Fomites

Objects on which pathogens are transported from source to host, i.e. bedding, towels.

Chapter 6

Infectivity and exclusion period of infections

Infection	Infectious	Exclusion
Chickenpox and herpes zoster	2 days before to 6 days after spots develop	Until all spots have crusted
Hepatitis A	Several days while asymptomatic until 7 days after onset of jaundice	Until 7 days after onset of jaundice and the patient feels well
Hepatitis B	Not infectious under normal work/ school conditions	Until patient is well
Impetigo	While spots discharging pus	Until spots have healed
Measles	A day before onset of symptoms and until 5 days after rash appears	Until the child feels well—minimum 4 days from onset of rash
Mumps	7 days before and until 9 days after the swelling appears	Until child feels well—minimum 9 days from onset of swelling
Pertussis	4 days before and until 21 days after the start of cough or until 6 days after antibiotic therapy started	5 days from starting antibiotic therapy
Rubella	1 week before and until 1 week after onset of rash	Until 7 days after rash appears
Scarlet fever	As sore throat starts, until the second day after antibiotic therapy started	Until the second day after antibiotic therapy started
Tuberculosis	When sputum cultures are positive. After 2 weeks of antibiotic therapy	After 2 weeks of antibiotic therapy

As a general rule, food handlers presenting in general practice with diarrhoea should be excluded from work until they are symptom-free and for 48 h afterwards.

Chapter 7

Immunization in practice

Immunization coverage

The immunization coverage represents the proportion of people that have been vaccinated. The WHO target for immunization coverage of children at 2 years of age is 95%.

The fifth objective of the Health for All in the Year 2000 programme of WHO-Europe states: 'By the year 2000, there should be no indigenous cases of poliomyelitis, diphtheria, neonatal tetanus, measles, mumps and congenital rubella in the region, and there should be a sustained and continuing reduction in the incidence and adverse consequences of other communicable diseases, notably HIV infection.' This objective has not been met. All 15 countries of the European Union have ratified this objective. Figure 7.1 shows the reported immunization coverage in Western European countries. This figure was prepared with kind assistance from Aventis Pasteur MSD and the source is the vaccine-preventable disease monitoring system of the WHO.

Fig. 7.1 Immunization coverage (percentage) of children aged less than 2 years in Western European countries. DTP (diphtheria/ tetanus/whole-cell pertussis combined vaccine), POL, (poliomyelitis), both 3 doses and one dose of measles vaccine, 1996– 1998.

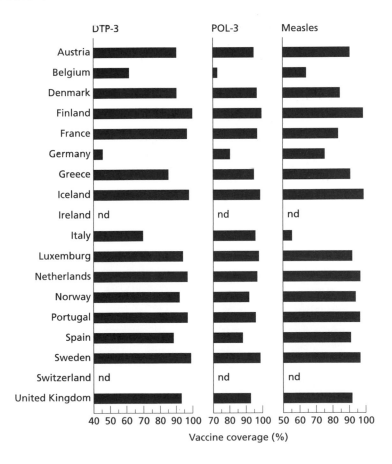

25

As yet, there is no standardization of measuring techniques in practice in all the countries of the European Union. This is particularly a problem in countries where vaccination is also carried out by the private sector.

Uptake of childhood immunization

Uptake of childhood immunization reached its highest level ever in England in 1996/97. Uptake of three doses of DT was 97%, three doses of pertussis 94%, *Haemophilus influenzae* b 94% and MMR 92%. The 'MMR scare' (see Chapter 22) has had a negative effect on the uptake of childhood immunizations in the UK with an overall drop. In the year 1997/98 the uptake among those reaching their second year of life was 96% for DT and polio, 95% for Hib, 94% for pertussis and 91% for MMR. The uptake for MMR in England continued to fall and was at its lowest level (87.6%) in the first quarter of 1999. It then rose for the first time in 2 years to 88% in the second quarter of 1999, still well away from the necessary 95%.

The achievement of high standards of immunization coverage depends on many factors, as shown in Fig. 7.2.

The aim of the Primary Healthcare Team

The aim through immunization is to protect the community as well as the person vaccinated from infectious diseases. This we try to achieve as early as possible, hence the DTP–OPV–Hib-MenC course is started in the UK at the age of 2 months old.

Sometimes the benefit of immunization is only to the vaccine recipient as in the case of tetanus. Most of the time immunization of individuals aims to achieve sufficiently higher coverage (*herd immunity*) to interrupt transmission into the community. This way both immunized and non-immunized individuals benefit.

Herd immunity is the basis on which all national immunization programmes are designed. The concept here is that not everyone in a population needs to be immunized in order to protect that population. As long as sufficient numbers of children are immunized against a specific disease the protection can extend to everyone. What is important is to find the percentage of the population that must be immunized for herd immunity to be created. This depends on:

● the infectivity of the disease (protection against the highly infectious measles will require a higher percentage of children to be immunized than for the less infectious mumps);
● the susceptibility of the population (has the infectious disease been circulating in the community and for how long?);
● vulnerability of the population (overcrowded inner city against a sparsely populated rural area);
● environmental factors (the disease may be more prevalent during one season of the year than

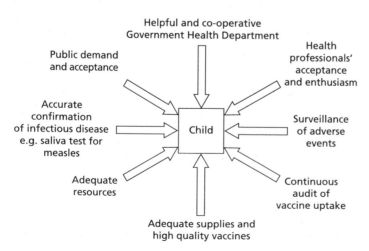

Fig. 7.2 Factors influencing the achievement of high immunization coverage.

another, i.e. meningitis and influenza during the winter months);

• the degree of protection a vaccine offers to its recipients (for measles this is around 90%).

In the case of measles and in order to create herd immunity, it is estimated that the immunization uptake in the UK must be about 95%. By comparison, for India this figure is about 99%.

Over time, as more children are immunized, less cases of the disease are seen. If, however, enough parents refuse immunization and the percentage of coverage drops, the infectious disease can start circulating again in the community. As the MMR vaccine uptake has dropped to 88% (second quarter of 1999), a new measles epidemic can be expected in the UK within the next 2 years, as this level of vaccine coverage is below the 95% level necessary to create herd immunity.

The Primary Healthcare Team is often called to advise on the interests of an individual and the public as a whole. The interests of both are served well when the disease incidence is high and the relative rate of vaccine-adverse effects low. However, as the vaccine programme becomes more successful in eradicating the disease, public and individual interests may diverge unless the vaccine has no adverse effects or the immunization programme is so successful that the disease is eliminated and the vaccine programme can be discontinued, as in the case of smallpox.

The UK has achieved higher standards of immuni-zation coverage without resorting to legal compulsion. It is my view that such a compulsion, in any form, acts against the spirit of the epidemiological attempt to control infectious disease. We can achieve high standards of immunization coverage by giving parents the choice as well as correct and up-to-date information. None the less, in a voluntary programme as with the one in the UK, it may become difficult to achieve elimination of an infectious disease because some individuals will perceive the risks of vaccination as outweighing the benefits and decline vaccination.

Why do parents refuse immunizations?

The challenges we face with vaccinations is the design and production of vaccines, the planning of the vaccination campaign (as well as its implementation and evaluation), the funding, the co-operation of the profession and the acceptance of any vaccination programme by the parents/population.

Apathy or parents' beliefs are occasionally reasons for refusal in the UK. Parents put forward from time to time some reasons which result in a child not receiving one or another vaccine. As immunization is not compulsory in the UK, parents who refuse their children vaccination take on their shoulders the full responsibility of their action. Unfortunately, the child, at that time, has practically no opinion.

Parents should be listened to and their worries recognized and addressed. Their prime concern is their children. The problem arises when their decisions are taken on the basis of religious beliefs, commercial newspaper reports, 'hearsay', etc. For the medical adviser, when in doubt doing nothing should not be an option. The parents should be referred to somebody else in or outside the practice who is in a position to advise them.

Some of the reasons parents put forward are cited below.

• *Religious beliefs.* Christian Scientists are the major group refusing immunization on religious grounds.

• *Homoeopathy.* Some parents believe immunization will adversely disturb the child's immune system. This is despite support for childhood immunization from the Faculty of Homoeopathy for the use of orthodox vaccines. There is no evidence that homoeopathic vaccines confer long-term or short-term protection.

• *Medical reasons—possible contraindications.* Sometimes the parents believe a vaccine is contraindicated, and on some occasions parents are incorrectly advised by a health professional. An example here is the 1996 court decision to award £825 000 damages to the parents of a child whose GP was alleged to have advised against immunization against measles in 1982, because the child had a suspected episode of convulsions as a baby. Five years later, she suffered 'catastrophic' brain damage after contracting measles. The GP maintains it was the parents who did not want their daughter immunized because of their fears over the potential vaccine side-effects. A health professional advising against a particular vaccine should follow the DoH guidelines on the contra-indications to that vaccine, should seek a second opinion, for example from a community paediatrician, and should record in the notes the reasons for his/her advice.

● *Belief that good hygiene and healthy living conditions make immunization unnecessary.* All children need to be immunized irrespective of their living standards.

● *Belief that the risks of vaccination are greater than the risk of the disease.* The opposite is true—refer to the various sections of this book to find comparisons.

● *Belief that because of herd immunity the risk to their child is very small.* If parents opt out of immunization, there will be increasing numbers of susceptible children among whom, as well as the 'vaccine failures', the infectious diseases could re-establish. These children are likely to be infected at a later age when the case fatality for most vaccine-preventable diseases is increased. The only time we can stop vaccinations is when we achieve global eradication of the particular disease as was the case with smallpox.

● *Belief that their children are too young and their immune system will be damaged by the injections.* They refer here mainly to the 2, 3, 4 months accelerated DTP/OPV/Hib/MenC schedule. Immune responses following early immunizations are the same as those following later immunizations. If anything, delaying immunization can increase the risks of adverse reactions occurring. In fact, the WHO recommends an even earlier start than in the UK, at 6, 10 and 14 weeks. By starting and completing earlier childhood immunizations in the UK, we have increased the vaccine uptake and decreased the 'drop outs' we used to see around the late third dose of DTP.

● *Belief that 'the system will be overloaded'.* This has arisen from the 'MMR controversy' in the UK. At the suggestion of a hospital doctor, some parents maintain that giving three live virus vaccines in one dose will 'overload the child's immune system'. There is no scientific basis or any evidence whatsoever that this is true. On the contrary, administering the three components individually (no longer an option in the UK) will delay protection and some children may catch the disease.

● *Belief that the child has had the disease, e.g. measles, therefore no need to have the vaccine.* History of the disease without laboratory evidence is not a reason for refusing to have the vaccine. Many viral infections can present with a similar rash to measles. The introduction of the saliva test for measles has made the situation clearer. In 1996, there were 5614 notified cases of measles disease. Of them, 3326 cases were saliva tested and only 63 cases were confirmed as measles infection, giving a rate of true disease of approximately 1.9% of those tested.

● *Concern about the preparation of the vaccine material.* Concerns were raised in the UK, particularly during the 1994 measles/rubella campaign. The concern was about the fact that when the rubella vaccine was developed, the rubella virus was grown on tissue that originated from an aborted fetus, although the abortion was performed for ethical medical reasons. Parents should be assured that vaccine production today does not involve fetal material. Leading religious authorities, such as the Roman Catholic Church, consider it ethical to use the rubella vaccine. Also, parents can be reassured that vaccines used for the UK childhood immunization schedule do not contain UK bovine or UK human albumin.

● *Belief that the vaccines do not always protect.* No vaccination protects all children the first time. It is known that a number of children do not produce antibodies in response to one injection of a vaccine. The evidence is that those few children not responding to the first injection will, overall, respond to a second injection, hence the second MMR dose. For those already protected, the second dose acts as a booster. The aim is to increase the herd immunity as much as possible.

● *Belief that the vaccines are not safe.* No vaccine is licensed in the UK without proper controlled trials. Vaccines are among the safest drugs we have.

● *The experience of emotional distress at the pros-pect of inflicting pain on the baby.* An empathetic approach by the nurse and the doctor can be very helpful. In some circumstances we offer to hold the baby so that the parent can have the option of going outside the room.

If we can identify the reasons some parents

refuse or are reluctant to allow their children to be vaccinated, we may be able to give correctly consistent and up-to-date advice to parents.

We should ensure that we enter in the notes the reasons why parents refuse immunization, and the advice we give them.

Factors which may adversely influence seroconversion of vaccines in children

- Age in relation to circulating maternal antibodies, e.g. measles vaccination postponed until after the first birthday.
- Fever above 38 °C at the time of vaccination.
- Immunosuppression by disease or treatment.
- Impaired immunological mechanism, e.g. hypogammaglobulinaemia.
- Human normal immunoglobulin given less than 3 months before a live vaccine is injected.
- A live vaccine injected less than 3 weeks from the injection of another live vaccine.
- Incorrect storage of vaccine, for example:
temperatures outside the recommended 2 to 8 °C range,
freezing the vaccine/diluent,
leaving the vaccine outside the pharmacy refrigerator,
storing the vaccines on the shelves or storage compartments of the refrigerator door,
storing the vaccines too tightly in the refrigerator, without allowing air to circulate around them.
- Incorrect transport of vaccines.
- Using out-of-date vaccines.
- Long exposure of vaccines to direct sunlight or heat.
- Reconstituted vaccines used beyond the manufacturer's recommended period.
- Non-completion of the primary immunization course or boosters—it is not necessary to recommence an interrupted schedule of immunization; it should simply be completed.
- Alcohol or other disinfecting agent not being allowed to evaporate before injection of a live vaccine.
- Injection into the fatty tissue of the buttock in the case of, for example, hepatitis B, hepatitis A and rabies vaccines.
- Incorrect injection technique.
- Route of administration other than the one recommended by the manufacturer, for example, intradermal injection of a vaccine recommended for intramuscular administration.
- Incorrect dose of the vaccine in relation to the child's age.
- Adding the diluent too fast so that frothing is created.
- Using multidose vials kept from a previous immunization session—they should be discarded after each session.

Chapter 8

Expanded programme on immunization

The WHO-suggested national immunization schedule for infants

The WHO recommends that children be immunized as early in life as possible to protect them against vaccine-preventable diseases in their country. Because the epidemiological situation varies from country to country, the model schedule below (Table 8.1) has been adapted in some way by most countries so that it more closely meets their needs. None the less, it provides a useful guide to the reader.

Table 8.1 WHO-recommended national immunization schedule for infants.

| Age | Vaccine | Hepatitis B vaccine* (two schemes) | |
		Alternative A	Alternative B
Birth	BCG, OPV-0	HB-1	
6 weeks	DTP-1, OPV-1	HB-2	HB-1
10 weeks	DTP-2, OPV-2		HB-2
14 weeks	DTP-3, OPV-3	HB-3	HB-3
9 months	Measles, Yellow fever†		

Abbreviations: OPV, oral poliomyelitis vaccine; DTP, diphtheria/tetanus/pertussis triple vaccine; HB, hepatitis B vaccine; BCG, vaccine against tuberculosis.

*Scheme A is recommended in countries where perinatal transmission of HBV is frequent (e.g. SE Asia), and scheme B in countries where perinatal transmission is less frequent (e.g. sub-Saharan Africa).

†In countries where yellow fever poses a risk. Measles vaccine is usually given at 12–15 months of age in industrialized countries where the threat of the disease comes after the first year of life. Such a policy benefits from the increased vaccine efficacy after 1 year of age. The vaccine is often combined with rubella and/or mumps vaccine when it is referred to as MR or MMR vaccine. Specific inquiries about a country's immunization schedule should be referred to the national or local authorities.

National immunization schedules

United Kingdom

Table 8.2 shows the UK immunization schedules for the year 2000.

Table 8.2 United Kingdom—2000 schedule of routine immunization for children.

Age	Vaccine	Dose/route	Comment
2 months	Triple (DTwP)*	0.5 mL IM/SC	If whole-cell pertussis vaccine is
	Hib†	0.5 mL IM/SC	contraindicated, consider monovalent
	Polio	3 drops orally‡	acellular pertussis vaccine (if indicated)
	MenC†	0.5 mL IM/SC	and/or DT, or DTaP
3 months	Triple (DTwP)*	0.5 mL IM/SC	
	Hib†	0.5 mL IM/SC	
	Polio	3 drops orally‡	
	MenC†	0.5 mL IM/SC	
4 months	Triple (DTwP)*	0.5 mL IM/SC	
	Hib†	0.5 mL IM/SC	
	Polio	3 drops orally‡	
	MenC†	0.5 mL IM/SC	
12–15 months	MMR	0.5 mL IM/SC	
4–5 years	DT	0.5 mL IM/SC	Nursery or primary school entry
	Polio	3 drops orally‡	
	MMR	0.5 mL IM/SC	Booster
10–14 years or infancy	BCG	0.1 mL ID	If tuberculin negative
		0.05 mL ID	At birth for babies in danger of contact with tuberculosis
13–18 years	Tetanus low-dose diphtheria vaccine for adults and adolescents (Td)	0.5 mL IM/SC	Booster for school leavers
	Polio	3 drops orally‡	

Abbreviations: DTwP, diphtheria/tetanus/whole-cell pertussis combined vaccine; Hib, *Haemophilus influenzae* b; MenC, meningococcal C conjugate vaccine; MMR, measles/mumps/rubella combined vaccine; DT, diphtheria/tetanus combined vaccine; BCG, Bacillus Calmette–Guérin vaccine; Td, tetanus and low-dose diphtheria vaccine.

*If DTwP is not available (i.e. supply problems), the diphtheria tetanus acellular pertussis combined vaccine (DtaP) can be used instead at any point but the schedule should be continued with DTwP as soon as it becomes available.

†One dose, if presenting for the first time after the age of 12 months (MenC two doses if presenting between five and 11 months of age).

‡Three drops or one monodose.

United States of America

Table 8.3 United States of America—Year 2000 schedule of routine immunization for children.

Age	Vaccine
Birth	Hep B$_1$
2 months	Hep B$_2$, DTaP$_1$, Hib$_1$, IPV$_1$
4 months	DTaP$_2$, Hib$_2$, IPV$_2$
6 months	Hep B$_3$ DTaP$_3$ Hib$_3$
12–15 months	Hib$_4$ MMR$_1$
6–18 months	IPV$_3$
15–18 months	DTaP$_4$
12–18 months	Varicella
4–6 years	DTaP$_5$ IPV$_4$ MMR$_2$
11–16 years	Td booster
'Catch-up vaccines' 11–12 years	Hep B, MMR, Varicella
2–12 years	Hep A in selected states and/or regions

Source: American Academy of Paediatrics, American Academy of Family Physicians

Hepatitis B

• Infants born to HBsAg-negative mothers should receive the first dose of the vaccine by age of 2 months, with the second dose 1 month after the first, and the third dose at least 4 months after the first and at least 2 months after the second but not before 6 months of age.
• Infants born to HBsAg-positive mothers should receive the vaccine plus 0.5 mL hepatitis B immunoglobulin (HBIG) within 12 h of birth at separate sites, with the second dose of vaccine at 1 month and the third dose at 6 months of age.
• Infants born to mothers whose HBsAg status is unknown should receive the vaccine within 12 h of birth. A sample of the mother's blood should be taken at the time of delivery, and if HBsAg positive, the infant should receive HBIG as soon as possible (not later than 1 week of age).

• All children and adolescents (up to the age of 18 years) should be vaccinated at any visit.

Tetanus and low-dose diphtheria

Boosters are recommended every 10 years after the fifth dose that is given at 11–16 years of age.

Pertussis

The exclusive use of acellular pertussis vaccine for all doses is now recommended. The fourth dose may be administered as early as the age of 12 months, provided 6 months have elapsed since the third dose and the child is unlikely to return at 15–18 months of age.

Haemophilus influenzae type b

Three conjugate vaccines are licensed for infant use. If Pedvax HIB or ComVax (Merck) is given at ages 2 and 4 months, a dose at 6 months is not required. As lower immune response to the Hib vaccine component may occur when using some combined vaccines, DTaP/Hib combination products should not be used for primary immunization in infants at 2, 4 or 6 months of age unless the vaccine is FDA-approved for these ages.

Poliomyelitis

In order to eliminate the risk of vaccine-associated paralytic polio (VAPP) the inactivated poliomyelitis vaccine (IPV) is now recommended for all children. They should receive four doses of IPV at 2, 4, 6–18 months and at 4–6 years of age.

The oral poliomyelitis vaccine (OPV) should be used only for the following special circumstances:
• mass vaccination campaigns to control outbreaks of paralytic polio;
• in unvaccinated children who will be travelling in less than 4 weeks to areas where polio is endemic or epidemic;
• in children of parents who do not accept the recommended number of vaccine injections. These children may receive OPV only for the third or fourth dose or both; the risk of VAPP should be discussed with the parents or guardians.

MMR

The second dose of MMR is recommended routinely at 4–6 years of age but may be administered during any visit, provided at least 4 weeks have elapsed since receipt of the first dose (vaccinations beginning at or after 12 months of age).

Varicella

This should be given at any visit after the first birthday for susceptible children, i.e. those with no reliable history of chickenpox (as judged by a healthcare professional) and who have not been immunized. Susceptible persons 13 years and over need two doses, given at least 4 weeks apart.

Hepatitis A

This is only necessary in selected states and regions.

The National Childhood Vaccine Injury Act requires that all healthcare providers, whether public or private, give to parents of patients copies of Vaccine Information Statements before administering each dose of the vaccines listed in the schedule above (except Hep A). Vaccine Information Statements developed by Centers for Disease Control and Prevention (USA) (CDC), can be obtained from state health departments and CDC's web site: http://www.cdc.gov/nip/publications/VIS.

CDC's Advisory Committee on Immunization Practices (ACIP) statements for each recommended childhood vaccine can be viewed, downloaded, and printed at CDC's National Immunization Program World Wide Website: http://www.cdc.gov.nip/publications/acip-list.htm.

On 22 October 1999, the ACIP recommended that Rotashield (rhesus rotavirus vaccine-tetravalent (RRV-TVI)) Wyeth Laboratories Inc., the only US-licensed rotavirus vaccine, no longer be used in the USA. Parents should be reassured that children who received rotavirus vaccine before July 1999 are not now at increased risk of intussusception.

In February 2000, the US Food and Drug Administration (FDA) approved Prevnar (Wyeth-Lederle Vaccines), a 7-valent pneumococcal conjugate vaccine. In a large-scale clinical trial in the USA, this vaccine was shown to have 100% efficacy (95% CI 75.4–100%) in preventing invasive pneumococcal disease, caused by the seven serotypes included in the vaccine, after immunization at 2, 4, 6 and 12–15 months of age. It is hoped that widespread use of this vaccine could possibly reduce the spread of drug-resistant pneumococci in the future. The ACIP recommends the use of Prevnar for all infants up to the age of 23 months, and in certain older children aged 24–59 months belonging to high-risk groups.

The current US schedule of childhood immunizations can be found on the website of the American Academy of Paediatrics: http://www.aap.org (see Chapter 64).

Table 8.4   United States of America—2000 schedule of routine immunization for adults.

Vaccine	Recommendations
Tetanus/diphtheria (Td)	Completion of the three-dose primary immunization schedule followed by either Td boosters every 10 years or a single booster at around age 50 years for those who have completed their full paediatric series and the young adult booster
Hepatitis B	Sexually active young adults; high-risk groups.
Influenza	Yearly for all aged 50 years and over. For younger adults with risk factors. May be offered to other healthy, younger adults
Pneumococcal	All adults aged 65 years and over; younger adults with risk factors. Re-immunize at 65 if 6 or more years have passed since first pneumococcal immunization

Australian Capital Territory

Table 8.5 Australian Capital Territory—1999 schedule of routine immunizations.

Age	Vaccine
2 months	DTwP or DTaP OPV Hib (HbOC or PRP–OMP)
4 months	DTwP or DTaP OPV Hib (HbOC or PRP–OMP)
6 months	DTwP or DTaP OPV Hib (HbOC)*
12 months	MMR Hib (PRP-OMP)†
18 months	DTaP or DTwP Hib (HbOC)
Pre-school (4–5 years)	DTaP or DTwP OPV MMR
10–16 years 1 month later 6 months after first dose	HBV–1‡ HBV–2 HBV–3
School leaving (15–19 years)	Td OPV
Every 10 years	Td
Post partum for nonimmune women	Rubella vaccine or MMR
Over 50 years (Aboriginal and Torres Strait Islander people)	Pneumococcal (every 5 years) Influenza (annually)
Over 65 years	Pneumococcal (every 5 years) Influenza (annually)

* HbOC is HibTITER; given at 2, 4, 6, 18 months.
† PRP–OMP is Pedevax HIB given at 2, 4, 12 months.
‡ HBV is hepatitis B vaccine for infants of parents who request it, infants of HBsAg-positive mothers and infants of groups with a hepatitis B carrier rate of over 2%—given at birth, 1 month and 6–12 months of age.

Please note the use of trade names and commercial sources is for identification only and does not imply endorsement.

New Zealand

Table 8.6 New Zealand—1999 schedule of routine immunizations.

Age	Vaccine
6 weeks	Hep B DTP Hib Polio
3 months	Hep B DTP Hib Polio
5 months	Hep B DTP Hib Polio
15 months	DTP Hib MMR
11 years	Polio MMR Td

Europe

Table 8.7 shows the immunization schedules for children in Europe. These tables were prepared with kind assistance of Aventis Pasteur MSD.

Table 8.7(a) Immunization schedules for children in Europe (birth to 11 months).

	Birth	1 month	2 months	3 months	4 months	5 months	6 months	7 months	8 months	10 months	11 months
Austria			DTP(27)–IPV–Hib1(14)+HB1(18)	DTP(27)–IPV–Hib2(14)	DTP(27)–IPV–Hib3(14)+HB2						
Belgium				DTwP1 + Hib1 + OPV	DTwP2 + Hib2 + HB1	DTwP3 + Hib3 + HB2 + OPV2					
Denmark				DTaP–IPV + Hib1		DTaP–IPV2 + Hib2					
Finland	BCG			DTwP1	DTwP2 + Hib1	DTwP3	IPV1 + Hib2				
France	BCG(1)		DTwP–IPV1–Hib1 + HB1	DTwP–IPV2–Hib2 + HB2	DTwP–IPV3–Hib3				HB3		
Germany	HB1(23)	HB2(23)	DTaP1 + Hib1 + IPV1 + HB1(5)	DTaP2 or DTaP2–Hib2–IPV2(24)	DTaP3 + Hib2 + IPV2 + HB2(5) or DTaP3–Hib3–IPV3(24)		HB3(23)				DTaP4 + Hib3 + IPV3 + HB3 or DTaP4–Hib4–IPV4(24) + MMR1:11/14m
Greece		BCG(1)	DT(a or w)P1 + OPV1 + Hib1 + HB1: 2/3m		DT(a or w)P2 + OPV2 + Hib2 + HB2: 4/5m		DT(a or w)P3 + OPV3 + Hib3: 6/7m		HB3: 8/9 m		
Iceland	BCG(6)			DTwP1 + Hib1	DTwP2 + Hib2		DTwP3 + Hib3 + IPV1	Polio			MMR1: 11/14m
Ireland			DTaP1 + OPV1 + Hib1		DTaP2 + OPV2 + Hib2		DTaP3 + OPV3 + Hib3				
Italy			DTaP1 + IPV1 + Hib1 + HB1		DTaP2 + IPV2 + Hib2 + HB2					Hib3 and DTaP3 + OPV3 + HB3: 10/11m	
Luxemburg		HB1 / BCG(1)	DTaP1–Hib1–IPV1: 2/3m	DTaP2–Hib2–IPV2 + HB2: 3/5m	DTaP3–Hib3–IPV3: 4/6m						DTaP4–Hib4–IPV4 + HB3: 11/12m
The Netherlands			DTwP1–IPV1 + Hib1	DTwP2–IPV2 + Hib2	DTwP3–IPV3 + Hib3						DTwP4–IPV4 + Hib4
Norway				DTaP1 + IPV1 + Hib1		DTaP2 + IPV2 + Hib2					DTaP3 + IPV3 + Hib3: 11/12m
Portugal	BCG: 0/1m + HB1		DTwP1 + OPV1 + Hib1 + HB2		DTwP2 + OPV2 + Hib2		DTwP3 + OPV3 + Hib3 + HB3				
Spain	HB1(6)		DTwP1(6) or DTaP1(6) + OPV1 + Hib1 + HB2(6): 2/3m		DTwP2(6) or DTaP2(6) + OPV2 + Hib2: 4/5m		HB3(6) + DTwP3(6) or DTaP3(6) + OPV3 + Hib3: 6/7m				
Sweden				DTaP1 + IPV + Hib1		DTaP2 + IPV2 + Hib2					
Switzerland			DT(a or w)P1 + Hib1 + IPV1		DT(a or w)P2 + Hib2 + IPV2		DT(a or w)P3 + Hib3 + IPV3				
United Kingdom	BCG(1)		DTwP1 + OPV1 + Hib1 + conjMenC1	DTwP2 + OPV2 + Hib2 + conjMenC2	DTwP3 + OPV3 + Hib3 + conjMenC3	conjMenC1 and 2(5): 5/12m					

continued p. 36

Table 8.7(b) Immunization schedules for children in Europe (12 months to 4 years).

	12 months	13 months	14 months	15 months	16 months	18 months	20 months	2 years	3 years	3 1/2 years	4 years
Austria		MMR1	DTP(27)–IPV–Hib4(14) + HB3: 14/17m								
Belgium		DTwP4(26) + Hib4 + OPV3 + HB3: 13/18m	MMR1: 14/18m								
Denmark	DTaP-IPV3 + Hib3			MMR1							OPV3
Finland	IPV2		MMR1 + Hib3: 14/18m				DTwP4 + IPV3: 20/24m	OPV1	OPV2		
France	MMR1 + HB3(22)				DT(a or w)P–IPV4–Hib4 + HB3(22): 16/18m				MMR2: 3/6y		
Germany											
Greece	MMR1: 12/15m					DT(a or w)P4 + OPV4 + Hib4					DT(a or w)P5 or DT5 + OPV5: 4/6y or MMR2: 4/8y or 11/12y
Iceland			DTwP4 + Hib4 + IPV							IPV	
Ireland	MMR1: 12/15m					MMR1					DT4 + OPV4: 4/5y
Italy								OPV4			DTaP4: 4/5y MMR2: 4/5y or 10/11y
Luxemburg											
The Netherlands			MMR1								
Norway				MMR1							DT IPV5
Portugal				MMR1: 15/18m		DTwP4: 18/24m + Hib4					
Spain years	MMR1: 12/15m (11)			MMR1			DTwP4 or DT4(6) or DTaP(6) + OPV4 + Hib4				MMR2(6): 4–6
Sweden	DTaP3 + IPV3 + Hib3					MMR1					DTaP5 + OPV5 or IPV5 + MMR2: 4/7y
Switzerland				Hib4 + MMR1 DT(a or w(16)) P4 + OPV4 or IPV4: 15/23m					MMR2		
United Kingdom	MMR1: 12/15m ConjMenC1(5): 1/5y								MMR2 DT4 + OPV4: 3/5y		

Austria: Bundesministerium für Arbeit, gesundheit und Soziales. Belgium: Direction générale de la santé. Denmark: EPI-News-Statens Serum Institut. France: Conseil supérieur d'hygiène publique de France. Direction générale de la santé. Germany: Robert-Koch-Institut (STIKO). Ireland: Immunization guidelines for Ireland. National immunization committee. Royal College of Physicians of Ireland. Italy: Ministero della Sanità. Luxemburg: Secretariat general de la direction de la santé. Netherlands: Staatstoezicht op de volksgezondheid. Norway: Meldingsystem for Smittsomme Sykdommer Statens Institutt for folkehelse. Sweden: Socialstyrelsen. SOSFS: Smittskyddssektionen Folkhälsoenheten (Swedish National Board of Health, Section for Infectious Diseases, Unit of public health). Switzerland: Office fédéral de la santé publique et Commission suisse pour les vaccinations.
w: weeks m: months y: years /: between -: combination (1): at risks infants only (2): girls only (3): boys only (4): if Mantoux test is negative (5): if not vaccinated before (6): in some districts only (7): booster if vaccinated before or primoimmunization (8): according to physician's decision (9): the need for a booster will be rediscussed in the light of further data (10): doses at 0, 1, 6 months (11): in case of special risk only: 1 dose at 9 months or earlier (12): all children vaccinated before or not (13): if travel in an endemic country (14): as soon as vaccine available (15): if did not receive a second dose (16): preferably aP (17): or primoimmunization if not done before (18): vaccination can begin later: should be done between 3 months and 13 years. Schedule can be 2 + 1 or 3 + 1 (19): at this age or before (20): catch up for aP (21): To finish an incomplete schedule (22): if not given before (23): if the mother is HBsAg positive or not tested for HBsAg (24): if pentavalent vaccine is/was used (25): if the last vaccination was less than 12 months ago, the vaccination can be omitted (26): aPer in the Flemish community (27): aPer only available through national tender 1 month means at 30 days of life (and not during the first month) 2/3 months means between the 60th and the 90th day of life. A '+' between vaccines means association whereas a '−' stands for combination.

Chapter 9

Vaccine damage payment scheme

Under this scheme, any person over the age of 2 years immunized against one or a group of the diseases below, in the UK, from the Isle of Man or in the Armed Forces, and who was immunized before his/her eighteenth birthday (except for polio or rubella during an epidemic or during an outbreak where the vaccine is given in the UK or the Isle of Man), and who has suffered severe mental and/or physical disablement of 80% or more as a result of the immunization, may apply for compensation. The said diseases are the following:

- diphtheria;
- tetanus;
- pertussis;
- poliomyelitis;
- tuberculosis;
- measles;
- mumps;
- rubella;
- *Haemophilus influenzae* b;
- smallpox.

A claim can also be made if a person is severely disabled as a result of his/her mother being immunized against any of the above diseases while she was pregnant. Also if the disability results from being in close contact with a person who has been immunized using the oral polio vaccine.

The claim must be made within 6 years of the date of immunization or of the child reaching the age of 2 years. Such a payment is not compensation and the amount payable is £30 000 for claims made on or after 15 April 1991. Direct claims should be addressed to: Vaccine Damage Payments Unit, Department of Social Security, Palatine House, Lancaster Road, Preston PR1 1HB, UK.

During summer 2000 the Government had announced that it will be passing through Parliament new legislation in order to introduce changes to the 1979 Vaccine Damage Payment Act. It proposes to raise the 6-year limit on making a claim to any time up to the age of 18 years old. It will also be raising the level of compensation to £100 000.

Chapter 10

Information sheet for parents

(This sheet may be copied and given to parents.)

Any parents would wish their child to grow up healthy. One of the most important tasks of a parent is to ensure that their child has received all immunizations at the recommended ages. We ought to consider ourselves very lucky in the UK, as we are able to afford a superb immunization programme that aims to prevent our children from contracting certain infectious diseases. The fact that nearly all children in the UK are immunized means that infectious diseases are rare. Our children could be in danger if fewer children were to be immunized. Also, when travelling abroad or when foreigners come to this country, children can come into contact with infectious diseases. It is therefore very important that every single child in the UK receives the full range of vaccinations, at the right age, as advised by the Department of Health. Here is some information that may be helpful to you.

• Immunization is the process of making a person resistant to a disease without suffering its symptoms. This is usually achieved by inoculation (injecting vaccine into the body) or by drops (oral polio vaccine).

• Immunization of a child not only protects that child but it helps prevent the infectious diseases from spreading to the rest of the family and the community.

• Vaccines usually give well over 90% protection if a full course of immunization is given. If a vaccinated child still catches the disease, he or she will usually have a mild form. The efficacy of routinely used vaccines in the UK's immunization programme for children is as follows: diphtheria 87–96%; tetanus over 90%; whooping cough over 90%; oral polio 90–100%; *Haemophilus influenzae* b 94–100%; meningococcal C over 98%; measles 90–95%; mumps 90–95%; rubella 97–99%; BCG (tuberculosis) about 80%.

Before having your child immunized, ask yourself:

(a) Is my child ill with a raised temperature?

(b) Has my child reacted to any previous immunization?

(c) Has my child ever had any kind of fit or convulsions?

(d) Does my child react to eggs or any antibiotics with swelling of the mouth and throat, difficulty in breathing and collapse?

If your answer to any of these questions is 'yes', or if you are unsure, talk it over with your doctor or nurse. He or she may advise postponement or avoidance of a particular vaccine.

Table 10.1 shows the timetable for routine immunization.

Table 10.1 Timetable for routine immunization.

Age	Vaccine
2 months	Diphtheria, tetanus, whooping cough, polio, *Haemophilus influenzae* b, Meningococcus C
3 months	Diphtheria, tetanus, whooping cough, polio, *Haemophilus influenzae* b, Meningococcus C
4 months	Diphtheria, tetanus, whooping cough, polio, *Haemophilus influenzae* b, Meningococcus C
12–18 months	Measles/mumps/rubella (MMR)
4–5 years	Diphtheria, tetanus, polio, MMR booster
13 years or infancy	Turberculosis (BCG)
15–19 years	Diphtheria, tetanus, polio

● Allergic conditions such as eczema, asthma or hay fever are not contraindications to immunizations. Some vaccines contain traces of some antibiotics, hens' eggs, etc. These vaccines are contraindicated in children who experience an anaphylactic reaction (swelling of the upper airways, collapse) and not just a dislike or rash when they ingest these antibiotics, hens' eggs, etc.

● Your child needs to be immunized against measles, mumps and rubella even if you think your child has already had one or more of these diseases. This is because there are many childhood illnesses which look like measles or German measles (rubella), so it is impossible to be sure that your child has indeed had them.

● The second dose of the measles/mumps/rubella (MMR) vaccine is given with the other preschool vaccinations, not only to boost your child's immunity but also to ensure that the vaccine takes if it did not do so the first time the MMR was given.

● If your child has not been immunized and comes into contact with a child with measles, he or she can still be protected if the MMR vaccine is given within 3 days of contact.

● If your child vomits soon after receiving the oral polio vaccine, a further dose may be necessary. Inform your doctor or nurse.

Reactions to vaccines

● All medicines have some risks but the vaccines used to immunize children against infectious diseases are among the safest but not without risk of side effects.

● The infectious diseases themselves can cause the same problems as the vaccines. The risk of side-effects from vaccines is much smaller than complications from infectious diseases.

● The current UK infant and childhood immunization programme confers vastly more benefit than possible harm. It is important, therefore, that uptake of vaccinations is maintained and, for MMR in particular, improved.

● Many children for whom immunization is perfectly safe can experience mild, harmless side-effects. A child might cry a bit more than usual, become slightly feverish and irritable for a few hours after the injection. Some children may have a fever and a measles rash 5–10 days after receiving the MMR combined vaccine. The rash lasts for 2–3 days and it is not transmissible to unvaccinated children. Occasionally a child may develop swollen glands on the face like mumps, about 2–6 weeks after vaccination with MMR. Rarely, others may complain of joint aches.

● The measles vaccine does not cause autism or bowel disease. The Department of Health as well as the World Health Organization and other countries such as Sweden and Finland, have repeatedly looked into this question and found no evidence to support this hypothesis.

● Delaying vaccination in order to administer the three components of the MMR vaccine separately (this option is not available in the UK) can be dangerous as the child could catch the disease while waiting, and it is without any scientific foundation.

● The chances of more serious side-effects are very rare indeed, and they occur much less frequently after immunization than if the child were to catch the disease. Febrile convulsions after measles are eight to ten times more common than after the measles vaccine. If brain damage from whooping cough vaccine occurs at all, it occurs so extremely rarely that it is difficult to prove. In fact, whooping cough vaccine may be protecting your child from brain damage by preventing whooping cough disease, which can be complicated by brain damage.

● If your child has a tendency to convulsions, you should discuss with the doctor the management of any fever and/or convulsions possibly developing after immunization. This could happen in the first 72 h after whooping cough immunization or 5–10 days after MMR immunization. In case of fever, it is recommended that you give the baby paracetamol, extra fluids, dress them in thin clothing, cool the room and even perform tepid sponging and consider having the child seen by the GP if you judge it necessary.

● Children receiving their oral polio vaccine can continue excreting the vaccine virus in their faeces for 30 or more days after vaccination. We would recommend adherence to strict personal hygiene for anybody who changes the nappies and in particular washing hands after nappy changes and safe disposal of the nappies. If any member of the family has not been immunized against polio, they should also receive the vaccine at the same time as the baby. (Mass immunization with oral polio vaccine was introduced in the UK in 1962.) It is safe to take the baby to swimming pools at any time.

• Please report to the doctor any symptoms your child experiences after immunization that worry you.

• Call your doctor right away if you notice more serious symptoms, such as:

(a) very high fever (39.5 °C (103 °F) or above);

(b) crying without stopping for 3 h or more;

(c) an unusual, high-pitched cry;

(d) hoarseness with difficulty in breathing, convulsions.

• We would advise you stay at the surgery for 20 min after vaccination. Severe reactions immediately after immunizations are very rare indeed (once in every 600 000 vaccinations).

Important websites for information on vaccines:

• UK: http://www.medinfo.co.uk/immunizations/mmr.html

• USA: http://www.ecbt.org/parents.htm#guide

• Canadian Immunization Awareness Program (CIAP): general, easy to understand information about vaccines and vaccine safety: http://www.immunize.cpha.ca/

• The National Vaccine Information Center: http://www.909shot.com

• People Advocating Vaccine Education: http://www.vaccines.bizland.com

• The National Immunization Program of the USA Centers for Disease Control: http://www.cdc.gov/nip

• The Institute of Vaccine Safety of John Hopkins University: http://www.vaccinesafety.edu/

• The Immunization Action Coalition: http://www.immunize.org

• The Department of Vaccines and Biologicals: http://www.who.ch/gpr-safety

• The National Immunization Information Network of the Infectious Disease Society–USA: http://www.idsociety.org

• Canadian Paediatric Society: http://www.cps.ca

Every child has the right to vaccination. To deny vaccination can be to deny the child its health. Your help in protecting your child and all children against infectious diseases is greatly appreciated and welcomed.

Chapter 11

Viral and bacterial vaccines

	Viral vaccines	Bacterial vaccines
Live	Measles Mumps Rubella Oral poliomyelitis Yellow fever Varicella	BCG Typhoid—oral
Inactivated	Influenza Hepatitis A Injectable poliomyelitis Rabies Tick-borne encephalitis Japanese B encephalitis Anthrax	Pertussis Cholera* Typhoid* Plague
Toxoids		Diphtheria Tetanus
Bioengineered	Hepatitis B	
Polysaccharide extracts		*Haemophilus influenzae* b conjugate Meningococcal A & C Meningococcal C conjugate Pneumococcal Typhoid—Vi antigen

* These two parenteral vaccines are no longer available in the UK.

Chapter 12

Special precautions for all vaccines

- All immunizations should be postponed if the patient is suffering from any acute febrile illness, particularly respiratory, until fully recovered. A minor infection without fever is not a reason to delay immunization; this is particularly true for well babies who chronically seem snuffly.
- In general, it is not necessary to recommence a primary course of immunization, however long a period has elapsed since the last dose was given. In infants whose basic course, for example DTP or poliomyelitis vaccine, has been interrupted, a single dose later in infancy (or two doses where only the first dose of the basic course had been given) is adequate to establish immunity, regardless of the time elapsing between the initial and subsequent doses. So, we do not repeat the missed dose but we continue the course regardless of time lapse. There is evidence that where there was an interruption of the course of immunization, higher titres were obtained when the missed dose was given late.

In the USA, the Public Health Service Recommendations advise that except for oral typhoid vaccine, it is unnecessary to restart an interrupted series of a vaccine or toxoid or to add extra doses.

In the UK, the manufacturer of the rabies vaccine (Aventis Pasteur MSD) recommends repeating an interrupted course of rabies vaccine in certain circumstances because rabies is such a fatal disease. The following therefore should apply to the rabies vaccine cultured on human diploid cells (HDCV) interrupted courses:

Three-dose course (0, 7, 28)

If interruption after the first (day 0) dose is less than 3 months: restart course.

If interruption after first and second (days 0 and 7) doses is over 6 months: restart course.

If over 5 years have elapsed since the three-dose primary course: restart course.

Two-dose course (0, 28)

If more than 2 years have elapsed since the 6–12 month missed booster was due: restart course.

- Recent vaccination (including OPV) is not a contraindication to surgery.
- No immunization should be given to a site showing signs of skin infection.
- Vaccines must be stored under the conditions recommended by the manufacturers, usually at a refrigerator temperature of between 2 and 8 °C. Do not freeze vaccines as this could cause deterioration of the product or breakage of the diluent container or glass syringe. Heat also causes deterioration of vaccines.
- Add the diluent slowly. Injecting with too much pressure will result in frothing with possible adverse effects on the vaccine efficacy.
- Multidose vials should be discarded after a vaccination session. This is because there is a risk of contamination with bacteria and moulds, which may result in a reduction of vaccine potency.
- Some vaccines contain traces of antibiotics or elements of hens' egg. Severe sensitivity to a particular antibiotic or hen's egg means an anaphylactic reaction and not just a rash.
- Premature babies should have their first injection 2 months from the actual rather than expected date of birth, i.e. they should be immunized at the same chronological age as full-term babies.
- In adults, avoid the left arm where possible as ischaemic heart pain radiating to the left upper limb may be considered by a patient as pain resulting from his or her recent vaccination. I have witnessed such a case personally.
- In the UK there is a popular belief that babies should not be taken to their local swimming pool until they have completed their first three im-

munizations. This is yet another myth about immunization that needs to be dispelled.

• The site of vaccination is important. Injection of a vaccine into a buttock may be associated with a reduced antibody level production. There is evidence of sciatic nerve damage from vaccinations given into the buttock, and reduced efficacy of immunizations given into the plentiful adipose tissue—reduced absorption and often suboptimal take up, as in the case of hepatitis A and B vaccines. The buttock is also a 'dirty' area with a risk of infection, and a greater chance of subcutaneous fibrous nodule formation. The British Paediatric Association recommends either the lateral thigh or deltoid. The deltoid in older children and adults (do not pinch and do not go too low), and the anterolateral thigh (high up, not too low) in infants under 1 year of age are the preferred sites for vaccinations. Ninety per cent of local reactions in infants are from injections given too low down the thigh.

• If alcohol or other disinfecting agent is used to clean the skin, it should be allowed to evaporate before injection. It is better to avoid using them as their use increases the rate of local reactions and can inactivate the live vaccine. For any bleeding just use cotton wool and pressure.

• A fever of 39.5 °C or greater within 48 h of vaccination constitutes a severe reaction and should be reported to the CSM (see below).

• Suggestions that immunizations may increase the risk of children developing type 1 diabetes mellitus (insulin-dependent) have been refuted. A working party of the US Institute for Vaccine Safety concluded that no vaccines have been shown to increase the risk of type 1 diabetes. There is some evidence, although not conclusive, that the opposite may be the case [(1999) *Paediatr. Infect. Dis. J.* 18, 217–22].

• Warfarin and vaccination. Provided the patient on warfarin has international normalized ratio (INR) within the therapeutic range, there should be no significant risk from injections—a small risk of haematoma does exist. Patients on warfarin because of artificial heart valves have to keep their INR to between 3.0 and 4.5. Their chance of a haematoma is proportionally higher. On balance, patients well controlled on warfarin should have their vaccinations performed after they have been informed of the small risk of a haematoma developing.

• Children with unknown immunization history (e.g. those immigrating to the UK) should be fully immunized as follows:

Under the age of 10 years
DTP, OPV: three doses at monthly intervals.
DT, OPV: booster 5 years later.
Hib: three doses if under 1 year of age, one dose if 1–4 years, no vaccination if over 4 years.
MenC: three doses if under 5 months, two doses if 5–12 months, one dose if older children.
MMR: two doses separated by three or more months. If it was given before first birthday, re-immunize.

Over the age of 10 years
Td, OPV: three doses at monthly intervals, booster 5 years later.
MMR: one dose.
BCG: if tuberculin negative.
MenC: one dose.
Child returning abroad within 1 year: keep to schedule of that country.
If in doubt: start a complete immunization programme as above according to age.

Report reactions to vaccines to the Committee on Safety of Medicines, FREEPOST, 1 Nine Elms Lane, London SW8 5BR, UK, or by phone on 020 7273 3000. Yellow Cards for reporting such events are available at the back of the British National Formulary (BNF), the Association of British Pharmaceutical Industry (ABPI) Data Sheet Compendium and directly from the CSM. Consider reporting reactions to the manufacturer.

Chapter 13

Special precautions for live vaccines

- Live virus vaccines (see table of viral and bacterial vaccines on p. 41) are inactivated by any pre-existing antibodies and therefore may be ineffective if given within a few weeks of administration of immunoglobulin (see below) or a blood transfusion.
- Live virus vaccines can also be inactivated if given to infants of mothers who at the time of pregnancy were immune (except OPV)—this is why the MMR vaccination is delayed until the child is over 1 year old.
- Reconstituted vaccines should be discarded if not used within the reconstituted life of the vaccine as recommended by the manufacturer, usually 1 h—some up to 4 h.
- A single injection of live virus vaccine, if it 'takes', produces long-term immunity and is not normally given more than once (except yellow fever for travel purposes). Oral poliomyelitis vaccine, however, contains three different components and is given more than once to ensure an adequate response to each component. The main purpose of the booster MMR dose is to induce serocon-version in the nonresponders.
- Live virus vaccines that are not combined preparations may be given simultaneously and in different sites. If not given simultaneously, their administration should be separated by an interval of at least 3 weeks. If a live virus vaccine is given soon after another live virus vaccine has been given, it is possible that the replication and the 'take' of the second vaccine could be interfered with by interferon or other inhibitory effects of the first vaccination. No live vaccine interferes with the activity of any 'dead' vaccine; therefore, in these cases no interval needs to be observed.
- Separate administration of the oral viral poliomyelitis vaccine from the oral bacterial typhoid vaccine by 3 weeks (see pp. 81 and 221).

- A 3-week interval is recommended between the administration of live virus vaccines and the giving of BCG (live bacterial vaccine) but they may be given simultaneously at different sites.
- A 3-week interval is also recommended between live virus vaccines (especially containing measles vaccine) and tuberculin testing (this may result in a false-negative result).
- With the exception of yellow fever and a special consideration for OPV and 'immediate travellers' (see p. 81), live vaccines should not be given within 3 months following the administration of human normal immunoglobulin (HNIG) (Fig. 13.1).

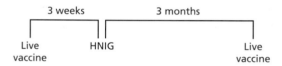

Fig. 13.1 Administration sequence of live vaccines and human normal immunoglobulin (HNIG).

- The parents of children with a tendency to have convulsions because of personal or family history of convulsions should be counselled on the management of any fever developing after immunization. Febrile convulsions may occur 5–10 days after measles immunization (MMR), whereas they may take place in the first 72 h after pertussis immunization, especially when the third dose is given after the age of 6 months. Suggestions may include giving paracetamol, sponging with tepid water, giving extra fluids, dressing in thin clothing and placing in a cool room. In high-risk children, an antipyretic drug may be suggested routinely for the first 24–72 h after immunization. Where the tendency is severe, the parents may be instructed on rectal diazepam administration.

• Seek specialist advice before continuing with any immunization if febrile convulsions occur after the administration of any vaccine.

• Live vaccines should not be administered to pregnant women, particularly early in pregnancy, because of possible harm to the fetus. However, where there is significant risk of exposure to such serious conditions as poliomyelitis or yellow fever, the importance of vaccination may outweigh the possible risk to the fetus.

Immunodeficiency and live vaccines

• Live vaccines should not be administered to persons whose ability to respond to infection is reduced for one reason or another. They could suffer from severe manifestations of the disease, e.g. paralytic poliomyelitis with oral polio, or dissemination of infection with BCG. These vaccines should not be given to persons suffering from malignant disease, gammaglobulin deficiency or to those with impaired immune responsiveness, whether idiopathic or as a result of treatment with steroids, radiotherapy, cytotoxic drugs or other agents. Children with malignancy but whose treatment has stopped for more than 6 months may be immunized. Close contacts of immunodeficient children and adults must be immunized, particularly against measles, mumps, rubella and polio. They should not be given the oral vaccine (OPV), and the inactivated/injectable polio (IPV) vaccine should be used to confer immunity.

• *An immunodeficient child is the child:*
(a) with serious conditions of the reticulo-endothelial system (leukaemia, lymphomas, etc.);
(b) with primary immunodeficiency conditions—for human immunodeficiency virus (HIV) infection (see p. 350);
(c) on doses of systemic steroids equivalent to 2 mg/kg/day or more of prednisolone, for over 1 week, or 1 mg/kg/day for over 1 month. Postpone vaccination until 3 months after stopping the steroid. A child on lower daily doses of systemic steroids may be immunosuppressed so seek a specialist's advice;
(d) receiving chemotherapy or generalized radiotherapy. Postpone vaccination until at least 6 months after completion of treatment;
(e) after organ transplantation and receiving immunosuppressive treatment.

• *An immunodeficient adult* is a patient with malignancy or primary immunodeficiency condition, or receiving chemotherapy, or radiotherapy, or on immunosuppressive treatment after organ transplant, or within 6 months of terminating such treatments. In addition, adults who receive 40 mg or more of oral prednisolone daily for more than 1 week.

• Give the vaccine 6 months after chemotherapy has finished, or 3 months after treatment with systemic steroids or other immunosuppressive treatment has stopped. Use immunoglobulin in case of exposure to a virus such as measles or varicella.

• The patient with human immunodeficiency virus (HIV positive) and immunization: see p. 324.

Chapter 14

Treating anaphylaxis

Anaphylaxis means a severe systemic allergic reaction. It involves one or both of two severe features: respiratory difficulty and hypotension. Other features may be present. Anaphylaxis is treatable and patients can make a full recovery.

Although an anaphylactic reaction following vaccination is rare, any healthcare personnel administering a vaccine should know what action to take on occurrence.

Anaphylactic reaction may occur within seconds or minutes of injection. The patient suddenly sweats profusely and loses consciousness. Alternatively, the onset may be gradual with urticaria, angio-oedema (hoarseness, stridor, dyspnoea) tachycardia with hypotension, bradycardia, nausea and vomiting, pallor and collapse. It can be delayed for 72 h or more (even days—as in the case of Japanese B encephalitis vaccine).

A strong central pulse (carotid and femoral) is more likely to indicate a simple faint (common in older children and adults, rare in younger children), while a weak or absent pulse may indicate anaphylaxis, in which case the following instructions should be followed.

• Call for help without leaving the patient.
• If conscious, make comfortable and elevate the legs if hypotensive.
• If unconscious, place the patient in the left lateral ('recovery') position.
• Insert airway (if unconscious).
• Administer oxygen at 10–15 L/min.
• Administer adrenaline (epinephrine) 1 : 1000 (1 mg/mL) by deep IM (slow absorption if given SC) injection and repeat in 5 min if required, up to a maximum of three doses, in a dose of 0.01 mL/kg bodyweight or in the doses listed in Table 14.1. Adrenaline (epinephrine) should not be given intravenously. Children should receive the IM injection slowly, over 10–15 s. As an α-receptor agonist, it reverses peripheral vasodilatation and reduces oedema. Its β-receptor activity dilates the airways, increases the force of myocardial contraction, and suppresses histamine and leukotriene release.

Table 14.1 Recommended doses of adrenaline (epinephrine) (1 : 1000—1 mg/mL) intramuscularly in the treatment of anaphylaxis.

Age (yr)	Dose	
	(ml)	(μg)
< 1	0.05	50
1	0.1	100
2	0.2	200
3–4	0.3	300
5	0.4	400
6–10	0.5	500
> 10	0.5–1	500–1000

• Children or adults, in severe cases (inspiratory stridor, wheeze, cyanosis, tachycardia), may also need to receive hydrocortisone IV (Table 14.2), although corticosteroids can take up to 4–6 h to have an effect (even when given IV). They may help in the emergency treatment of an acute attack, and they may also have a role in preventing or shortening protracted reactions.

Table 14.2 Recommended doses of hydrocortisone IV in the treatment of anaphylaxis.

Age (yr)	Dose (mg)
< 1	25
1–5	50
6–11	100
> 11	100–500

Table 14.3 Recommended doses of chlorpheniramine intramuscularly in the treatment of anaphylaxis.

Age (yr)	Dose (mg)
1–5	2.5–5
6–11	5–10
> 11	10–20

• In adults, chlorpheniramine maleate (Piriton) by slow IV (to avoid drug-induced hypotension) or IM injection may be given at doses listed in Table 14.3.

• Monitor pulse and blood pressure.

• Replace volume with crystalloid solution if blood pressure is low. A rapid infusion of 1–2 L may be needed. Give children 20 mL/kg rapidly, followed by another similar dose if there is no clinical response.

• In the case of bronchospasm, administer via a nebulizer a ß-2 agonist such as salbutamol or terbutaline.

• Commence cardiopulmonary resuscitation if appropriate.

• Be prepared to perform emergency tracheostomy if necessary.

• It is recommended that all cases of anaphylaxis are admitted to hospital for observation.

• Report the reaction to the CSM (yellow cards at the back of the BNF) and, if possible, to the manufacturer.

• The adrenaline (epinephrine) injection solution deteriorates, particularly when exposed to light; replace ampoules annually (my policy is to do this every Christmas) or at expiry date, whichever is earlier, and follow the manufacturer's instructions. Store adrenaline (epinephrine) at room temperature and protect from light.

• The reported rate of anaphylaxis resulting from immunization of children and adults in primary and secondary care in the UK is one case in 632 000 vaccinations.

• Experience from the Measles and Rubella Immunization Campaign in the UK in 1994, when children aged 5–18 years were vaccinated, has shown a rate of anaphylaxis of one case in 100 000 vaccinations (more frequently among children aged 9 years and over, and in females).

• No deaths were reported in the UK between 1992 and 1995 in the individuals that developed anaphylaxis as a result of vaccination.

Waiting time after vaccination: there is no universal agreement on the length of time (if any) an individual should remain within the medical centre after receiving a vaccine. Some centres recommend 20 min for everybody, others vary the time according to the vaccine (e.g. MMR—20 min, yellow fever—30 min, Japanese B encephalitis—30 min). In any case, all vaccinees should remain under observation until it is evident that they are in good health and experiencing no immediate adverse reaction. It is extremely unlikely that a child who appears completely well 30 min after vaccination will subsequently develop a severe reaction.

On reviewing 'yellow card' data from the Medicines Control Agency, there have been two fatal anaphylactic reactions (one after DTP and another after influenza vaccine) in the 27 years between July 1963 and February 2000.

The Resuscitation Council (UK) updated its guidelines in 1999. These can be found on http://www.resus.org.uk.

Part 2

The UK National Immunization Programme Vaccines

Chapter 15

Complications of infectious diseases and vaccines: an *aide-mémoire*

Diphtheria

Diphtheria infection

- Acute infection of the upper respiratory tract and occasionally the skin, sore throat, fever with:
  respiratory obstruction;
  inflammation of larynx and trachea;
  loss of function of the vocal cords;
  persistent skin ulcers.
- WHO data: $\sim 100\,000$ cases per year and up to 8000 deaths.
- Reduction in immunization (e.g. in Russia), leads to resurgence of diphtheria

Diphtheria vaccine

- Swelling and redness at injection site.
- Occasionally painless nodule at injection site— usually disappears without sequelae.
- Transient fever, headaches, malaise, myalgia.
- Rarely urticaria, anaphylactic reaction.
- Very rarely neurological reactions.

Tetanus

Tetanus infection

- Bacterial infection—spores found in many places, e.g. soil, faeces, etc.
- Used to be known as 'lockjaw'.
- The toxin reaches the spinal cord and brain via the blood and peripheral nerves.
- Increases reflex excitability in motor neurones.
- Muscle spasms.
- Kills 500 000 babies worldwide every year.

Tetanus toxoid vaccine

- Soreness, swelling and redness at injection site for up to 10 days postinjection.
- Transient pyrexia, headaches, malaise, myalgia.
- Rarely urticaria, anaphylactic reaction.
- Extremely rarely Guillain–Barré syndrome and brachial neuritis.

Pertussis

Pertussis infection

- Starts as a mild upper respiratory tract infection.
- Progresses to severe paroxysms of cough, followed by vomiting.
- Characteristic 'whoop' (inspiratory attempt to breathe in after the child is out of breath in a coughing spasm).
- Lasts 1–3 months.
- Complications in infants are:
  1 in 8 progress to pneumonia;
  1 in 20 progress to encephalopathy;
  seizures;
  permanent brain damage;
  1 in 200 die.

Pertussis vaccine

Acellular vaccines result in significantly fewer side-effects than whole-cell vaccines. Incidences shown below are for whole-cell vaccines.
- Soreness, swelling and redness at injection site.
- 1 in 100 cry for 3 h or longer.
- 3 in 100 have a high fever.
- 1 in 1750 exhibit hypotonic–hyporesponsiveness (collapse) without any lasting sequelae.
- 1 in 1750 get seizures (first 48 h) without any lasting sequelae.

Haemophilus influenzae type b (Hib)

Haemophilus influenzae type b infection (Hib)

- Bacterial infection occurring mostly in children under 5 years of age.
- Complications are:
  6 in 10 contract Hib meningitis;
  between 1 and 3 in 10 develop long-term sequelae including seizures, intellectual impairment, vision/hearing loss, motor dysfunction, behaviour alterations;
  15 in 100 get epiglottitis;
  1 in 10 get septicaemia;
  1 in 20 die.

Haemophilus influenzae type b vaccine

- Soreness, swelling and redness at injection site in approximately 10% of vaccinees.
- Transient fever, headaches, malaise, myalgia.
- Irritability, inconsolable high-pitched crying.
- Very rarely, seizures.

Meningococcal

Meningococcal disease

- Occurs most frequently in children under 5 years of age.
- Next highest risk group is young people aged 15–19 years.
- Onset is abrupt usually, or insidious.
- Symptoms are:
  headaches, malaise, nausea, vomiting, fever, joint aches, photophobia, drowsiness or confusion, stiff neck, raised anterior fontanelle tension in infants, coma;
  rash:
  (a) petechial or purpuric (does not blanche) in 8 out of 10 cases;
  (b) maculopapular (13 in 100);
  (c) no rash (7 in 100).
- Meningitis usually, but septicaemia in 15–20 in 100.

- Death in 1 in 10 (meningitis 7 in 100, septicaemia 1 in 5).

Meningococcal C conjugate vaccine

- Soreness, swelling and redness at injection site.
- Low-grade fever (<5 in 100 in the under-2-year-olds, up to 3 in 100 in older children).
- Headaches (~1 in 10 in those over 2 years of age).
- Irritability (5 in 10: infants under 1 year; 2 in 10: those 1–2 years).

Meningococcal polysaccharide A + C vaccine

- Soreness, swelling and redness at injection site in approximately 1 in 10 of vaccinees.
- Irritability and fever in first 48 h after vaccination, more commonly in young children than adults.
- Very rarely, anaphylaxis.

Poliomyelitis

Poliomyelitis infection

- 80–90% of cases in under-3-year-olds.
- Asymptomatic in 90–95% of cases.
- 1 in 10 have pyrexia without paralysis.
- 5 in 100 have headaches, vomiting, photophobia, neck stiffness, paralysis.
- 1–5 in 100 progress to poliomyeloencephalitis.
- 1 in 100 suffer paralysis of the lower motor neurones.

Oral poliomyelitis vaccine

Vaccine-associated paralysis:
- vaccinees: after first dose—1 in 1.5 million doses;
- contacts of first-dose vaccinees: 1 in 2.2 million doses, which will be eliminated if all children and adults are immunized;
- risk after subsequent doses is lower;
- overall risk of vaccine-associated poliomyelitis: 1 in 2.4 million doses.

Measles

Measles infection

- More than 1 million children die worldwide each year from measles infection.
- Almost all children have rash and fever.
- 1 in 20 have ear infections.
- 1 in 200 suffer convulsions.
- 1 in 1000 progress to encephalitis; 15 out of 100 will die from it.
- Between 1 in 2500 and 5000 die.

Measles vaccine

Side-effects from the combined MMR vaccine are similar to those from monovalent vaccines.
- 1 in 1000 suffer a febrile convulsion.
- Serious reactions are extremely rare.
- Complications such as meningoencephalitis are very rare, around 1 in 1.8 million doses.

Mumps

Mumps infection

- Fever.
- 1 in 25 have hearing impairment.
- 1 in 4 boys/young men suffer painful inflammation of the testicles.
- Risk of miscarriage in pregnancy.
- Rarely, sterility in boys.

Mumps vaccine

- Serious reactions are extremely rare.
- Complications such as meningoencephalitis are very rare, around 1 in 1.8 million doses.

Rubella

Rubella infection

- Known as 'German measles'.
- Low-grade fever.
- Transient polyarthralgia.
- 7 in 3000 have thrombocytopenia.
- 1 in 6000 progress to encephalitis.
- Asymptomatic in 25–50% of cases.
- Congenital rubella syndrome: 9 in 10 rubella infections in the first term of pregnancy will cause fetal damage.

Rubella vaccine

- 5 in 100 have a rash.
- 5–15 in 100 have fever, 5–12 days after vaccination.
- 1 in 200 children suffer mild episodes of joint pain.
- Up to 1 in 4 adults have transient arthralgia.

Chapter 16

Diphtheria/tetanus/pertussis (DTP) combined and diphtheria/tetanus (DT, Td) combined

Contraindications to vaccination

Those of the individual components of the combined vaccines are described under diphtheria vaccine (p. 57), tetanus vaccine (p. 61) and whole-cell pertussis vaccine (p. 65).

Possible side- and adverse effects

Local reactions

Swelling and redness at the site of injection can appear within the first 48–72 h, and may last up to 1–2 weeks. A painless lump can appear under the skin within 1 week, especially when the injection was not given deeply enough. It may persist for several weeks.

General reactions

The reader is referred to the section on general reactions of the monovalent vaccines (pp. 51, 61, 65). Here, a brief summary is provided of a report from the Institute of Medicine (USA) on DTP vaccine-

related adverse events [(1992) *J. Am. Med. Assoc.*, 267, 3].

- *Acute encephalopathy*: the range of excess risk of acute encephalopathy following DTP immunization is consistent with that estimated for the British National Encephalopathy Study: 0.0–10.5 per million immunizations.
- *Shock and 'unusual shock-like state'*: the evidence did not provide for reliable estimates of excess risk following DTP immunization. Reported incidence in the literature varies from 3.5 to 291 cases per 100 000 immunizations.
- *Anaphylaxis*: in the absence of formal studies of incidence, rates of anaphylaxis are estimated to be approximately two cases per 100 000 injections of DTP (six cases per 100 000 children given three doses of DTP).
- *Protracted, inconsolable crying*: incidence rates are estimated to range from 0.1 to 6% of recipients of a DTP injection and vary with type and dose of vaccine and with immunization site.

Table 16.1 shows the UK schedule of DTP immunization.

Table 16.1 UK schedule of DTP immunization of children.

Vaccine	2 months	3 months	4 months	4–5 years	15–19 years
Adsorbed DTP†	0.5 mL	0.5 mL	0.5 mL	–	–
Adsorbed DT (first three doses only if pertussis is to be omitted)	(0.5 mL)*	(0.5 mL)*	(0.5 mL)*	0.5 mL (all children)	–
Adsorbed Td vaccine for adults and adolescents BP	–	–	–	–	0.5 mL

* If whole-cell pertussis vaccine is contraindicated.
† Use the combined DTP-Hib vaccine where possible (see p. 78).

Table 16.2 Administration specifications for adsorbed tetanus and low-dose diphtheria vaccine for adults and adolescents BP (Td) for children over 10 years of age and unimmunized adults.

Dose (ml)	Route	Primary immunization	Boosters
0.5	IM/SC	Three doses at monthly intervals (nonimmunized children over 10 years of age and adults only)	Every 10 years or more*

*Further 10-yearly boosters are not recommended in the UK, other than at the time of injury. Consider further boosters for travel to high-risk areas or for continuous exposure.

The vaccines

• *Adsorbed DTP vaccine* is an aqueous suspension containing a mixture of purified diphtheria and tetanus toxoids and killed *Bordetella pertussis* organisms, adsorbed onto aluminium hydroxide. Thiomersal is added as a preservative. Each 0.5-mL dose has a potency of not less than 30 IU of diphtheria toxoid, not less than 60 IU of tetanus toxoid, and not less than 4 IU of *Bordetella pertussis* cells.

• *Adsorbed DT vaccine* is similar to DTP but without the pertussis component and with a reduced content (not less than 40 IU) of tetanus toxoid. It can only be used in the under 10 year olds.

• *Adsorbed tetanus and low-dose diphtheria vaccine for adults and adolescents BP* (Td) (Table 16.2) has been available in the UK since the summer of 1994. It contains not less than 4 IU of diphtheria toxoid and not less than 40 IU of tetanus toxoid, both adsorbed onto aluminium hydroxide with thiomersal added as a preservative. It is available for the immunization of adults and children over the age of 10 years.

• The triple adsorbed DTP vaccine is recommended for the primary course for infants from 2 months of age. The course consists of three doses with an interval of 1 month between each dose. Where the pertussis component is to be omitted, adsorbed DT is used instead. Each dose is 0.5 mL and is given by IM or deep SC injection. The container should be shaken before withdrawing the vaccine suspension.

• A booster dose of adsorbed DT (pertussis omitted) is given at the age of 4–5 years, at school entry.

• DTP and DT should not be used in children over the age of 10 years.

• School-leavers aged 15–19 years receive a booster of the adsorbed tetanus and low-dose diphtheria vaccine for adults and adolescents BP (Td).

• If the primary course of DTP or DT is started later than 2 months of age (in the under 10 year olds), the booster dose of DT should be given 3 or more years later. Although a minimum of 5 years is normally recommended between tetanus boosters, there is no evidence that giving a booster a year or two early in these very early years of life is associated with any increased risk of a severe reaction. Once a child has reached age 10 years, any completion of primary course or booster should be with Td.

• Immunization with three doses of triple vaccine (DTP) at monthly intervals completed before 6 months of age probably provides adequate protection against diphtheria, tetanus and whooping cough which will persist until the age of the preschool booster [Ramsay *et al.* (1991) *Br. Med. J.* 302, 1489–91]. A booster dose of DTP at 18 months and pertussis at 4–5 years is not recommended in the UK, while children in the USA receive boosters of DTP or DTaP at 18 months and 4–6 years. Long-term follow-up of antibody concentrations in infants immunized on accelerated schedules introduced in 1990 are necessary to determine whether the present British immunization policy should change.

• The coverage of completed DT (three doses) immunization by the summer of 1999 in the UK was 95.9% (England 94.7%, Wales 95.6%, Northern Ireland 96.4% and Scotland 97%).

• The UK coverage of pertussis immunization (three doses) in children under 2 years of age in the summer of 1999 was 94.6% (England 93.7%, Wales 93.3%, Northern Ireland 96.3% and Scotland 96.7%).

• The general practice now is to administer the combined DTP/Hib vaccine (see p. 78). Studies show such a combined vaccine elicits a greater immune response than the two vaccines given separately, although there is also a higher incidence of local reactions [(1992) *J. Am. Med. Assoc.* 268(24)].

• From the summer of 1994, the adsorbed tetanus and low-dose diphtheria vaccine for adults and adolescents BP (Td) became available. This vaccine is suitable for:

(a) immunization of children over 10 years of age if primary immunization and/or reinforcing dose were not previously given;

(b) to booster the immunity of school-leavers as part of the UK schedule of routine immunization for children;

(c) for the primary immunization of unvaccinated adults;

(d) for boosters for adults at risk, e.g. those travelling to endemic areas.

The dose is 0.5 mL given IM or SC.

Vaccine availability

• Adsorbed DTP vaccine BP (Aventis Pasteur MSD) available in prefilled syringes of 0.5 mL and 0.5-mL single-dose ampoule (pack of five).

• DTP Vaccine Behring (manufactured by Chiron Behring GmbH & Co, made available in the UK by Wyeth Laboratories) available in 0.5 mL suspension in ampoules (pack of 10 ampoules).

• Adsorbed diphtheria and tetanus vaccine BP (CHILD) (Medeva Pharma Ltd) available in 0.5-mL single-dose ampoule (pack of five) as well as multidose vials of 5 mL fill (10 doses).

• Adsorbed diphtheria and tetanus vaccine BP (Aventis Pasteur MSD) available in 0.5-mL single-dose prefilled syringe (pack of 10) and 0.5-mL single-dose ampoule (pack of five).

• Adsorbed diphtheria and tetanus vaccine BP manufactured by Chiron Behring (supplied in the UK by Aventis Pasteur MSD), in packs of 5 0.5 mL ampoules.

• Adsorbed diphtheria and tetanus vaccine for adults and adolescents BP (Aventis Pasteur MSD) available in 0.5-mL single-dose ampoule (pack of five) and 10-dose vial. It should be used only as part of the UK childhood immunization programme for school leavers.

Farillon, Scottish Healthcare Supplies Division of Common Service Agency, and Regional Pharmacist, Procurement Coordinator, Eastern Health and Social Services Board, Belfast distribute all the above childhood immunization vaccines free to GPs, on behalf of the DoH.

• Diftavax—adsorbed diphtheria and tetanus vaccine for adults and adolescents BP (Aventis Pasteur MSD) available in 0.5-mL single-dose prefilled syringe unit pack. Shake the syringe to obtain a homogeneous suspension. This vaccine should be used for primary immunization and boosters for adults and travellers. It should not be used for the immunization of school leavers who should receive the vaccine in ampoule or vial (see above). Diftavax can be purchased directly from the manufacturer or other suppliers.

Storage. Between 2 and 8 °C. Do not freeze. Protect from light.

For DTP + Hib combined vaccines see p. 78.

Note: Because of vaccine shortages, the Chief Medical Officer (PL/CMO/99/5) authorized in December 1999, the use of the triple acellular pertussis-containing vaccines (DTaP and DTaP-IPV) in order to ensure continuous availability of vaccines for the UK childhood immunization programme— see acellular pertussis vaccines on p. 69.

As the DTaP-IPV contains also inactivated polio vaccine that does not form part of the UK immunization programme, it will be kept in reserve. Children that receive this vaccine should not receive the oral polio vaccine (OPV) at the same time. A course started with OPV can be completed with IPV and vice versa.

The DTaP can be used interchangeably with DTwP. A course started with DTwP can be completed with DTaP and vice versa.

The DTaP vaccine of a manufacturer can be mixed with the same manufacturer's *Haemophilus influenzae* b vaccines, e.g. DTaP-IPV with Act-Hib (Aventis Pasteur MSD). *Infanrix* (SmithKline Beecham) is available in one pack with the SKB *lyophilized Hib* vaccine (two vials for mixing). They can be given at the same immunization session as meningococcal C conjugate vaccine but at different sites.

Chapter 17

Diphtheria

Contraindications to vaccination

- Acute febrile illness (except in the case of an outbreak).
- Severe reaction such as a neurological or anaphylactic reaction to an earlier diphtheria immunization.
- Severe hypersensitivity to aluminium and/or thiomersal.
- Pregnancy—there are no data on the use of diphtheria vaccine in pregnancy. Do not use in pregnancy unless the mother is at high risk.
- Do not use the paediatric diphtheria vaccine on anybody over the age of 10 years.

Possible side- and adverse effects

Local reactions

- Swelling, redness and pain.
- A small, painless nodule may form at the injection site, but usually disappears without sequelae.

General reactions

- Transient fever, headaches, malaise, rarely urticaria, pallor and dyspnoea.
- Neurological reactions occur very rarely.

The vaccine

- The adsorbed diphtheria vaccine BP is a suspension of highly purified toxoid from the exotoxin of *Corynebacterium diphtheriae*, adsorbed onto hydrated aluminium phosphate. Thiomersal is added as a preservative. The immunizing potency of each 0.5-mL dose is not less than 30 IU (the old

system of flocculation units, Lf, merely expressed the quantity of toxoid present). The low-dose diphtheria vaccine must be used for children over 10 years of age and adults. Each 0.5-mL dose contains 1.5 Lf of diphtheria toxoid.

- *Indications*: for active immunization against diphtheria of children under the age of 10 years, where a combined DTP or DT vaccine was not used. Three doses of 0.5 mL are given 1 month apart by IM or deep SC injection. Children receiving their primary course in infancy should receive a reinforcing dose of 0.5 mL at about 5 years of age (at least 3 years after the previous dose). The next reinforcing dose is given on leaving school (at 15–19 years of age) with tetanus and low-dose diphtheria (adults) vaccine (Td) or low-dose monovalent diphtheria vaccine.
- An interrupted primary course should not be repeated but continued.
- Diphtheria vaccine is available in the following combinations:

  adsorbed diphtheria vaccine—child, currently not available in the UK (D);

  adsorbed low-dose diphtheria vaccine for adults (d);

  adsorbed DTP vaccine;

  adsorbed DT vaccine;

  adsorbed tetanus and low-dose diphtheria vaccine for adults and adolescents BP (Td).

- For primary immunization or boosters of children over the age of 10 years and adults: when a monovalent diphtheria vaccine is necessary, the adsorbed low-dose diphtheria vaccine for adults BP should be used. The dose is 0.5 mL both for boosters and the primary immunization course, which consists of three doses of the vaccine, given by deep SC or IM injection at intervals of 1 month.
- When receiving the school-leaving booster, if a documented fifth dose of tetanus vaccine exists,

the low-dose monovalent diphtheria vaccine (d) should be given. If this is not available, the combined tetanus and low-dose diphtheria for adults vaccine (Td), in the ampoule formulation, should be given as long as at least 1 month has elapsed since the last dose of tetanus toxoid was given.

• Where the low-dose diphtheria vaccine (d) is not available for vaccination of a child over 10 years of age, or an adult, the paediatric diphtheria vaccine (D) can be used, but only 0.1 mL of the vaccine should be injected instead of 0.5 mL. This recommendation, originally made by the DoH Chief Medical Officer, falls outside the vaccine licence.

• Travellers to epidemic or endemic areas should be immunized or receive a booster if necessary.

• Nonimmunized contacts of a case of diphtheria should be immunized and should receive a prophylactic course of erythromycin or penicillin. If previously immunized, they should receive a booster.

• HIV-infected patients may be immunized against diphtheria.

• Diphtheria antitoxin is used in suspected cases of diphtheria infection.

• The minimum level of diphtheria antitoxin titres necessary for protection is 0.01 IU/mL and above. Levels below this figure are not protective. Levels above 0.1 IU/mL give good protection. Serotesting 3 months after the primary course is necessary for individuals exposed to diphtheria, e.g. in the course of their work.

• *Boosters*: Immunity is over 10 years. For those remaining at risk (e.g. exposed to diphtheria in the course of their work), regular boosters (Td or d) every 10 years after completion of the initial immunization series will assure continued immunity.

• Control of diphtheria depends on widespread acceptance of immunization in order to create herd and individual immunity. Vaccine-induced immunity tends to wane. With a large vaccine uptake as in the UK (95.9% of 2 year olds in the summer of 1999 in the UK), there is decreased frequency of exposure to the organism and therefore decreased maintenance of immunity secondary to community contact. In published reports, at least 70% of the adults who receive a booster dose of diphtheria toxoid achieve protection [Galazka

A.M. & Robertson S.E. (1996) Immunization against diphtheria with special emphasis on immunization of adults. *Vaccine* 14, 845–57]. This means that about 30% of subjects do not respond to a booster. About 38% of UK adults are susceptible to diphtheria. The USA also faces a similar problem. There is therefore a case for recommending regular booster injections of diphtheria toxoid every 10 years after completion of the primary immunization. As yet, this recommendation has not been put forward by the DoH. On the other hand, the DoH recommends including diphtheria when performing the school-leavers' booster (Td). This vaccine may be used for primary immunization of the unvaccinated patient, or as a booster for previously immunized adults when travelling to at-risk areas or when exposed to diphtheria in the course of their work.

Vaccine availability

• The adsorbed diphtheria vaccine, BP (CHILD) (Medeva Pharma Ltd) is no longer available in the UK. The combined DT/DTP should be used when appropriate. As an alternative, children under 10 years of age who require single antigen diphtheria can be boosted using the low dose adult diphtheria vaccine.

• Diphtheria vaccine adults (adsorbed) (Swiss Serum Vaccine Institute, Berne, Switzerland) available in 0.5-mL ampoules. Distributed by Farillon Ltd and MASTA. In Scotland, these vaccines are available from the Scottish Healthcare Supplies Division of the Common Services Agency.

• For combined diphtheria/tetanus with or without pertussis vaccines, see p. 54.

Storage. Between 2 and 8 °C. *Do not freeze*. Protect from light.

Diphtheria antitoxin

Diphtheria antitoxin is obtained from the serum of horses that have been immunized with diphtheria toxoid. Because of the risk of provoking a hypersensitive reaction to the horse serum, it is no longer used in the UK for diphtheria prophylaxis. Nonimmunized contacts are given the vaccine and antibiotic prophylaxis instead.

Where diphtheria is suspected, or for treatment of confirmed cases, diphtheria antitoxin is given. Ensure antihistamines and adrenaline are available in case of allergic reactions or anaphylaxis.

Diphtheria antitoxin is given by SC or IM injection. It is available in 10-mL (10 000 IU) and 20-mL (40 000 IU) ampoules.

Dosage

- Laryngopharyngeal signs for less than 48 h: 20 000–40 000 IU.
- Characteristic nasal–pharyngeal lesions: 40 000–60 000 IU.
- Severe disease for 3 days or more: 80 000–120 000 IU.

Children under 10 years of age receive half of the above adult doses.

The entire dose is given in a single IM injection.

- For very severe diphtheria, 40 000–60 000 IU by slow IV drip, diluted in 500 mL of physiological saline. In order to allow for desensitization, give the infusion at a slow rate over the first 30 min. The active dose should not be given in less than 90 min. Observe the patient closely. The diphtheria vaccine (for the nonimmunized or inadequately immunized person) should be administered on a different limb.

Diphtheria antitoxin availability

Pasteur diphtheria antitoxin is supplied by the PHLS Communicable Disease Surveillance Centre, except in Northern Ireland, where the Public Health Laboratory, Belfast City Hospital supply it.

Diphtheria infection

Diphtheria infection is caused by *Corynebacterium diphtheriae*, a Gram-positive, club-shaped rod that produces a greyish membrane in the throat of infected patients. It is an acute infection of the upper respiratory tract and occasionally it involves the skin. Life-threatening complications of diphtheria include obstructive laryngotracheitis, myocarditis, thrombocytopenia, paralysis of the vocal cords, and ascending paralysis similar to that of Guillain–Barré syndrome, causing death in 1 in 20 cases. The bacterium also causes infections of the skin, mainly in the form of persistent ulcers.

There are two strains of the bacterium: one toxigenic and the other nontoxigenic. The former is responsible for the classical manifestations of the disease. Humans are the only reservoir of the bacterium. Transmission results from touch or intimate contact with a patient or carrier and by airborne droplets. The incubation period is 2–5 days, but occasionally longer, and the infectivity period in untreated persons lasts for 2–4 weeks. Occasionally, carriers can shed the organism for several months. The characteristic symptoms are sudden onset fever, malaise, sore throat, muffled voice, together with a thick, grey, tonsillar exudate and difficulty in swallowing. Its toxins may cause polyneuritis and myocarditis. The organism is sensitive to penicillin and erythromycin, which are also given to contacts. Consider diphtheria antitoxin in respiratory disease.

Diphtheria vaccine was introduced in the UK in 1940. It has had a dramatic effect on the incidence of diphtheria and has virtually eliminated the disease in the UK (Table 17.1). None the less, sporadic cases do occur, although most of them are imported.

Table 17.1 Rates of diphtheria infection in the UK. Data for 1996–98 refer to England and Wales.

| Period | Notifications | Isolates of | | Deaths |
		Non-toxigenic	Toxigenic *C. diphtheriae*	
1940	46 281			2480
1957	37			6
1986–95	38			1
1996	12	10	3	0
1997	22	20	5	0
1998	23	21	3	0

Sources include Notifications of Infectious Diseases (NOIDS), Office for National Statistics (ONS), Public Health Laboratory Services (PHLS), Diphtheria Reference Unit.

Finally, it is important to remember that although diphtheria is most severe in non-immunized or inadequately immunized persons, it can also infect people who have been immunized in the past according to the schedule recommended by the DoH.

Among UK blood donors, 37.6% are susceptible to diphtheria. This susceptibility increases with age. While 25.2% of those aged 20–29 years were found to be susceptible, among the 50 to 59 year olds it was 52.8% [(1995) *Lancet* 345, April 15].

Worldwide, the WHO estimates that there are about 100 000 cases a year and up to 8000 deaths.

The epidemics of diphtheria in the Russian Federation, Ukraine and other countries of the former Soviet Union in the 1990s (Table 17.2) have shown how this disease can make a comeback if immunization coverage rates are not maintained. Prior to the epidemic, vaccination rates in children had fallen from 80% of Russian children in 1980 to 68% in 1990 (desirable coverage to prevent the epidemic is 95%). Between 1990 and 1996, more than 110 000 cases and 2900 deaths from diphtheria were reported in the Russian Federation.

Table 17.2 Incidence of diphtheria in the former Soviet Union area between 1991 and 1995.

Year	Number of cases
1991	3100
1992	5700
1993	19 500
1994	46 000
1995	52 000

The resurgence of diphtheria in the Russian Federation and Eastern Europe can be attributed to:
- a decrease in vaccine coverage in young children;
- a waning immunity to diphtheria in adults;
- large movements of the civil population;
- the disorganization of health services;
- the irregular supply of vaccines.

The disease is now thought to be under control.

Diphtheria is a notifiable disease.

Chapter 18

Tetanus

Contraindications to vaccination

- Acute febrile illness, unless the patient has a tetanus-prone wound, in which case the vaccine is positively indicated.
- Severe general reaction (fever > 39.4 °C within 48 h of injection, peripheral neuropathy, anaphylaxis) to a previously administered dose of the vaccine.
- Severe hypersensitivity to aluminium. Also thiomersal (except Clostet, Medeva Pharma Ltd—as it does not contain thiomersal).
- Caution is necessary during the first year after a primary course or a booster (a hypersensitivity reaction may be provoked—see 'Arthus phenomenon' below).
- May be used in pregnancy if necessary.

Possible side- and adverse effects

Local reactions

Swelling, redness and pain may develop up to 10 days after injection. An insufficiently deep or intradermal injection may result in a persistent nodule at the site of injection.

General reactions

Pyrexia, headaches, malaise and myalgia are general reactions. Urticaria and acute anaphylactic reaction occasionally occur. Peripheral neuropathy is rare. Brachial neuritis and Guillain–Barré syndrome are very rare.

The vaccine

- Adsorbed tetanus vaccine is a suspension of purified tetanus toxoid, adsorbed onto aluminium to increase its immunogenicity. Each 0.5-mL dose has an immunizing potency of not less than 40 IU. It stimulates the production of antitoxin, which provides immunity against the effects of the tetanus toxin.
- The available adsorbed tetanus vaccines are monovalent, or combined with diphtheria (DT), diphtheria and pertussis (DTP), or with low-dose diphtheria (Td).

Tetanus vaccine in simple solution (plain) has not been available in the UK since July 1994. It was less immunogenic than the adsorbed vaccine and had no advantage in terms of reaction rates.

Administration

- The dose for all ages is 0.5 mL, given by deep SC or IM injection.
- Children under the age of 10 years should receive DTP (or DT if pertussis is contraindicated) at the age of 2, 3 and 4 months and a DT booster prior to school entry. A second booster is given before leaving secondary school with low-dose diphtheria combined with tetanus vaccine (Td).
- Adults and children over 10 years who have not previously been immunized should be immunized according to the schedule outlined in Table 18.1.
- If a course is interrupted, it should be continued and not restarted.
- Avoid too frequent tetanus vaccination as this can cause intense local reaction as a result of the 'Arthus phenomenon' (inflammatory skin reaction after injection of antigen in a subject with pre-existing high levels of antibody).

Table 18.1 shows the immunization schedule for tetanus monovalent vaccine in the UK.

- After vaccination with tetanus toxoid, immunological memory may persist for life, although an

Table 18.1 Immunization schedule for tetanus monovalent vaccine in the UK for nonimmunized adults and children over 10 years of age.

Dose (ml)	Route	Primary immunization course*	Boosters
0.5	Deep SC or IM	At 0, 1 and 2 months (three doses)	Every 10 years for two doses†

* If there is also no record of diphtheria immunization, consider tetanus/low-dose diphtheria vaccine (Td).
† Further 10 yearly boosters are not recommended in the UK other than at the time of injury. Consider further boosters in the case of travel to very high-risk areas.

injury with potential infection necessitates a single booster if due. The results can be a 10- to 100-fold increase in circulating antitoxin within 24 h.

• HIV-infected children and adults should be considered for tetanus immunization.

• Tetanus vaccine became available for use with armed forces personnel in 1938. Male patients who were in the British forces during World War II were fully immunized. A considerable number of male teenagers would have received tetanus immunization during their National Service in the years immediately following the war. While many local authorities had provided vaccination previously, it was not until 1961 that childhood immunization against tetanus was recommended nationally by the DoH. Tetanus immunization was also offered to members of groups who were at particular risk, e.g. farm workers.

• The UK average coverage of tetanus immunization in children under 2 years of age was 95.9% in the summer of 1999.

• Unlike diphtheria, tetanus control does not depend on herd immunity because *Clostridium tetani* is widely distributed in the soil and animal excreta. The object of immunization is to protect each individual directly.

• About 10% of babies born to mothers with a placenta heavily infected with *Plasmodium falciparum* parasites may fail to acquire passively a protective level of tetanus antibody despite adequate maternal antibody concentrations.

• Statistics show that the highest risk group is the elderly, particularly women. Of all tetanus cases notified in England and Wales between 1985 and 1991, 53% of cases were in people over the age of 65 years. Serological studies in the USA indicate that at least 40% of people over the age of 60 do not have a protective serum level of antitoxin. Similarly, 11% of adults aged 18–39 years lack

protective levels of antitoxin. Inadequate immunity may result from failure to receive primary immunization or to have boosters at the recommended intervals.

• Antibody levels decline over time among the elderly as well as schoolchildren.

• Protective antibody titre is accepted as being between 0.01 mIU/mL and above.

• A wound or burn is considered tetanus-prone if:
  (a) it is a puncture-type wound;
  (b) it has come into contact with soil or manure;
  (c) clinical evidence of sepsis is present;
  (d) surgical treatment of the wound or burn has been delayed (unattended) for more than 6 h.

In the event of such a wound occurring on a patient who has not fully completed the primary course, this should be completed. If the last booster was given 10 or more years previously, another booster should be given. If the patient is not immunized or uncertain, a full three-dose course should be given.

In all the above cases, a dose of *antitetanus immunoglobulin* should be given IM and at a different site to the vaccine in the following doses (adults and children):

• within 24 h of the injury occurring, 250 IU (1-mL ampoule);

• over 24 h from the injury occurring, 500 IU (2 mL).

The dose should be given to fully immunized persons (who have received three primary plus two booster doses) if the wound is contaminated, e.g. with soil or stable manure. Thorough cleansing of the wound is essential, whatever the immunization history.

• In the event of the *antitetanus immunoglobulin* being used for the treatment of tetanus, the dose is

150 IU per kilogram bodyweight, given IM, in multiple sites.

Vaccine availability

● Clostet—adsorbed tetanus vaccine (Medeva Pharma Ltd—manufactured by Chiron Behring, Germany) in 0.5-mL prefilled syringe.
● Adsorbed tetanus vaccine BP (Medeva Pharma Ltd) in 1-mL capacity (0.5-mL fill) single-dose ampoule (pack of five), and multidose 8-mL (5-mL fill) vial.
● Adsorbed tetanus vaccine BP (Aventis Pasteur MSD) in a single-dose, prefilled syringe (unit pack and pack of 10), single-dose ampoule (pack of five).

Storage. Between 2 and 8 °C. *Do not freeze.* Protect from light. Vials should be stored upright. Discard partly used, multidose vials.

Antitetanus immunoglobulin availability

● Antitanus immunoglobulin is available from the PHLS.
● Human Tetanus Immunoglobulin intramuscular (Bio Products Laboratory) is supplied as a vial containing a minimum of 250 IU of tetanus antibody.
● Tetabulin—tetanus immunoglobulin BP (Hyland Immuno—Baxter Healthcare Ltd) in a prefilled syringe containing 250 IU of human tetanus antitoxin in 1 mL.

Storage. Between 2 and 8 °C. *Do not freeze.* Protect from light.

Tetanus infection

Tetanus is caused by *Clostridium tetani*, a Gram-positive bacillus that grows under anaerobic conditions. Soil is its natural habitat. Its spores can also be found in the faeces of domestic animals and even in human faeces. It is transmitted to humans by the introduction of spores into wounds or burns. Tetanus is not transmissible from person to person. It is distributed worldwide and is more frequent in warmer months and climates.

Clostridium tetani produces two toxins: tetanospasmin and tetanolysin. Only the former is significant as it reaches the spinal cord and brain via blood and peripheral nerves. It increases reflex excitability in motor neurones by blocking the function of inhibitory neurones. It can affect the medullary centres and can pass along sympathetic fibres leading to overactivity of the sympathetic nervous system.

The incubation period is between 2 and 60 days, usually 10–14 days. The onset is gradual and progresses to rigidity and severe muscular spasm, which can lead to respiratory failure and death (3 in 100).

Tetanus is mainly diagnosed clinically as there are no specific diagnostic laboratory tests and differential diagnosis of the characteristic features is limited. The development of tetanus despite full immunization is extremely rare—it is estimated at 4 per 100 million immunocompetent vaccinated subjects [Band J.D. & Bennet J.V. (1983) Tetanus. In: Hoeprich P.D. (ed.) *Infectious Disease.* Harper and Row, Philadelphia, PA]. The mechanism of immunization failure is unclear. Partially immunized subjects remain at risk. Nonimmunized people are at risk.

Neonatal tetanus, resulting from infection of the baby's umbilical stump, is a common cause of neonatal mortality in many countries in Africa and Asia. It is rare in Europe, although cases still occur in countries such as Turkey. It kills 0.5 million babies every year and in some countries it accounts for half of neonatal mortality. It is preventable by immunizing women who are of reproductive age or pregnant with tetanus toxoid, by clean delivery, proper cord care, and postpartum care.

In 1989, the WHO adopted a goal of eliminating neonatal tetanus from the world by 1995. As a result, the proportion of women in developing countries who received at least two doses of tetanus toxoid rose from 18% in 1986 to 48% in 1994 (60% excluding China). Neonatal tetanus is second only to measles as the leading cause of vaccine-preventable deaths in children. Passive protection of the young infant through tetanus toxoid immunization of the mother will prevent approximately 70% of neonatal tetanus deaths.

The number of maternal deaths as a result of tetanus is approximately 50 000 per annum.

Tetanus is a rare disease in the UK. Nevertheless, sporadic cases (including deaths) do occur, mainly among elderly people, who are at greatest risk. Between 1984 and 1996, 153 cases were notified to the Communicable Diseases Surveillance Centres (CDSC) in England and Wales. Between 1996 and 1998 seven cases were notified each year (Table 18.2). Nonimmunized or partially immunized sections of the population remain at risk. Over half of all deaths are in people over 65 years of age, two out of three of these being women.

Table 18.2 Tetanus notifications and deaths in England and Wales.

	Notifications	Deaths
1990	9	1
1991	8	3
1992	6	1
1993	8	3
1994	3	0
1995	6	1
1996	7	0
1997	7	2
1998	7	1

Sources include NOIDS and ONS.

In the UK, as in other developed countries, tetanus is a disease of the elderly. Immunity to tetanus deteriorates with age, but also in the presence of systemic disease. The antibody titres of the elderly with underlying disease are, on average, 20% below their healthy elderly counterparts. Elderly women are at greater risk. Most cases of tetanus occur among adults who are unvaccinated or whose history of vaccination is unknown. The disease is rarely seen among ex-service personnel who did their National Service in the years immediately following World War II—hence the predominance of tetanus in women. Up to 60% of the elderly are not immune. It is therefore important that tetanus immunization is discussed with the elderly.

Tetanus is a notifiable disease.

Chapter 19

Pertussis

No whole-cell monovalent pertussis vaccine is available in the UK. Information on the acellular pertussis-containing vaccines can be found on pp. 69–72.

Whole-cell pertussis vaccine

Contraindications to vaccination

- Acute febrile illness.
- Severe hypersensitivity to aluminium and thiomersal.
- Severe local reaction to a previous pertussis or pertussis-containing vaccine (extensive redness and hard swelling involving much of the circumference of the limb at the injection site).
- Severe general reaction to a previous pertussis or pertussis-containing vaccine:

    (a) fever > 39.5 °C within 48 h of vaccination not resulting from another identifiable cause;

    (b) prolonged unresponsiveness (hypotonic-hyporesponsiveness episode);

    (c) prolonged inconsolable or high-pitched screaming for more than 4 h (DoH)—the manufacturers advise 3 h;

    (d) convulsions or encephalopathy occurring within 72 h of vaccination;

    (e) any of the following: anaphylaxis, bronchospasm, laryngeal oedema, generalized collapse.
- Unstable or evolving neurological problem—defer until the condition is stable (administration of pertussis vaccine may coincide with or hasten the recognition of inevitable manifestations of the progressive disorder, with resulting confusion about causation, e.g. uncontrolled epilepsy, infantile spasms, progressive encephalopathy).
- Pregnancy, unless a young mother is at great risk, in which case her risk may outweigh the theoretical risk to the fetus.

Children with a problem history

- *The child with immediate family (parents and siblings) history of epilepsy*: although the risk of seizures in such children is increased, these are usually febrile in origin and have a generally benign outcome. Subsequent developmental progress in these children has not been found to have been impaired. Immunize and advise on management of fever (see p. 44). Consider antipyretic prophylaxis, such as paracetamol every 4–6 h, for the first 24 h.
- *The child with personal history of epilepsy*: there is an increased risk of convulsions after pertussis immunization, and this is probably simply a reflection of the pyrogenic nature of pertussis cellular (whole-cell) vaccine. In the UK, pertussis vaccine is rarely given to children when they are of an age to have a confirmed diagnosis of epilepsy. Defer vaccination until a progressive neurological disorder is excluded. Immunize as soon as epilepsy is under good control and advise on management of fever. Some parents may have to be supplied and instructed on the use of rectal diazepam to use if convulsions occur, while awaiting the arrival of the ambulance or general practitioner (GP). In the older child (where vaccinations were not started at the age of 2 months), the GP may wish to discuss the use of the acellular pertussis-containing vaccine (DTaP) DT or Td, with the community paediatrician.
- *The child with personal or family history of febrile convulsions*: immunize, but advise on management of fever and appropriate medical care in the event of a seizure.
- *The child with stable neurological conditions*: these patients should be immunized (examples include children with cerebral palsy or spina bifida).
- *HIV-positive individuals* may receive the vaccine.
- In advising parents of children with a problem

history, the GP should inform them of the risks and benefits of pertussis immunization and should give advice on how to manage the child's fever or seizure should it occur. A nonvaccinated child will remain susceptible to pertussis infection. If in doubt, seek advice from the hospital or community paediatrician.

Possible side- and adverse effects

Adverse effects (especially local reactions and pyrexia) are fewer when the new British accelerated schedule for immunization (starting at 2 months of age) is used compared with the extended schedules, which used to last into the second half of the first year of life, when febrile convulsions are more common.

Local reactions

Local reactions are swelling, redness and pain. A small painless nodule may form at the injection site, but usually disappears without sequelae.

General reactions

● Transient low fever, anorexia, limpness, crying, vomiting.
● Fever of 40.5 °C or greater within 48 h in 0.3% of vaccinees—significantly less with the acellular pertussis vaccine (APV).
● Crying, screaming and irritability may occur after pertussis vaccination and also when pertussis is omitted and DT vaccine only is given. Inconsolable screaming or crying (sometimes high-pitched) can occur within the first 48 h (1 in 100 doses—significantly less with APV). This side-effect occurs with other vaccines and is not associated with sequelae. Whole-cell pertussis vaccine is contraindicated if such crying/screaming lasts for over 4 h (DoH; the manufacturers suggest ≥3 h).
● Transient urticarial rashes, unless appearing within minutes of vaccination, are unlikely to be anaphylactic in origin.
● Seizures occurring within 48 h of administration of whole-cell-containing pertussis vaccine are rare (incidence put at 1 in 1750—substantially less with

APV [American Academy of Paediatrics (2000) *Red Book*, p. 444]). They occur usually in febrile children, are brief, generalized and self-limiting (usually febrile convulsions). Predisposing factors are personal and/or family history of convulsions. They have not been shown to result in the subsequent development of recurrent afebrile seizures (such as epilepsy) or other neurological sequelae. No further whole-cell pertussis vaccine should be given. These seizures are seen less frequently with APV.
● Episodes of hypotonic-hyporesponsiveness (collapse) can occur in about 1 in 1750 vaccines [American Academy of Paediatrics (2000) *Red Book*, p. 444]). Earlier work from the UK has found the rate to be 1 in 6000 [Pollock T. *et al.* (1984) Symptoms after primary immunization with DTP and DT vaccine. *Lancet* ii, 146–9]. There is no evidence of subsequent serious neurological damage or intellectual impairment occurring. Collapse after pertussis vaccine (hypotonic-hyporesponsiveness episode) remains a contraindication to further doses. Researchers from the Netherlands described 101 children who experienced such an episode, of whom 84 subsequently received further doses of whole-cell pertussis-containing vaccine; none experienced a recurrence or other adverse event. In contrast, one of the 17 children who remained unvaccinated had severe pertussis [Vermeer-de Bond P.E., *et al.* (1998) Rate of recurrent collapse after vaccination with whole-cell pertussis vaccine: follow up study. *Br. Med. J.* 316, 902–390]. The acellular pertussis vaccine may be associated with a reduced risk for collapse (see p. 73, The Canadian experience).
● Anaphylactic reactions are rare (approximately 2 cases per 100 000 injections).
● Encephalopathy, permanent neurological disability (brain damage) and even death have in the past been considered as rare sequelae of pertussis immunization. Such adverse events and illnesses can occur in immunized and nonimmunized children from a variety of causes, particularly in the first year of life. As there is no specific test, determination of whether pertussis vaccine is the cause is not possible. Avoid further whole-cell pertussis vaccine if encephalopathy occurs within 72 h of administration of the vaccine.

• Public and professional anxiety about the safety of pertussis vaccine resulted from the UK National Childhood Encephalopathy (NCE) study contacted between 1976 and 1979. This study, at the time, indicated that the risk of encephalopathy was 1 in 140 000 doses of pertussis vaccine and that the risk of permanent brain damage was 1 in 330 000. Of the 1182 children aged 2–36 months with acute neurological illness reported to this NCE study, only 39 had a history of recent (within 7 days) pertussis vaccination. Six of these children were found to have infantile spasms not attributed to DTP. Further and later analysis of these data indicated that the above encephalopathy rate was developed by, among others, adding in a number of children with febrile convulsions, which are not usually associated with permanent sequelae. If those subjects are excluded, the remaining numbers are too small to show conclusively whether or not the vaccine can cause such adverse effects. The conclusion is therefore that although the data do not prove pertussis vaccine can never cause encephalopathy/brain damage, none the less they do indicate that if it does so, such occurrences must be exceedingly rare. There are no specific tests available to identify cases which may have been caused by pertussis vaccine. Interestingly, one case of encephalitis (190 days after vaccination and, therefore, unrelated) occurred among 82 892 children who received pertussis vaccine in a Swedish trial [Olin P, Rasmussen F, Gustafsson L *et al.* (1997) Randomised control trial of two-component, three-component, and five-component acellular pertussis vaccines compared with whole-cell pertussis vaccine. *Lancet* **350**, 1569–1577]; three cases occurred among the 17 607 children who did not participate—all three resulted from a confirmed pertussis infection. The benefits of pertussis vaccine far outweigh any possible risks.

• Three American studies have re-examined the risks of febrile seizures and other neurological events after immunization with pertussis-containing vaccines (1990) *J. Am. Med. Assoc.* 263, 1641–5. The total number of subjects was 230 000 with more than 700 000 immunizations. There were no proven vaccine-induced permanent central nervous system injuries. J. Cherry, in an editorial [Cherry J. (ed.) (1990) *J. Am. Med. Assoc.* 263, 1679–80] com-

menting on these studies, indicated that 'the myth of encepha-lopathy should end'.

• Pertussis vaccine has not been found to be linked with the development of asthma—as has been suggested. A study in the *British Medical Journal* [(1999) *Br. Med. J.* 318, 1173–6] has concluded that there is no evidence to support a proposed link between pertussis vaccination and wheezing illness in young children. Neither is it linked to cot deaths (they most commonly occur during the first year of life). On the contrary, immunized infants are less likely to suffer from cot death.

• Health professionals counselling parents about pertussis immunization may wish to have in mind the following review 'Pertussis vaccine and injury to brain' by Dr G.S. Golden, an American paediatric neurologist [Golden, G. S. (1990) *J. Paediatr.* 116, 854–61]. His conclusions are as follows:

(a) population studies, particularly the UK National Childhood Encephalopathy study, do not provide evidence of permanent neurological sequelae resulting from pertussis vaccine;

(b) there is no convincing evidence that children with a personal history of neurological disease or family history of convulsions will deteriorate more rapidly if they receive triple vaccine, although caution is usually advised;

(c) pertussis vaccine does not cause epilepsy, although about 1 in 10 000 children will have a febrile seizure;

(d) there is no convincing evidence to link pertussis vaccine with infantile spasms;

(e) there is no convincing evidence of a causal link between pertussis immunization and sudden infant death syndrome (cot death);

(f) in cases where pertussis vaccine has been blamed for causing neurological damage, there are no specific neuropathological findings.

• Finally, the reader may wish to be aware of the case of Kenneth Best against Wellcome. The case was heard in the Irish Supreme Court in 1992. The Court found Wellcome's batch 3741 of pertussis vaccine 'liable' (and the company negligent) for severe brain damage to Best, who was immunized in 1969. It found the batch failed laboratory tests for potency and toxicity, yet was released. Evidence showed it was eight times more potent than the recommended dose and toxic to an infant. Best was awarded IR£2.75 million in damages and legal fees thought to be IR£4 million. A further lesson we learn from this case is that we should never forget to record the vaccine batch number of a vaccine we administer.

The vaccine

• Pertussis vaccine is a suspension of inactivated *Bordetella pertussis*. It is given as part of the triple vaccine combined with diphtheria and tetanus vaccines. The estimated potency is not less than 4 IU in each 0.5 mL. The vaccines contain aluminium and thiomersal.

• The whole-cell, pertussis-containing vaccine, currently used in the UK childhood immunization programme, is effective and has an established safety record. The introduction of the accelerated immunization schedule in the UK (first triple at 2 months of age) has been associated with fewer minor reactions such as fever, further decline in disease incidence and deaths, and an improvement in vaccine uptake. Therefore, the case for replacing the existing whole-cell DTP vaccine for children under 1 year of age with acellular preparations needs to be convincing and, in particular, it requires evidence of better immunogenicity, reduced adverse reactions (already accepted as a fact) and potentially better vaccine uptake. The evidence is currently being evaluated.

There is a good case for substituting DT at preschool age with DTaP.

Administration

For administration of combined DTwP vaccine, see p. 54.

• After the primary course of three doses at 2, 3 and 4 months, respectively, no boosters are recommended in the UK. Vaccination against pertussis, *Haemophilus influenzae* b and meningococcal C are the only immunizations in infancy in the UK that are not reinforced when children first attend school at the age of 4–5 years.

• Children presenting for their preschool DT booster, and who have not had their third dose of pertussis, can have the DTaP, which is licensed for up to and including 6 years of age, rather than the DTwP.

• If the primary course is interrupted, it should be resumed from where it was stopped and not repeated.

• HIV-positive individuals may receive the vaccine.

• If a febrile convulsion occurs after a dose of pertussis-containing vaccine, the GP is advised to seek the advice of the hospital or community paediatrician before considering further vaccinations.

• An increased incidence of reactions may occur as a result of failure to shake the container to resuspend the vaccine before withdrawing the dose, inadvertent intravenous injection, or over-rapid injection.

• An inadequately immunized 1-year-old child has a 1 in 6 chance of developing pertussis before the age of 10 years. Protection is likely after the second dose of vaccine.

• The estimated efficacy of the pertussis vaccine is in excess of 70% (50–90%) after a full primary course (three doses).

• Vaccine-induced immunity persists for at least 3 years and diminishes thereafter. Several years after vaccination, the efficacy is less than 50%. As adults lose their immunity they become a huge reservoir for the nonimmunized. Falls in immunization rates can lead to local outbreaks. No reinforcing doses are as yet recommended in the UK, while American babies receive two further reinforcing doses, one at 18 months and another around 5 years (as DTwP or DTaP).

• Pertussis infection in those immunized is usually mild.

• Whole-pertussis vaccines can give good protection against both clinical disease and transmission of infection. In the 1990s the overall notification rate for all ages has continued to show a downward trend. Unfortunately, the same cannot be said for the notification rate in infants younger than 3 months. The most probable source of these infant infections would seem to be undiagnosed infection in older vaccinated, but also infection in nonvaccinated people.

• The UK coverage of pertussis immunization (three doses) in children under 2 years of age in the summer of 1999 was 94.6% (England 93.7%, Wales 93.3%, Northern Ireland 96.3% and Scotland 96.7%).

Vaccine availability

No monovalent whole-cell pertussis vaccine is available in the UK. Whole-cell pertussis vaccine is only available as a component of the combined DTP.

Acellular pertussis vaccines

Contraindications to vaccination

These contraindications are to the monovalent acellular pertussis vaccine (APV) and the combined DTaP and DTaP-IPV.
- Acute febrile illness.
- Severe localized or generalized reaction to a preceding dose of the acellular pertussis vaccine.
- Severe generalized reaction to a previously administered dose of the whole-cell pertussis vaccine
- Severe hypersensitivity to thiomersal (for the monovalent APV)—DTaP contains 2-phenoxyethanol as preservative. For DTaP-IPV severe sensitivity to thiomersal, neomycin, streptomycin and polymyxin B.
- Any neurological condition in which there are changing developmental or neurological findings (e.g. uncontrolled epilepsy, infantile spasms and progressive encephalopathy).
- Encephalopathy of unknown aetiology occurring within 7 days following previous administration of pertussis-containing vaccine.
- Pregnancy and lactation: these vaccines are intended only for paediatric use.
- DTaP (Infanrix) and DTaP-IPV (Tetravac) should not be used in subjects over 10 years of age because of the high-dose (paediatric) diphtheria component in these vaccines, as recommended by the DoH. Infanrix has a licence up to and including 6 years and Tetravac up to 12 years of age.

The following events that will normally be a contraindication to pertussis immunization, can now be considered to be general precautions for an acellular pertussis-containing vaccine. This especially when there may be circumstances, such as high incidence of pertussis, in which the potential benefits of pertussis immunization outweigh possible risks, particularly because these events are not associated with permanent sequelae.

- Temperature of $\geqslant 40.5$ °C ($\geqslant 40$ °C for DTaP-IPV) within 48 h of vaccination (not as a result of another identifiable cause).
- Collapse or hypotonic-hyporesponsiveness episode occurring within 48 h of vaccination.
- Persistent inconsolable crying lasting $\geqslant 3$ h and occurring within 48 h of vaccination.
- Convulsions (febrile or afebrile) occurring within 72 h of vaccination.

A severe local reaction to the whole-cell pertussis-containing vaccine is not necessarily a contraindication to the APV as the likelihood of such a reaction after APV is small.

Possible side and adverse effects

Local reactions

Local reactions are soreness, erythema, swelling and induration at the injection site. They usually improve within 48–72 h.

General reactions

Less general reactions occur when the vaccine is administered at 2, 3 and 4 months of age.

Mild, transient fever can be experienced by some children. Less commonly vaccinees may complain of restlessness, drowsiness, crying, some degree of anorexia, diarrhoea and vomiting.

Very rarely they may experience headaches, fatigue, malaise, myalgia (flu-like illness), arthralgia, urticaria, allergic reactions including anaphylactic reactions.

Extremely rarely collapse (hypotonic-hyporesponsiveness episode) and convulsions within 48–72 h of vaccination. In all reported cases recovery was spontaneous and full without any sequelae. High fever > 40 °C in $< 0.1\%$ of vaccinees.

Because APV (and DTaP, DTaP-IPV) causes high fever less frequently than DTP, convulsions are anticipated to be much less likely after APV (and DTaP, DTaP-IPV).

The vaccines

According to a DoH circular (letter from the Chief Medical Officer of 2 December 1999), there appears to be an association between higher efficacy and the vaccine having more antigen components.

The monovalent acellular pertussis vaccine (APV)

Single-antigen, acellular pertussis vaccine adsorbed is an unlicensed product. It was available by the DoH under Crown Immunity (the Medicines Act 1968), via its official suppliers, i.e. Farillon Ltd, on a 'named-patient' basis. Due to production difficulties this vaccine was no longer available in the UK from September 2000. The DoH was making every effort to secure supplies from alternative sources. Success is very unlikely.

The vaccine contains the following components: pertussis toxoid, filamentous haemagglutinin, pertactin (69 kDa outer membrane protein) and fimbriac type 2. Thiomersal has been added as a preservative.

Administration (Table 19.1)

● *Indications*
 (a) for primary immunization of children aged 2 months and over who are not to receive the whole-cell vaccine;
 (b) for the completion of pertussis immunization in children whose primary immunization did not include three doses of pertussis vaccine, that is children who have not received, or partially completed their pertussis immunization (they may have received DT);
 (c) for the immunization of older children who have not received pertussis vaccine;
 (d) if local reaction/pyrexia has occurred following earlier DTP.
● APV should not be used in the UK as an alternative to the existing whole-cell pertussis-containing vaccine (combined with diphtheria and tetanus). Members of the primary healthcare team should promote the existing trivalent DTwP vaccine and should counsel worried parents. Any baby whose pertussis immunization is delayed in the first years of life is in danger of infection. The APV can be used for pertussis 'catch up'.
● If at the preschool vaccination a child is found not to have received pertussis vaccination earlier, one dose of DTwP should be given, and a further two doses of APV at monthly intervals.
● A primary course of immunization started with whole-cell, pertussis-containing vaccine can be completed with APV. If interrupted, there is no need to recommence the primary course and it should be completed.
● Children with stable central nervous system disorders, including well-controlled seizures or satisfactorily explained single seizures, may receive the APV. The GP should assess the individual's potential risks and benefits. The community paediatrician may be consulted. It should be noted that a family history of seizures is not a contraindication to immunization with APV.
● The APV should be shaken vigorously before administration. It should only be given by deep SC or IM injection. Exercise caution when giving it to a child with thrombocytopenia or any coagulation disorder that would normally contraindicate IM injection.
● As the APV is not available in the UK, an extra dose of DTaP can be given between 12–18 months of age, or at least 6 months after the previous dose of DT/P, and the preschool booster can be given in the form of DTaP (instead of DT) if there is a need to complete interrupted pertussis immunization.

Vaccine availability (APV)

Monovalent acellular pertussis vaccine (APV), adsorbed, is manufactured by Wyeth Laboratories and was distributed under Crown Immunity, free of charge and on behalf of the DoH by

Table 19.1 Administration specifications for acellular pertussis monovalent vaccine ('named-patient' basis).

Dose (ml)	Route	Primary course	Boosters
0.5	IM or deep SC	Three injections at monthly intervals from two months of age	None (in the UK)

its officials distributors, i.e. Farillon Ltd, on a 'named-patient' basis. In Scotland, it was supplied through the Scottish Healthcare Services Division of the Common Services Agency. In Northern Ireland, it was available from the Regional Pharmacist, Procurement Co-ordinator, Eastern Health and Social Services Board. It was not available as of September 2000 because of production problems.

Single-dose 0.5-mL suspension in vials. Shake well before use in order to obtain a homogeneous suspension.

Storage. Between 2 and 8 °C. *Do not freeze.*

The diphtheria-tetanus-acellular pertussis vaccines (DTaP)

Two DTaP vaccines are licensed in the UK:
1 Infanrix (SB) is trivalent and contains DTaP. This vaccine has three antigen components: pertussis toxoid, filamentous haemagglutinin and pertactin (69 kDa outer membrane protein), adsorbed on to aluminium salts.
2 Tetravac (Aventis Pasteur MSD) which additionally contains inactivated polio vaccine—DTaP-IPV. It has two antigen components: pertussis toxoid and filamentous haemagglutinin.
● The whole-cell, pertussis-containing vaccine (DTwP) is the recommended vaccine for the UK childhood immunization programme and should always be used unless there are specific contraindications to its use.
● As a result of vaccine supply difficulties and in order to ensure UK immunization programmes continue uninterrupted, the DoH has made available (December 1999) the above vaccines to be used when the DTwP is not available. The DTaP can also be used when parents refuse to accept the whole-cell pertussis component but will agree to

have the acellular component (instead of having to use DT plus APV in two injections).
● Where the DTwP is not available, the acellular pertussis vaccine (DTaP) can be used interchangeably with DTwP. Courses started with DTwP can be completed with DTaP and vice versa.
● The DTaP vaccines can be mixed with the same manufacturer's *Haemophilus influenzae* b (Hib) vaccine: e.g. Infanrix with Hiberix (SB) as Infanrix-Hib; Tetravac with Act-Hib (Aventis Pasteur MSD).
Very rare reactions have been reported in the form of lower limb oedema with cyanosis or transient purpura, occurring within the first hours following immunization with vaccines containing *Haemophilus influenzae* b. There were no cardiorespiratory signs and they resolved spontaneously without sequelae. One such case was reported during clinical trials of Tetravac and conjugate Hib that were administered simultaneously and at different sites.
● Because Tetravac contains inactivated polio vaccine (IPV) which does not form part of the UK immunization schedule (the oral polio vaccine is used exclusively), the DoH has advised that this vaccine will be kept in reserve. If it is used, the OPV should not be given too. In such a situation IPV and OPV can be used interchangeably through a course of immunization. Courses started with OPV can be completed with IPV and vice versa.
● Acellular pertussis vaccine can be given safely at the same time as meningococcal C conjugate vaccine.

Administration

Infanrix (Table 19.2)

Infanrix is licensed for children up to and including 6 years of age. It is indicated as a booster dose for children who have previously received a full primary course with DTwP or DTaP, according to the national policy in effect at the time.

Table 19.2 Administration specifications for Infanrix (DTaP).

Dose (ml)	Route	Primary course (up to age six)	Boosters
0.5	Deep IM	Three injections at monthly intervals	None (in the UK)

In the UK, the Chief Medical Officer has recommended that this vaccine be used when the DTwP is not available (PL/CMO/99/5) as a result of vaccine shortage.

The vaccine (0.5 mL) is given by deep IM injection. The primary course consists of three doses, 4 weeks apart, starting from the age of 2 months (Table 19.2). No booster doses are recommended in the UK.

There are no immediate plans to revise the UK's immunization schedule to include a DTaP booster (instead of just DT) at preschool age, although this issue is being kept constantly under review. We have been witnessing a rise in the proportion of pertussis notifications in infants less than 3 months of age since 1990, when the accelerated immunization schedule for diphtheria, tetanus, pertussis and polio vaccines (2, 3 and 4 months) was introduced in the UK. Between 1991 and 1998, the proportion of cases occurring in infants under 3 months of age has risen from 2.3% to 13.3%. Introduction of a preschool booster for pertussis could reduce transmission to very young, unvaccinated siblings and neighbours.

Some countries (USA is an example) have introduced a pertussis booster in the second year of life. Following administration of Infanrix booster in the second year of life to Infanrix-primed infants, the antibody titres were >0.1 IU/mL to both diphtheria and tetanus. The booster response to the pertussis antigens was observed in more than 96% of these children.

Tetravac (Table 19.3)

Tetravac is licensed for primary vaccination of infants and for booster in children who have previously received a primary course of DTwP or DTaP. It can be administered to children up to the age of 12 years who were previously immunized with a whole-cell vaccine. The reader should observe the DoH recommendation that the high-dose paediatric diphtheria vaccine should be given up to the age of 10 years. It has particular application in specialist units such as Special Care baby units.

Vaccine availability

● Infanrix (SmithKline Beecham) is available in 0.5-mL single-dose presentation in 1-mL prefilled syringe. Shake the vaccine well in order to obtain a homogeneous, turbid suspension. This vaccine is available directly from the manufacturer. If it were to be used as a preschool booster in the UK, it would have to be paid for privately as this booster does not form part of the UK's immunization programme.

● Tetravac (Aventis Pasteur MSD) is available in 0.5-mL single-dose prefilled syringe. Shake before use to obtain a homogeneous, white turbid suspension.

Storage: Between 2 and 8 °C. Protect from light.

Pertussis immunization in Europe and Canada

All countries currently use combined DTP either with whole-cell (DTwP) or acellular (DTaP) vaccines, except the French-speaking community of Belgium, which uses whole-cell pertussis vaccine alone (wP). Whole-cell pertussis vaccines have been withdrawn in the second half of the 1990s in six European countries (Austria, Denmark, Germany, Ireland, Luxembourg, Norway) and replaced by acellular vaccines. Sweden discontinued the whole-cell vaccine in 1979 and introduced acellular vaccines in 1996. Some countries (France, Greece, Italy, Spain and the Flemish community of Belgium) use both whole-cell and acellular vaccines.

Table 19.3 Administration specifications for Tetravac (DTaP-IPV).

Dose (ml)	Route	Primary course* (up to age 10)	Boosters*
0.5	IM	Three injections at monthly intervals, at 2, 3 and 4 months of age	None (in the UK)

*The DoH has specified that this vaccine will be used where DTwP or DTaP are not available because of vaccine shortages.

The most widely used acellular vaccine is Infanrix (DTaP). Seven countries also use tetravalent (Denmark, Spain) and/or pentavalent (Austria, France, Germany, Italy, Luxembourg) vaccines with *Haemophilus influenzae* b and/or inactivated polio (DTaP-Hib, DTaP-IPV, DTaP-Hib-IPV). Austria is planning to introduce a hexavalent vaccine that will include hepatitis B.

The acellular monovalent pertussis vaccine forms part of the trivalent DTaP vaccine used for childhood immunization in the USA. Acellular pertussis vaccines have been in routine use for some time now in Japan.

Canadian researchers examined every admission resulting from febrile seizures or hypotonic-hyporesponsive episodes for those that may have been related to recent immunization against pertussis. They found that admissions for febrile seizures following DTwP/DTaP immunization declined by 87%, and hypotonic-hyporesponsive episodes by 75% from 1996 to 1998, after introduction in 1997 of the DTaP vaccine. They presented their findings at the annual meeting of the Infectious Diseases Society of America in Philadelphia, Pennsylvania in 1999 (reporter Dr David Scheifele, Vancouver).

Pertussis infection

Pertussis is caused by *Bordetella pertussis*, a small, aerobic, Gram-negative pleomorphic bacillus. Some cases are also attributed to *Bordetella parapertussis*. The bacillus adheres to the cilia of human respiratory tract epithelial cells where it multiplies and releases toxic substances.

Humans are the only known reservoir. It is transmitted by aerosol droplets from the respiratory tract of an infected patient. The incubation period is 1–3 weeks, usually 7–10 days.

The disease affects any age, but especially infants. It begins with mild, upper respiratory tract symptoms and cough (catarrhal stage), when the patient is most infectious. Within 7–10 days the cough progresses to severe paroxysms of cough followed by vomiting (paroxysmal stage) that last usually about 6–10 weeks, followed by a decrease in symptoms (convalescent stage).

The characteristic whoop, when present (may be absent in young infants), results from an attempt to breathe in after the child is out of breath in a coughing spasm. It is more severe at night when the child can sound as if he or she is choking. During these spasmic periods, apnoea can occur. In the attempt to clear the thick mucous, the child with whooping cough vomits. There is little fever. The duration of the illness is 6–12 weeks and, in spite of the above symptoms, the child can appear well most of the time. The Chinese call it the '100-day cough' disease. A negative nasal swab does not preclude the diagnosis.

Infants under 6 months of age may not experience whoop but apnoea is a common manifestation.

Complications that can arise in infants are weight loss because of vomiting, pneumonia (22%), encephalopathy (0.9%), seizures (3.0%), permanent brain damage and death (1.3% in infants under 1 month, 0.3% in those aged 2–11 months). The younger the child, the more common the complications.

● Treatment with erythromycin decreases the likelihood of infection. The infected children usually become culture-negative within 6 days and most will not relapse if the treatment course is continued for 14 days (the recommended duration of therapy to prevent bacteriological relapse). Best results are achieved when this antibiotic is started within 21 days of onset of symptoms. The macrolides, azithromycin and clarithromycin, are alternatives. They may be effective in shorter courses of 5–7 days, however, their efficacy is currently unproven. Exclude the patient from school or work for 5 days after starting treatment.

● Close contacts of patients with pertussis may need erythromycin prophylaxis if they are unvaccinated, partially vaccinated, or immunosuppressed, provided the patient's illness had started not more than 21 days previously. The prophylactic dose of erythromycin is 50 mg/kg body weight per day in three divided doses for children under 12 years, and 500 mg three times daily for adults, for 10–14 days.

While the UK immunization programme does not include a pertussis booster dose at preschool age (four and a half years), the prophylactic dose is recommended for close (family) contacts age 5 years and over because of the possibility of reduced post-vaccination pertussis antibody by this age.

Caution should be exercised when prescribing

Table 19.4 The 1970s pertussis contraindications myths. These conditions are not contraindications to immunization.

Asthma, eczema, hay fever
Prematurity low attained weight
Breast-feeding
Antibiotic treatment
Congenital heart disease
Chronic lung disease
Cerebral palsy and other neurological conditions
Chromosomal abnormalities
Topical or inhaled steroids
Pregnancy in mother
Family history of convulsions in distant relatives
Family history of immunization reaction
Previous mumps, measles or rubella infection
Jaundice after birth
'Snuffles'

erythromycin to neonates as this may place them at higher risk of developing infantile hypertrophic pyloric stenosis (IHPS). In 1999, a US health department identified a cluster of 200 infants with pertussis who had been born at a community hospital, and recommended that these infants should be treated with oral erythromycin. However, the following month, seven cases of IHPS, which is characterized by nonbilious, projectile vomiting, were reported to the state health department. A team of experts from the Centres for Disease Control and Prevention were sent in to investigate. Using ultrasonographic data, the investigators diagnosed the index cases and compared them with historical cases of IHPS. They found that all seven index cases vs. none of the comparison cases had received at least 10 days of erythromycin as prophylaxis for pertussis [Honein M. *et al.* (1999) Infantile hypertrophic pyloric stenosis with erythromycin: a case review and cohort study. *Lancet* 354, 2101–5]. They noted that an increase in the duration of erythromycin therapy led to an increase in the risk of IHPS. Since alternative therapies are not as well studied, the American Academy of Paediatrics continues to recommend the use of erythromycin for prophylaxis and treatment of pertussis infection. It urges physicians who prescribe erythromycin to newborn infants to inform parents about potential risks of developing IHPS and signs of IHPS.

Pertussis morbidity and mortality are strongly correlated with socioeconomic conditions. It is a major public health problem, particularly for poor, malnourished infants in whom the mortality rates are far higher than among infants in developed countries. In the developing world, the mortality rate is as high as 1 in 100 cases. More than 355 000 annual deaths worldwide are a result of pertussis infection, with probably over 40 million cases of pertussis occurring every year. Countries with high immunization rates among infants have seen the virtual elimination of the disease.

In the UK, the pertussis vaccine was introduced in 1953 and was soon to have a dramatic effect on the number of cases notified. However, a few cases of alleged neurological damage associated with pertussis immunization were widely publicized by the media in the 1970s. Among the medical profession there was also disagreement, especially after the publication of the paper 'Neurological complications of pertussis inoculation' by Kulenkampff *et al.* (1974) (*Arch. Dis. Child.* 49, 46–9). Some doctors started inventing contraindications (Table 19.4) and the public lost its confidence in the vaccine. This resulted in a huge drop in vaccine acceptance from 80 to 30%. Pertussis infection became widespread with the number of cases notified matching the prevaccine era and deaths rising. These events provided the clearest evidence that the benefits of pertussis immunization outweighed the possible risks associated. Once the public's (and doctors') confidence was restored in the late 1980s, the rate of notifications and deaths again dropped dramatically. The restored high uptake of the vaccine has also seen the virtual disappearance of the characteristic 2-year peaks and troughs (Table 19.5).

Although the mass immunization programmes against *Bordetella pertussis* infection that started in the 1950s have led to a decrease in frequency, it was not previously thought to prevent transmission. Asymptomatic pertussis reinfections indicate the disease may persist despite immunization. Researches from Cambridge assessed the duration of the period between epidemics from a large dataset. They demonstrated that the onset of pertussis vaccination coincided with a significant lengthening of the interval between epidemics from 2 to 2.5 years to almost 4 years, in 10 large

Table 19.5 Immunization rates and pertussis notifications (England and Wales).

Year	Immunization rate (%)	Pertussis notifications	Comment
1952	0	> 100 000	Year before vaccine introduction. Death rate: 1 in 1000 cases notified
1973	80	2400	Year before 'pertussis scare'
1975	30	> 100 000	After 'pertussis scare'
1978		> 65 000	Twelve deaths from whooping cough
1986	65	36 506	After misinterpretation of UK National Encephalopathy study (NES) results. 3 deaths
1987		15 203	5 deaths
1988		5117	NES clarified. No deaths
1989		11 646	Still 2-year peaks and troughs present. 1 death
1990		15 286	7 deaths (6 in infants under 4 months of age). Timing of pertussis vaccination accelerated to start from 2 months
1991	88	5201	First year of immunization targets in the GP contract. No deaths
1992	92	2309	1 death
1993		4091	Peaks twice yearly. No deaths
1994		3964	3 deaths
1995	94	1869	Coverage rising. 2 deaths
1996	94	2387	2 deaths
1997	94	2989	1 death
1998	94	1577	4 deaths

Sources include NOIDS, ONS.

cities in England and Wales. They concluded that the lengthening of the interval between epidemics demonstrates that a substantial reduction in transmission of the bacteria has occurred. It is accepted that the increase in interval between epidemics is compatible with a reduction in transmission. The investigators also studied the pattern of 'fade-outs'—the frequency and duration of reports of no cases in particular locations. They found that both the number and the duration of 'fade-outs' had increased since the introduction of pertussis immunization. The conclusion is that the present paediatric immunization scheme in England and Wales is successfully reducing pertussis infection transmission, as well as the incidence of the clinical disease [Rohani P. *et al.* (2000) Impact of immunization on pertussis transmission in England and Wales. *Lancet* 355, 285–6].

A study in Birmingham [Miller, E. & Flemming,

D. (2000) Serological evidence of pertussis in patients presenting with cough in general practice in Birmingham. *Communicable Disease and Public Health* 3 (2), 132–4] showed that 40 out of 145 patients with prolonged cough that provided blood for serological testing had evidence of recent infection with *Bordetella pertussis*. During the study a further 18 patients (mostly younger patients who presented early) had a diagnosis of pertussis confirmed by culture. This study demonstrates that pertussis circulates in the community, therefore pertussis infection should be considered in the differential diagnosis. It also highlights the need to introduce at least one booster of pertussis vaccine. Practically, this booster dose could be given during the preschool vaccinations. As yet, the DoH has not decided to make such a recommendation.

Pertussis is a notifiable disease.

Chapter 20

Haemophilus influenzae b

Contraindications to vaccination

- Acute febrile illness.
- Hypersensitivity to tetanus protein (ACT-Hib) or diphtheria toxoid (HibTITER).
- Severe local redness and swelling involving most of the circumference of the limb, at the site of the injection.
- Severe general reaction to a previously administered *Haemophilus influenzae* b (Hib) vaccine—see adverse reactions below.
- Pregnancy—no data available. The vaccine is intended for paediatric use.

Possible side- and adverse effects

Local reactions

Local reactions are swelling, redness and pain soon after vaccination and lasting up to 24 h in up to 10% of vaccinees, mainly after the first dose. The incidence of such local reactions declines with subsequent doses.

General reactions

General reactions include malaise, headaches, fever, irritability, inconsolable and high-pitched crying, vomiting, diarrhoea and restless sleep. Very rarely, anaphylactic reaction, erythema multiforme, Guillain–Barré syndrome and convulsions are seen, although a cause and effect relationship has not been established. The vaccine can be generally considered as very safe.

The vaccine

The polysaccharide capsule of *Haemophilus influenzae* type b (polyribosylribitol phosphate, PRP) forms the basis of the Hib vaccine (Table 20.1). Unfortunately, PRP alone provokes a poor antibody response in younger children (under 18 months of age), who are at greatest risk. The present conjugate vaccine involves linking the capsular polysaccharide to a protein such as diphtheria or tetanus toxoid. This linking improves considerably the immunogenic response, especially in children less than 1 year of age. It provokes higher titres of antibody (predominantly IgG) and a longer lasting immune response because of stimulation of memory cells.

Administration (Table 20.2)

- The primary course consists of three doses of the vaccine with a 4-week interval between each dose starting from the age of 2 months. This vaccine should be given by deep SC or IM injection.
- No booster is recommended for children who have received all three injections.
- The vaccines are interchangeable between themselves (ACT-Hib with HibTITER). If children under the age of 1 year are started on a course with one

Table 20.1 *Haemophilus influenzae* **b vaccines.**

Trade name	Abbreviation	Carrier protein	Manufacturer
ACT-HIB	PRP-T	Tetanus toxoid	Aventis Pasteur MSD
HibTITER	HbOC	Mutant diphtheria toxin	Wyeth

Table 20.2 Administration specifications for Hib vaccine.

Age at first immunization (years)	Dose (ml)	Route	No. of doses	Interval (weeks)	Booster
< 1	0.5	SC/IM	3	4	None
> 1	0.5	SC/IM	1	—	None

vaccine and the course is interrupted, it should be resumed irrespective of the interval and with the same vaccine. If that brand of vaccine is not available, a different brand of vaccine should be used.

- The Hib vaccine (ACT-HIB, HibTITER) can be given at the same time as the MMR, or polio and triple vaccination (DTP), but should be given in the opposite thigh (the site at which each vaccine has been given should be recorded).
- It is more convenient to mix or use combination vaccines.
- They may be mixed before injection as follows: Aventis Pasteur MSD ACT-HIB with Aventis Pasteur MSD DTP (combined volume 0.5 mL); or Tetravac (see p. 72).
  Wyeth HibTITER with Behring DTP (combined volume 1.0 mL—such a volume is well tolerated).
- An alternative is to use the Hib and DTP combination vaccines (ACT-HIB DTP).
- The addition of the Hib vaccine does not increase the risk of febrile convulsions occurring within 72 h of vaccination.
- Action in the case of a major reaction following the administration of a combined DTP and Hib vaccine: continue immunizations but separate the two components and give them on different limbs. If severe, do the same but omit pertussis.
- Routine immunization of older children and adults with the Hib vaccine is not currently recommended in the UK—the incidence of the disease declines over the age of 4 years.
- Vaccination of babies at 2, 3 and 4 months is included in the GP target payments.
- Vaccine efficacy is estimated at 98–99% for infants immunized from 2 months of age and receiving three doses of the vaccine. Antibody titres greater than 1μg/mL are thought to correlate with long-term protection. Vaccine failure is extremely rare, especially because community circulation of

the disease has substantially diminished with vaccination.

- The Hib vaccine has been estimated to prevent approximately seven deaths and between 7 and 26 cases of severe disability per 100 000 children who have been immunized [*Br. Med. J.* (1999) 319, 1133].
- Nonimmunized asplenic patients of all ages over the age of 1 year should receive a single dose of the vaccine.
- The Hib vaccine is only effective against encapsulated strains of *H. influenzae* type b, therefore it will not protect against conditions such as otitis media and acute exacerbations of chronic bronchitis caused by nonencapsulated strains. It has been shown to protect children against pneumonia [*Lancet* (1997) 349, 1191–7].
- The tetanus and diphtheria proteins in the vaccine do not replace the need for routine tetanus and diphtheria immunization.
- Premature babies should be given Hib vaccine at 2, 3 and 4 months of age without adjusting for prematurity.
- The vaccine may be given to HIV-positive patients.
- The DoH advises the following action in the case of contact with a patient with invasive Hib disease.

  (a) In a nursery, playgroup or crèche, all non-immunized children under 4 years of age should be immunized.

  (b) Nonimmunized household contacts under 4 years of age should be immunized; rifampicin prophylaxis should be given to all household contacts (except pregnant women and immunized children under 4 years)—dosage is 20 mg/kg once daily (with a maximum daily dose of 600 mg) for 4 days.

  (c) The index case should also be immunized, irrespective of age.

  (d) Nonimmunized contacts should receive

three doses of the vaccine if under the age of 1 year, or one dose if aged 1–4 years.

• The UK coverage of *Haemophilus influenzae* b immunization (three doses before 13 months or one dose thereafter) in the summer of 1999 was 95.7% (England 94.3%, Wales 95.4%, Northern Ireland 96.3% and Scotland 96.7%).

• It has been suggested that there may be a link between Hib immunization and type 1 diabetes. A Finnish paper published in 1999 found that there was no difference in the risk of developing type 1 diabetes after 10 years in children not vaccinated against *Haemophilus influenzae* type b, compared with children who received the vaccine [Karvonem M. *et al.* (1999) Association between type 1 diabetes and *Haemophilus influenzae* type b vaccination: birth cohort study. *Br. Med. J.* 318, 1159–72].

• Immunizing infants against *Haemophilus influenzae* type b with conjugate vaccines has reduced rates of invasive disease in the developed world. Reports from the Gambia suggest a similar potential for the developing world [(1997) *Lancet* 349, 1191–7]. Some consider a second dose of the conjugate vaccine in the second year of life necessary for long-term immunity. This may limit the use of the conjugate vaccines in the developing world. In the UK, infants immunized at 2, 3 and 4 months of age receive no booster. We have evidence of the effectiveness of this scheme [(1997) *Lancet* 349, 1197–202], although its success may be related to the immunization of nearly all children under 5 years of age. Such mass immunization may have abruptly reduced nasopharyngeal carriage and modes of transmission. Immunological memory induced by this accelerated primary schedule may provide long-term protection even when circulating antibody titres are low [(1998) *Br. Med. J.* 316, 1570–1].

Vaccine availability (monovalent)

• ACT-HIB (Aventis Pasteur MSD) available as single vial of lyophilized vaccine plus a 0.5-mL ampoule of diluent. Use within 1 h of reconstitution.

• HibTITER (Wyeth Laboratories) available as monodose vials containing the 0.5-mL dose in packs of 1 and 10. Shake well before administration. Use within 30 min of withdrawing.

All vaccines for childhood immunization are distributed free of charge to GPs by Farillon Ltd, on behalf of the DoH.

Storage: Between 2 and 8 °C. *Do not freeze.*

The *Haemophilus influenzae* b and diphtheria/tetanus/pertussis combined vaccines

After the introduction of effective Hib conjugate vaccines, clinical practice has driven the development of combination vaccines comprising Hib conjugate with DTP.

In the spring of 1997, the combined DTwP-Hib vaccines were introduced into the UK. They are replacing the existing separate Hib and DTwP, which will remain available in case of vaccine shortages and for those infants who need to receive them separately.

The primary course remains unchanged: three doses, with an interval of 1 month between them, starting at 2 months of age (see Table 16.1). Each dose consists of 0.5 mL of the vaccine and is given by IM injection.

The combined DTwP-Hib vaccine should not be used for preschool children (over the age of 4 years). It should never be administered to anybody over the age of 10 years, when the low-dose diphtheria-containing vaccine should be used.

Combination with Hib vaccines containing an acellular pertussis component (DTaP-Hib) may result in the antibody response to Hib being lower than that with separate injections. This is the reason why the USA immunization programme (see Table 8.3 on p. 32) does not recommend DTaP-Hib combination products for use in primary immunization in infants. Although the mechanism of this interference needs to be studied further, there is a body of opinion that believes that this finding does not have major clinical implications and that the lower antibody concentrations are not associated with altered priming of memory function.

Following some vaccine shortages, the DoH has made available a combined vaccine containing the acellular pertussis component. This vaccine is Infanrix-Hib for use in children from 2 months of age. It is given by deep IM injection, of 0.5 mL, in three doses at monthly intervals.

The contraindications and side-effects applying to the separate vaccines will apply to the combined vaccine.

Vaccine availability

DTwP-Hib

- ACT-HIB DTP dc (Aventis Pasteur MSD). Supplied in a prefilled dual chamber (dc) syringe. The rear chamber contains liquid DTP and the front chamber lyophilized ACT-HIB. Depressing the plunger pushes the liquid DTP in the rear chamber through the bypass into the front chamber for reconstitution with freeze-dried ACT-HIB, resulting in 0.5 mL of vaccine. Shake well to form a cloudy/white suspension throughout.
- HibTITER, and Behringwerke DTP vaccine from Wyeth Laboratories is available as two separate vaccines that can be mixed in one syringe with the total volume of 1 mL.

DTaP-Hib

Infanrix-HIB combines diphtheria/tetanus/acellular pertussis vaccine (DTaP) and *Haemophilus influenzae* b (Hib) vaccine (SmithKline Beecham). The entire contents of the container of the DTaP vaccine should be added to the vial containing the Hib pellet. Shake the mixture well until the pellet dissolves completely. Use within 1 h of reconstitution.

Storage: Between 2 and 8 °C. *Do not freeze.* Protect from light.

Haemophilus influenzae type b infection

Haemophilus influenzae is a Gram-negative coccobacillus with six antigenically distinct capsular types (a–f) as well as nonencapsulated strains. It was discovered by Pfeiffer in 1892.

The nonencapsulated strains (75–95% of the carriage strains) cause infections that are nonpreventable, such as otitis media and bronchitis. They can be found as asymptomatic in the throat of over 60% of children. Only 5–25% are encapsulated strains (about half are type b).

Type b accounts for more than 95% of the encapsulated *H. influenzae* disease. It is an important cause of life-threatening infection in early childhood, when it is the dominant cause of nonepidemic bacterial meningitis and a major cause of pneumonia. It is estimated by the WHO to account for more than 3 million cases of serious disease and 700 000 deaths annually worldwide.

Haemophilus influenzae b infection causes meningitis (60% of cases), epiglottitis (15%), septicaemia (10%), septic arthritis, pneumonia, empyema, pericarditis, osteomyelitis and cellulitis. About 2–8% of meningitis cases end in death and 10–30% in long-term neurological sequelae such as seizures, intellectual impairment, vision and/or hearing loss, motor dysfunction and behavioural alterations.

More than 85% of Hib disease cases occur in children under the age of 5 years, with peak incidence of Hib meningitis occurring in children between 6 and 12 months and epiglottitis in children aged 2–4 years. The death rate is put at 4–5%.

The source of infection is the upper respiratory tract where type b organisms used to be recovered from 1–5% of children before vaccine introduction—much less now. The incubation period is unknown and the case fatality rate is 5% (1 in 20).

In England and Wales, there were 869 laboratory reports of Hib disease in 1983, rising steadily

Table 20.3 Notifications of *Haemophilus influenzae* b, and deaths from *Haemophilus* meningitis in England and Wales.

	Notifications	Deaths from *Haemophilus* meningitis
1992	484	21
1993	168	6
1994	52	1
1995	51	0
1996	57	0
1997	33	1
1998	29	1

Source: PHLS Communicable Disease Surveillance Centre.

to 1259 reports in 1989. The Hib vaccine was introduced into the UK in October 1992. During that year, there were 627 laboratory reports of Hib infection in England and Wales (229 in babies under 1 year of age), while in 1993 the number of reports dropped to 168 (65 in babies under 1 year of age). In 1995, the number was 39 (nine under the age of 1 year) and only one death. Notifications of *H. influenzae* meningitis in England and Wales have declined from 484 in 1992 when the vaccine

was introduced to 29 in 1998, an overall fall of a remarkable 94% (Table 20.3).

Countries where Hib vaccine has been introduced into routine immunization schedules, such as Finland, have seen a dramatic reduction in cases of Hib disease and the sequelae from it. This success is being repeated in the UK thanks to widespread acceptance of immunization against the disease.

Chapter 21

Poliomyelitis

Oral poliomyelitis vaccine (OPV)

Contraindications to vaccination

- Acute febrile illness.
- Diarrhoea and vomiting as they may interfere with replication (take rate) of the vaccine.
- Severe reaction to a previously administered dose of OPV.
- Severe hypersensitivity to penicillin, streptomycin (as they are derived from Sabin seed) and neomycin; in addition, to polymyxin B for the Medeva Pharma OPV.
- Immunodeficiency resulting from disease or treatment, and malignancy.
- Human immunodeficiency virus- (HIV) positive symptomatic (or asymptomatic for the Medeva Pharma product) individuals.
- Household contacts of patients who are immunocompromised for any reason (viable poliomyelitis vaccine virus may be excreted in the faeces of the recipient—see below)—give the inactivated (injectable) polio vaccine.
- Within 3 weeks of administration of a live viral vaccine—they can be given simultaneously.
- Within 3 weeks of administration of the live bacterial BCG, but may be given simultaneously. When BCG is given to infants, the primary polio immunization schedule starting at 2 months of age should not be delayed.
- Within 3 weeks from administration of the oral typhoid vaccine because of possible interference of the immune response in the gut.
- At 3 weeks before and 3 months after an injection of human normal immunoglobulin (HNIG). In the case of immediate travel, this contraindication may be ignored in the UK and OPV given. Where the vaccine is given as a booster, the possible inhibiting effect of immunoglobulin is less important.
- Pregnancy, although if there is a significant risk of exposure to poliomyelitis, as in the case of travel to an endemic area, the importance of vaccination may outweigh the theoretical risk to the fetus. If it is at all possible, postpone vaccination until after the sixteenth week of pregnancy (DoH advice). The WHO advises that oral immunization against poliomyelitis is not contraindicated in pregnancy [WHO, *International Travel and Health*, (1999) 88]. A safer solution is to use the injectable polio vaccine instead.

Previous vaccination with the inactivated (injectable) polio vaccine is not a contraindication; the two vaccines, although given by different routes, are interchangeable.

Possible side- and adverse effects

OPV has been associated with paralysis in vaccine recipients and their contacts. The risk is very small and can be expressed numerically as follows:
- among first-dose recipients—one case in 1.5 million doses;
- among contacts of first-dose recipients—one case in 2.2 million doses;
- the overall risk of vaccine-associated poliomyelitis is one case in 2.4 million doses;
- immunodeficient individuals—the risk is 3200- to 6800-fold higher than that in immunocompetent persons.

After the first dose, the risk with subsequent doses is considerably lower (about one-third of the risk with the first dose). It is important to ensure that contacts of children receiving OPV are fully immunized in order to reduce or even eliminate recipient contact cases.

A British review of all cases of paralytic poliomyelitis in England and Wales between 1985 and 1991 [(1992) *Br. Med. J.* 305, 79–82] estimated the risk of vaccine-associated paralysis to be 1.46 per million for the first dose, 0.49 for the second, 0 for the third and fourth doses, and 0.33 for the fifth.

In England and Wales, an average of one recipient and one contact case is reported every year in relation to over 2 million doses of the vaccine distributed.

The vaccine

OPV is a trivalent vaccine, containing live attenuated strains of poliomyelitis viruses types I, II and III, grown in cultures of human diploid cells (Medeva Pharma Ltd) or on monkey kidney cells (SmithKline Beecham Pharmaceuticals).

Viable poliomyelitis vaccine virus is excreted by healthy vaccinees and may persist in the faeces for up to 6 weeks—this is a possible risk for infection in immunocompromised household members as the OPV virus has the ability to spread from vaccinees to susceptible contacts. Although it can also induce immunity in unvaccinated immunocompetent contacts, it should not be relied upon to do so—immunity to poliovirus can be assured by immunizing each and every child directly. Nonimmunocompetent individuals can excrete the virus for longer.

Administration

A dose is the entire content of a monodose tube or three drops of vaccine from the 10-dose tube (Table 21.1). To enhance the taste, in some schools it is given on a sugar lump.

In the UK, OPV is given in infancy at the same time as routine immunization against diphtheria, tetanus, pertussis, *Haemophilus influenzae* b and meningococcal C.

- If a child vomits within 1 h of receiving the vaccine, that dose should be repeated. If the repeat dose is not retained, repeat the dose at a later visit.
- Seroconversion: 95% of recipients. Breastfeeding does not interfere with antibody response to OPV.
- Duration of immunity: after full immunization, in most people immunity is lifelong.
- In the primary course, all three doses should be given in order to ensure that each type of vaccine poliovirus is given an opportunity of establishing immunity. The OPV prevents circulation/infection of the natural (wild) poliovirus by inducing local immunity in the gut. IPV vaccine induces immunity but it does not induce gut immunity. The OPV is used in preference when aiming to eliminate wild polio infection.
- If the primary course is interrupted, it should be resumed from where it was left and not repeated.
- Babies in Special Care Units: while in the unit, use IPV. If vaccinated at the time of discharge, give the OPV complete immunization with OPV.
- Carers of recently immunized babies should be advised of the need for strict personal hygiene (washing hands after nappy changes) and safe disposal of soiled nappies. Having the vaccine in the intestines also means that it can be passed from the child to other household members.
- There is no reason to exclude a recently immunized baby from swimming pools.
- Nonimmunized parents and household contacts of children receiving primary OPV immunization should be immunized against poliomyelitis at the same time as their children (Table 21.2). If they have been fully immunized in the past, there is no need to give a booster.
- The DoH advises that HIV-positive, asymptomatic individuals may receive OPV (Medeva Pharma advise this as a contraindication for their preparation). It is important to note that such

Table 21.1 Childhood immunization with OPV in the UK.

Primary immunization	First booster	Second booster	Further boosters
Age 2, 3, 4 months (three doses at monthly intervals)	At school entry (age 4–5 years)	At school leaving (age 15–19 years)	Not recommended, except for those at risk, every 10+ years

individuals continue to excrete the vaccine virus in their faeces for longer than immunocompetent individuals and this will apply to adults as well as infants (wash hands after nappy changes, dispose of soiled nappies safely). The IPV may be given instead.

● HIV-positive, symptomatic individuals should receive the IPV.

● A person who has been immunized with OPV may receive the injectable inactivated poliomyelitis vaccine (IPV) as a booster and vice versa.

● Individuals born before 1962 (UK introduction of OPV), and especially before 1956 (UK introduction of IPV), may not have been immunized and no opportunity should be missed to immunize them (see Table 21.2).

● Particular care should be taken to provide immunization to those travelling abroad to areas where poliomyelitis is endemic (developing countries).

Vaccine availability

● Poliomyelitis vaccine live (oral) PhEur (Sabin strains) (SmithKline Beecham Pharmaceuticals) available in 10-dose dropper tubes as well as individual plastic monodose tubes. Discard any remaining vaccine at the end of a vaccination session as contamination with bacteria and moulds is possible—vaccine potency may be reduced). The manufacturer advises that the multidose use can be the same morning or afternoon only. The DoH advises up to 4 weeks when stored at appropriate cold chain conditions—check expiry date.

● OPV poliomyelitis vaccine live (oral) BP trivalent (Sabin type) (Medeva Pharma Ltd) in monodose tubes. This vaccine was withdrawn by the DoH in October 2000. This was necessary because the manufacturer had used a growth medium containing material of UK-sourced bovine origin despite guidance to the contrary by the Committee on Safety of Medicines in 1989. European guidance (1999) also makes it clear that oral medicinal products should not use bovine materials in the manufacturing process from countries in which there are known cases of BSE.

All vaccines for childhood immunization programmes and adults are distributed free of charge to GPs by the appointed vaccine distributors (Farillon Ltd in England and Wales) on behalf of the DoH.

Storage: Between 2 and 8 °C. Protect from light.

Inactivated poliomyelitis vaccine

Contraindications to vaccination

● Acute febrile illness.
● Anaphylactic reaction to a previously administered dose of the vaccine.
● Severe hypersensitivity to neomycin.

Possible side- and adverse effects

No serious adverse effects to IPV have been documented.

The vaccine

IPV Salk is a trivalent vaccine containing strains of poliomyelitis viruses types I, II and III which have been inactivated with formalin. The enhanced potency inactivated poliomyelitis vaccine (eIPV) is produced in human diploid cell cultures and is highly immunogenic.

Administration (Table 21.3)

● Boosting with IPV leads to very much higher levels of polio antibodies than boosting with OPV, irrespective of whether the patient has previously been immunized with OPV or IPV.

● Indications:
(a) for anybody who has refused OPV immunization, but will accept IPV;
(b) for anybody for whom the OPV is contraindicated and in particular for: (i) persons with compromised immunity who are unimmunized or partially immunized; (ii) siblings and other household contacts of immunosuppressed individuals; (iii) HIV-positive, symptomatic individuals; or (iv) healthcare personnel in close contact with immunosuppressed patients.

● There is now evidence that the incidence of OPV-associated poliovirus faecal excretion rates in

Table 21.2 Adult immunization with OPV in the UK.

Primary immunization	Boosters
Three doses at monthly intervals	Not recommended, except for those at risk, every 10 + years*

* Includes travellers to areas where polio is endemic or epidemic, healthcare workers, and laboratory workers likely to be exposed to the polio virus.

Table 21.3 Administration specifications for IPV.

Dose (ml)	Route	Primary immunization	Boosters
0.5	Deep SC or IM injection	Three doses at monthly intervals	Every 10 + years for those at risk

children can be reduced by administering IPV for their first dose in the childhood primary immunization schedule and then using OPV for their subsequent doses. IPV provides some degree of mucosal immunity. This reduces excretion of the OPV virus when given.

• In the early years of polio immunization, Salk (injectable) vaccines were cultured on kidney tissue taken from dead monkeys. This may have resulted in the contamination of the vaccine with a monkey virus known as SV40 that may (although not absolutely certainly) be associated with the development of certain forms of cancer such as mesothelioma (primarily linked to exposure to asbestos), and possibly brain tumours and bone cancer. The SV40 monkey virus was detected in 1963 and screened out. Since then all injectable polio vaccines have been vigorously checked for safety and efficacy and have been free from SV40 virus.

• In countries where the wild poliovirus is under control, such as the UK and USA, current debate concerns whether IPV should be adopted in place of OPV. This could prevent the small number of vaccine-associated paralysis cases in recipients and contacts. The UK will continue with the OPV for the time being, but will use the combined DTaP-IPV (Tetravac) in case of vaccine shortage. In Italy, the first two doses of Sabin attenuated OPV given to children at 2–4 months of age will be replaced by two doses of intramuscular Salk IPV vaccine. These will be followed, as previously, by two doses of OPV at 15–18 months and at 4–6 years of age. Germany in 1999 and the USA (6–8 vaccine-associated paralytic polio cases per year in the

absence of natural transmission) in January 2000 have made a total switch in their childhood recommendations, from OPV to IPV.

Vaccine availability

IPV, produced by Connaught, is available in 0.5-mL ampoules. Distributed for the DoH by Farillon Ltd in England, the Welsh Health Common Service Authority, the Common Services Agency in Scotland, and the Regional Pharmacist Procurement Coordinator in Belfast.

An unlicensed IPV (Imovax) is available from Aventis Pasteur MSD on a 'named-patient' basis. It is available in 0.5-mL prefilled syringes.

Storage: Between 2 and 8 °C. *Do not freeze.*

Poliomyelitis infection

The infection is caused by polioviruses, which are enteroviruses of which there are three types (I, II and III). Humans are the only reservoir for the virus. It is spread by contact with infected faeces or pharyngeal secretions, contaminated food and water. Perinatal transmission from mother to newborn infant can occur. Eighty to 90% of individuals who contract polio are under the age of 3 years.

The incubation period is 4–21 days. The patient is most infectious 7–10 days before and after the onset of clinical illness when the virus has colonized the throat and is excreted in large amounts in the faeces for up to 6 weeks or longer. Over 95% of children will be asymptomatic. About 4–8% of children will develop pyrexia without paralysis and 5% will progress to suffer headaches, vomiting, photophobia, neck stiffness and paralysis. Polio-myeloencephalitis can follow in 1–5% of cases. One in every 250 children develops paralysis of the lower motor neurones (paralytic poliomyelitis; Table 21.4).

As time progresses the patient can enter a second, slowly progressive phase, unrelated to normal ageing. The onset of symptoms is slow. On occasions it develops suddenly and progresses at an irregular pace. It may follow physical or emotional strain or surgery. The patient lacks strength and endurance, with increased weakness, fatigue, muscle weakness, myalgia, arthralgia and respiratory difficulties. This second phase is called 'post-polio syndrome'. It becomes apparent 30 or 40 years after the initial infection in about 25–40% of people infected during the era of wild poliovirus circulation.

The WHO has declared the UK as one of the countries where the indigenous poliomyelitis resulting from wild virus has been eliminated (the same applies to the whole of northern Europe, where it is now impossible to contract the disease indigenously). In England and Wales in 1955, before the introduction of the first polio vaccine in the UK, 4000 cases of poliomyelitis were notified. Between 1985 and 1995, there were only 28 cases reported, of which six were contracted abroad, 19 were vaccine-associated and three were of unknown source.

In the year of 1996–7 (summer to summer), the vaccine uptake in the UK in children under 2 years of age was maintained at 96%. Coverage in adults is not as high, therefore no opportunity in general practice should be missed to immunize all susceptible adults. Vaccine-associated contact cases could be eliminated if GPs could ensure polio immunization of all children and non-immunized adults.

Poliomyelitis is still prevalent in many developing countries where it occurs in epidemics. Up to 25 000 children a year in 50 countries still contract the virus. Ten of these countries face serious problems where poor immunization coverage has left large pools of infected people. To stop transmission, 80–90% of households in a community need to be immunized. India is one of the five 'polio reservoirs', the others being Pakistan, Bangladesh, Nigeria and Ethiopia. India alone 'consumes' up to 45% of the WHO immunization programme's resources. Corporate sponsorship, such as that from the diamond trading multinational company De Beers, which donated $2.7 million to help fund the 1999–2000 Angola programme, is helping offset some of the programme's resource shortfall. Three vaccine manufacturers (SmithKline Beecham, Aventis Pasteur Connaught, and Chiron-Behring) have provided 100 million free vaccine doses during 1997–99, worth $10 million.

As mentioned before, people infected with HIV, particularly those with AIDS, should not be given live vaccines, e.g. OPV. However, eradication of poliomyelitis globally requires the use of oral, live attenuated vaccine. Thus, complications after vaccination with live OPV vaccine might be expected to be more common in children infected with HIV, especially in countries where the prevalence of HIV infection is high. Such cases are known to have occurred. Nevertheless, the huge benefits of the polio eradication programme far outweigh the risk of such complications.

In 1988, the WHO declared its intention to eradicate poliomyelitis by December 2000. This is now more likely to happen by the year 2005 and

	1970–84	1985–95	1996	1997	1998
Unknown source	30	3	0	0	0
Contracted abroad	11	6	0	0	0
Vaccine-associated:					
Recipients	17	14	1	1	1
Contacts	12	5	0	1	0

Table 21.4 Poliomyelitis rates for England and Wales.

Sources include ONS and PHLS Communicable Disease Surveillance Centre.

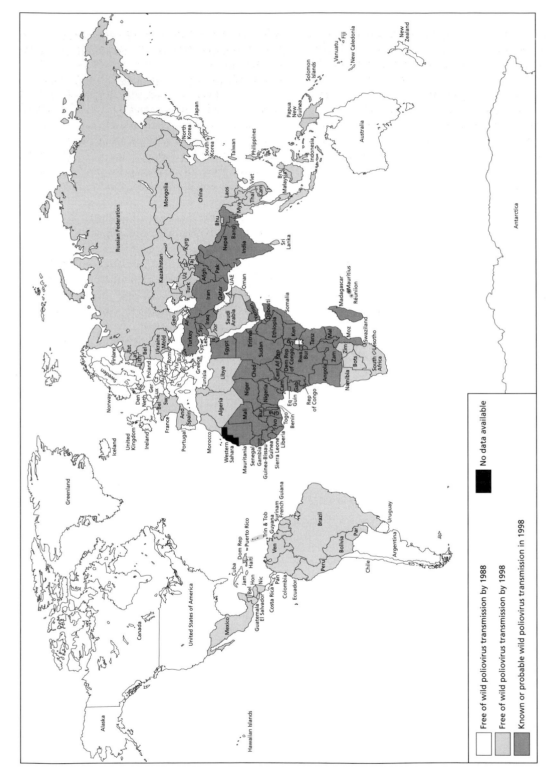

Fig. 21.1 Reductions in wild poliovirus transmission between 1988 and 1998—data according to the WHO World Health Report 1999 *Making a difference.*

Legend:

Free of wild poliovirus transmission by 1988

Free of wild poliovirus transmission by 1998

Known or probable wild poliovirus transmission in 1998

No data available

immunization is expected to stop by the year 2010. In 1974, less than 5% of children in developing countries were receiving polio immunization. By 1991, 85% of children worldwide were receiving three doses of polio vaccine. During 1997, 450 million children under the age of 5, in the polio-endemic world were given two doses of the OPV regardless of their previous immunization history. Unfortunately, because of local political conflicts, important countries such as Sierra Leone, Liberia and the Democratic Republic of Congo did not benefit from this campaign. In 1999, 147 million doses of polio vaccine were given.

Poliomyelitis has been eliminated from the USA since 1974 and from the rest of the continent since 1991. The Americas (from Argentina to Alaska) have been certified by an international commission to have eliminated wild virus poliomyelitis (defined as 'no case for a period of at least 3 years'—the last case was reported in Peru on 23 August 1991). The Western Pacific Region and the European Region appear to be free of indigenous wild poliovirus transmission, according to the WHO. The Indian subcontinent is one of the two remaining major reservoirs of wild poliovirus in the world; the other is sub-Saharan Africa.

In 1999, there were approximately 6000 cases of paralytic poliomyelitis worldwide. The global number of cases is actually much higher as some parts of Africa had not reported cases. Two-thirds occur in the Indian subcontinent. Other affected areas are West and Central Africa, the horn of Africa, and some countries in the Middle East (Fig. 21.1).

Progress Toward Global Poliomyelitis Eradication: http://www.cdc.gov/epo/mmwr/preview/mmrhtm/mm4916a4.htm

● Disease and vaccine information from the CDC: http://www.cdc.gov/nip/publications/acip-list.htm

● British Polio Fellowship: information for patients who have had polio. Eagle Office Centre, The Runway, South Ruislip, Middlesex HA4 6SE. Tel.: 0800 108 0586.

Poliomyelitis is a notifiable disease.

Chapter 22

Measles/mumps/rubella combined vaccine

Contraindications to vaccination

- Acute febrile illness (mild illnesses such as otitis media, diarrhoea, upper respiratory tract infection with cough and coryza are not a contraindication).
- Within 3 weeks of administration of another live virus vaccine or the live bacterial BCG vaccine.
- Within 3 months of administration of blood or plasma transfusion or HNIG (if the vaccine is given, check seroconversion 8 weeks later).
- Malignancy and immunodeficiency by disease or therapy. It should not be given to an immunodeficient person. HIV is not a contraindication unless the patient is severely immunocompromised (low CD4 + T-lymphocyte counts or percentage of total lymphocytes).
- Untreated tuberculosis patients with active tuberculosis should at least be on treatment if vaccination is administered. If there is a need for tuberculin skin testing, it should be performed on the day of MMR vaccination or 4–6 weeks later—measles vaccination can temporarily suppress tuberculin reactivity and render the test temporarily negative.
- Pregnancy and at least 1 month before (the manufacturer of MMR II (Aventis Pasteur MSD, Maidenhead, Berks, UK) advises 3 months before, the DoH and the manufacturer of Priorix (SmithKline Beecham Pharmaceuticals, Welwyn Garden City, Herts, UK) advise 1 month before). No data are available for the period of lactation so vaccinate if the benefit outweighs the risk and ensure the mother is using a reliable method of contraception for the next 1–3 months (depending on vaccine used).
- Severe reaction to a previously administered dose of the vaccine.
- History of thrombocytopenia occurring within 6 weeks of the first dose of MMR vaccine.

- Severe hypersensitivity to neomycin and/or gelatine (a vaccine stabilizer)—the most common cause of immediate hypersensitivity reactions. Contact dermatitis to neomycin is not a contraindication.
- Anaphylactic hypersensitivity to hens' eggs. A leading article by Dr R. Lakshman (Sheffield Institute for Vaccine Studies) that appeared in *Archive of Childhood Diseases* in February 2000, maintains that 'children allergic to eggs (including those who have had anaphylactic reactions to egg) do not appear to be at greater risk for anaphylaxis to MMR vaccine than other children'. The amount of egg in the vaccine appears to be too small to provoke an allergic reaction. Adverse reactions to MMR might be caused by the presence of gelatine or neomycin. Only children with a known egg allergy, who have had a life-threat-ening reaction, or who have egg allergy and chronic severe asthma, may be at risk of adverse effects from MMR vaccination.
- Children below 12 months of age in the UK should not normally be vaccinated as persisting, passively acquired, maternal antibodies can interfere with their ability to respond to the vaccine and they may not develop sustained antibody levels when later reimmunized. If it is necessary to give the vaccine to a child under the age of 12 months (e.g. when exposure to natural measles is likely as in the case of a local epidemic or travel abroad to an endemic area), a second dose should be given at 15 months and a third at preschool entry.

Possible side- and adverse reactions

Local reactions

Local reactions are swelling, redness and pain,

burning and/or stinging at the injection site. Wheal and flare reactions at the injection site are usually a result of traces of neomycin and/or gelatine in the vaccine. Only a small number of children are affected (less than 7.2% with Priorix) and reaction lasts for a short time.

General reactions

General reactions are similar to those expected from administration of monovalent vaccines given separately. The attenuated vaccine viruses are not thought to be transmissible to contacts when a rash or other side-effects occur in a vaccinee.

Reactions to the measles component of the vaccine

● Transient rash in 5% of vaccinees.
● Fever over 39.4 °C in 5–15% of vaccinees, between 5 and 12 days after vaccination, lasting 1–2 days (on occasions up to 5 days).
● Rash, fever and malaise (just like measles, but not transmissible) appear 5–12 days after vaccination in 5% of vaccinees and last for 2–3 days. Ensure you warn parents.
● Malaise, pharyngitis, headaches, nausea, vomiting and diarrhoea. Erythema multiforme and urticaria are rare.
● Febrile convulsions, usually at 6–11 days, in 1 in 1000 doses of the vaccine. It may be higher in children with previous or family history of idiopathic epilepsy or febrile convulsions. No long-term sequelae of post-vaccination febrile convulsions have been reported (incidence of febrile convulsions in natural measles is about 1 in 200). Such children should be immunized and the parents should be warned about the timing and the risks, and advised on ways to control fever, including consideration for the use of paracetamol in the period of 5–10 days after immunization. Parents of very susceptible children may have to be supplied with, and instructed in the use, of rectal diazepam to administer while awaiting arrival of the GP in cases where post-vaccination convulsions occur. Do not refuse immunization, but seek specialist paediatric advice if necessary. Children with personal histories of seizures or children whose first-degree relatives have histories of seizures may be at a slightly increased risk of seizures. They should be immunized as the benefits greatly outweigh the risks.
● Encephalitis and encephalopathy occurring within 30 days after vaccination have been reported in less than 1 in 3 million doses of measles vaccine. In no cases has it been shown that reactions were a result of the vaccine. The true incidence therefore is probably none. The incidence of encephalitis of unknown aetiology is much higher than this. After natural measles is 1 in 1000–5000 cases.
● Subacute sclerosing panencephalitis (SSPE) is a neurodegenerative disease caused by persistent infection of the brain by an altered form of the wild measles virus. It is now thought not to occur after measles vaccine. The wild measles virus rather than the vaccine virus has been isolated at necropsy, even when the vaccine has been the suspected cause. Some of these children may have had unrecognized measles disease before vaccination. SSPE can affect children who have had measles infection in the past (1 in 25 000 cases, and 1 in 5500 in children under the age of 1 year). In the great majority of cases the onset is in the first two decades of life, or about 8 years from measles infection—insidious onset, intellectual (school work) deterioration, particularly in reading and writing, deterioration of vision, rigidity, spasticity and death within a year or two. The wild measles virus persists in an altered form in the brain causing chronic inflammation with chronic consequences. Four cases of SSPE were reported in 1998 in the UK, in patients aged 5, 6, 11 and 15 years. All four had a history of probable measles infection and all four had been vaccinated. Gene sequencing from a frozen brain specimen from one case revealed evidence of wild but not vaccine-like measles virus infection. It can be concluded that measles vaccine protects children from SSPE by preventing measles infection. Indeed, the incidence of SSPE has fallen dramatically since the introduction of the MMR vaccine. The importance of a second dose of MMR vaccine is emphasized so as to achieve 99% protection—see below.
● Guillain–Barré syndrome is probably not caused by MMR vaccination—there is no evidence that it is.
● Thrombocytopenia within 2 months (mostly 2–

3 weeks) of MMR vaccination in 1 per 25 000–40 000 vaccinees receiving the first dose. The risk after the second dose of the vaccine is considerably less. Children at increased risk of thrombocytopenia are those with a history of thrombocytopenia or thrombocytopenic purpura. The risk of this complication from measles disease is much greater: 1 in 3000).

For comparison of complications resulting from measles infection and vaccine, see Table 22.1 on p. 95.

Reactions to the mumps component of the vaccine

- Parotitis in about 1% of vaccinees, 3 weeks or more after vaccination.
- Orchitis may rarely occur, and retrobulbar neuritis very rarely.
- Meningoencephalitis occurring 14–30 days after immunization is mild and the sequelae are rare. At present, only the Jeryl Lynn mumps strain-containing MMR vaccine is licensed in the UK. Such a complication is expected extremely rarely and put at 1 in 1.8 million doses. The DoH withdrew all MMR vaccines containing the Urabe Am 9 strain in September 1992 as the rate of meningoencephalitis was reported in 1 in 300 000 doses among those vaccinees (this complication after natural mumps infection is reported to occur at a rate of 1 in 400 cases).

Reactions to the rubella component of the vaccine

differing in kind

- Rash in 5% of vaccinees.
- Fever in 5–15% of vaccinees, 5–12 days after vaccination.
- Lymphadenopathy less commonly.
- Thrombocytopenia is seen rarely (see Reactions to the measles component, above).
- Transient peripheral neuritis, paraesthesiae and pain in the upper and lower limbs can rarely occur 3 days to 3 months after immunization.
- Mild episodes of joint pain, usually in small peripheral joints, in 0.5% of children.
- Arthritis and arthralgia occur in up to 25% of adults receiving the vaccine. Joint involvement

begins 7–21 days after vaccination and is generally transient. Adults seldom have to limit their work activities. Symptoms may persist for months or, on rare occasions, for years, but the aetiological relationship to vaccination is unclear.

Controversies associated with MMR immunization

Claims have been made, mainly in the UK, of an association between measles-containing vaccines, such as the MMR, and inflammatory bowel disease (Crohn's disease, ulcerative colitis). This hypothesis was postulated in a paper published in the *Lancet* by researchers from the Royal Free Hospital, London [Thompson N.P., Mongomery S.M., Pounder R.E. & Wakefield A.J. (1995) Is measles vaccination a risk factor for inflammatory bowel disease? *Lancet* 345, 1071–74]. This study compared the prevalence of Crohn's disease, ulcerative colitis, coeliac disease and peptic ulcer in one vaccinated cohort, their partners (assumed to have been immunized later or to have had natural measles infection) and an unvaccinated cohort. The relative risk of developing Crohn's disease in the vaccinated group was found to be 2.95 and that of ulcerative colitis 2.05 (nonsignificant) compared with those in the unvaccinated group.

This study did not prove a link. It attempted to draw our attention to epidemiologically based evidence. On the other hand, the study was characterized by serious problems of study design.

- The vaccinated and control cohorts were drawn from disparate populations, with substantial differences in geographical location, age and other covariates that may have influenced the risk for inflammatory bowel disease.
- The vaccinated cohort had a history of measles disease and vaccination well documented; they were also specifically asked about inflammatory bowel disease. The control group was assumed not to have received the measles vaccine and cases of inflammatory bowel disease were picked up passively from a more general survey conducted for an unrelated purpose.
- No standardized criteria were used for the diagnosis of inflammatory bowel disease.
- The researchers made the assertion that the

only obvious difference (between cohorts) was that one group only received measles vaccine.

- The difference in reported measles infection among controls (89%) and vaccinated subjects (0%) was not addressed in this study. However, a link between natural measles infection and inflammatory bowel disease has also been proposed [Ekbom A., Wakefield A.J., Zack M. & Adami H.O. (1994) The role of perinatal measles infection in the aetiology of Crohn's disease: a population-based epidemiological study. *Lancet* 334, 508–10].

- The Royal Free Hospital Bowel Disease Study Group suggested that measles virus can be shown to be present in inflammatory bowel tissues affected by Crohn's disease [Wakefield A.J., Pittilo R.M. & Sim R. (1993) Evidence of persistent measles virus infection in Crohn's disease. *J. Med. Virol.* 39, 345–53].

Using reagents provided by the above group at the Royal Free Hospital, an independent group could not replicate the above results [Liu Y. *et al.* (1995) Immunocytochemical evidence of *Listeria*, *Escherichia coli* and *Streptococcus* antigens in Crohn's disease. *Gastroenterology* 108, 1396–404].

Using the most sensitive and specific molecular techniques (reverse transcriptase–polymerase chain reaction), three groups of researchers, including the Royal Free Hospital Bowel Disease Study Group, have not been able to detect measles virus genetic material in either Crohn's disease-affected tissues, normal bowel tissue, or in peripheral blood lymphocytes [Afzal M.A. *et al.* (1998) Absence of measles-virus genome in inflammatory bowel disease. *Lancet* 351, 646–7; Haga Y. *et al.* (1996) Absence of measles viral genomic sequence in intestinal tissues from Crohn's disease by nested polymerase chain reaction. *Gut* 38, 211–15; Iizuka M. *et al.* (1995) Absence of measles virus in Crohn's disease. *Lancet* 345, 199; Iizuka M. & Masamune O. (1997) Measles vaccination and inflammatory bowel disease. *Lancet* 350, 1775].

One large international case–control study reported no association between measles vaccination and inflammatory bowel disease [Gilat T., Hacohen D., Lilos P. & Langman M.J.S. (1987) Childhood factors in ulcerative colitis and Crohn's disease. *Scand. J. Gastroenterol.* 22, 1009–24].

In 1997, a British, case-control study looked at 140 patients with inflammatory bowel disease (83 with Crohn's disease) and 280 controls matched for sex, area and age (all born in or after 1968, when measles vaccination was introduced). They had measles vaccination rates of 56.4 and 57.1%, respectively. The researchers concluded that their findings were incompatible with the hypothesis that measles vaccination in childhood predisposes to the later development of any form of inflammatory bowel disease [Feeny M., Clegg A., Winwood P. & Snook J. for the East Dorset Gastroenterology Group. (1997) A case–control study of measles vaccination and inflammatory bowel disease. *Lancet* 350, 764–6].

In view of the great interest shown by the British media and the negative reporting in the press, the available evidence was then thoroughly scrutinized by the Joint Committee on Vaccination and Immunization on behalf of the DoH, and by the WHO. The alleged link between the MMR vaccine and inflammatory bowel disease was not found to be supported by the available evidence.

In 1994, around 7 million children in the UK received the combined measles/rubella (MR) vaccine. National data from hospital episode statistics show no increase in new cases or exacerbation of existing cases of Crohn's disease following the immunization campaign.

The alleged association between MMR and autism was derived from a television programme in Denmark in 1993 in which the mother of twins, one of whom developed autism, claimed the MMR vaccine was responsible. This claim of association was thoroughly investigated by the Danish National Department of Epidemiology, and the UK Joint Committee on Vaccination and Immunization. There was no biological or epidemiological evidence available to support a link.

The National Autistic Society has stated that, in their opinion, there has been no increase in the incidence of Autistic Spectrum Disorders but there is increased recognition of the range of the condition. About one-third of children with autistic disorder exhibit regression after apparently normal development in the first year of life [Mauk J.E. (1993) Autism and pervasive developmental disorders. *Paediatr. Clin. N. Am.* 40, 567–78]. The mean age at which the parents of children with autism first report concern about their child's development is 18–19 months, and 14 months for experienced parents [Siegal B. *et al.* (1988) How children with autism are diagnosed: difficulties in identification of children with multiple developmental delays. *J. Dev. Behav. Paediatr.* 9, 199–204]. Each year over 600 000 British children receive MMR vaccine after their first year of life and before their second birthday, so the probability of parents first noticing abnormal behaviour shortly after MMR vaccination in a child previously thought to be developing normally is considerable.

A Swedish study has looked at the incidence of autism over a 10-year period [Gillberg C. *et al.* (1991) Is autism more common now than 10 years ago? *Br. J. Psychiatry* 158, 403–9]. This study had good and consistent data. It looked at the incidence of autism in Gothenburg over a 10-year period during which the MMR vaccine was introduced into their childhood immunization programme. The incidence of autism was unaffected by the introduction of the MMR vaccine.

In 1998, the Royal Free Hospital published a paper in which they claimed to have identified associated gastrointestinal disease and developmental regression in a group of children [Wakefield A. *et al.* (1998) Ileal-lymphoid-nodular hyperplasia, nonspecific colitis, and pervasive developmental disorder in children. *Lancet* 351, 637–41]. The condition described is benign and disappears over time spontaneously, with no long-term sequelae. It is a common condition, occurring in 24% of barium follow-through examinations when investigating for suspected childhood inflammatory bowel disease. It is not therefore surprising that the 12 children (aged 3–10 years) examined in this paper had this condition, as there was cause for concern for them to be referred to a London specialist paediatric gastroenterology unit. Their parents or GP attributed their bowel condition and developmental regression to MMR vaccine in eight children, measles infection in one and otitis media in one child. Four children were said to have abnormally low levels of some immunoglobulins and this observation was used to propose an increased susceptibility to the effects of the attenuated viruses in MMR. At least four of the 12 children had behavioural problems prior to the onset of symptoms of inflammatory bowel disease,

the supposed mechanism for autism after the MMR vaccination. Subsequent examination of their work showed they were using the wrong reference range—that for adults and not for children. When the appropriate paediatric standards were used, only one child had a low IgA level. No scientific analyses were presented to substantiate their claim, and factors such as referral bias and the small sample size were not considered. Additionally, the theory that autism in the 12 patients is caused by poor absorption of nutrients is not supported by this study's own clinical data. The researchers admitted they 'did not prove an association between measles, mumps, and rubella vaccine and the syndrome described'.

Researchers from Finland found no evidence for a causal association between MMR, inflammatory bowel disease and autism in a surveillance study of all adverse reactions to 3 million doses of MMR vaccine administered between 1982 and 1996 [Peltola H. *et al.* (1998) No evidence for measles, mumps, and rubella vaccine-associated inflammatory bowel disease or autism in a 14-year prospective study. *Lancet* 351, 1327–8].

1999 saw the publication of two important studies. The first, carried out by researchers from the Public Health Laboratory Service (PHLS) and a team from the Royal Free Hospital, investigated the history of all 498 known autistic children born in the North Thames region since 1979, thus covering the period before and after the introduction of MMR in 1988 [Taylor B., Miller E., Farrington C. *et al.* (1999) Autism and measles, mumps and rubella vaccine: no epidemiological evidence for a causal association. *Lancet* 353, 1987–8]. The age at diagnosis of autism was not different in those vaccinated before or after the age of 18 months and those never vaccinated. There was a steady rise in cases from 1979 onwards but no sudden change in trend following the MMR vaccine introduction. The researchers concluded that there was no association found between MMR immunization and onset of developmental delay.

The second study, by a working party set up by the Committee on Safety of Medicines (CSM), examined the records of 92 children with suspected autism and 15 with suspected Crohn's disease, that arose in temporal association with MMR or MR vaccines, attributed by parents and reported to a firm of solicitors [CSM (1999) Report of the working party on MMR vaccine. *Curr. Probl. Pharmacovigilance* 25, 9–10]. The committee of experts examined all data put to them and found no evidence to support the suggested causal association between MMR and MR vaccines and autism or inflammatory bowel disease. Nor there was any cause for concern about the safety of these vaccines.

A similar situation concerns asthma. The DoH has found no evidence from any well-controlled studies to support a link between asthma and the MMR vaccine.

Some mothers request that their children receive the three monovalent vaccines separately, one each year as suggested but not substantiated by Dr Andrew Wakefield, instead of the combined MMR vaccine, in order 'to reduce the viral load'. There is no published evidence that proves or indicates this is a safer or more effective way of administering the MMR vaccine and the DoH supports and recommends the administration of the trivalent MMR, which contains attenuated (weakened) and not wild viruses. The fact is, splitting MMR into separate doses may prove harmful for some children as it exposes them unnecessarily to potentially serious diseases—the completion of vaccination and the process of acquiring immunity will take longer. In the UK, having the MMR in three monovalent vaccines is no longer an option as the monovalent measles and mumps vaccines are no longer available. Some parents have resorted to going abroad in order to obtain the vaccines. Others have resorted to the dangerous and irresponsible practice of the 'measles parties', where they bring their children into contact with other children who are thought to have the infection. These are very sporadic cases and hopefully, with better parent education, will soon cease.

Some parents have cited Japan as an example where the Government promotes single antigen immunization against measles, mumps and rubella. Japan manufactures its own vaccines and had a problem with the mumps strain of their MMR after its introduction in 1989. Their mumps strain was found to be associated in some cases with aseptic mumps virus meningitis. They therefore 'temporarily suspended' their MMR vaccine

in April 1993. Because of the problem with the mumps strain in their MMR vaccine, mumps immunization is voluntary, while measles and rubella immunization is mandatory. Japan is hoping to have another MMR available soon.

A recent study from Japan examined intestinal biopsies from 20 patients with Crohn's disease, 20 with ulcerative colitis, 11 with noninflammatory bowel disease, and nine controls, looking for the presence of measles virus in the bowel mucosa. They found there was no difference between the three groups with bowel disease, but all three were significantly more likely to have 'measles-related antigen'. The same researchers have recently shown that the 'measles-related antigen' present in the intestinal mucosa of patients with Crohn's disease is not in fact measles virus, but an as yet unidentified human protein, not unique to Crohn's disease. Previous studies, which have supported the link between measles virus and Crohn's disease, have drawn this conclusion because of the presence of measles antibodies in the intestine. The authors of this study suggest that this may actually have been an antibody not to the measles virus itself, but to a human protein, the 'measles-related antibody'. If the authors are right in their conclusion that this antigen is not measles virus at all, then the theory that attempts to link Crohn's disease and measles virus would be further discredited [Iizuka M *et al.* (2000) Immunohistochemical analysis of the distribution of measles related antigen in the intestinal mucosa in inflammatory bowel disease. *Gut* 46, 163–9].

A US Congressional hearing in April 2000 heard evidence about possible links between MMR vaccination and autism. The chair of the Congressional Committee, Senator Dan Burton (Rep. Indiana) is reported to believe his grandchild's autism was caused by MMR. Professor John O'Leary (Dublin) and Dr Andrew Wakefield (Royal Free Hospital, London) reported to the Committee that they had examined bowel tissue obtained by Dr Wakefield from 25 children with evidence of a condition described by Dr Wakefield as 'autistic enterocolitis'. Wakefield presented uninterpretable fragments of results only and concentrated on refuting studies that had contradicted his findings. His conclusions were noncommittal: 'the virological data indicate that this may be measles virus in some children'.

Professor O'Leary reported evidence of measles virus in 24 of the cases, and evidence of measles virus in 1 of 15 normal children controls—although it is not clear whether these controls are appropriate. Nor is it clear whether the presence of measles virus would indicate a causal link with autism. If Professor O'Leary had tested his material for measles virus by immunohistochemistry with the anti-measles monoclonal antibody, the possibility that samples from children with autism showed a false positive result might be high since the samples probably had inflammations, namely autistic enterocolitis. It is crucial to determine the nucleotide sequence of the fragment and compare it with that of the measles virus. This work has not been published and therefore remains scientifically unscrutinized.

The UK's DoH comments were that 'this is a highly selective sample, carried out with incorrect and inappropriate controls and unverifiable by the usual scientific means'. During the Congressional hearing Professor Brent Taylor (Royal Free Hospital, London) outlined his research in 498 autistic children, published in *The Lancet* (see above), showing no relation between MMR vaccination dates and onset of the condition.

Following this hearing, a spokesman from the Royal Free Hospital, London (where Dr Wakefield works) said: 'Recently published work has strongly suggested that Dr Wakefield's original observation resulted from an immunological cross-reaction. There appears to date no work by any other expert group that has substantiated Dr Wakefield's thesis. Dr Wakefield has been strongly urged to undertake a further study which would include blind testing of subjects, appropriate controls and independent testing by disinterested expert laboratories. Dr Wakefield agreed to do this in December 1999 and the outcome is awaited.'

British researchers announced in March 2000 a two-year Medical Research Council (MRC) review of 2 million GP records at 300 practices in a bid to explain the rise in autism. This study, which will be led by Professor Andrew Hall of the London School of Hygiene and Tropical Medicine, will investigate whether autistic children have a history of other medical problems, and will consider the impact of viral infections in the uterus or soon after birth. It will also examine any possible links between autism and the MMR vaccine. Already, the MRC had carried out a 2-year monitoring of research into inflammatory bowel disease and autism. They concluded that 'between March 1998 and September 1999 there has been no new evidence to suggest a causal link between MMR and inflammatory bowel disease/autism' (http://www.mrc.ac.uk/Autismreport.html).

MMR vaccine has been used around the world for the past 27 years. Over 300 million doses of the MMR vaccine have been distributed worldwide (over 200 million doses in the USA alone) and no association with bowel disease or autism has been found. In the UK, about 12 million doses have been given since the MMR vaccine was introduced in 1988.

While advising parents about the possible side-effects of the MMR vaccine, we must not forget the frequent and devastating consequences of measles infection (nearly 1 million children killed every year around the world), and the millions of lives the vaccine has and is saving. Table 22.1 gives a comparison of complications between measles infection and measles vaccine.

For those parents interested in obtaining information on the Internet, I would recommend the Medinfo UK website: http://www.medinfo.co.uk

The vaccine

The MMR II vaccine contains the attenuated Enders Line of the Edmonston measles vaccine strain, and Priorix vaccine the attenuated Schwarz measles vaccine strain. Also, MMR II contains the Jeryl Lynn Level B mumps vaccine strain, and Priorix the RIT 4385 (Jeryl Lynn-derived) mumps vaccine strain. Both MMR II and Priorix contain the Wistar RA 27/3 strain of live attenuated rubella vaccine.

Administration (Table 22.2)

● The vaccine should be reconstituted only with the diluent supplied and should be used immediately after reconstitution (within 1 h MMR II, 3 h Priorix). Protect it from light at all times.

- The injection site is the upper arm, although infants receive it at the anterolateral thigh.
- Seroconversion after a single dose of MMR vaccine generally occurs in 95% for measles, 95% for mumps, and 97–99% for rubella, although it is possible that higher seroconversion is achieved with the newer vaccines. Immunity is at least 27 years for measles, 14 years for mumps, and 27 years for rubella—although because of immunological memory, immunity is probably for life.
- An immunization coverage of at least 95% is necessary to form 'herd' immunity, which goes a long way in protecting nonimmunized children and those who do not seroconvert to the vaccine, as long as they remain within their community and don't travel or mix with travellers (probably an impossibility in the 21st century).
- Incorrectly stored vaccine and exposure of the vaccine to light (which can inactivate the measles component) may cause failure of the vaccine to protect. Overall, protection in recipients after a single dose of MMR vaccine is achieved in around 90% for measles, 90% for mumps and 95% for rubella. At the time when immunization coverage in England and Wales was 92%, it was estimated that only 83% of children vaccinated each year were protected, hence one of the reasons for the need for a booster at school entry. It also gives the doctors' practices another chance to immunize those who were not immunized in their second year of life. This increases seroprotection among vaccinees to 99% or more against all three diseases.
- In the Canadian experience, during an epidemic of measles in Quebec City in 1989, 41 of 441 (9%) vaccinated children developed measles (vaccine efficacy 91%), while 17 unvaccinated children (100%) developed measles.
- It can be concluded therefore that the level of the MMR vaccine effectiveness after the first dose of the vaccine given during the second year of life is:

  90–95% against measles;
  90–95% against mumps;
  97–99% against rubella;

Table 22.1 Comparison of complications between measles infection and measles vaccine.

	Measles infection	MMR or measles vaccine monovalent
Rash and pyrexia	Almost 100%	5–10% (day 5–12)
Ear infection	1 in 20	None
Diarrhoea	1 in 6	None
Chest infection	1 in 25	None
Convulsions	1 in 200	1 in 1000 (day 6–11)
Thrombocytopenia	1 in 3000	1 in 29 000
Encephalitis	1 in 1000/5000	< 1 in 3 million
	15% fatal; 20–40% residual neurological sequelae	(probably none)
Subacute sclerosing panencephalitis (SSPE)	1 in 25 000	None (it protects against SSPE)
	1 in 8000 in the < 2-year-olds	
	1 in 5500 in the < 1-year-olds	
Anaphylaxis	None	1 in 100 000 (after 1st MMR)
Death	1 in 2500–1 in 5000	None

Table 22.2 Administration specifications for MMR vaccine.

Age	Dose (ml)	Route	Reimmunization	Boosters (UK)
Children over 12 months and susceptible adults	0.5	SC or IM	Only if given before 12 months of age (monovalent or combined)	At school entry (usually age 4–5 years)

≥ 99% after the second (preschool) dose against all three infections

• In a USA/Canadian study, over 80% of measles seronegative children after a first dose of MMR vaccine seroconverted after a second dose. It is most important that high vaccination coverage is achieved for a first and second dose of MMR vaccine.

• Administration of the MMR vaccine under the age of 12 months is avoided in the UK because of the possible interference in the uptake of the measles vaccine by persisting passively acquired maternal antibodies against measles. However, up to 30% of African children contract measles before 9 months of age, therefore the WHO recommends that in countries with a high incidence of measles in infancy, measles vaccine should be given at 6 months of age. Immunization against measles causes a spectacular reduction of 30–86% in child mortality in developing countries. This benefit is greatest in the 6–12 months after immunization, and in infancy (44–100%).

• MMR should be given to children irrespective of history of previous measles, mumps or rubella infection. Vaccination is not harmful to individuals already immune.

• The MMR vaccine is protective if given within 72 h of contact with measles. The same is not observed for mumps and rubella, as the antibody response to them is too slow for effective prophylaxis after exposure.

• *Indications*: in the UK, the MMR vaccine is recommended for:

(a) children aged 12–15 months; a second dose at school entry (age 4–5 years);

(b) children of any age not previously immunized and especially children with chronic conditions such as cystic fibrosis, congenital heart or kidney disease, Down's syndrome, failure to thrive or in residential or day care;

(c) unimmune adults who request it, especially those in long-term institutional care or unimmunized travellers;

(d) HIV-infected individuals in the absence of contraindications.

• Symptomatic HIV-infected patients who are exposed to measles should receive HNIG prophylaxis regardless of vaccination status (vaccination may not provide protection). Patients receiving HNIG at regular intervals are covered if they have received HNIG within 3 weeks from exposure.

• Missed MMR vaccination:

(a) before school entry: give the first dose and arrange for the second dose to be given at school entry age;

(b) at school entry: give the first dose (at the same time as DT and OPV), then give the second dose 3 months after the first;

(c) after school entry vaccinations have been given: recall these children and give MMR vaccine;

(d) at school leaving: give MMR at the same time as Td and OPV;

(e) nonimmune adults (students, travellers at risk, etc.): offer MMR vaccination.

• MMR vaccine uptake among 2-year-olds in England and Wales was 93% in 1993, 92% in 1996, 91% in the year 1997–98, falling to 87.35% in the summer of 1999 (Table 22.3).

• In order to stop the occurrence of outbreaks of

Table 22.3 Completed MMR vaccination by 24 months and 5 years in England, Wales and Northern Ireland: July to September 1999.

	Coverage at 24 months*	Coverage at 5 years	
	MMR-1 (%)	MMR-1 (%)	MMR-2 (%)
England	87.3	93.3	77.1
Wales	87.4	93.7	74.2
Northern Ireland	90.0	97.2	84.2
England, Wales and Northern Ireland	87.3	93.4	78.5

Source: *Communicable Disease Report Weekly* (2000) 10, 31.
* The figure for Scotland is 92.3%, giving a UK average of 88.5%.

measles, the level of immunity required in the UK is at least 85% in preschool children, 90% in primary school pupils and 95% in secondary school children. As the uptake of MMR has declined in recent years, the proportion of the population susceptible to measles infection has increased. An epidemic of measles infection may be inevitable by the year 2001/2.

● We are witnessing small outbreaks of measles infection in areas of low vaccination rate. Unfortunately, some already immunized children develop the disease for the reasons explained above. Between the end of the years 1998 and 1999, 103 cases of measles were notified from a religious community in Salford, UK, where the average MMR coverage in those under 24 months of age was 77.5% (range 70–85%). Most were unvaccinated children under 9 years of age. Three children had to be admitted to hospital because of complications. Of the 85 notified cases whose immunization histories were available, eight had been vaccinated with the MMR vaccine. Several clinical cases of measles were notified in 1999 from a similar community in East London. An outbreak of measles in the UK in 1997 affected unvaccinated children in several Rudolf Steiner communities, which discourage vaccination against measles on philosophical grounds. A total of 293 clinical (150 confirmed) cases were identified in 9 months. Only two confirmed cases had been vaccinated against measles, and 90% were under 15 years of age. The Salford measles strain was shown to be the same as the Steiner outbreak strain, a genotype known to be circulating widely in Europe. In Holland, 2300 cases of measles, including three fatal cases and almost 20% with serious complications, were reported from April to December 1999 in communities who refuse vaccination for religious reasons. Although the national coverage of MMR vaccine in the Netherlands is 96%, only 3% of the 2300 Dutch cases had been vaccinated [source of all above information: *Communicable Disease Report Weekly* (2000) 10, 29].

In 2000, the Republic of Ireland suffered its worst measles outbreak for seven years as a result of the low uptake (average 76%, range 68–86%) of the MMR vaccine. During the first half of the year, a total of 1220 cases of measles were reported (compare this to the 148 cases reported during the whole of 1999). Two children died as a result of measles infection.

● On the international scene, measles is so infectious that immunization rates of over 95% would be required over many years, in order to head towards measles infection elimination. No animal reservoir is known (humans are the only reservoir) and available vaccines are very effective.

● For 1998, the WHO estimates that approximately 30 million measles cases and 888 000 measles-related deaths occurred worldwide; an estimated 85% of these deaths occurred in Africa and the South-East Asia region [The WHO report (1999) Making a difference. WHO, Geneva, Switzerland]. Failure to deliver at least one dose of measles vaccine to all children remains the primary reason, despite widespread availability of an effective vaccine. Before the measles vaccine was introduced, around approximately 5.7 million people worldwide died each year of measles. During the twentieth century in England and Wales measles killed a quarter of a million children.

● It is important to consider measles immunization for young travellers abroad. Even in many areas in Europe and some Mediterranean countries, many families cannot afford to have the vaccine or the MMR vaccine uptake is poor. The situation is even worse in countries further afield. In a feasibility study in 1993/94 in the UK, the measles vaccine was given to babies aged 1–11 months, in order to assess the protection expected in case of an outbreak or travel abroad. It was found that measles vaccine would protect 30% of infants at 5 months and that a second dose at 13 months results in almost universal seroconversion [Ko, B. *et al.* (1999) Neutralizing antibody responses to two doses of measles vaccine at 5 and 13 months of age in the UK. *Communicable Disease and Public Health* 2 (3), 203–6].

● Measles, once a common rite of passage for children, has all but been wiped out in the USA. In 1998, there were only 100 cases reported to the CDC, most of them believed to have originated outside the USA. This achievement was attributed in large part to a concerted push in recent years to raise immunization rates and the addition of a second dose of the vaccine for young schoolchildren.

Antibody	Measles	Mumps	Rubella
IgM (indicates recent infection or vaccination)	Yes	Yes	Yes
IgG (indicates past infection or vaccination)	Yes	Not available	Yes

Table 22.4 Saliva antibody test interpretation and availability.

• *Measles, mumps, rubella saliva antibody diagnostic test*: noninvasive confirmation of measles, mumps and rubella using a single saliva sample is routinely available in the UK. It is an accurate test and samples should be taken between 2 and 4 weeks after the onset of the first symptom, although a range of 1–6 weeks is acceptable. When a case of measles or mumps or rubella is suspected, the GP should request a kit from the local Consultant in Commun-icable Disease Control at the Health Authority. This is sent by post. Once the saliva specimen is taken, it is sent by post (prepaid) to the Public Health Laboratory (Colindale), which, in turn, notifies the practice by post of the result within 2 weeks. The result of the test does not affect the payment of the fee for notification. For interpretation of the results see Table 22.4.

Vaccine availability

MMR II (Aventis Pasteur MSD)

The vaccine is distributed to GPs on behalf of the DoH, free of charge, by its appointed suppliers. Available as single-dose vials of freeze-dried vaccine powder with diluent. Use within 1 h of reconstitution.

Storage: Between 2 and 8 °C. *Do not freeze diluent.* Protect from light. During transport, maintain temperatures of 10 °C or less, but no lower than 2 °C. Although no other temperatures but these are recommended for storage, it is known that the vaccine retains at least eight times the minimum immunizing dose even after 6 weeks at 22 °C or 1 week at 37 °C.

PRIORIX (SmithKline Beecham Pharmaceuticals)

The vaccine is distributed to GPs on behalf of the DoH, free of charge, by its appointed suppliers. Available in glass vials with diluent in an ampoule. Use within 3 h from reconstitution.

Storage: Between 2 and 8 °C. *Do not freeze diluent.* Protect from light.

• Already a measles vaccine has been developed that is delivered by aerosol generated from a nebulizer. This is not available in the UK and could help in future immunization campaigns, especially when administering the second dose.

Immunoglobulin

• Children and adults with contraindications to the MMR vaccine, such as those with malignancies or immunosuppressed by disease or treatment, children under 12 months, or susceptible pregnant women, should receive human normal immunoglobulin (HNIG) IM (Table 22.5), as soon as possible and not later than 6 days after exposure to measles. If MMR is not further contraindicated, 3 months should be allowed to pass before vaccination is undertaken.

• HNIG should also be given to pregnant women with confirmed rubella infection, for whom therapeutic abortion is unacceptable. It must be given as soon as possible after exposure at the dose of 750 mg IM.

• HNIG can be obtained from the Central Public Health Laboratory Services, Baxter Healthcare Ltd—Hyland Immuno (Gammabulin—not expected to be available after the summer of year 2000), Pharmacia and Upjohn Ltd (Kabiglobulin), The Laboratories, Belfast City Hospital and the

Blood Transfusion Services, Scotland (see p. 399 for addresses).

- HNIG is supplied in 250- and 750-mg single-dose vials.

- For more information on the latest published research on MMR: http://www.bmj.com
- For disease and vaccination information from the CDC (USA): http://www.cdc.gov/nip/publications/acip-list.htm
- From the John Hopkins University, Institute of Vaccine Safety: http://www.vaccine safety.edu/cc-mmr.htm
- Information on MMR for parents: http://www.medinfo.co.uk

Storage: Between 2 and 8 °C.

Table 22.5 Dosage of HNIG in measles.

Age (years)	Dose (mg)
To modify an attack:	
< 1	100
⩾ 1	250
To prevent an attack:	
< 1	250
1–2	500
⩾ 3	750

Chapter 23

Measles

A measles monovalent vaccine is no longer available in the UK in line with the Chief Medical Officer's advice that 'children should receive MMR vaccine and should not be given the separate component vaccines since there is no evidence that doing this has any benefits and it may even be harmful.'

The monovalent measles vaccine is retained here for the benefit of readers in those European countries where it is still available.

At the end of this chapter readers can find information on measles infection.

Contraindications to monovalent measles vaccine

Contraindications to monovalent measles vaccine are described under the MMR vaccine (see p. 88) with the addition of a history of severe hypersensitivity to kanamycin.

Possible side- and adverse effects

See MMR vaccine (pp. 88–90).

The vaccine

Monovalent freeze-dried preparation of live attenuated virus of the Schwarz strain, prepared on chick embryo cell cultures by the Institute Mérieux.

Administration

The vaccine requires reconstitution with diluent (0.5 mL) provided by the manufacturer. Once reconstituted, it should be used immediately or within 7–8 h. Alcohol should not be used, but if it is necessary for the skin to be cleaned prior to injection, the alcohol should be allowed to evaporate dry before the vaccine is given.

Adults and children over 12 months should be given 0.5 mL of the reconstituted vaccine by deep SC or IM injection. If given to a child under 12 months, a second dose of monovalent measles vaccine or MMR should be given at 15 months. The multidose vial can be adapted for mass vaccination programmes in developing countries with an IMOJET type injector.

After the first dose, seroconversion is 90–95% and immunity lasts for about 27 years—probably for life.

Indications

● Susceptible, nonimmunized adults or children exposed to measles should receive the vaccine within 72 h of exposure. An acceptable alternative for individuals in whom measles vaccine is contraindicated is to use HNIG (see p. 98). HNIG can prevent or modify measles infection if given within 6 days of exposure. HNIG should not be given with measles vaccine.

● Nonimmunized, susceptible adults or children with chronic conditions such as cystic fibrosis, congenital heart or kidney disease, failure to thrive, Down's syndrome, and those patients in residential or day care.

● Susceptible travellers abroad.

● Children whose parents refuse to allow vaccination with the rubella and/or mumps components of MMR vaccine, but will allow vaccination against measles.

● In the case of a measles epidemic where there is a decision to vaccinate children under 12 months, if MMR is not used. Such children should receive the MMR vaccine at the age of 15 months and over.

• MMR (therefore measles) vaccine is currently recommended for HIV-infected children or adults.

Vaccine availability (none in the UK)

ROUVAX (Aventis Pasteur), single-dose vial with syringe and diluent (0.5 mL). When freeze-dried, the vaccine is cream in colour, becoming yellowish after reconstitution.

Storage: Between 2° and 8°C. *Do not freeze diluent.* At these temperatures, the vaccine can be kept for 2 years. It is a stable vaccine for field work, where it can be stored for at least 4 months at 20–25 °C, 1 month at 37 °C and 5–6 days at 45 °C.

'Egg-free' measles vaccine (no longer available in the UK)

This is for use in cases of severe anaphylaxis to eggs, and where the physician wishes to use a measles vaccine that does not contain traces of egg proteins. TRIVIRATEN (Berna) is available in single-dose vials of lyophilized vaccine, with diluent in a syringe. The dose is 0.5 mL by SC injection. The reconstituted vaccine should be used within 1 h (8 h if refrigerated) after reconstitution.

Storage: Between 2° and 8 °C. *Do not freeze diluent.* Protect from light.

The future

A synthetic measles peptide vaccine is being developed at the London School of Hygiene and Tropical Medicine. The vaccine is still under development. Possible advantages over the live measles vaccine may be oral or nasal administration, and the fact that it can be given as early as 6 months of age because the vaccine is not recognized by maternal antibodies.

Measles infection

Measles is an acute, highly transmissible viral infection, has a worldwide distribution, and humans are the only reservoir. It is a single-stranded RNA virus with one antigenic type, classified as a morbillivirus. It is transmitted by direct contact with infectious droplets. The incubation period is 8–12 days from exposure to onset of symptoms and 14 days to appearance of the rash. Patients are contagious for 1–2 days before the onset of symptoms and for 3–5 days before the rash.

Clinical features include the pathognomonic Koplik spots, conjunctivitis, coryza, pharyngitis, fever and rash. Complications can occur in 1 in 15 cases of measles infection (see Table 22.1) and include otitis media (5%), chest infection (3–7%), febrile convulsions (1 in 200), encephalitis (1 in 1000–5000) and SSPE (4 in 100 000, and 18 in 100 000 in those under 1 year of age)—further information on SSPE can be found on p. 89. Complications are reported in the UK in 5–10% of cases. The fatality rate from measles is 1 in 2500–5000 cases. Measles killed a quarter of a million children in England and Wales during the twentieth century but such deaths in the UK are now rare.

Because many deaths from measles in young children are caused by bacterial pneumonia, consider co-amoxiclav for severe cases and/or in high-risk cases, e.g. a malnourished child.

Measles infection during pregnancy increases the risk of miscarriage, premature labour and low birthweight. Pregnant women are 6.4 times as likely to die of measles complications than non-pregnant women with measles. HNIG should be considered for unvaccinated/susceptible pregnant women in contact with measles (see p. 98).

Notification of measles began in England and Wales in 1940 and measles vaccine was introduced in 1968. This was associated with a dramatic reduction in notifications to the Office of Population Censuses and Surveys (OPCS) of cases and deaths from measles. Further improvement was seen when the MMR vaccine was introduced in 1988 (Table 23.1).

The introduction of the simple saliva test for detection of specific IgM for measles (rubella and mumps as well) has shown the diagnosis of measles infection to be wrong in most cases. In 1996, of the 5614 cases notified, 3328 were saliva tested and measles was confirmed in 63 (1.9%) of those tested

Table 23.1 Measles notifications and deaths in England and Wales.

Year	Notifications	Deaths
1940–67	160 000–800 000	(1940) 1000
1968	400 000	90
1970s	50 000–180 000	13
1985	97 400	10
1986	82 061	10
1987	42 165	6
1988	86 001	16
1989	26 222	3
1990	13 302	1
1991	9680	1
1992	10 268	2
1993	96 12	4
1994	16 375	1
1995	7447	1
1996	5614	0
1997	3692	3
1998	3728	3

Sources include PHLS Communicable Disease Surveillance Centre.

Table 23.2 Measles notifications and confirmed cases by saliva test in England and Wales.

Year	Measles cases notified (*n*)	Cases saliva was tested (*n*)	Measles cases confirmed by saliva test (% of those tested)
1996	5614	3328	63 (1.9)
1997	3692	2598	147 (5.7)
1998	3728	2308	43 (1.9)

Source: ONS, PHLS-CDSC, Enteric and Respiratory Virus Laboratory (ERVL).

(Table 23.2). Does this mean the UK is nearing elimination of measles? If it is not measles, what is it?

Studies have been investigating the causes of cases notified but not confirmed as measles and also 'vaccine failures'. A study in Finland [Davidkin I. *et al.* (1998) Aetiology of measles- and rubella-like illness in measles, mumps and rubella-vaccinated children. *J. Infect. Dis.* 178, 1567–70] found that the disease caused was mainly a result of infection with parvovirus, enteroviruses, adenoviruses, and human herpes virus 6 (HHV-6). Four per cent of children were found to have double infections. Other agents that may be responsible are cytomegalovirus, Epstein–Barr virus, group A streptococci and others. An appreciable number of 'imported' cases of confirmed measles are reported: 12 cases in 1994/95 and five cases in 1996.

In the early 1990s measles infected 42 million globally and killed 1.1 million children every year. Before the vaccine was introduced in the 1960s, it used to kill about 5.7 million a year and caused over 135 million cases a year. Malnutrition is an important contributory factor. Others are poor socioeconomic status, low immunization coverage, immunosuppression (including HIV and AIDS) and vitamin A deficiency. Administration of vitamin A (two doses in hospital and a third 4–6 weeks later) to children with vitamin A deficiency (e.g. with xerophthalmia) has been shown significantly to reduce morbidity and mortality; when given prophylactically, it reduces mortality.

According to the WHO, the number of measles cases in 1998 is estimated to have been 30 million worldwide with 888 000 measles-related deaths. In developing countries about 10% of all deaths in children under 5 years are measles related. In 1990, the World Summit for Children adopted a goal of vaccinating 90% of children by the year 2000. Despite this undertaking, global coverage actually declined from 79% in 1997 to 72% in 1998—16 countries reported coverage below 50% in 1998.

The WHO has put forward advice to health workers in developing countries with the aim of reducing the severity of measles. The basic principles of management according to the WHO are:

- admit severely ill children to hospital;
- anticipate complications in high-risk groups;
- give paracetamol if temperature > 39 °C;
- treat with high dose of vitamin A;
- provide nutritional support to all children;
- encourage breast-feeding;
- use antibiotics for clear indications only;
- give oral hydration solution for diarrhoea;
- treat eyes promptly to prevent blindness;
- treat multiple complications at the same time;
- monitor growth regularly.

Measles is a vaccine-preventable disease. Countries are encouraged to achieve and maintain a measles vaccine coverage that exceeds 95%. Only then can herd immunity be achieved.

- Disease and vaccine information from the CDC: http://www.cdc.gov/nip/publications/acip-list.htm. Measles is a notifiable disease in the UK.

Chapter 24

Mumps

A mumps monovalent vaccine is no longer available in the UK in line with the Chief Medical Officer's advice that 'children should receive MMR vaccine and should not be given the separate component vaccines since there is no evidence that doing this has any benefits and it may even be harmful.'

The monovalent mumps vaccine is retained here for the benefit of readers in those European countries where it is still available.

At the end of this section readers can find information on mumps infection.

Contraindications to monovalent mumps vaccine

These are described under the MMR vaccine (see p. 90).

Possible side- and adverse effects

See MMR vaccine (pp. 88–90).

The vaccine

Monovalent, live attenuated, virus vaccine, prepared in chick embryo cell culture from the Jeryl Lynn strain (so named after the daughter of Dr Maurice Hillman, who 'supplied' the virus to her father for culture).

The vaccine should be reconstituted with the diluent provided. Shake gently to mix and withdraw the entire vial content into a syringe. Use within 1 h of reconstitution. Protect from light.

Administration

● Adults and children over 12 months: the total volume of reconstituted vaccine (0.5 mL) injected SC, preferably into the outer aspect of the upper arm.

● It is not recommended for children under 12 months of age as persisting, passively acquired maternal mumps antibodies can interfere with the immune response to the vaccine.

● Seroconversion occurs in approximately 97% of susceptible children and 93% of susceptible adults.

● Duration of immunity is long-lasting, at least 14 years, and probably lifelong. There is no need to give boosters other than the second dose of MMR. Revaccination is only recommended if there is evidence that initial immunization was ineffective. If given to a person who already has naturally acquired or vaccine-induced immunity, it is not associated with adverse effects.

● The vaccine will not protect when given after exposure to mumps infection.

● Human normal immunoglobulin (HNIG) is not recommended for postexposure protection (there is no evidence that it is effective). Mumps-specific HNIG is no longer available in the UK.

Indications

● For unvaccinated children over 12 months of age whose parents refuse to allow immunization against measles and/or rubella, but will allow vaccination against mumps to be given.

● Susceptible children and adults (lack of documented mumps vaccination or infection, lack of serological evidence of immunity), particularly those approaching puberty.

● Susceptible travellers abroad.

● MMR (therefore mumps) vaccine is currently recommended for HIV-infected children.

Vaccine availability (none in the UK)

MUMPSVAX (Aventis Pasteur) available as a single-dose vial of lyophilized vaccine with an ampoule containing diluent.

Storage: Between 2 and 8 °C. *Do not freeze diluent.* Protect from light.

Mumps infection

Mumps is a generalized infection caused by the mumps virus, which is a paramyxovirus. 'To mump' is an old word meaning to look glum and weary, which patients with parotid swelling do.

Humans are the only reservoir of the virus, which is transmitted by direct contact with infectious drop-lets. The incubation period is 14–21 days and mumps is transmissible from 7 days prior to 9 days after the onset of parotid swelling. It lasts for 7–10 days.

Approximately one-third of infections do not cause parotid gland enlargement. Parotitis is usually accompanied by fever. The most serious aspects of mumps are the complications:

- epididymo-orchitis in as many as 25% of post-pubertal boys and men with clinical illness, but sterility rarely occurs. It is unilateral in 85% and appears as other signs settle;
- meningoencephalitis in 1 in 300–400 cases;
- pancreatitis;
- myocarditis;
- arthritis;
- thyroiditis;
- mastitis;
- oophoritis;
- renal involvement;
- hearing impairment in 1 in 25 cases;
- facial palsy, Guillian–Barré syndrome, transverse myelitis;
- miscarriage in pregnancy.

During the first trimester of pregnancy, it can increase the rate of miscarriage up to 27%. Epidemics of mumps have occurred at 3-yearly intervals in England and Wales.

Before the introduction of the MMR vaccine, mumps was the most common cause of viral meningitis in children, a common cause of permanent unilateral deafness at any age, and was responsible for about 1200 hospital admissions each year in England and Wales. Following the introduction of MMR, hospital admissions for mumps fell by 92% to a rate of 0.2 per 100 000 population per year.

Mumps was made a notifiable disease in the UK in October 1988 to coincide with the introduction of the MMR vaccine. There was a marked impact on the incidence of mumps notified to the Office of Population Censuses and Surveys (OPCS) following the introduction of the MMR vaccine, with a 79.4% drop in notifications during 1990 compared with 1989 figures. The 3-yearly epidemic cycle was also interrupted (Tables 24.1 and 24.2). On the other hand, the dramatic fall in the incidence of mumps as a consequence of vaccination in children increases the susceptibility in other unvaccinated people. A resurgence of mumps can be expected in students and the military.

Table 24.1 Notification of mumps infection in England and Wales.

Year	No. of cases notified
1989	20 713
1990	4277
1991	2924
1992	2412
1993	2153
1994	2494
1995	1936
1996	1747
1997	1914
1998	1587

Sources include ONS and PHLS-CDSC.

Table 24.2 Deaths as a result of mumps infection in England and Wales.

Year	Deaths
1962–81	4.7
1982–85	2.9
1986	4
1987	3
1988	2
1989	1
1990–96	0
1997	1
1998	2

Sources include ONS and PHLS-CDSC.

The success of the British campaign has been highlighted by the WHO [*Bulletin of the WHO* (1999) 77, 3–14]. Its report shows that the introduction of the MMR vaccine into the childhood immunization schedule in 1988 has resulted in an 88% reduction in the incidence of mumps in England and Wales. Mumps incidence fell to five cases per 100 000 population in 1993/1995, compared with 40 per 100 000 during 1983/1985. Furthermore, the number of hospital admissions fell by 92%.

Despite receiving MMR at approximately 15 months of age, up to 15% of 2- to 6-year-olds have no detectable antibodies, compared with 8% for measles and 10% for rubella. A second dose of MMR at school entry, introduced in October 1996, will reduce further the susceptibility to infection, but also will provide another opportunity to immunize the 8–12% who do not receive the first dose at 15 months.

It is recommended that the saliva test is always performed on all cases suspected of mumps infection. For information about this test see p. 98. Table 24.3 shows the results of the saliva tests in recent years.

● Disease and vaccine information from the CDC: http://www.cdc.gov/nip/publications/acip-list.htm.

Mumps is a notifiable disease in the UK.

Table 24.3 Mumps notifications and confirmed cases by saliva test in England and Wales.

Year	Mumps cases notified (*n*)	Cases saliva tested (*n*)	Mumps cases confirmed by saliva test (% of those tested)
1996	1747	967	101 (9.2)
1997	1914	1103	67 (6.1)
1998	1587	998	228 (22.8)

Source: ONS, PHLS-CDSC, Enteric and Respiratory Virus Laboratory (ERVL).

Chapter 25

Rubella

Contraindications to monovalent rubella vaccine

Contraindications are described under MMR vaccine (see p. 88) with the exception of anaphylactic hypersensitivity to hen eggs, which does not apply—the vaccine is not prepared on chick embryo cell cultures, but in human diploid cells.

Possible side- and adverse effects

See MMR vaccine (p. 90).

The vaccine

The rubella vaccine available in the UK contains the Wistar RA 27/3 strain grown in human diploid cells and comes with diluent.

Administration

Once reconstituted using the diluent provided, the monovalent vaccine should be used within 1 h. The dose for all ages is 0.5 mL given by SC or IM injection.

- Seroconversion occurs in 95–98% of vaccinees. True vaccine failure rate is estimated at less than 2% if the vaccine is stored and administered correctly.
- Vaccine-induced antibodies to rubella are detectable 18–20 or more years after immunization in the UK. Immunity for those who seroconvert is probably lifelong. On the other hand, the potential consequences of rubella vaccine failure are substantial (i.e. congenital rubella), therefore pregnant women should be screened early in the first trimester, irrespective of previous positive rubella antibody tests.
- The administration of rubella vaccine to a person with either vaccine-induced or naturally acquired immunity is not associated with an increased risk of adverse reactions
- It is not recommended for children under 12 months of age, as persisting, passively acquired maternal rubella antibodies can interfere with the immune response to the vaccine.
- The vaccine will not protect when given after exposure to rubella infection.
- Human normal immunoglobulin (HNIG) should be given to pregnant women in whom rubella infection has been confirmed by laboratory tests. It must be given as soon as possible after exposure at a dose of 750 mg IM. Such action could reduce the likelihood of clinical symptoms and possibly reduce the risk to the fetus. (For HNIG availability see p. 98.)
- Rubella vaccination should be avoided during pregnancy and 1 month before pregnancy. The current advice is that the risk of rubella-associated damage following inadvertent rubella vaccination in pregnancy, or shortly before, is low therefore termination of pregnancy should not be routinely recommended in these circumstances. The maximum theoretical risk of fetal damage following rubella vaccination in the critical period (1 week before and 1 month after conception) is estimated at 4.4%. In the cases of inadvertent rubella vaccination during pregnancy that continued to delivery, notified between 1981 and 1992, no child was born with defects attributable to congenital infection, although in four out of 14 infants rubella-specific IgM antibody was detected (similar findings in the USA). 1990 saw the lowest rate of termination because of rubella immunization in pregnancy, just five cases (738 in 1972).
- In the USA the maximal theoretical risk for the occurrence of congenital rubella when the vaccine was given within 3 months of pregnancy has been

estimated at 1.6%. This is based on data accumulated by the Centres for Disease Control and Prevention (CDC) from 226 susceptible women who received the current RA27/3 strain vaccine during the first trimester. Of the offspring, 2% had asymptomatic infection but none had congenital defects. Receipt of rubella vaccine in pregnancy is not therefore considered to be an indication for termination of the pregnancy.

• During the 1994 measles and rubella campaign (designed to help avert a predicted measles epidemic), nine girls aged 14–16 years were in-advertently vaccinated while pregnant (between 2 and 12 weeks)—their rubella status was unknown at the time of vaccination. The nine pregnancies resulted in eight live births and one intrauterine death (cord around baby's neck at delivery). All eight live babies were negative for rubella-specific IgM antibody at birth. Viral studies on the baby who died *in utero* were also negative.

• Since 1996, children in the UK have been receiving a second dose of the MMR vaccine at preschool age (around four and a half years of age).

• *Screening for rubella immunity.* In the USA, the recommendation is that patients who do not have a documented history of vaccination should be given the choice of serological test or vaccination. In the UK, the DoH recommends a different approach, whereby all women of childbearing age should be screened (serotested) for rubella antibody and immunized where necessary. Screening can be undertaken at every opportunity, such as at family planning, antenatal care, infertility clinics, and so on. Furthermore, it is recommended that women be screened at every pregnancy and on request when pregnancy is contemplated, irrespective of a previous positive rubella antibody result. It is important to note that apart from possible laboratory errors where a negative result is reported as positive, 25% of the small number of women infected during pregnancy had been reported to be rubella-immune in the past.

• Anti-D immunoglobulin, if required by a rhesus-negative, postnatal, patient who also requires rubella vaccine, could be given at the same time, although using a different site and a separate syringe (although it has been established that it does interfere with the antibody response to the vaccine

in 50% of the cases). Blood or plasma transfusion could also inhibit antibody response, therefore it is necessary to check antibody response 8 weeks after vaccination and/or transfusion.

• Nursing mothers immunized with live attenuated RA 27/3 strain rubella vaccine may transmit the virus via breast milk. In those babies with serological evidence of rubella, none showed clinical disease.

• Although some vaccinees shed small amounts of vaccine virus from the pharynx, such virus is not transmissible, therefore there is no need to defer immunization of the contacts of pregnant women.

• Rubella reinfection can occur in women with both natural and vaccine-induced antibody. When it occurs in pregnancy, the risk to the fetus cannot be calculated precisely, but it is considered to be low. The criteria for confirming a diagnosis of maternal rubella reinfection requires evidence of either two or more previous antibody-positive laboratory reports, or a documented history of rubella immunization followed by at least one antibody-positive report. Between 1990 and 1992, there were 37 women with confirmed rubella infection in pregnancy. Of these, nine were considered to have a confirmed or probable reinfection according to the above criteria. Eight of these women continued with their pregnancies and no evidence of fetal infection was found in the six infants tested (two were not followed up) [(1993) *Commun. Dis. Rep.* 30].

• An 'immune' result after routine antenatal testing does not preclude recent or current infection, and all pregnant women with suspected symptoms or exposure in the first 4 months of pregnancy should be offered diagnostic investigations.

• The decline in reports of congenital rubella has resulted in a higher proportion of cases associated with infection acquired abroad or occurring in women with a history of previous vaccination or infection (neither of which confers absolute protection). Immigrant women are more susceptible than the indigenous population, therefore targeting them for immunization may be appropriate.

• If the decline in MMR vaccine uptake seen in the last 3 years of the 1990s is not reversed and a high uptake not maintained, rubella could once again circulate among young children and ultimately among pregnant women.

Indications

- For all school-leaving boys and girls who have not previously received the rubella or MMR vaccine. A history of rubella should be ignored. Give the rubella or MMR vaccine with Td and oral polio.
- Nonpregnant women of childbearing age who are seronegative. They should avoid becoming pregnant for at least 1 month after vaccination.
- Postnatal patients who have been found to be seronegative at the antenatal clinics. Vaccination should take place in the postnatal ward or during the immediate postnatal period. The mother should be warned of the need to use adequate contraception for 1 month after vaccination.
- All healthcare staff, both male and female, who work in antenatal clinics, GP surgeries or anywhere else where they may come into contact with pregnant patients.
- MMR (therefore rubella) vaccine is currently recommended for HIV-infected children or adults in the absence of other contraindications.
- Children whose parents refuse to allow vaccination with the measles and/or mumps component of MMR vaccine, but will allow vaccination against rubella.
- A group of women who health professionals are well advised to target are Asian and Oriental women. Of the women giving birth to congenitally infected infants between 1987 and 1992, 24% were Asian or Oriental, of whom at least three (out of 22) acquired the infection abroad. Remember to target young immigrant women coming to the UK after school age. Forty per cent of children born with congenital rubella syndrome in the early 1990s were Asian.

Vaccine availability

Ervevax (SmithKline Beecham Pharmaceuticals). Available in a single-dose vial of freeze-dried vaccine with diluent. The reconstituted vaccine should be used immediately and not later than 1 h from reconstitution.

Storage. Between 2° and 8°C. *Do not freeze diluent.* Protect from light.

Rubella infection

Rubella is also known as German measles. The word German is probably derived from the word 'germane', meaning something akin to or very like something else. In this sense, German measles means something very like ordinary measles.

Rubella is a mild disease characterized by an erythematous, maculopapular, discreet rash (not always present), cervical lymphadenopathy, low-grade fever and transient polyarthralgia. Thrombocytopenia (7 in 3000) and encephalitis (1 in 6000) may follow infection, which in 25–50% of cases is asymptomatic.

Rubella has a worldwide distribution, with humans as the only reservoir. It is transmitted through direct or droplet contact from naso-pharyngeal secretions. The incubation period is 14–21 days and the infectivity period from 1 week before until 5–7 days after the onset of rash. The peak incidence of infection is in late winter and early spring.

The significance of rubella lies almost entirely in its ability to cause miscarriage, fetal malformation or intrauterine death if contracted by susceptible pregnant women—congenital rubella syndrome (CRS).

The risk of fetal damage from rubella infection is estimated at 90% in the first 10 weeks of pregnancy. It then declines to 10–20% by 16 weeks. In the second half (after the 17th week) of pregnancy, the risk of fetal damage is negligible (very rare). Susceptibility to rubella among pregnant women in the UK in 1994/95 was 2% in nulliparous and 1.2% in parous women.

Possible fetal defects are:
- cardiac—patent ductus arteriosus, atrial or ventricular septal defects, pulmonary artery stenosis;
- auditory—sensorineural deafness;
- ophthalmological—cataracts, glaucoma, microphthalmia, pigmentary retinopathy;
- neurological—mental retardation, meningo-encephalitis, microcephaly.

Other findings can be purpuric-like skin lesions, thrombocytopenia, jaundice, hepatomegaly, splenomegaly and growth retardation.

Infants with CRS can continue to shed virus in

nasopharyngeal secretions and urine for a year or more and therefore can transmit infection. Even in those infants not clinically affected at birth, the virus can persist in the lenses of the eyes and in the ears, leading to cataracts and progressive deafness.

Attempts at elimination of rubella in the UK, Europe and North America depend upon an ability to immunize most, and if possible all, young children of both sexes and, thus, create conditions of herd immunity. This should stop the rubella virus circulating and, thus, prevent nonimmune women acquiring the infection. This policy relies on sufficient numbers of children (over 90%) being immunized.

Preventing fetal infection and consequent CRS is the primary objective of rubella immunization. Rubella vaccination was introduced in the UK in 1970, primarily for schoolgirls aged 11–13 years. In October 1988, the MMR vaccine was introduced for all children, with primary immunization at 15 months. By 1992, the MMR vaccine uptake in England and Wales reached 92% among 2-year-olds, and has remained around 91–92%. Since 1996 an additional dose of MMR vaccine has been given to children at school age.

The high uptake of MMR vaccine has had a major impact on rubella susceptibility in children under 5 years old, with interruption of the epidemic cycle as well as the occurrence of congenital fetal infection. There were 200–300 babies born with CRS every year before the vaccine introduction in 1970, 75 cases between 1987 and 1989 and none between 1997 and 1999.

The rubella vaccine, which was introduced in the USA in 1967, was very effective in reducing the annual number of babies with CRS from an estimated 20 000 in 1964 to just 7 in 1983.

Susceptibility to rubella in children aged 5–16 years, targeted in the November 1994 UK measles and rubella campaign, has fallen from 15.7% to 3.4%. On the other hand, susceptibility among males aged 17–24 years (not included in the campaign) was about 16% in the mid-1990s and therefore a source of infection for susceptible women and others—it is expected to fall to 7% by the year 2000 when the cohorts vaccinated in the MMR campaign reach this age. The decline in MMR uptake seen in the late 1990s may reverse this success.

Rubella became a notifiable disease in the UK in October 1988 to coincide with the introduction of the MMR vaccine. There has been a dramatic reduction in rubella cases notified to the OPCS (Table 25.1) as well as a reduction in the number of CRS cases (Table 25.2).

Table 25.1 Number of notified rubella cases in the UK.

Year	No. of cases
1988	Not notifiable
1989	24 570
1990	11 491
1991	7174
1992	6212
1993	9724
1994	6326
1995	6196
1996	9081
1997	3260
1998	3208

	CRS (E, W, SC)	TOP (E, W) because of:		
		Disease	Contact	Vaccination
1990	12	10	3	5
1991	3	8	9	8
1992	7*	3	0	10
1993	3	11	2	9
1994	7	6	2	5
1995	1	3	2	6
1996	12	7	2	0
1997	0	0	2	4

Source: National Congenital Rubella Surveillance (NCRSU).
*Includes a set of triplets.

Table 25.2 Number of cases of congenital rubella syndrome (CRS) in England (E), Wales (W) and Scotland (SC), and terminations of pregnancy (TOP) because of rubella infection, contact or vaccination, in England (E) and Wales (W).

Year	Cases notified (n)	Cases saliva tested (n)	Rubella cases confirmed by saliva test (% of those tested)
1996	9081	4227	36 (0.9)
1997	3260	2037	27 (1.3)
1998	3208	2206	44 (2.0)

Table 25.3 Rubella notifications and confirmed cases by saliva test in England and Wales.

Rubella, like measles and mumps, should be confirmed by a saliva test. For information about this test see p. 98. Table 25.3 shows the results of the saliva tests in recent years.

Preventing fetal infection and CRS are the primary objectives of rubella immunization.
● Disease and vaccine information from the CDC: http:/www.cdc.gov/mp/publications/acip-list.htm.
Rubella is a notifiable disease in the UK.

Chapter 26

Meningococcal infection

Meningococcal C conjugate vaccine

Contraindications to vaccination

- Acute febrile illness.
- Severe reaction to a previously administered dose of the vaccine.
- Hypersensitivity to any components of the vaccine, including diphtheria toxoid (Meningitec—Wyeth, Menjugate—Chiron) and tetanus toxoid (Neis Vac-C—Baxter Hyland Immuno).
- Pregnancy, unless there is a significant risk of infection in the mother.

Possible side- and adverse effects

Local reactions

Redness (> 3 cm in 3–4% of infants and toddlers, 26–29% in older children), swelling, tenderness and pain are common but not usually clinically significant.

General reactions

Irritability in 50% of infants and 19% of toddlers. Pyrexia above 38.0 °C (rarely above 39.1 °C) in 2–4% of infants, 5% of toddlers and up to 2.5% of older children. Headaches in about 10–14% of older children. There is evidence that the younger the baby, the fewer the side-effects.

The vaccine

The meningococcal C conjugate vaccine (MenC) uses the same technology as with the Hib vaccine. In this case, the carrier protein, a nontoxic derivative of either diphtheria toxin CRM_{197} (Meningitec and Menjugate) or tetanus toxoid (NeisVac-C) is attached (conjugated) to the polysaccharide antigen formed from the coat of the bacterium. The vaccine is able to induce T-cell-dependent antibody response as well as immunological memory. It is therefore immunogenic in children under the age of 2 years. It selectively protects against group C disease.

Administration

- The vaccine is given by IM injection, in the anterolateral thigh in infants and deltoid in older children and adults. Patients with bleeding diathesis can receive the vaccine SC.
- The vaccine does not confer immunity to diphtheria (Menjugate, Meningitec) or tetanus (Neis-Vac-C).
- Immunization with MenC was introduced as part of the routine Childhood Immunization Programme in the UK in March 1999 and commenced in October 1999. In fact, the UK was the first country to introduce MenC. Infants under 4 months receive three doses of the vaccine at monthly intervals, starting at 2 months of age (together with DTP/Hib/polio vaccines). Babies aged 4–12 months receive two doses, while older children receive one dose of the vaccine (Table 26.1).

A second MenC vaccine, Menjugate (Chiron Vaccines, Germany), was licensed in the UK in March 2000, initially for the immunization of children over the age of 12 months (0.5 mL IM). The licence for infant indication was expected to follow. A third MenC vaccine NeisVac-C (Baxter Hyland Immuno) was licensed in August 2000 for children over the age of 12 months and adults. It will also be used in the school immunization programme.

Table 26.1 Administration specifications for meningococcal C conjugate vaccines.

Age	Dose (ml)	Route	Course	Booster
Under 4 months*	0.5	IM	At 2, 3 and 4 months (3 doses)	None
4–12 months*	0.5	IM	Two doses at monthly intervals	None
Over 12 months and adults*†	0.5	IM	One dose	None

*Meningitec
†Meningitec, Menjugate and Neisvac–C (2000)

The three available vaccines can be considered as interchangeable.
• In the UK a booster dose will not be recommended unless subsequent surveillance shows a booster dose to be required. Immunity is estimated to last for 20 years.
• If an infant still under 4 months of age presents (for the first time after 2 months of age) for MenC immunization, it should receive three doses of the MenC vaccine at monthly intervals, even if this takes the infant beyond his/her fourth month of age.
• Any infant presenting for the first time at 4–11 months of age should receive two doses of vaccine. If presenting at 1 year of age or older, the child should receive only one dose.
• An Item of Service fee is payable to GPs for MenC immunization. At 2, 3 and 4 months, fees are paid at A, A and B rate. Between 4 and 12 months fees A and B are paid, while immunization of older children attracts fee B (other than those immunized by the school services).
• Seroconversion: < 1 year is near to 100%; 12–24 months is 92%; 15–17 years is 97%. Protective serum bacteriocidal antibody is present in 1 in 8 people in the UK.
• Infants and older children who receive the MenC vaccine remain susceptible to infection by the other (B and A) serogroups of the organism.
• The 1999/2000 campaign in the UK aimed at immunizing students, school children and pre-school children, in parallel to MenC introduction in the Childhood Immunization Programme starting at 2 months of age.
• MenC should not be mixed with any other vaccine in the same syringe.
• For travellers to at-risk areas, the meningococcal plain polysaccharide vaccine should be given to cover the A serogroup, even if the MenC has been given before. Observe the following gap between the two vaccines:

(a) MenC given first: allow at least 2 weeks (ideally 1 month) before administering the plain polysaccharide A + C vaccine;
(b) plain polysaccharide A + C vaccine given first: allow 6 months before administering the MenC vaccine, except in the case of children under 5 years of age for whom a gap of at least 2 weeks (ideally 1 month) may be appropriate as they are not expected to have responded well to the earlier administration of the C component of the polysaccharide vaccine.
• MenC can be given to HIV-positive individuals in the absence of contraindications.
• If the success of Hib is repeated, we should expect MenC not only to eliminate disease caused by serogroup C organisms, but also to reduce carriage. By immunizing the age groups with the highest carriage rates we could create sufficient herd immunity to block transmission and thereby protect age groups that are not immunized. During the last six months of 2000 (7 months after the start of the vaccination campaign) there was a 90% reduction of cases of meningococcal C infection amongst 15–17 year olds, and a reduction of 82% among the under one year olds. The overall reduction across all age groups was 75%. It is estimated that 500 cases of meningococcal C infection were prevented and 50 deaths were avoided.

DoH—Use of meningococcal group C conjugate vaccine—key pharmaceutical/technical issues: http://www.doh.gov.uk/meningitis-vaccine/keypharm.htm.

Vaccine availability

• Meningitec (Wyeth Laboratories). Suspension in a single-dose vial, pack sizes of 1 and 10. Shake the vaccine in order to obtain a homogeneous white suspension. Supplied directly and free by the DoH's agents.

• Menjugate (Chiron Vaccines, Germany). It is supplied as lyophilized powder for injection and one vial and the adjuvant, aluminium hydroxide as a suspension for injection. Mix the contents of the two vials and gently shake to reconstitute the vaccine. It is available in single- and 10-dose vials.

• NeisVac-C (Baxter Hyland Immuno) suspension in a single-dose glass syringe. Pack size of 20. Shake well before use.

Storage: 2 to 8 °C. *Do not freeze.*

Meningococcal plain polysaccharide A + C vaccine

Contraindications to vaccination

• Acute febrile illness.
• Severe reaction to a previously administered dose of the vaccine.
• In children under the age of 2 months as they do not generally respond to the vaccine.
• Pregnancy, unless there is a significant risk of infection, in which case the importance of vaccination may outweigh the possible risk to the fetus.

Possible side- and adverse effects

Local reactions

Local reactions are swelling, redness and pain, lasting for 1–2 days in approximately 10% of vaccinees.

General reactions

General reactions are irritability, fever and rigors in the first 24–48 h and more commonly in children than in adults. Anaphylaxis is very rare.

The vaccine

An inactivated polysaccharide vaccine against *Neisseria meningitidis* serogroups A and C. Each 0.5-mL dose of reconstituted vaccine contains at least 50 µg of each purified bacterial capsular polysaccharide.

Administration

• Neither of the two vaccines available is effective against meningococcus group B, the strain most commonly found in the UK. Currently, no vaccine is marketed that will cover strain B.
• After a single injection, the earliest protective antibodies can appear is 5–7 days—important when travelling or attempting to control an epidemic (Tables 26.2 and 26.3). About 67% of children aged 2–3 years seroconvert, 85–93% in 3- to 9-year-olds, and 90% in adults.
• The vaccine may not induce an effective response in the immunosuppressed.
• Children under 18 months of age show poor response to the group C strain of the vaccine, while infants under 3 months of age show poor or no

Table 26.2 AC VAX (SmithKline Beecham).

Age	Dose (ml)	Route	Seroconversion (older children/adults)	Booster (age)	
				<5 years	>5 years
Adults and children from 2 months	0.5	Deep SC or IM	> 90% within 14–21 days	1–2 years	5 years

Table 26.3 Meningivac A + C (Aventis Pasteur MSD).

Age	Dose (ml)	Route	Seroconversion (older children/adults)	Booster
Adults and children from 18 months	0.5	Deep SC or IM	> 90% within 5–14 days	> 3 years

response to group A. In case of travel to areas where the risk of meningococcal meningitis A is high, such children should be vaccinated, but another dose of the vaccine should be given at the age of 18 months or 3 months afterwards, whichever is first (Meningivac A + C) or 1–2 years afterwards for those under 2 years of age (AC Vax). For the C strain, children should receive the MenC.

● The vaccines are available on NHS prescription.

Indications

● Routine vaccination of children against A and C strains is not recommended other than for travel to endemic areas. The conjugate C vaccine is now used in preference. Vaccination should be considered in children who are in high-risk groups for both strains A and C.

● Students have been recommended to receive the polysaccharide A + C vaccine while stocks of the conjugate C vaccine are not sufficient. They should receive later the conjugate C vaccine—allow at least 6 months in between the two vaccines to ensure a good response but may be given sooner in certain situations, such as in an outbreak, or a close contact of a recent case.

● Postsplenectomy or patients with functional asplenia should receive the vaccine before travelling to areas at risk.

● Close contacts of cases of meningococcal meningitis caused by group A or C should be given the vaccine in addition to chemoprophylaxis. It is ineffective in cases where the group B organism has caused the disease.

● In outbreaks of meningococcal disease caused by group A and/or C in schools, playgroups, colleges, universities, military camps, etc., immunization of contacts should be considered as well as chemoprophylaxis.

● It can be given to people who are HIV-positive. To access the DoH's current 'Questions & Answers' sheet for pharmacists connect onto the DoH's website: http://www.doh.gov.uk/meningitis-vaccine/keypharm.htm

● Travellers to endemic areas should receive vaccination. These areas are mainly countries in the 'meningitis belt' of Africa, running from Kenya in the east to Senegal in the west: Kenya, Uganda, Central African Republic, Cameroon, Nigeria, Ivory Coast, Liberia, northern parts of Sierra Leone, Gambia, Guinea, Togo, Benin, southern Senegal, Mali, Niger, Chad, Sudan and south-west Ethiopia (Fig. 26.1)—countries whose borders are between the Equator and latitude 15°N.

In addition to the above countries, immunization is advisable for travellers to Burundi, Tanzania and Zambia, reflecting a southwards extension of the high-risk areas. Most at risk are travellers staying for over 1 month and/or backpackers or those working/living with local people. The risk is highest in the Savannah in the dry season December/January to April–June. Travellers should receive the polysaccharide A + C vaccine even if they have received the conjugate C vaccine in the past, in order to cover the A strain.

Information concerning geographic areas for which immunization is recommended for travellers can be obtained on: http://www.cdc.gov/travel/

● Travellers to Mecca, Saudi Arabia, for the purpose of 'Umra', or pilgrimage, during the Haj season are recommended vaccination and certification as these are required (since 1988) by the Saudi Arabia authorities. The certificate of immunization needs to be issued not more than 3 years and not less than 10 days before arrival in Saudi Arabia. It should be on official doctor's or clinic paper and should show the type of vaccine given, date of administration, patient's date of birth, and should be signed by the individual who administered the vaccine. The Ministry of Health of Saudi Arabia issued new specific requirements in 2000. These are that:

(a) adults and children over 2 years of age should be given one dose of meninitis A and C vaccine;

(b) children between 3 months and 2 years of age should be given two doses of meningitis A and C vaccine with a 3-month interval between the two doses. In the UK, children within this age would have entered the National Programme of Immunization, which includes the conjugate meningococcal C (MenC) vaccine. The manufacturers advise a 1 month delay after completing the course of MenC before administering the polysaccharide A and C vaccine. It is important that such immunizations at this age are planned well in advance, as the time needed to complete both courses can be prolonged.

- In the spring of year 2000, a number of cases of serogroup W-135 were reported throughout Europe but also in other areas, in association with the Haj in Saudi Arabia. In the UK and immediately after the Haj, there were 13 cases, including four deaths; eight of the cases have been in pilgrims who had returned from the Haj, and five cases in close contacts. For a full report on reported cases in Europe see *Eurosurveillance Weekly* (http://www.eurosurv.org). The European countries use the bivalent A + C meningococcal vaccine, which does not protect against group W-135 infection. In the USA, the quadrivalent A/C/Y/W-135 vaccine is the only vaccine licensed. This vaccine (Mencevax—SmithKline Beecham Pharmaceuticals) is available in the UK, if required (see below). Serogroup W-135 Meningococcal Disease Among Travellers Returning from Saudi Arabia—USA: http://www.cdc.gov/epo/mmwr/preview/mmwrhtml/mm4916a2.htm.
- Sporadic outbreaks or small epidemics have been reported in Nigeria, Niger, Chad, Burkina Faso, Tanzania, Kenya, Burundi in Africa, Mongolia, Nepal, Pakistan, Bhutan and northern India (Delhi region). Particular care should be exercised when advising travellers to the area around Delhi, Nepal, Bhutan and Pakistan.
- In 1995, 33 047 and in 1996, 153 655 cases of cerebrospinal meningitis in Africa were reported to the WHO.

Vaccine availability

- AC Vax (SmithKline Beecham Pharmaceuticals), available in monodose and 10-dose vials, each with a separate ampoule of diluent. Ensure the vaccine pellet completely dissolves in the diluent.
- Meningivac A + C (Aventis Pasteur MSD) available as a single-dose vial of lyophilized vaccine with a syringe of diluent (0.5 mL).
Storage: Between 2 and 8 °C. *Do not freeze diluent.* Use within 1 h from reconstitution. Shake before use.

Quadrivalent Meningococcal Polysaccharide Vaccine (A/C/Y/W-135)

Contraindications and adverse effects

Contraindications are as for the plain polysaccharide A + C vaccine (above).

The vaccine

Each 0.5-mL dose of the A/C/Y/W-135 meningococcal polysaccharide vaccine Mencevax contains at least 50 µg each of meningococcal polysaccharides serogroups A, C, W_{135} and Y in a lyophilized form.

Administration

The vaccine should be administered by deep SC injection (Table 26.4). Reconstitute the vaccine by adding the entire contents of the diluent to the vaccine vial. Ensure the vaccine pellet completely dissolves in the diluent and use immediately, or within 1 hour from reconstitution.

Table 26.4 Administration specifications for A/C/Y/W-135 Mencevax vaccine (on 'named-patient' basis).

Age	Dose (ml)	Route
Adults and children from 2 months	0.5	Deep SC

Vaccine availability

'ACWY Vax' Meningococcal Polysaccharide (Mencevax) vaccine (SmithKline Beecham Pharmaceuticals) is currently an unlicensed vaccine. It is available on a 'named-patient' basis directly from the manufacturer. A letter containing the name(s) and date(s) of birth of the patient(s), the name and signature of the doctor wishing to prescribe, as well as the clinical indication should be faxed to the SmithKline Beecham Medical Department on 020 8913 4425. The vaccine can be dispatched to a hospital pharmacy if so requested.

It is available in a 1-dose vial, as well as 10- and 50-dose vials with diluent.

Storage: 2 to 8 °C.

Future meningococcal vaccines

Unconjugated polysaccharide vaccines are thought not to induce T-cell-independent immunity and therefore do not induce immunological memory. Without repeated immunization, antibodies to group A antigens decline within 8 years to levels found in nonimmunized adults. Considerable work has been undertaken on group A and C conjugate vaccines which, when available, are likely to replace the polysaccharide vaccine. Because group B polysaccharide does not elicit an adequate antibody response even in adults, a number of alternative vaccines have been developed in Cuba, Norway and elsewhere.

Cuba is believed to be the first country in the world to have licensed a meningitis B vaccine (Vamengoc-BC, developed by the state-run Finlay Institute) and conduct a successful mass immunization programme. It has shown 83% efficacy against serogroup B in Cuba and Brazil in teenagers when vaccinated with a purified total outer membrane protein (OMP) and high molecular weight OMP vaccine for meningitis B. However, this vaccine has shown low efficacy in children aged 3–23 months during outbreaks. The vaccine's immunogenicity was limited in studies in Iceland and Chile.

The Cuban vaccine seems to be strain-specific. It may therefore have a role in controlling epidemic disease in older children and adults when a single strain predominates. In Cuba there is only one strain of meningitis B and the vaccine has been tailored to this. In the UK there are more than a dozen strains (heterogenous organism) and scientists need to overcome this problem. In 1999, the USA authorities gave SmithKline Beecham Pharmaceuticals permission to licence the Cuban Finlay Institute meningitis B vaccine.

A vaccine based on OMP in vesicles has shown 57% efficacy in teenagers in Norway. A yet to be published study of a genetically engineered Dutch strain B OMP vaccine in 100 Gloucestershire children given at 2, 3 and 4 months, with a booster at 14 months, is reported to have shown 'promising results'.

Chiron announced in November 1999 that it will codevelop with the Norwegian Institutes of Public Health (NIPH) a combination vaccine against *Neisseria meningitidis* B and C. The vaccine will combine Chiron's Menjugate vaccine against meningococcus C disease with the NIPH's meningococcal B vaccine.

Meningococcal infections

Neisseria meningitidis, the causative organism, is a Gram-negative diplococcus with 13 antigenically distinct groups identified as A, B, C, X, Y, Z, W135, 29E, H, I, K, L and Z. These are further subdivided by serotype and sulphonamide sensitivity. The relative importance of the causative serogroups also varies with age—70% of cases under 5 years are attributable to group B in the UK, but this falls to 50% in those over 10 years of age [Williams & Burnie (1987) *Bacterial Meningitis*, pp. 93–115. Academic Press, London]. An effective vaccine against this strain remains elusive—its genome has only recently been sequenced.

Serogroups A, B, and C account for more than 90% of all cases. In developed countries, around 60% of cases are caused by group B and 40% by group C but in a few countries in Europe group C now predominates.

Of all (1459) isolates submitted to the British PHLS Meningococcal Reference Laboratory in 1995, group B strains accounted for 63%, group C for 32%, and other groups including A for 5%. [*PHLS Communicable Disease Report* (1997) 7—Review no. 4]. Generally in the UK, group B strain accounts for about half the cases, the group C contribution is about one-third, while group A (important for travellers) is approximately less than 1%. Other sero-groups usually account for about one-fifth of all cases (Table 26.5).

Meningococcal disease affects about 2500 children every year in the UK. In the year of July 1998 to June 1999 this figure was 2962, while in 1994/95 it was 1555. In 1998/99 in England and Wales, 1530 cases of group C, with 150 deaths were

Table 26.5 Laboratory confirmed cases, notifications and deaths caused by meningococcal infection: 1997–98 in England and Wales.

Meningococcal serogroup	1997 Laboratory confirmed cases (% of total)	Notifications (All)	Deaths (All)	1998 Laboratory confirmed cases (% of total)	Notifications (All)	Deaths (All)
Group A	2 (< 0.1)			0		
Group B	1157 (47.1)			1193 (49.2)		
Group C	813 (33.1)			811 (33.4)		
Other Groups	483 (19.7)			421 (17.4)		
Total	2455	2660	243	2425	2661	210

Source: ONS, Meningococcal Reference Unit (MRU), PHLS-CDSC

reported. Forty of the deaths occurred in young people, aged 15–19 years of age.

Infection is acquired by inhaling infected droplets of respiratory secretions from the nose and throat or by direct contact (especially kissing) with a patient or carrier. About one in four (25%) young adults may be carriers at any one time, while the rate in the general adult population is 1%. Meningococcal disease may occur, usually within days, after the new acquisition of *N. meningitidis* in the nasopharynx. The incubation period is from 1 to 10 days, most commonly less than 4 days.

Humans are the only known carrier of the meningococcus (in the upper respiratory tract) and act as a reservoir for transmission of the disease. Meningococcal disease shows marked seasonal vari-ation: peak level in the winter, low level in the summer. The winter seasonal onset of the disease usually coincides with that of influenza.

Meningococcal infections occur most frequently in children younger than 5 years, especially under 1 year, with peak incidence at 3–5 months. The onset can be insidious (particularly in young infants) or fulminant, as in the case of septicaemia. Headaches, nausea, vomiting, fever, joint aches, photophobia, drowsiness or confusion, raised anterior fontanelle tension in infants, stiff neck, coma and a petechial or purpuric rash that does not blanche are the classical signs of meningococcal disease. Kernig's sign (the patient's leg cannot be straightened because of hamstring spasm) may be present and/or the patient may be unable to touch the chin to the chest. Both these signs may

be absent in mild meningism. The tripod sign is a more subtle test; the patient cannot sit up from lying down without making a tripod with their two hands behind themselves on the bed. Although two in three adults have the classical triad of fever, meningism and change in mental status, all have at least one of these symptoms.

The absence of a petechial or purpuric rash (both haemorrhagic and hence nonblanching) does not preclude meningococcal infection. It is present in 80% of cases, while 13% have a maculopapular rash and 7% may have no rash. The classical signs of neck stiffness and a bulging fontanelle are absent in more than 50% of infants below 3 months of age. In this age, watch for irritability and seizures (the most common presenting features), lethargy and poor feeding.

Major sequelae of all types of bacterial meningitis include sensorineural hearing loss (10.5%), severe learning disability (4%), seizures (4.2%) and spasticity with or without paresis (3.5%). About 83.6% of patients recover with no detectable sequelae. The usual presentation is meningitis but in 15–20% of cases septicaemia predominates.

In Africa, rates of meningococcal disease recorded are more than $800/10^5$ with an overall mortality rate of 10%. For those with meningitis it is 7%, and for those with meningococcal septicaemia 20%.

The death rate in Europe is 6%. The majority of deaths occur within the first 24–48 h. About 150–200 deaths registered in England and Wales each year are attributed to meningococcal disease.

In recent years, group C disease has been on the

Table 26.6 Recommended dose of rifampicin chemoprophylaxis.

Age	Dose (mg) twice daily for 2 days
0–2 months	20 (1 mL syrup) or 5 mg/kg BW
3–11 months	40 (2 m 1 syrup) or 5 mg/kg BW
1–2 years	100 (5 mL syrup) or 10 mg/kg BW
3–4 years	150 (7.5 mL syrup) or 10 mg/kg BW
5–6 years	200 (10 mL syrup) or 10 mg/kg BW
7–12 years	300 (1 capsule) or 10 mg/kg BW
> 12 years/adults	600 (2 capsules) or 10 mg/kg BW
Contraindications to rifampicin	Allergy to rifampicin
	Liver disease (hepatotoxic). May inhibit drug metabolism such as anticonvulsants, anticoagulants (of which higher doses may be needed). Red dye in rifampicin excreted in urine, sputum and tears— may permanently stain contact lenses

BW, body weight.

increase, mainly because of its spread among teenagers and young adults, among whom the case fatality rates are high. Young adults aged 15–19 years are the second highest risk group (after infants under 1 year). Close contacts of patients with meningococcal disease are at increased risk of developing the infection. It is estimated that 50% of group C cases occur in teenagers over 14 years. Compared to group B disease, group C infection is thought to have a higher fatality rate.

• Any suspected meningococcal infection case should be immediately admitted to hospital and, if practicable, benzylpenicillin should be given before admission, by the GP, unless there is a history of anaphylactic reaction to penicillin. The IV route is preferable to the IM whenever this is possible. It comes in 600 mg powder in a vial. Unfortunately, no diluent is made available with this preparation, so ensure you have water for injection available for the emergency. The dose is as follows:

< 1 year: 300 mg;

1–9 years: 600 mg;

⩾ 10 years and adults: 1200 mg.

If previous penicillin anaphylaxis, cefotaxime: child 100 mg/kg BW; adult 2 g IV/IM.

Close contacts of cases of meningococcal infection should receive appropriate chemoprophylaxis, although they remain at risk. The recommended chemoprophylaxis is rifampicin, which, in the absence of contraindications, may be used in all age groups. It is available in 300-mg capsules and syrup containing 100 mg in 5 mL. The recom-

mended dosage is given in Table 26.6. All doses are given twice daily for 2 days.

Alternatives are ciprofloxacin as a single dose of 500 mg (not licensed for this purpose, contraindicated in pregnancy, in children and growing adolescents under 16 years of age, except where benefits exceed risks), and 250 mg ceftriaxone in adults (including pregnant women), 125 mg in children under 12 years, by IM injection (not licensed in the UK for this purpose).

• Once it is certain the strain in the index case is group C, a decision should be taken with the local consultant in communicable disease control on appropriate chemoprophylaxis and immunization. Occasionally group A disease occurs, when the meningococcal A + C vaccine may have to be used too. The quadrivalent 'ACWY Vax' meningococcal (Mencevax) vaccine is available from the manufacturer SmithKline Beecham on a 'named-patient' basis (see above). It contains serogroups A, C, W_{135} and Y. There is no need to give the vaccine to contacts of group B cases.

• Chemoprophylaxis is indicated for people who have been in close personal and prolonged contact with the index case during the previous 7 days (the average time it takes for the invasive disease to develop).

• Pregnant women in contact with a case of meningococcal disease may receive no chemoprophylaxis, or receive rifampicin, or ceftriaxone, or have a nasopharyngeal swab and receive rifampicin or ceftriaxone if the swab shows the same strain as the index case.

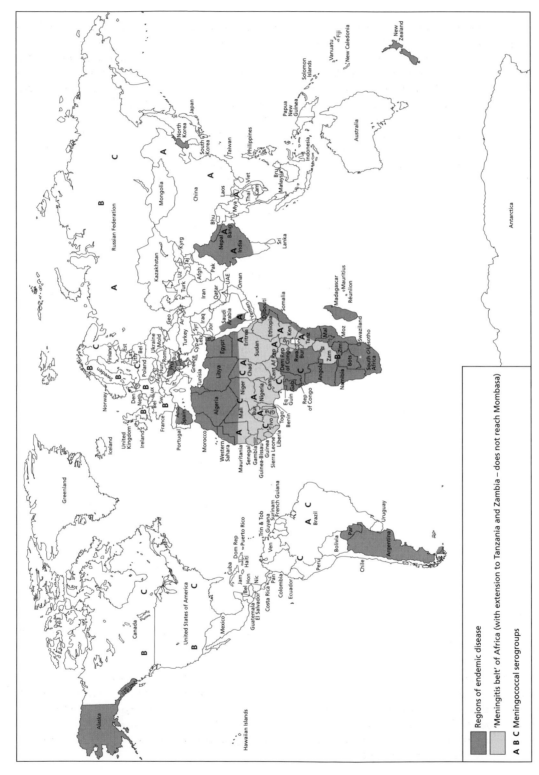

Fig. 26.1 Worldwide distribution of meningococcal disease and most prevalent serogroups. (This map generalizes available data.)

Epidemics occur worldwide, and in recent years we have seen such occurrences in the 'meningitis belt of Africa' (see Fig. 26.1) where the outbreaks are generally in the hot dry season, that is, in the first 4 months of the year. There have also been outbreaks in the Americas, Asia and even Europe. The reasons may be large population movements, overcrowded households and poor living conditions. Other contributory factors are acute respiratory infections, dry seasons and dust storms.

The WHO figures show that some 500 000 people a year suffer from meningitis with about 35 000 deaths. Meningococcal meningitis ends fatally in as many as 80% of untreated cases, and in up to 10% of those treated. About half a billion of the six billion people in the world carry *N. meningitidis* in the nasopharynx—lowest in young children and highest in adolescents and young adults. Carriage may last a long time in about 25% of carriers, be intermittent in 35%, and transient or infrequent in the remaining 40%. Rates of transmission are higher among populations living in confined areas (military recruits, dormitories), and they are exacerbated by factors such as cigarette smoking and upper respiratory infections. Meningococcal carriage is an immunizing process that can result in systemic protective antibody response.

The risk of invasive meningococcal disease in children is strongly influenced by parental smoking and unfavourable socioeconomic circumstances, according to new research [Kritz P., Bobak M. & Kritz B. (2000) Parental smoking, socioeconomic factors, and risk of invasive meningococcal disease in children: a population-based case-control study. *Archives of disease in Childhood* 83, 117–121]. The largest increase in risk—more than eightfold—was among children of parents who both smoked, with lower risk if only one parent smoked. They also identified several socioeconomic factors, notably maternal education, ownership of a car, non-crowded housing, ownership of a weekend cottage and spending time out of town, as being important in determining risk of the disease. The authors from the Czech Republic state that exposure to smoke causes direct damage to the nasopharyngeal mucosa.

Passive smoking is associated with increased risk of respiratory disease in young children.

Current UK guidance for healthcare workers coming into contact with patients advise that only those participating in mouth-to-mouth resuscitation of an affected patient should receive antibiotic prophylaxis. This guidance excludes some individuals whose exposure to the organism may have been considerable. It is good practice to advise chemoprophylaxis for healthcare workers exposed to airway secretions of patients with fulminant meningococcal disease. Furthermore, healthcare workers with clear exposure to oropharyngeal secretions in the first 24 h after presentation, who participate in endotracheal intubation, examining the oropharynx, and initial resuscitation of meningococcal patients, may be at an increased risk of acquiring the organism. Exposure to airway secretions may be reduced by wearing a mask for routine care, and a mask and visor for intubation and examination of the oropharynx. Healthcare workers who do not have direct contact with the airway secretions but handle the patient or are just in the same room are at negligible risk.

- For further information from the DoH on the Internet visit: http://www.doh.gov.uk/meningitis-vaccine/htm).
- National Meningitis Trust: Fern House, Bath Road, Stroud, Gloucestershire, GL5 3TJ. Tel.: 01453 768 000.
- Meningitis Research Foundation, 13 High Street, Thornbury, Bristol, BS12 2AE. Tel.: 01454 413 344 and 0845 6000 800. 24-h support line (calls charged at local rates): 0345 538 118. http://www.meningitis-trust.org.uk.
- Prevention and control of Meningococcal Disease: Recommendations of the Advisory Committee on Immunization Practices (ACIP): http://www.cdc.gov/epo/mmwr/preview/mmwrhtm/rr4907a1.htm.
- Geographic areas for which vaccination is recommended on: http://www.cdc.gov/travel/.
- Disease and vaccination information from the CDC: http://www.cdc.gov/nip/publications/acip-list.htm.

Meningococcal meningitis is a notifiable disease.

Chapter 27

Tuberculosis

Contraindications to bacillus Calmette–Guérin vaccination

- Acute febrile illness.
- Septic skin conditions or burns at the proposed vaccination site.
- Generalized eczema—may be given during remission or to an eczema-free arm. Immunization of children with active atopic dermatitis should be deferred until remission, as the vaccine may exacerbate this skin condition.
- Malignancy.
- Immunodeficiency by disease or treatment (including oral steroids) or deficiency (e.g. hypogammaglobulinaemia).
- AIDS patients. HIV-positive individuals, including infants born to HIV-positive mothers—such infants can be immunized provided they are found to be HIV-negative. In countries where the risk of tuberculosis is high, the WHO recommends that asymptomatic HIV-infected children should receive BCG at birth or shortly afterwards.
- Tuberculin-positive reactors (apart from Heaf grade 0 and 1 reactors, as well as Mantoux responders of 0–4 mm induration who can be regarded as tuberculin-negative).
- Within 3 weeks of administration of another live vaccine, but may be given simultaneously and at a different site.
- Pregnancy, particularly at early stages. However, where there is a significant risk of infection, the importance of vaccination may outweigh the possible risk to the fetus. If possible, postpone vaccination until after delivery.
- Patients who are receiving prophylactic doses of antituberculous drugs.
- The ID route must not be used for the percutaneous BCG vaccine.
- No further immunization should be given in the arm used for BCG vaccination for at least 3 months because of the risk of regional lymphadenitis.

Possible side- and adverse effects

Local reactions

A papule is expected at the site of the vaccination within 2–6 weeks. Over time, the papule flattens and widens with some scaling and crusting. A discharging ulcer may occur at the vaccination site, usually as a result either of inadvertent SC injection or excessive dose. If allowed to dry without irritation from clothes or dressings/plasters, the ulcer usually heals, leaving only a small scar. Rarely, an abscess may form.

At 6 weeks after BCG vaccination, there should be a scar of a diameter measuring at least 4 mm. Perform a post-BCG tuberculin test on any vaccinee who shows unsatisfactory or no reaction and, if negative, revaccinate. Healthcare personnel who show no satisfactory reaction after reimmunization need to reconsider their place of work.

Some individuals (especially of some racial groups) are more prone to keloid formation even when given at the recommended site for vaccination (middle of the upper arm at the insertion of the deltoid muscle). Sites higher than those recommended or elsewhere are associated with a higher risk of keloid formation.

Most of the local complications (about 70%) are abnormal primary complexes, either lesions at the injection site or, more commonly, suppurative lymphadenitis. Lesions at the injection site are either ulcers, subcutaneous abscesses, or necrotic lesions resulting from excessive delayed hypersensitivity reactions. Fewer than 1 in 1000 vaccinees develops significant local reactions.

General reactions

Occasionally general reactions include dizziness and vertigo. Adenitis (usually minor), with or without suppuration and discharge, is not uncommon. Very rarely lupoid skin reaction and anaphylaxis may occur.

The risk of BCG vaccine-disseminated infection is very rare indeed, estimated at less than 1 in 1 million, and suppurative adenitis 100–4300 in 100 000 vaccinees. The risk of post-BCG vaccination osteitis is put at 25 in 100 000.

The vaccine

Two BCG vaccines are available and they both contain a live attenuated strain derived from *Mycobacterium bovis* (known to protect against tuberculosis). The potency of the ID BCG vaccine is 10 times less than that of percutaneous BCG vaccine.

Administration

ID BCG vaccine (Table 27.1)

The ID BCG vaccine is available freeze-dried in rubber-capped vials with diluent in a separate ampoule. The vaccine suspension is prepared by adding 1 mL of diluent (sodium chloride injection BP) to the 10-dose vial and the 20-dose vial, and 5 mL to the 50-dose vial. Only the diluent supplied with the vial should be used (not water for injections BP). Do not shake or mix. Allow to stand for 1 min, and then draw into the syringe (a disposable tuberculin syringe and needle are ideal) twice to ensure homogeneity. It should then be protected from light and used within 4 h.

If alcohol is used to swab the skin and/or the rubber bung of the vial, it should be allowed to evaporate.

All children over the age of 3 months should be tuberculin tested before inoculation.

Percutaneous BCG vaccine

Percutaneous BCG vaccine is used only for neonates, infants and very young children (not recommended for children older than 5 years) as an alternative to the ID route. A modified Heaf gun is used. Such a multiple puncture apparatus is equipped with no less than 18–20 needles to give reliable penetration of the skin to a depth of 2 mm in mid-dermis, and is properly sterilized each time after use according to the manufacturer's instructions, or a new disposable head is used every time.

The same precautions about the use of alcohol on the skin and rubber bung of the vial apply as mentioned above.

Water (0.3 mL) for injection Ph. Eur. or sodium chloride injection BP is added to the 1 multidose vial, or the 5 multidose vial, or the 10 multidose vial and the suspension, without being shaken, is allowed to stand for 1 min. With a glass rod, platinum loop or spatula, or a syringe (with the needle removed) a small amount (about 0.1 mL) is transferred onto the skin and immediately punctured with the multiple puncture apparatus. The vaccine suspension should be protected from light and used within 4 h.

A tuberculin test must be carried out before BCG immunization in any child older than 3 months.

General

- The site of injection of both vaccines is the insertion of the deltoid muscle onto the humerus near the middle of the upper arm.
- Post-BCG active immunity is evident (Mantoux 5 mm or over—positive) after 8–14 weeks from vaccination.

Table 27.1 Administration specifications for ID BCG vaccine.

Age	Dose (ml)	Route
Adults and children over 3 months (prior tuberculin skin test mandatory)	0.10	Strictly ID
Infants under 3 months	0.05	Strictly ID

- Protection lasts for about 15 years. The WHO does not recommend reimmunization, as it is of unproven benefit and may possibly cause more severe local reactions.
- BCG is not usually recommended for individuals over the age of about 45 years. There is no clear age limit, so if the risk is high and the skin test negative, BCG can be given.
- If after a Heaf test the BCG vaccine has not been given for 3 months, the skin test should be repeated. Also, repeat earlier if the individual has been exposed to tuberculosis.
- Disposal of vaccine material should be by incineration at a temperature not less than 1100 °C at a registered waste disposal contractor.
- BCG has been used extensively since 1921, but its contribution to disease control has been limited for two reasons. First, its protective efficacy differs considerably around the world, from 0% to about 80%. Secondly, when it is effective it protects well from the serious, but usually noninfectious forms of primary tuberculosis, but gives little or no protection against the postprimary forms of the disease, because of endogenous reactivation or exogenous reinfection, which are responsible for transmission of the disease.
- The efficacy in British children is approximately 70–80% (80% observed in the British Medical Research Council trial).
- In a 15-year follow-up of a large randomized trial of BCG vaccine undertaken in Chingleput district, India, it was found that BCG offers no overall protection to adults, and only a low degree of protection (about 27%) against pulmonary tuberculosis among children [(1999) *Ind. J. Med. Res.* 110, 56–69].

Indications: in the UK, the DoH recommends BCG immunization for the following groups provided BCG immunization had not been carried out before (check for the characteristic scar), and they are tuberculin-negative (except babies under 3 months of age who may be immunized without prior skin testing):

At 'normal' risk:
(a) schoolchildren aged 10–14 years (the main target group, about 70% of which receives the vaccine);

(b) newly born babies and children whose parents request BCG immunization;
(c) adults who request BCG immunization.
At higher risk:
those at higher risk include,
(a) healthcare staff who may come into contact with infectious patients or material;
(b) veterinary and other staff;
(c) contacts of cases with active tuberculosis;
(d) immigrants from countries with high prevalence of tuberculosis, their children and their infants born subsequently in the UK;
(e) those intending to stay in Asia, Africa, Central or South America for more than 1 month.
About 50 000 neonates are vaccinated each year in these selective programmes.

- In addition to the above groups recommended by the DoH, other at-risk groups are people who live in poor and overcrowded conditions, vagrants (alcohol appears to predispose to tuberculosis) and IV drug users.
- Neonatally administered BCG is highly effective in preventing severe tuberculosis infection in children. The British Paediatric Association and DoH recommend vaccination of the following groups:

(a) babies of Asian and other immigrant families with high rates of tuberculosis;
(b) infants who reside in or travel to areas of high risk;
(c) infants with a family history of tuberculosis in the past 5 years;
(d) infants in contact with active pulmonary tuberculosis.

- Patients with tuberculosis infection should be tested for HIV after counselling. The BCG vaccine should not be given to HIV-positive individuals or infants born to HIV-positive mothers, unless the infant is subsequently confirmed to be HIV-negative.

Tuberculin testing and BCG

- Patients develop cell-mediated immunity 6–8 weeks after *M. tuberculosis* infection, which can be demonstrated using ID injection of purified tuberculin protein. This shows whether the patient

Table 27.2 Interpretation of tuberculin tests.

Heaf test grade	Mantoux response (mm)
0*	1 < 4*
1* (four or more indurated papules)	< 4*
2 (indurated rings, clear centre)	5–14
3 (uniform disc of induration)	15–19
4 (solid induration > 10 mm in diameter, sometimes with vesiculation or ulceration)	> 20

*Heaf grades 0 and 1 or Mantoux response of 0–4 mm induration are regarded as negative.

has ever come into contact with a *Mycobacterium* species and has developed sensitivity.

● Skin tests for tuberculosis now used in the UK are the Mantoux and Heaf tests. Induration around the site of injection at 48–72 h is the key outcome of the test. The DoH in its book *Immunization Against Infectious Disease* (HMSO, 1996) provides instructions on the performance and interpretation of tuberculin tests. Table 27.2 provides a guide to the interpretation of tuberculin tests.

● With the exception of infants up to the age of 3 months, all other individuals intended to receive the BCG vaccine should first be tuberculin skin tested and found to be negative.

● The test should not be carried out within 3 weeks of receiving live viral vaccines as they can suppress the test.

● Conditions that can suppress the reaction to tuberculin protein include viral infections (e.g. measles, rubella, glandular fever), sarcoidosis, Hodgkin's disease, immunosuppressing disease (including HIV) and corticosteroid therapy. If the skin test is negative, it should be repeated 2–3 weeks after clinical recovery.

● In individuals who have received the BCG vaccine, it is not possible to determine whether a positive tuberculin skin test is caused by myco-bacterial infection or by the BCG vaccination itself.

● Immunotherapy with BCG vaccine has been shown to be an effective treatment for superficial urine bladder carcinoma, interstitial cystitis, prostate cancers, malignant melanomas, small-cell lung cancers, visceral leishmaniasis and chronic hepatitis B infection.

● The intradermal BCG isoniazid-resistant vaccine is no longer available in the UK.

Vaccine availability

● Intradermal BCG vaccine BP (Medeva Pharma Ltd) available in 3-mL 10- and 20-dose vials (packs of 5 and 10) and 5-mL 50-dose vials (pack of 5) with appropriate diluent.

● Percutaneous BCG vaccine BP Percuvac (Medeva Pharma Ltd) available in 1, 5 and 10 multidose vials (pack of 10). Water for injection Ph. Eur. is included.

● Tuberculin purified protein derivative (PPD) BP (Medeva Pharma Ltd), available in 10, 100, 1000 (for Mantoux test) and 100 000 (for Heaf test) dilutions.

Any remaining vaccine after an immunization session should be discarded and incinerated or treated with a disinfectant such as strong hypo-chlorite solution. The appropriate disposal is by incineration at a temperature not less than 1100 °C at registered waste disposal contractors.

BCG vaccines are distributed to users by Farillon in England and Wales, and Unichem in Scotland, on behalf of the DoH. In Northern Ireland, they are distributed through the Hospital Pharmaceutical Service.

The BCG vaccines are not routinely available to GPs.

Storage. Between 2 and 8 °C. *Do not freeze diluent. Protect from light.*

Tuberculosis infection

Almost all cases of human tuberculosis are caused by *M. tuberculosis*, discovered by Robert Koch in 1882. It is an aerobic 'acid and alcohol-fast bacillus' (AAFB). The form of tuberculosis suffered by cattle, as a result of infection with *M. bovis*, is rarely seen nowadays because of tuberculosis eradication programmes in farming practice (transmitted via ingestion of infected raw milk).

The transmission of tuberculosis is by inhalation of droplets from a patient with active pulmonary or laryngeal tuberculosis, with cavities in the lungs, who coughs or sneezes; such droplets are sputum-positive for the bacillus. These droplets need to be small enough (1–2 μm across) to be suspended in the air, sometimes for hours. The bacteria are sensitive to UV light, which can kill them, while they grow best at a temperature of about 27 °C. Factors that affect person-to-person transmission include a genetic susceptibility to infection, the individual's health as well as poverty and overcrowding.

The incubation period from infection to development of a positive reaction to the tuberculin skin test is about 2–10 weeks. However, months or years may elapse from infection to development of disease and, in most instances, infection becomes dormant and never progresses to clinical disease. Only about 10% of infected people develop a clinical disease that can become infectious; 5% within 2 years from infection and another 5% at some point in their lifetime. Reactivated tuberculosis is the most common clinical manifestation. Most tuberculosis cases are 'pulmonary', while 15% present with the 'extra-pulmonary' form where any part of the body can be involved.

Tuberculosis caused by bacteria that are not resistant to a range of drugs is curable in virtually all cases. It kills over half of people who receive no treatment.

Factors that promote reactivation of tuberculosis are old age, malnourishment, concomitant pulmonary disease, alcoholism, diabetes mellitus, gastric resection, corticosteroid therapy and immunosuppression, including HIV disease. Risk groups for tuberculosis are patients with the above conditions, close contacts of smear-positive patients, immigrants and people from ethnic minorities, the homeless and those living in poor, overcrowded conditions, older white people, and travellers (especially long-term) to areas of high prevalence.

In the absence of HIV infection or other cause of immunosuppression, only about 10% of people infected by *M. tuberculosis* develop overt tuberculosis, indicating that the immune response to this pathogen is usually good. There is evidence that the immune response in those who do develop TB is not weak but wrongly regulated. T-lymphocytes mature along two pathways to form Th1 and Th2 cells, distinguished between them from the cytokinins (chemical messengers) they release. Glucocorticoids and dehydroepiandrosterone may be influencing regulation of Th1 and Th2. The protective immune response in tuberculosis is mediated by Th1 cells, which activate macrophages. A Th2 or a mixed Th1/Th2 response renders cells very sensitive to killing by the cytokinin tumour necrosis factor. This results in gross tissue destruction, which is characteristic of progressive tuberculosis.

The immune response may be programmed to respond in a certain way by past experience, including past exposure to the antigens of mycobacteria present in the environment. Stress and gluco-corticoids have a tendency to recruit T-cells towards Th2. At the same time they inhibit the ability of macrophages to limit the growth of *M. tuberculosis*. Vaccinating a person whose immune response is inappropriately programmed may therefore not lead to protection. This may explain why protection from BCG differs in different areas around the world.

In 1921, the French workers Albert Calmette and Camille Guérin of the Pasteur Institute produced the first human vaccine against tuberculosis. Half of the world's population has been injected with BCG vaccine since 1948, but its effectiveness differs, being more effective in some countries than in others. While in Britain it has been shown to be 70–80% effective, BCG has not been found to be so effective in some American trials and in India (27% effective against pulmonary tuberculosis among children—see above). Because of scepticism about its benefits, BCG is not routinely used

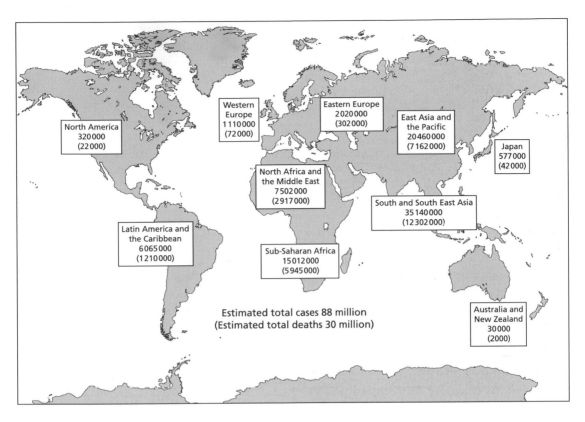

Fig. 27.1 Cumulative tuberculosis cases and (in parentheses) deaths for the decade of 1990–2000. Data from the World Health Organization (WHO) forecast [Dolin P.J., Raviglione M.C. & Kochi A. (1994) Global tuberculosis incidence and mortality during 1990–2000. *Bulletin of the WHO* 72(2), 213–20]. Adapted with permission from the Global Tuberculosis Programme of the WHO.

in the USA; however, its cheapness, safety and ability to stimulate a long-term immune response has made it the most widely used vaccine in the world. While BCG may not always protect against tuberculosis, it may suppress the development of some of the more serious complications, particularly in children. BCG protection tends to decrease with age.

About 1.8 billion people are infected with the tuberculosis bacillus, which may lie dormant for many years.

The WHO reports about 8 million new cases of tuberculosis every year; Asia 1.8 million, Africa 0.7 million, Latin America 0.2 million, Middle East 0.2 million, and industrialized countries 0.1 million. The largest number of cases and the largest increases have been reported in South-East Asia and western Pacific regions. Some of these increases have undoubtedly been the result of improved case finding and reporting. (Figs 27.1 and 27.2) More than 30 000 people in the Russian Federation leave prison infected with tuberculosis every year.

Tuberculosis is the leading infectious cause of death worldwide, with 98% of deaths occurring in the poorer developing countries. About 2 million people die each year from tuberculosis—the most common infective cause of death among adults. The WHO has calculated that unless urgent action is taken, the annual number of deaths could rise to 4 million by the year 2004.

The disease is most prevalent among poor people. Ninety eight per cent of annual deaths from tuberculosis and 95% of new cases are in developing countries. Incidence of the disease, which affects primarily men and women in their most productive years, age 15 to 54, is increasing worldwide.

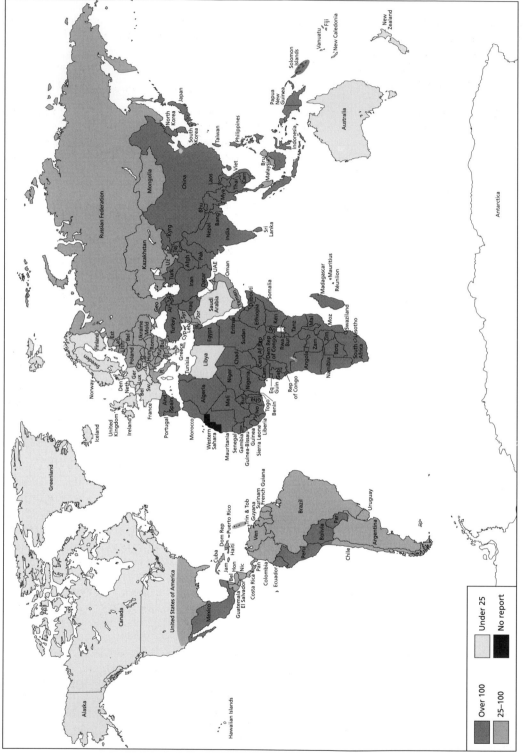

Fig. 27.2 Estimated prevalence of *Mycobacterium tuberculosis* per 100 000 population in the year 2000 by the WHO.

Early diagnosis and delivery of effective treatment are most important. Among those aged over 5 years, tuberculosis kills more people than malaria, diarrhoea, AIDS, leprosy and other diseases in the tropics put together. More than 250 000 children die of tuberculosis every year.

The risk of tuberculosis in long-term travellers to high-endemicity countries, even if not engaged in health care work, is substantial and of similar magnitude to the average risk for the local population. The risk of infection is 7.9 per 1000 person-months of travel for health care workers, and 2.8 per 1000 person-months of travel for non-health-care workers [Cobalens, F. *et al.* (2000) Risk of infection with *Mycobacterium tuberculosis* in travellers to areas of high tuberculosis endemicity. *The Lancet* **356**, 461–65]). Long-term travellers increase their individual risk.

Reactivation of tuberculosis is a common presentation. The infection does so in one-third of cases and causes the disease all over again. Elderly people, white or those from ethnic minorities, who were exposed to higher levels of tuberculosis when they were young, may present with symptoms that should alert us to consider the possibility of tuberculosis.

Improvement in living standards, pasteurization of milk, the development of a vaccine and antituberculous chemotherapy, have all contributed to a fall in the incidence of infection in the developed countries worldwide. On the other hand, the global incidence of tuberculosis is growing according to the WHO.

Recent research has shown that people who travel frequently by plane and those who visit countries where tuberculosis is endemic are at greater risk of contracting the disease than those who do not. Such travellers may wish to have a tuberculin test. Persons who show a positive skin test are unlikely to be reinfected website: http://www.who.int/h tb.htm).

Tuberculosis in the UK

The incidence of tuberculosis fell steadily from 1922, when official figures commenced, to 1987. In 1950, approximately 50 000 cases were reported. By 1953, BCG vaccination was in general use, and soon after effective chemotherapy became available. This accelerated the annual fall in the number of cases reported—about 10% drop every year. A significant number of people arrived in the UK in the 1960s and 1970s from the Indian subcontinent and West Africa. None the less, the incidence continued to fall at a lower rate of about 5% a year.

In the 1990s we witnessed small year-on-year increases in the number of tuberculosis notifications (Table 27.3). The incidence of tuberculosis in the UK is higher in the inner city areas, in ethnic groups that originate in high-risk countries or situations such as African refugees. White and Indian subcontinent ethnic groups each account for 38% of cases, and the Black African ethnic group for 13%. More than half the cases in 1998 were born outside the UK and very high rates of disease continue to be seen in non-White ethnic groups, particularly among those who have recently arrived from countries where the prevalence of tuberculosis is high.

The incidence of tuberculosis in England and Wales was 10.1 per 100 000 in 1993 and 10.9 per 100 000 in 1998. Although this is fairly stable, the concern is travel. Members of families from ethnic minorities often travel abroad, usually back to their homeland to stay with relatives. Under these circumstances, the chances of acquiring the TB infection increase considerably. In addition, mil-

Year	1987	1993	1994	1995	1996	1997	1998
Notifications	5087	5921	5591	5608	5654	5859	6087
Deaths	430	423	419	448	416	385	392

Table 27.3 Number of tuberculosis deaths and disease notifications in England and Wales.

Source: ONS, PHLS-CDSC.

lions of British people travel abroad to areas where the risk of acquiring the infection exists.

Tuberculosis in the USA

There are no recommendations in the USA for routine BCG vaccination for prevention of tuberculosis. Efforts for such control are directed towards early identification and treatment of infected persons, preventive therapy with isoniazid and prevention of transmission to others.

Between 1962 and 1985, the prevalence of tuberculosis was declining in the USA by an average of 6% each year, but since then there has been a steady climb, with an overall increase of 20% between 1985 and 1992. The largest annual increase, 9.4%, was recorded in 1990. In some urban centres, the rise has been more marked. Frieden *et al.* [(1993) *New Engl. J. Med.* 328, 521–6] reported a 132% increase in tuberculosis notifications between 1980 and 1990 in New York, mainly among the 25–44 years age group, immigrants and ethnic minorities. This has been attributed largely to the increase in tuberculosis among those infected with HIV or diagnosed as having AIDS, an increase in homelessness in inner city areas, increases in alcohol and IV drug use, and the recent emergence of multidrug-resistant strains of *M. tuberculosis*. These phenomena are also seen in Asia, Africa and the Pacific region.

New York City has seen in the past three times as many new cases of tuberculosis annually as any other city in the USA but, as a result of great efforts, New York City saw a 15% fall in the number of new cases reported in 1993—a drop from 3811 new cases in 1992 and 3235 in 1993.

Treatment

Short courses of rifampicin and isoniazid are highly effective. However, drug resistance to these drugs can develop. Prolonged treatment with less effective (and often more expensive) drugs is required. The DoH recommends that drug treatment of tuberculosis should be supervised by a hospital physician with a special interest in the disease. The WHO recommends 'directly observed treatment short course' (DOTS) in the commu-

nity. A new initiative (The Amsterdam Declaration-2000) by the WHO, the World Bank and 20 countries most burdened by tuberculosis, aims to increase coverage of these highly effective DOTS programmes from 25% of patients with tuberculosis to 70% in 5 years (by 2005) . Only 21% of tuberculosis patients globally were treated in DOTS programmes in 1998.

Drug-resistant tubercle bacilli have become an important problem in the fight against tuberculosis. Among patients who had not been treated previously, resistance to at least one drug worldwide is between 2 and 42% (median 9.9%). Some strains are resistant to multiple drugs (MDR TB): isoniazid (7.3%), streptomycin (6.5%), rifampicin (1.8%), ethambutol (1.0%)—England and Wales 1.1%. Among patients who had been treated before, a median of 36% of strains (range 5.3—100%) are resistant to any one of the four drugs, while MDR is 2.2% (range 0 –21%). In England and Wales it is 1.9% [(1998) *N. Engl. J. Med.* 338, 1641–9]. Data from the UK Mycobacterial Resistance Network show a 6.1% resistance to isoniazid and 1.3% MDR across the UK in 1998. Between 1993 and 1998, there was a 30.6% increase in drug resistant tuberculosis, according to the Mycobacterium Reference Laboratory.

The American Thoracic Society (ATS) and the US Centres for Disease Control and Prevention (CDC) issued new guidelines in April 2000, for the treatment of latent tuberculosis infection (LTBI). They call for targeted testing of high-risk populations and clinical monitoring of those with LTBI, at least at monthly intervals. This should be supplemented with patient education on adverse drug effects, and questioning about drug adherence. Recent CDC data show that only 60% of patients complete at least 6 months of drug therapy. Routine laboratory monitoring is not generally recommended but it should be a consideration for those with abnormal liver function tests and for those at risk of hepatic disease. With regard to treatment, the current choices include 9 months of isoniazid; 6 months of isoniazid; 2 months of rifampicin and pyrazinamide; or rifampicin for 4 months.

Tuberculosis and HIV

Worldwide, we are experiencing considerable problems with drug-resistant tuberculosis, breakdown of tuberculosis control programmes, mainly because of lack of funds, but above all we are witnessing a lethal partnership between tuberculosis and HIV. In 1990, 4.2% of tuberculosis cases were attributed to HIV infection. By 1998, 8–10% of all cases of tuberculosis worldwide were related to HIV infection, but the association is much more common in many African countries, often 20% or more.

HIV is increasingly contributing to increases in notifications in the UK. In one study in 1993, 7% of tuberculosis cases in London were among HIV-positive persons. However, a more recent study of 157 patients starting treatment for tuberculosis at an inner-city London hospital in 1996 and 1997 showed that 25% were coinfected with HIV; among them 44% Europeans, 49% Africans and 3% Asians [Marshall B. *et al.* (1999) HIV and TB in an inner London Hospital—a prospective anonymous sero-prevalence study. *J. Infection* 38, 162–6].

According to the WHO (http://www.who.int), tuberculosis is the leading cause of death among people who are also HIV-positive.

UK guidance on the prevention and control of transmission of HIV-related and drug-resistant tuberculosis

Current recommendations are that major HIV units should ideally site negative-pressure facilities and any single rooms for nursing HIV-infected patients with tuberculosis physically separated from the HIV ward. In all hospitals, patients with suspected or confirmed infectious tuberculosis (regardless of HIV status) should be admitted to single isolation rooms until they have provided three consecutive sputum specimens negative of acid-fast bacilli. Those with tuberculosis that is only 'potentially infectious' (sputum negative but culture positive or results of culture not yet known) need not necessarily be isolated unless they are likely to be close to patients with HIV infection.

Patients with pulmonary tuberculosis whose infection is likely to be or is confirmed as MDR TB should be required to stay in negative-pressure isolation rooms until negative sputum smears have been obtained on three occasions over 14 days or MDR TB has been excluded. Patients with MDR TB being cared for in rooms contiguous with a ward or wing housing patients with severely impaired immunity, such as patients with HIV infection, should be in negative-pressure isolation with automatically controlled air pressure and continuous automatic monitoring until they are no longer considered infectious. The guidance includes details on discontinuation of isolation, treatment, discharge, follow-up and re-admission of such patients.

WHO guidelines on tuberculosis and air travel

The WHO stresses that while transmission of tuberculosis during air travel has been documented, the risk is low. They recommend tracing and informing passengers and crew members who were on a commercial flight with an infectious person, if the flight, including ground delays (during which passengers remain on board the aircraft with little or no ventilation), lasts more than 8 hours. This is the procedure if less than 3 months have elapsed between the flight and notification of the case to the health authorities.

In addition, maximum efficiency air filters should be installed and properly maintained on all aircraft, and ground delays kept to a minimum. Anyone with infectious tuberculosis should postpone travel until they become noninfectious. Boarding can and should be denied to persons known to have infectious tuberculosis.

Modern aircraft use 'high efficiency particulate air' (HEPA) filters for recirculation of air in the cabin (see Air Travel on p. 294). Such filters should capture material as small as 0.3 µm. *Mycobacterium tuberculosis* is between 0.5 and 1.0 µm, so any tubercle bacilli should be removed from cabin air during the recirculation process. The potential risk from a person with infectious tuberculosis in an aircraft with recirculation should therefore be limited to droplet spread to a small number of seats in the immediate vicinity of the infected passenger (unless the infectious person is a flight attendant) before recirculation takes place.

Map

Government scientists are said to have found *M. avium paratuberculosis* (Map) in 129 out of 1000 pasteurized milk samples they tested in a survey and reported in the UK's lay press in 1999. Standard milk pasteurization until the 1960s in the UK involved heating the milk to 63 °C and maintaining it at that temperature for 30 min. This method was superseded by a high-temperature, short-time technique, where milk is heated to 72 °C for 15 s. Some of the big milk producers are said to have increased the time to 25 s because of such findings. This may not be long or high enough to eliminate wild strains of Map, which has been implicated in

chronic inflammatory disease of the bowel, such as Crohn's disease. (For further information see: Hermon-Taylor J. (1998) Commentary: the causation of Crohn's disease and treatment with antimicrobial drugs. *Ital. J. Gastro-enterol. Hepatol.* 30, 607–10.)

Disease and vaccine information from the CDC: http://www.cdc.gov/nip/publications/acip-list.htm.

Tuberculosis is a notifiable disease in the UK.

Table 27.4 Deaths of the famous from tuberculosis.

King Amenophis IV and his wife Nefertiti	1360 BC
Henry Purcell	1659–1695
Nicolo Paganini	1721–1764
Emily Bronte	1818–1848
Anne Bronte	1820–1849
Robert Louis Stevenson	1850–1894
Anton Chekhov	1860–1904
Edward Grieg	1843–1907
D.H. Lawrence	1885–1930
George Orwell	1903–1950
Igor Stravinski	1882–1971

Part 3

The Other Vaccines

Chapter 28

Anthrax

Contraindications to vaccination

- Acute febrile illness.
- Severe hypersensitivity to a previously administered dose of the vaccine.
- Severe hypersensitivity (anaphylactic reaction) to thiomersal contained in the vaccine.
- Pregnancy, unless the mother is at increased risk.

Possible side- and adverse effects

Local reactions

Local reactions include swelling and redness, which may occur for 24–48 h.

General reactions

General reactions are mild febrile reactions, regional lymphadenopathy, and urticaria may rarely develop.

The vaccine

The human anthrax vaccine contains alumprecipitated anthrax antigens and is the product of the growth of the Sterne strain of *Bacillus anthracis*, rendered sterile by filtration and preserved with thiomersal.

Administration (Table 28.1)

- The primary course consists of four doses of 0.5 mL of the vaccine, given IM, preferably into the deltoid muscle. The first three doses are given at intervals of 3 weeks, followed by a fourth dose 6 months later.
- A booster of 0.5 mL IM is given annually.
- Anthrax is almost entirely an occupational disease. Immunization is therefore recommended for workers at risk of exposure to infected hides, wool, hair, bristle, bone, bonemeal and carcasses.

Vaccine availability

The human anthrax vaccine is available from the Public Health Laboratory Services.

Storage: Between 2 and 8 °C. Shake well before use. *Avoid freezing.*

Anthrax infection

Anthrax is a rare acute bacterial infection caused by *B. anthracis*, a Gram-positive organism. Most commonly it affects the skin, rarely the lungs and/or the gastrointestinal tract. Humans become infected through occupational exposure to infected animal products such as meat, bone, hide, wool. The spores of the bacterium can also contaminate soil where they can survive for years.

The drug of choice is penicillin IV for 7 days. In

Table 28.1 Administration specifications for the anthrax vaccine.

Age	Dose (ml)	Route	Schedule	Booster
Children and adults	0.5	IM	0, 3, or 6 weeks, 6 months after dose 3 (4 doses)	Annually

case of penicillin allergy, tetracycline, chloramphenicol or erythromycin can be used.

Anthrax is rare in the UK because of carefully supervised sterilization and disinfecting of imported animal products.

It is one of the greatest infections of antiquity. The fifth and sixth plagues in the Bible book of *Exodus* may have been outbreaks of anthrax in cattle and humans, respectively. The 'Black Bane', a disease that swept through Europe in the 1600s causing large numbers of human and animal deaths, was probably anthrax. In 1876 anthrax became the first disease for which a microbial aetiology was established, and in 1881 the first bacterial disease for which a vaccine was available. Today, anthrax represents the single greatest biological warfare threat.

Surveillance for Adverse Events Associated with Anthrax Vaccination—US Department of Defence: http://www.cdc.gov/epo/mmwr/preview/mmwrhtml/mm4916a1.htm.

Anthrax is a notifiable disease.

Chapter 29

Cholera

The whole-cell parenteral cholera vaccine is no longer available in the UK. The WHO gives preference to the oral vaccines as 'the traditional parenteral cholera vaccine conveys an incomplete, unreliable protection of short duration and its use therefore is not recommended'.

Two vaccines are available in some countries in Europe and some Latin American countries. Where available, these vaccines are not meant for short-term travellers. The risk of contracting cholera is estimated to be around 1 in 100 000 travellers, with a case fatality rate of <2%. They should be considered for the frequent traveller or long-term resident in developing countries. For now, the main recipients are disaster relief workers and refugees in high-risk areas.

The oral cholera vaccines

None of the new oral vaccines are available in the UK. Where they are used, they are replacing the parenteral whole-cell vaccine because they are better tolerated and more immunogenic.

Inactivated oral cholera vaccine (Dukoral)

The oral, whole-cell, inactivated *Vibrio cholerae* 01 plus recombinant B-Subunit cholera toxin (WC/rBS), representing the classic Inaba and Ogawa serotypes and El Tor biotypes, was originally produced in Sweden and codeveloped with Smith-Kline Beecham Biologicals. In field trials, it was shown to have a protective efficacy of 86% when given in two doses (nothing should be eaten or drunk for 1 h before and after vaccination), 1 or 2 to 6 weeks apart, with the protection being evident within 7 days after the second dose. There is no lower age limit. No serious adverse reactions have been reported. The booster dose is so far undetermined, but is probably indicated after 1 year. After 3 years there was still a protective efficacy of 40%. The vaccine should be stored at 2 to 8 °C.

Dukoral is now licensed in Sweden and Norway. It is also available in several Latin American countries. Of important relevance to travellers is the fact that Dukoral produces antitoxin immunity that gives short-lived protection (about 52%) against enterotoxigenic *Escherichia coli* (ETEC) diarrhoea. The duration of protection for Dukoral is 78% after 1 year in subjects of over 5 years of age. It does not give protection against *V. cholerae* 0139 (Bengal) serogroup. As this is an inactivated vaccine the only relative contraindication is pregnancy.

Oral cholera vaccine (CVD 103-HgR)

The second emerging, new cholera vaccine is the live attenuated, lyophilized oral *V. cholerae* 01 from the classic Inaba 569B strain vaccine (CVD 103-HgR). It is highly immunogenic, providing protective efficacy of 62% against El Tor or Ogawa, to 100% against classical biotype *V. cholerae* 01 (but in Indonesia field trials <20%). No protection is given against *V. cholerae* 0139 (Bengal) serogroup. Protection starts 8 days after a single dose (one sachet mixed with unchlorinated water, stirred and ingested immediately—no food or beverages for 1 h before and after vaccination).

The duration of protection is 6 months (probably more) when a booster dose may be given if it is necessary. It should be stored at 2 to 8 °C. It is licensed in Switzerland (Orochol, Swiss Serum and Vaccine Institute, Berne) and Canada (Mutacol Berna Products). It is contraindicated in children under 2 years of age and in pregnancy because of lack of data, also in immunodeficient persons. Mild diarrhoea occurs in 2% of cases. It does not give protection against ETEC diarrhoea.

Cholera infection

Cholera is an acute intestinal infection caused by the enterotoxin-producing *V. cholerae*, a Gram-negative, comma-shaped rod that has two biotypes: the El Tor (now predominant) and the classic. Inaba and Ogawa are serotypes based on 0 (or somatic) antigenic determinants. During the last few years, a new biotype has emerged in the Indian subcontinent and South-East Asia. It is the *V. cholerae* 0139, otherwise called the 'Bengal' strain, with pandemic potential.

Cholera is predominantly a disease of countries with poor sanitation and poor standards of personal and food hygiene (Fig. 29.1). It is transmitted via the faecal–oral route by ingestion of contaminated water or food. Person-to-person transmission is rare. Adequate cooking of food and boiling of water eradicates the organism. Humans are the only known natural host.

The incubation period ranges from a few hours to 5 days. The illness is characterized by the sudden onset of painless, profuse, watery diarrhoea (up to 1 L/h in the first day), which leads to dehydration, metabolic acidosis, hypokalaemia and hypovolaemic shock. Rarely patients may become persistent carriers. Mild or asymptomatic infection occurs. In El Tor infection, there are 50 mild or asymptomatic cases for each symptomatic case. Persons with the blood group O or hypochlorhydria are more likely to become symptomatic and be more severely affected.

In epidemics in Latin America, raw fish and seafood products, vegetables that had been irrigated with raw waste water, and inadequate chlorination of drinking water supplies were identified as main sources and causes. Beware of ice, ice cream, locally grown vegetables, raw fish and shellfish, as well as any food or drink sold by street vendors.

In 1991 and 1992, over 500 000 cases of cholera were reported each year to the WHO, of which approximately 70% occurred in Latin America and nearly 30% in Africa. In 1994, 384 403 cholera cases were officially reported, with 10 692 deaths, corresponding to a case fatality rate of 2.8%. In 1997, nearly 150 000 cases from 65 countries were reported to the WHO.

Thirty-two cases of cholera were reported in England and Wales in 1996, 33 in 1997 and 48 in 1998, reflecting travel overseas—the last documented indigenous case was in 1893.

Some recent events have raised international awareness about cholera and its importance among the other emerging infections in the 1990s. Cholera was reintroduced into Latin America in 1991. Outbreaks then followed from Peru to Mexico that have affected more than a million people and have caused more than 10 000 deaths in the Americas. In India and Bangladesh, a new epidemic strain emerged in 1992, the *V. cholerae* 0139. This is distinct antigenically from *V. cholerae* 01. There is a lack of cross-immunity in endemic areas and vaccines against *V. cholerae* 01 have proved ineffective. In Africa, there was a massive outbreak of cholera among Rwandan refugees at Goma in 1994. In the autumn of 1997, a cholera epidemic spread from rural areas in Nyanza province to Kisumu, an urban centre in western Kenya and further to the adjacent Rift Valley province as well as south into Tanzania. At the end of the last millennium, cholera epidemics were sweeping through east African cities, mainly in slums where no clean water is available (Table 29.1).

Table 29.1 WHO 1997 figures for cholera in the Horn of Africa.

Country	Cases	Deaths
Djibouti	1991	41
Kenya	17 200	555
Somalia	6724	248
Uganda	600	1
Tanzanian mainland	34 449	1720
Zanzibar	570	122

Cholera is undoubtedly a disease of poverty and the risk to travellers, especially on a package holiday, is very small. The WHO no longer recommends cholera vaccination for travel to and from cholera endemic areas. However, border officials acting unofficially (and sometimes officially) may insist on a valid International Certificate of

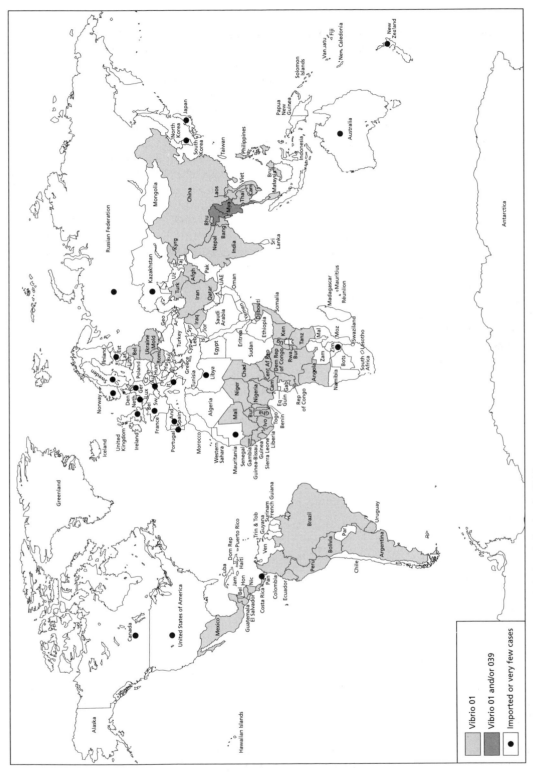

Fig. 29.1 Worldwide distribution of cholera infection in 1995.

Vibrio 01

Vibrio 01 and/or 039

• Imported or very few cases

139

Vaccination indicating cholera immunization within the previous 6 months. The traveller is advised to have an official letter from his GP stating that cholera vaccine is not indicated. In addition, he should carry a sterile syringe pack just in case the borderofficials proceed to vaccination. If the vaccine was to be available, it should be given at least 6 days prior to entry and recorded on an official travel document. Some officials may require proof of vaccination from people arriving from or travelling through endemic areas in the past 5 days. Mozambique is known to have required a cholera certificate from travellers. In some West African countries, a certificate may be requested when entering through a remote border post. Some cruise liners consider the vaccine a requirement for their crews to certain destinations.

Multidrug resistance of *V. cholerae* is now becoming a problem, not only for endemic areas/developing countries, but also for industrialized states bordering on epidemic or endemic areas. Such a problem arose, for example, during the Albanian cholera epidemic in 1994. There is now resistance of the organisms to cotrimoxazole, tetracycline, doxycycline, streptomycin and chloramphenicol, while cases may be susceptible to ciprofloxacin, gentamycin, tobramycin, ampi-

cillin, nalidixic acid and cefalotin. Treatment with ciprofloxacin, in a short course rather than a single dose, may be the best we can offer for multidrug-resistant cases or in the cases where microbiological antibiotic sensitivities are awaited or not available.

Taking antibiotics daily during a trip to prevent cholera may theoretically reduce the risk of infection, although antibiotics themselves can cause diarrhoea and increase the risk of the emergence of resistant strains. They could be considered in special cases:
● when cholera occurs in a closed group with a common exposure, such as on board a ship;
● for competitors in international sport events;
● for senior politicians on foreign visits.
Travellers can virtually avoid cholera by taking meticulous care in the selection of everything they consume during their trip. They should avoid any raw or undercooked seafood and tap water, including anything that is made from (e.g. ice cubes) or washed in it. Cholera vaccines, in the very few countries where they are available, offer additional safety.
● Disease and vaccine information from the CDC: http:www.cdc.gov/nip/publications/acip-list.htm
Cholera is a notifiable disease.

Chapter 30

Hepatitis A

Contraindications to vaccination

- Acute febrile illness.
- Severe reaction to a previously administered dose of hepatitis A vaccine.
- Severe hypersensitivity to any components of the vaccine such as aluminium hydroxide, phenoxyethanol and neomycin.
- Pregnancy and lactation, unless there is a definite risk of hepatitis A infection to the mother.
- Children under 1 year of age (Havrix, SmithKline Beecham) and 2 years (Vaqta, Aventis Pasteur MSD)—the vaccines are not licensed for this age.

Possible side- and adverse effects

Local reactions

Mild, transient soreness, redness and rarely induration can occur.

General reactions

Flu-like symptoms such as fever, malaise, fatigue, headaches, nausea, loss of appetite, diarrhoea, myalgia can occur, although not always necessarily related to the vaccine, lasting for 24–48 h. Mild, reversible elevation of liver enzymes has been reported.

The vaccine

There are three vaccines available in the UK.
- Havrix Monodose (SmithKline Beecham Pharmaceuticals) is formaldehyde-inactivated, prepared from the HM175 strain of hepatitis A virus (HAV) grown in human diploid cells. Each 1 mL of vaccine contains 1440 enzyme-linked immunosorbent assay (ELISA) units of HAV protein for adults, and 720 ELISA units in 0.5 mL for children.
- Avaxim (Aventis Pasteur MSD) is a formaldehyde-inactivated vaccine prepared from the GBM strain of HAV grown on human diploid cells. Each 0.5-mL adult dose contains 160 units of HAV antigen.
- Vaqta (Aventis Pasteur MSD) is a formaldehyde-inactivated vaccine. Each 1.0 mL contains 50 UL of HAV antigen for adults, and 25 U in 0.5 mL for children.

Administration

- The primary course of immunization for children and adults consists of one dose of the vaccine.
- Two to four weeks after the primary (first dose) immunization, the seroconversion rate is well over 95% (88% and over after 2 weeks), and provides anti-HAV antibodies for at least 1 year. Nearly all healthy, young people will have seroconverted by 1 month. It is prudent therefore to vaccinate travellers, where possible, at least 4 weeks before departure, in line with recommendations of the US Advisory Committee on Immunization Practices (ACIP) and the Centres for Disease Control (CDC).
- Peak antibody concentrations to HAV (anti-HAV) tend to be lower in immunocompromised patients than in healthy individuals.
- A reinforcing dose given at 6–18 months (depending on which vaccine is used) after the primary immunization will increase seroconversion to virtually 100% and extend immunity to at least 10 years (Table 30.1).
- The same vaccine used for the primary immun-

Table 30.1 Administration specifications for hepatitis A vaccine.

Age (yr)	Vaccine	Primary course Dose (ml)	Route	Reinforcing dose period (months)	Booster
1–15	Havrix Junior Monodose	0.5	IM	6–12	Every 10+ years
16 and over Adults	Havrix Monodose	1.0	IM	6–12	Every 10+ years
2–17	Vaqta Paediatric	0.5	IM	6–18	Every 10+ years
18 and over Adults	Vaqta Adult	1.0	IM	6–12	Every 10+ years
16 and over Adults	Avaxim	0.5	IM	6–12	Every 10+ years

ization should be used when administering the reinforcing dose. If this is not available or not known, any of the above hepatitis A vaccines can be used.

• The prefilled syringe should be shaken well before use and the vaccine given IM. In the case of patients with severe bleeding diathesis (i.e. patients with thrombocytopenia, haemophilia) in whom the SC route may be considered in the same dose—Avaxim is licensed for this purpose.

• The deltoid muscle is the recommended site of injection for all vaccines available. The gluteal region should not be used because vaccine efficacy may be reduced.

• The minimum protective antibody concentration is 20 mIU/mL. The levels of antibody produced by the primary course and reinforcing dose are similar to those seen after natural HAV infection and 100–300 times the level seen after a protective dose of human normal immunoglobulin (HNIG). Routine postvaccination serotesting is not indicated. Even if postvaccination antibodies are not detected, that person may still be protected (immunological memory).

• Adequate antibody titres may not be obtained after the primary course in patients on haemodialysis or with impaired immune system. Such patients may require additional doses of the vaccine if serotesting indicates a low response.

• The vaccine may be ineffective if given during the presence of hepatitis A infection (incubation time 15–50 days).

• There is evidence that active immunization gives good protection if administered shortly before, or immediately after exposure. Evidence from Alaska and Slovakia indicates that when hepatitis A vaccine is given to a defined population, it can interrupt an ongoing outbreak of the disease.

• Serotesting for anti-HAV IgG prior to vaccine administration is recommended in the UK for:

(a) those aged 50 years and over;

(b) individuals who were born and brought up in areas of high or intermediate HAV endemicity;

(c) persons who have a history of jaundice.

• Some individuals of ethnic minorities born in the UK may not be immune to HAV; older generations born overseas are more likely to be immune.

• Nonimmune travellers, for whom hepatitis A immunization is indicated, and who are expecting to travel in less than 2 weeks, should be given the first dose of vaccine as soon as possible—the HNIG is no longer recommended in the UK for travellers. If time before departure is short, the vaccine is still considered likely to prevent or at least modify the infection. There is some evidence of protection even when vaccine is given after exposure to HAV. The reinforcing dose of the vaccine should be given at the appropriate time on their return.

• HNIG given before departure (no longer recommended in the UK) cannot provide protection for travellers staying abroad for over 4–5 months. Hepatitis A immunization not only protects the traveller, but also removes the need to carry lyophilized immunoglobulin for repeat intramuscular doses in countries with no reliable source of refrigerated HNIG (needs to be kept at 2 to 25 °C and readers should note it is no longer available in the UK).

● All recipients of clotting factors derived from plasma pools should be tested for antibodies to hepatitis A and, if found to be susceptible, offered a course of the hepatitis A vaccine. In such cases, routine postvaccination seroconversion testing may not be necessary unless the recipient is known to be HIV-positive.

● The reinforcing dose is important for long-lasting protection, which is expected to last for at least 10 and maybe over 20 years.

● Hepatitis A immunization is recommended for those travelling to high-risk areas, that is all countries outside Western Europe, Scandinavia, North America, Japan, New Zealand and Australia, particularly those with poor sanitation and public hygiene.

Vaccine availability

● Havrix Monodose Vaccine and Havrix Junior Monodose Vaccine (SmithKline Beecham Pharmaceuticals) are available in single-dose prefilled syringes containing 0.5 mL (Junior Monodose) and 1 mL (Monodose for adults) suspension in packs of 1 and 10.

● Vaqta Adult and Vaqta Paediatric (Aventis Pasteur MSD) is available in single-dose prefilled syringes, containing 1.0 mL (Adult) and 0.5 mL (Paediatric) of the vaccine, in packs of 1 and 10 (Adult) and single pack (Paediatric).

● Avaxim (Aventis Pasteur MSD) is available in single-dose prefilled syringes containing 0.5 mL suspension in packs of 1 and 10.

Storage: Between 2 and 8 °C. *Do not freeze.* Do not dilute. Protect from light. Shake the syringe well immediately before use. Shelf-life of 2 years for Avaxim and 3 years for all other hepatitis A vaccines. Potency of the Vaqta preparations is not significantly affected after exposure to temperatures up to 28 °C for up to 3 months, however, this is not a storage recommendation.

Human normal immunoglobulin (HNIG)—hepatitis A

HNIG is prepared from the plasma of at least 1000 blood donors. Serum proteins are separated and concentrated so that the solution contains 100–800 g/L of human plasma protein, of which not less than 90% is IgG fraction.

There has been concern that failing prevalence of HAV infection in the UK general population might lead to HNIG not containing adequate levels of anti-HAV antibody. There have been no reported incidents where HNIG has failed to control outbreaks, and it is known that even low levels (10 mIU/mL) of neutralizing antibody are enough to prevent infection. None the less, there may soon be a need to use plasma from donors in high endemicity areas for the preparation of HNIG.

Each plasma donation, and the final product, is tested by validated procedures and found non-reactive for hepatitis B surface antigen and antibodies to HIV. The ethanol fractionation procedure used in manufacture has been shown to remove/inactivate viruses, including HIV. In addition, blood donors themselves are screened for HIV, hepatitis B and hepatitis C.

It is becoming more and more difficult to produce HNIG in the UK. The provision of clean water for drinking and washing, modern sewage disposal systems and greatly increased standards of personal hygiene have contributed to a reduction in the antibody to HAV among the population. It is thought that 40% of the population used to have antibodies following infection with HAV, while this has now dropped to possibly 10%.

HNIG may be given simultaneously with inactivated hepatitis A vaccine, at a different site. It does not appreciably affect the seroconversion rate, although the antibody levels achieved may be reduced.

When used for pre-exposure prophylaxis, it offers short-term protection (up to 4–5 months) against HAV infection, depending on the dose given. Travellers staying abroad in 'at-risk' areas for over 5 months have the option to carry lyophilized immunoglobulin for repeated intramuscular

Table 30.2 HNIG (with or without simultaneous administration of hepatitis A vaccine) could be considered in the following circumstances.

Travellers	To intermediate or high endemicity areas, who are nonimmune
Contacts	Of patients with hepatitis A infection. This group includes not only household contacts, but also household visitors—kissing contacts and those who have eaten food prepared by the patient. Contacts in child day-care centres in order to protect adult staff—children are likely to have a mild to subclinical infection
Outbreaks	In institutions, closed communities and schools (children—many of them would have been infected by the time HNIG is given—teachers and staff)
Newborn	Of a mother jaundiced at the time of delivery

doses, provided it can be stored during travel and kept at temperatures between 2 and 25 °C. This preparation is no longer available in the UK.

Administration of HNIG early in the incubation stage of hepatitis A infection can prevent or attenuate the illness, but may not prevent virus excretion. Postexposure HNIG prophylaxis is usually given to close contacts of patients with hepatitis A infection.

Before administration of HNIG, where practicable, serotesting for anti-HAV IgG may be worthwhile for those over 50 years of age, or for individuals who were born and brought up in areas of high or intermediate endemicity or who have a history of jaundice.

Active immunization by vaccination offers long-term immunity and is preferable. On the other hand, passive immunization with HNIG may be necessary in circumstances described in Table 30.2. It should be noted that HNIG does not guarantee protection against fatal, fulminant hepatitis A in travellers. None the less, when HNIG is given within 2 weeks after exposure to HAV, it is 85% effective in preventing symptomatic infection [American Academy of Paediatrics (2000) *Red Book* p. 282].

In the USA, HNIG is still recommended for children under 2 years of age, because the vaccine is licensed for this age group. Residual anti-HAV antibodies passively acquired from the mother may interfere with vaccine immunogenicity. These are likely to have disappeared by the end of the first year of life. In the UK, one of the vaccines (Havrix) is licensed from 1 year of age.

Contraindications to HNIG

- Severe reaction to a previously administered dose of HNIG.
- Within 3 weeks of administration of a live virus vaccine (e.g. measles, mumps, rubella, oral poliomyelitis), but not yellow fever, as HNIG obtained in the UK is unlikely to contain antibody to yellow fever virus. If HNIG has been administered first, the live virus vaccines (except yellow fever—see p. 231) should not normally be given for 3 months. This contraindication may be ignored in some circumstances, especially with regard to OPV (see pp. 44–81) when given to travellers with insufficient time for full immunization before they travel. The administration of hepatitis A vaccine should be considered instead.
- Pregnancy, unless there is a risk of hepatitis A infection to the mother. There is inadequate evidence of safety in pregnancy, but HNIG has been widely used for many years without apparent adverse consequence.

Possible side- and adverse effects

Local reactions

There may be short-term discomfort at the injection site.

General reactions

Very rarely anaphylactic reaction may occur, mainly in patients with hypoglobulinaemia who have antibodies to IgA, or in patients who have had atypical reaction to blood transfusion or treatment with plasma derivatives.

Table 30.3 Dosage of HNIG—hepatitis A.

Age	Low dose for 2 months travel	High dose for 3–5 months travel and for contacts
< 10 years	125 mg	250 mg
⩾ 10 years	250 mg	500 mg
All ages	0.02–0.04 mL/kg BW	0.06–1.12 mL/kg BW

Administration

HNIG is administered as a single dose strictly IM. It must not be given IV because it may cause severe generalized reaction. Recommendations and doses given in Table 30.3 refer to weight (mg) or volume (mL) of a 16% solution.

HNIG availability

- Kabiglobulin (Pharmacia & Upjohn Ltd, Milton Keynes, Bucks, UK) in 2- and 5-mL ampoules. Long term product problems—unlikely to be available on the market but still licensed in the UK.
- Gammabulin liquid (Baxter Hyland, Hyland-Immunodivision, Newbury, Berks, UK) available in 10-mL vials. No longer available for Hepatitis A prophylaxis.
- Blood Transfusion Service, Scotland.
- Public Health Laboratory, Belfast City Hospital.
- PHLS: for indications in Table 30.2. Not for travellers.

Storage: HNIG preparations should be stored at between 2 and 8 °C.

The lyophilized form of immunoglobulin is not available in the UK.

Hepatitis A infection

Hepatitis is one of the oldest diseases known to mankind. Hippocrates gave the first description of an epidemic of jaundice in the fifth century BC. The virus responsible for hepatitis A was identified in 1973 and was grown effectively in a laboratory in 1979. It is a single-strand ribonucleic acid (RNA) virus belonging to the family Picornaviradae. It replicates exclusively in the cytoplasm of the host cell. The virus is heat stable and will survive for up to a month at ambient tempera-

tures in the environment. It can be inactivated by ultraviolet radiation, autoclaving, sodium hypochlorite and iodine.

HAV causes a spectrum of infection ranging from silent or subclinical infection to clinical hepatitis with or without jaundice, to fulminant disease (0.1%) and death (mortality rate in excess of 2% in the over-60 age group, 1.1% in the 40–59, 0.3% in the 15–39 and 0.1% in those under 4 (including infants). Recovery from hepatitis A is gradual and may take 6–12 months.

Asymptomatic disease is common in children and the severity tends to increase with age. Symptomatic hepatitis is present in approximately 30% of infected children under 6 years old. Less than 10% of cases of acute HAV infection in children under the age of 6 years are associated with jaundice, increasing to 40–50% in the 6–14 age group, and 70–80% in adults.

Table 30.4 shows the UK DoH recommended risk groups for hepatitis A infection among nonimmune individuals. With regard to travellers, my personal opinion is that, irrespective of duration of stay, nonimmune travellers from countries of low HAV endemicity who visit high-endemicity regions (Africa, South and Central America, Mexico, Caribbean and south-east Asia) should be actively immunized before they travel.

Hepatitis A is transmitted by the faecal–oral route (over 95% of all cases—the rest via blood) and spread mainly by person-to-person contact. Common source outbreaks may occur as a result of faecal contamination of food and drinking or coastal water. Generally, HAV infection is related to poor housing conditions with poor hygiene and sanitary conditions, especially where sewage comes into contact with drinking water. The epidemiology of hepatitis A is closely related to the level of economic development in a country or region; as living standards improve, disease incidence and prevalence decline.

Table 30.4 UK DoH risk groups for hepatitis A infection among nonimmune individuals.

Travellers	To areas of intermediate or high endemicity therefore travellers to countries outside northern and western Europe, North America, Japan, New Zealand and Australia. This group includes frequent holiday and business travellers or those planning to stay for longer than 3 months, airline personnel, foreign aid workers, missionaries, professionals working abroad, immigrants visiting country of origin, armed forces and diplomatic personnel
Occupations	Any occupation that exposes an employee to the HAV. These may include: • sewerage workers • food handlers • healthcare workers such as doctors, nurses, laboratory workers, cleaning staff, laundry staff, food handlers • child day-care centre staff • staff of residential institutions for the mentally and physically handicapped • military personnel
Persons	• With chronic liver disease (hepatitis A more serious for them) • Recipients of clotting factors derived from plasma pool such as haemophiliacs (give the vaccine by SC injection—see text) • Homosexual men • Intravenous drug abusers, especially if living under conditions of poor hygiene • Family members and close contacts of patients infected with HAV • Carers of people whose personal hygiene may be poor • Those living in poor housing conditions with poor standards of hygiene and sanitation

Sewage has been implicated in outbreaks. A wide range of foods have been implicated in food-borne outbreaks, such as shellfish (from sewage-polluted waters eaten raw or poorly cooked), milk, orange juice, ice cubes in drinks, mineral water, salads, strawberries, bread, caviar, hamburgers, spaghetti, sandwiches, pasties, cream. An outbreak of infection can be imported from another country. An example is the outbreak of hepatitis A in Spain around Valencia, in the autumn of 1999, which was caused by consumption of previously frozen clams imported from Peru.

Sexual practice most likely to spread HAV is insertive anal intercourse. Oral–anal contact and digital–rectal intercourse are considered to be low-risk activities for the acquisition of infectious disease, and are practised widely by homosexual men. However, such practices expose them to pathogens that can be transmitted by the faecal–oral route, such as hepatitis A and HIV. Another significant risk factor is sharing contaminated needles. Casual contact, such as kissing or sharing of utensils, is not an efficient source of transmission.

Use of common toilets, such as in families or schools, can be a route of secondary transmission in outbreaks of hepatitis A. Person-to-person spread of HAV is well documented in child day-care centres. Between 16 and 30% of an inoculum of HAV placed onto the hands of volunteers was recovered from their hands after 4 hours. The virus was also recovered from clean surfaces after being touched by the volunteers' contaminated hands, confirming that transmission by fomites (objects) is possible [Mbithi J. *et al.* (1992) Survival of hepatitis A virus on human hands and its transfer on contact with animate and inanimate surfaces. *J. Clin. Microbiol.* 30, 757–63]. Sundkvist *et al.* [Sundkvist T. *et al.* (2000) *Commun. Dis. Public Health* 3, 60–2] describe an outbreak of 10 cases of hepatitis A in a public house where a barman had served drinks while incubating hepatitis A himself. In this outbreak, there were three potential routes of infection: food, contaminated surfaces in the toilets, and drinking glasses (sexual transmission was excluded).

Recipients of clotting factors derived from plasma pools have been reported to occasionally contract the disease. Transmission by blood transfusion is rare. On rare occasions, infection has been contracted from nonhuman primates living in captivity and having had previous contact with humans.

The disease is highly contagious because large numbers of viruses are excreted in the faeces dur-

Table 30.5 Markers of hepatitis A virus (HAV) infection.

Anti-HAV IgM	Indicates recent onset of HAV infection. Persists for about 12 weeks and occasionally for up to 2 years
Anti-HAV IgG	Indicates past infection or vaccination and immunity to HAV. It can be detected in serum, urine and saliva
Carrier state	Does not exist (but the diseases can relapse)

ing the incubation period of the disease (15–50 days, mean 30 days), especially during the last 2 weeks before the onset of illness, and for at least 1 week afterwards. Faecal excretion for several months has been reported in a few infected neonates and adults. In addition, the source of infection may not develop symptoms and, thus, may not be identified. The prodromal phase follows with pyrexia, headache, nausea, vomiting, fatigue, anorexia, abdominal discomfort, occasionally diarrhoea and arthralgia, lasting 2–7 days. The urine darkens and the stools may be noticeably pale.

The icteric phase then follows with jaundice first seen in the sclerae and later in the skin. The fever resolves, virus excretion ceases and the patient is no longer infectious. Jaundice begins to resolve within a few days but recovery can take several months. One in 10 children under 14 years and one in five young adults aged between 15 and 39 years are hospitalized for their symptoms. Patients do not become carriers of the virus. For markers of HAV infection, see Table 30.5.

A carrier state does not exist. On the other hand, the disease can relapse several months after the initial infection. Eventually, symptoms diminish over the course of 1–6 months and the prognosis in these cases is good. Patients with cholestatic hepatitis A have prolonged jaundice and pruritus. The alkaline phosphatase is raised.

In economically developing countries most infections occur by 5 years of age. In communities experiencing recurrent hepatitis A outbreaks, children aged 3–5 years seem to be important transmitters of infection. In developed countries, the main risk factors and sources of infection are large families, household crowding, poor education, inadequate human-waste disposal systems, mixing with other children in day-care centres, and children spending holidays in endemic countries.

There is no specific treatment and therefore therapy is supportive. Most patients show complete clinical and biochemical recovery within 3–6 months of the onset of the illness. Up to 20% of patients with acute hepatitis A will relapse 4–18 weeks after recovery. Other complications are fulminant hepatitis (up to 1%), cholestatic hepatitis and death (for mortality rates, please see above). Underlying liver disease may predispose to a more severe outcome. Lifelong immunity follows an attack.

In most developing countries, infection by HAV is usually acquired subclinically in childhood but, as standards of hygiene and sanitation improve, children escape early infection only to be infected clinically and in large numbers as young adults. The largest ever recorded outbreak of hepatitis A infection occurred in Shanghai, China in 1988 and was attributed to the consumption of sewage-contaminated clams. Clams are traditionally cooked in Shanghai by steaming or being soaked in boiling water, neither of which kills the HAV. More than 300 000 clinical cases of hepatitis A infection were reported, mostly in persons aged between 20 and 29 years. Before the outbreak, half of the population under 30 years were susceptible.

North-western Europe is an area of low endemicity. Spain, southern Italy, Turkey and Greece are considered to be areas of intermediate endemicity, while eastern and southern Mediterranean countries are areas of high endemicity (Fig. 30.1). Seroprevalence in those aged under 50 years in industrialized countries is <20%. The WHO recommends traveller immunization for Africa, Asia, Latin America and parts of eastern Europe.

While the number of notified hepatitis A cases in England and Wales fell by about 80% during 1990–98, the proportion accounted for by those with a history of travel abroad rose from 7.3 to 13.7% (the PHLS website—http://www.phls.co.uk). Table 30.6 shows the number of notifications of hepatitis A in

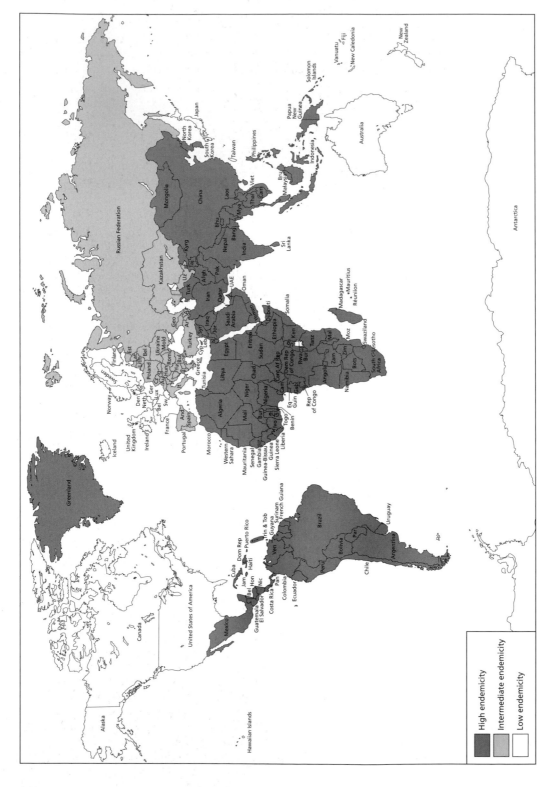

Fig. 30.1 Worldwide distribution of hepatitis A virus infection. (This map generalizes available data.)

High endemicity

Intermediate endemicity

Low endemicity

Table 30.6 Hepatitis A notifications and deaths in England and Wales.

Year	1988	1989	1990	1991	1992	1993	1994	1995	1996	1997	1998	1999*
Notifications	3190	5278	7316	7430	7856	4457	2715	2120	1339	1837	1515	1676
Deaths	12	6	14	14	11	13	10	9	5	2	0	4

Source: ONS, PHLS—Communicable Disease Surveillance Centre (CDSC).   *1999 Figures provisional

Table 30.7 Laboratory-confirmed cases and notifications of hepatitis A infection: 1996–98 England and Wales.

	History of travel			Number	
Year	Yes	No	No information	Notified	Laboratory-confirmed
1996	165	140	781	1339	1086
1997	185	133	992	1837	1310
1998	131	62	911	1515	1104

Source: ONS, PHLS-CDSC.

England and Wales. A marked increase in the numbers of HAV infections in young men (many known homosexuals) in London was being reported in 1997. In south-east England a total of 476 cases were reported in weeks 27–41 in 1997, compared with 249 cases in the same period of 1996. Table 30.7 shows the laboratory confirmed cases and notifications of hepatitis A infection, with history of travel, in England and Wales. The biggest destination 'contributors' are India and Pakistan.

About 1.4 million cases are reported worldwide every year. The true incidence, of course, is much higher and put at around 10 million cases every year. According to the WHO, in unprotected travellers hepatitis A is 1000 times more common than cholera, and 100 times more common than typhoid. It is the third most common disease after traveller's diarrhoea and malaria, and the most frequent vaccine-preventable disease in travellers.

In nonimmune travellers, the average incidence rate of HAV infection per month of stay in a high-risk area is 3 per 1000 (or one passenger on an average planeload of 333 unprotected tourists returning from an area at high-risk for hepatitis A), increasing to 20 per 1000 (1 in 50) for those nonimmune travellers facing unfavourable hygienic conditions, e.g. backpackers, aid workers in remote areas, missionaries per month of stay [Steffen & DuPont (1999) *Manual of Travel Medicine and Health*. B.C. Decker Inc, Hamilton, Ontario].

The risk of a British traveller contracting hepatitis A abroad has been calculated by Dr Ron Behrens and his coworkers (see Table 30.8).

Endemicity of hepatitis A mirrors economic development. In many newly developed and industrialized countries, the provision of clean water for drinking and washing, modern sewage disposal systems and greatly increased standards of personal hygiene have reduced HAV prevalence. Immunity to hepatitis A infection within these populations is therefore failing, leaving a growing pool of susceptible people. HAV continues to persist, putting nonimmune people at risk at a later age, when sequelae can be considerable.

At high risk are nonimmune travellers and workers in 'high-risk' jobs. Personal precautions are vital and include hand washing in clean water, avoidance of ice cubes added to drinks, the avoidance of tap water for drinking and cleaning teeth, and following the advice on food that says: 'boil it, cook it, peel it or forget it'. General hygiene and sanitary measures are the most important tools in preventing the spread of hepatitis A.

Indeed, the disease can be transmitted through contaminated water, ice, shellfish harvested from sewage-contaminated water, fruit, vegetables or any other uncooked food contaminated during handling. Cooked food is safe (the HAV is inactivated by boiling to 85 °C for at least 1 min), although it can be contaminated after cooking. Fruit that is peeled is not always safe—take the example where the producer injects his melons with (contaminated) water in order to increase their weight. Adequate chlorination of water in-

Destination	Risk relative to risk in France and Scandinavia
Country	
France	1
Scandinavia	1
Greece	4
Spain	5
Turkey	42
Mexico	612
Region	
European Union	3
Other countries in Europe	4
Eastern Europe	20
Australia and New Zealand	20
Middle East	85
Fast East	102
North Africa	110
Rest of Africa	235
South America and Caribbean	243
Indian Subcontinent **(Bangladesh, India, Pakistan, Nepal, Sri Lanka)**	
All travellers	1835
Age < 15 years	
• Visiting friends and relatives	2347
• Tourists or purpose of visit not known to researchers	295
Age > 15 years	
• Visiting friends and relatives	1083
• Tourists, or on business, or purpose of visit not known	1111

Table 30.8 Risk of a British traveller contracting hepatitis A relative to the risk in France and Scandinavia, which is taken to be 1 [adapted from Behrens *et al.* (1995) *Br. Med. J.* 311, 193].

activates HAV. Staying in a 5 star hotel, although recommended, cannot be considered as absolutely safe—the employees do not live in the hotel too!

Immigrants visiting their country of origin and their families are at greatest risk of contracting hepatitis A, especially children who may contract the disease, remain asymptomatic, but spread the disease to other children at school and people in the community on their return. Immunization is therefore recommended for children of immigrant parents, born in Western Europe (low endemicity) and visiting their parents' country of origin (high endemicity).

In the USA, the CDC and ACIP recommended in February 1999 that children living in states, counties and communities with consistently ele-

vated hepatitis A incidence should be routinely immunized. This includes areas where the average annual hepatitis A incidence rate during 1987–97 was at 20/100 000 population (approximately twice the national average). The 11 states covered under the recommendation are Arizona, Alaska, California, Idaho, Nevada, New Mexico, Oklahoma, Oregon, South Dakota, Utah and Washington.

Regular passive immunization (with HNIG) against HAV is an impracticable preventive measure. Active immunization by vaccination offers long-term immunity.

• Disease and vaccine information from the CDC: http://www.cdc.gov/nip/publications/acip-list.htm

Hepatitis A is a notifiable disease.

Chapter 31

Hepatitis A and typhoid combined vaccine

Contraindications to vaccination

- Acute febrile illness.
- Severe reaction to a previously administered dose of monovalent or combined hepatitis A and typhoid vaccine.
- Severe hypersensitivity to neomycin, phenoxyethanol or aluminium hydroxide.
- Persons under 15 years of age—the vaccine is not licensed for this age group.
- Pregnancy and lactation are relative contraindications. The combined vaccine should only be used when there is clear risk of hepatitis A and typhoid fever.

Possible side- and adverse effects

Local reactions

Mild transient soreness, redness and swelling may occur.

General reactions

Malaise, headaches and generalized aches occur in approximately 9% of vaccinees. Nausea (2.3%), itching (1.8%) and fever (1.1%). Some vaccinees may report vomiting and/or loss of appetite. Anaphylactic reaction is very rare.

The vaccine

The vaccine combines the existing inactivated hepatitis A (Havrix Monodose) and typhoid Vi antigen (Typherix) vaccines. Each 1 mL of vaccine contains 25 µg of the Vi capsular polysaccharide of *Salmonella typhi* and not less than 1440 ELISA units of inactivated hepatitis A viral antigen.

Administration

- The dose is 1 mL for adults and adolescents aged 15 years and older. It is administered IM as a single dose in the deltoid muscle (Table 31.1).
- In exceptional circumstances the vaccine may be administered by SC injection to patients with bleeding diathesis. Apply firm pressure to the injection site for at least 2 min. Do not rub.
- A reinforcing single dose of the monovalent hepatitis A vaccine is necessary between 6 and 12 months after the primary immunization with the combined hepatitis A and typhoid vaccine, in order to ensure long-term immunity. If more than 12 months have elapsed, do not restart but give the reinforcing dose of the monovalent hepatitis A vaccine.
- Boosters, when necessary, are given with the monovalent vaccines; at 3 years with the typhoid Vi polysaccharide vaccine and at 10 years with the monovalent inactivated hepatitis A vaccine.
- Two weeks after the primary immunization,

Table 31.1 Administration specifications for the combined hepatitis A and typhoid vaccine.

Age	Dose (ml)	Route	Primary immunization	Reinforcing dose	Boosters
15 years and over	1.0	IM	Single dose	Monovalent Hep A 6–12 months	With monovalent: Hep A 10+ years Typhoid Vi: 3 years

seroconversion is achieved in 90% (hepatitis A) and 97.5% (typhoid) of vaccinees. At 1 month, seropositivity is 99% (hepatitis A) and 96% (typhoid) in subjects aged 15–50 years.

• Immunosuppressed patients such as those with HIV, may not obtain adequate protective antibody from one dose of the combined hepatitis A and typhoid vaccine. They may require administration of additional doses of vaccine.

• It is not as yet known whether the combined vaccine will prevent hepatitis A infection in a patient already in the incubation period of the disease when vaccinated.

• The combined vaccine will not protect against paratyphoid fever as these bacteria do not posses the Vi antigen.

Vaccine availability

• Hepatyrix—combined inactivated hepatitis A and purified Vi polysaccharide typhoid vaccine (SmithKline Beecham) is available in single, glass, prefilled syringes, in packs of one and 10. Shake well before use to obtain a homogeneous, slightly opaque white suspension.

Storage: Between 2 and 8 °C. *Do not freeze.* Protect from light.

Chapter 32

Hepatitis B

Contraindications to vaccination

- Acute febrile illness.
- Severe reaction to a previously administered dose of hepatitis B recombinant yeast vaccine.
- Severe hypersensitivity to aluminium, thiomersal or yeast.
- Pregnancy, unless there is a risk of hepatitis B to the mother or she is in a high-risk category, in which case immunization should be considered.

Possible side- and adverse effects

Local reactions

Mild transient soreness, erythema, swelling and induration are evident in some vaccinees.

General reactions

There may be pyrexia (in the first 48 h) malaise, fatigue, headaches, nausea, dizziness, myalgia, vomiting, diarrhoea, hypotension, arthralgia, lymphadenopathy, abdominal pain, abnormal liver function tests, and rashes, including, rarely, erythema multiforme and urticaria. Some symptoms appear 1 week or more after injection. Neurological complications are very rare (paraesthesiae, neuropathy, neuritis, Guillain–Barré syndrome, optic neuritis, demyelinating disease), but no causal relationship with hepatitis B vaccine has been established.

Several reviews have been undertaken at the US Centres for Disease Control (CDS) and have not shown a scientific association between hepatitis B immunization and severe neurological adverse events such as optic neuritis and Guillain–Barré syndrome. As for sudden infant death syndrome

(SIDS), epidemiologically the CDS has noted a reduction of incidence, from 4800 in 1992 when the hepatitis B vaccine was introduced in the USA (coverage rate 8%), to 3000 in 1996 (coverage rate 82%).

During 1996, articles in the French popular press and television programmes raised concerns among the public that hepatitis B (HB) immunization may be linked to new cases or relapses of patients with multiple sclerosis. These concerns have led to a significant reduction in the uptake of hepatitis B vaccination in France. After examining the evidence, French authorities have concluded that there were no scientific data to support this link [*Weekly Epidemiological Record* (1997) 72, 149–56]. Under pressure from antivaccine groups and the media, on 1 October 1998, the French government suspended their recommendation for routine school-based vaccination of adolescents with hepatitis B vaccine, while continuing to support vaccination of all infants, adults at increased risk of infection and adolescents through their primary care physician. This decision was made despite advice to the contrary from the WHO and from a meeting of the Viral Hepatitis Prevention Board held in Geneva in September 1998. This meeting of experts reached a consensus that the data available, although limited, did not demonstrate a causal association between HB immunization and central nervous system demyelinating disease, including multiple sclerosis.

In British Columbia, Canada, HB vaccination has been offered annually to 11- to 12-year-old students (grade six) since October 1992. By September 1998, the programme participation averaged 92.3% and covered 267 412 grade six students. A total of 288 657 children attended grade six during 6.76 years before the introduction of HB immunization. Researchers examined the incidence of multiple sclerosis among those attending school during the vaccination period (289 651) of whom 92.3% were vaccinated (5 cases), and those in the prevaccination period (9 cases). These data provide no evidence for a relation between HB vaccination, at age 11–12 years and the subsequent onset of adolescent multiple sclerosis. The same researchers looked at the number of cases of postinfectious encephalomyelitis, because the French concerns included demyelinating diseases other than multiple sclerosis. They found no evidence for a link between HB vaccination and postinfectious encephalomyelitis [Sadovnick Dessa A. & Scheifele D. (2000) School-based hepatitis B vaccination programme and adolescent multiple sclerosis. *Lancet* 355, 549–50].

The National Institute of Public Health Surveillance in France conducted a risk–benefit analysis, weighing the risks of side-effects of the vaccine against the benefit of being protected against hepatitis B infection [(1999) *Viral Hepatitis*, (8, 1), December]. The results were firmly in favour of vaccination and the conclusions were that:

• the available data do not support any modification of vaccination strategies for infants or high-risk populations;
• under all scenarios considered, the risk of serious adverse events after HB vaccination, if real, appears very low, and less than 1 per 100 000 vaccinated;
• the balance for immunization of preteenagers, even in the worst-case scenario, is in favour of maintaining this strategy.

The use of more than a billion doses of hepatitis B vaccine since 1989 has shown an exceptional record of safety and efficacy.

The inactive ingredient aluminium hydroxide is probably responsible for the local side-effects. Some of the general side-effects such as urticaria may be a result of another inactive ingredient, thiomersal.

The vaccine

The recombinant vaccine is produced by yeast cells into which a plasmid containing the gene of the hepatitis B surface antigen (HBsAg) has been inserted. Each 1 mL of the vaccine contains 20 µg

(SmithKline Beecham Pharmaceuticals) or 10 µg (Aventis Pasteur MSD) of hepatitis B surface antigen (HBsAg) protein, adsorbed on aluminium hydroxide adjuvant. Thiomersal is used as a preservative.

Note: Vaccines that are preservative (thiomersal) free are already on the international market with the MERCK Recombivax HB and the SmithKline Beecham Engerix B Paediatric (already available in the USA).

The hepatitis B carrier plasma-derived vaccine is no longer available in the UK. Individuals immunized with this vaccine in the past can receive boosters using the recombinant yeast vaccine. This vaccine is predominant in the developing countries because it is cheaper to produce. The countries that produce/and use it (not always exclusively) are: China, Indonesia, Myanmar, North Korea, South Korea and Vietnam.

Plasma derived HB vaccine is prepared from purifying HBsAg particles from the plasma of HBsAg positive donors. It is then inactivated to insure that no infectious viral or other micro-organisms are present, and then aluminium adjuvented. Such a vaccine was available in the UK between 1982 and 1987.

The goal of the use of vaccine against hepatitis B is to provide life-long protection against the disease and the risk of persistent carriage, which may result in chronic liver disease, including primary hepatocellular carcinoma.

Administration (Table 32.1)

• The vaccine should be given by IM injection, except in patients with severe bleeding diathesis (i.e. haemophiliacs), in whom the SC route may be considered. The vaccine is not licensed for ID use and its administration by any route other than IM is not often associated with an effective antibody response. If the ID route is to be used, for example in patients with bleeding diathesis, the dose [of Engerix B suggested by the DoH (1996) *Immunization against Infectious Disease*, p. 103] is 1/10th of the normal dose, i.e. 0.1 mL—this is outside the product's licence. In patients with a bleeding diathesis, the risk of bleeding after IM injection of the vaccine can be minimized by administration

Table 32.1 Administration specifications for hepatitis B vaccine.

Age	Dose	Route	Primary immunization (all)	Booster*
0–12 years Engerix B Paediatric	10 μg (0.5 mL)	IM	0, 1, 6 months	5 years (single)
0–15 years HB-Vax II Paediatric	5 μg (0.5 mL)	IM		5 years (single)
Adults			(For both vaccines, all ages, accelerated course: 0, 1, 2, 12 months)	
Engerix B	20 μg (1 mL)	IM	(For Engerix B and in adults over 18 years: very accelerated course: 0, 7, 21 days plus booster at 12 months from first dose)	5 years (single)
HB-Vax II	10 μg (1 mL)			
Immunocompromised or dialysis patients: Engerix B	2 × 20 μg (2 mL)†IM			5 years (check antibody level periodically)
HB-Vax II 40	40 μg (1 mL)	IM		

* Single booster—for children and adults whose immune system is normal, the routine administration of boosters is not recommended in the UK. In those who continue to be at risk of infection, a single booster at 5 years after completion of the primary course is sufficient to retain immunity. However, patients at high risk, such as those on haemodialysis or the immunocompromised, should periodically have their anti-HBsAg titres checked and boosters given if they fall below 100 mIU/mL.

† This information is given in the DoH 1996 *Immunization against Infectious Disease*, p. 101—it is outside the vaccine's licence.

immediately after the patient receives replacement factor. Use a 23G (blue) or smaller needle, and apply direct pressure to the vaccination site for at least 2 min [American Academy of Paediatrics (2000) *Red Book*, p. 293].

● The deltoid muscle is the preferred site of injection in adults and the anterolateral thigh in infants and younger children. The gluteal region should not be used because vaccine efficacy may be reduced.

● Shake the prefilled syringe, and also the vial before withdrawing the vaccine suspension—once shaken, the vaccine is slightly opaque.

● The immunization regimen for both vaccines consists of three doses, the second dose at 1 month and the third at 6 months after the initial dose (0, 1 and 6 months). A study in Sicily [Mangione *et al.* (1995) *Lancet* 345, 1111–12] has confirmed it is not necessary to restart the schedule if delays between doses are longer than those recommended. Seroconversion in all ages occurs in ⩾ 96%.

● Where more rapid immunization is required

(i.e. following exposure to the virus, a newborn infant to an infected mother, 'imminent' travel, or travel to a very high endemicity area), the third dose may be given at 2 months after the initial dose, with a booster dose at 12 months (0, 1, 2 plus 12 months). Seroconversion is 15% after first dose, 89% after third, and 95.8% after the fourth (last) dose—data given for Engerix B.

● In some circumstances in adults over 18 years of age, where a more rapid induction of protection is required, e.g. persons travelling to areas of high endemicity and who commence a course of vaccination against hepatitis B one month prior to depart-ure, Engerix B is licensed to be given at 0, 7 and 21 days plus 12 months after the first dose. Sero-conversion occurs in 65.2% after 1 week, and in 76% 5 weeks following completion of the primary schedule (after the third dose), and 98.6% after the fourth (last) dose.

● The manufacturers make no suggestion that the two rapid schedules described above should be used routinely in the UK.

Table 32.2 Risk groups for hepatitis B—recommendations for pre-exposure immunization.

Healthcare workers	Doctors, dentists, midwives, nurses, ancillary staff working in dialysis, drug-dependency units, mental institutions
	Laboratory technicians, blood bank personnel
	Hospital workers at risk, e.g. laundry workers, theatre technicians
	Research workers at risk
	Medical/dental/nursing students
	Dental hygienists and nurses
	Acupuncturists
	On secondment to work in high-risk areas abroad
Patients	Requiring frequent blood transfusions, e.g. thalassaemia major, leukaemia
	Receiving blood products, e.g. haemophiliacs
	Haemodialysis, transplants
	Undergoing surgery that may require blood or blood products transfusion
	With severe learning disabilities (mentally handicapped) in institutions
	Infants of mothers who are chronic hepatitis B carriers or who had acute hepatitis B infection in pregnancy
Persons	Abusing drugs intravenously
	Homosexual and bisexual men
	Prostitutes (male and female), men or women with multiple sex contacts
	Long-term prisoners
	Carers, household and sexual contacts of patients with acute or chronic HBV infection
	Having tattoos, body piercing
	Immigrants from countries with high carrier rate
	Refugees from Eastern Europe, South-east Asia, Africa, South America and reception staff
	Families adopting children from high-risk areas (serotest children adopted from these areas)
Emergency services and high-risk workers	Selected police, ambulance, fire and rescue services
	Staff at custodial institutions
	Staff working with individuals with severe learning disabilities
	Morticians, embalmers
	Waste disposal workers
	Sewage plant workers
Travellers	Long-stay (over 1 month) in high-risk areas, e.g. aid workers, missionaries, healthcare workers, military personnel
	Likely to require medical/dental procedures in high-risk countries
	With sexual behaviour placing them at risk
	At higher risk of trauma
	Younger travellers, particularly aged 20–29 years
	Participants in adventure sports, e.g. climbers
	Motorcycle/car drivers or passengers in high-risk countries
	Likely to be injured, e.g. to be involved in fights
	Seafarers

- For serological markers of hepatitis B (see Table 32.9).
- For pre-exposure immunization for hepatitis B see Table 32.2.

Higher antibody level after primary vaccination increases the persistence of protective antibody titres. Initial antibody titres following a primary vaccination course correlate to the antibody response after the administration of a booster dose, therefore, the strength of immunological memory can be predicted from the initial antibody titres [Jilg W., Schmidt M.& Deinhardt F. (1990) Hepatitis B vaccination: strategy for booster doses in high risk population groups. In: *Progress in Hepatitis B Immunization* (Eds. Coursaget P., Tong M.J). pp. 419–27 John Libbey Eurotext Ltd].

- The duration of protection and the need for booster doses is not yet known precisely, but it is thought to be of the order of 5–10 years or more. Probably lifelong if the vaccinee responds with antibodies to HBsAg (anti-HBs) of ⩾ 100 mIU/mL. In most countries boosters are now considered unnecessary. On present evidence, in the UK a single booster dose 5 years after the primary course is recommended only for those who continue to be at risk of infection.

● *The European Consensus Group on Hepatitis B Immunity* published its recommendations in February 2000 [Are booster immunizations needed for lifelong hepatitis B immunity? *Lancet* 355, 561–5]. They point out that 'Post-vaccination immunological memory seems to last 15 years in immunocompetent individuals. To date there are no data to support the need for booster dose of HB vaccine in immunocompetent individuals who have responded to a primary course....Several countries and individuals have a policy of administering booster doses to certain groups. Boosters may be used to provide re-assurance of protective immunity against benign breakthrough infection. For immunocompromised patients, regular testing for anti-HBs, and a booster injection when the titre falls below 10 mIU/mL, is advised....All nonresponders to a primary course should continue to be studied.'

● Check antibody titres 2–4 months (in the USA 1–2 months) after completion of the primary course (the third dose), in persons whose subsequent clinical management depends on knowledge of their immune status, e.g. healthcare workers, patients on dialysis, with HIV infection, immunocompromised patients at risk of HB infection, regular sexual contacts of HBV carriers, infants born to HBsAg-positive mothers.

The primary course induces seroconversion in 99% of healthy young adults, with an adequate antibody response to the HBsAg (anti-HBs >100 mIU/mL) in more than 90%, and in more than 95% of infants, children and adolescents. The antibody levels decline logarithmically with time, and quantitative anti-HBs results vary significantly between laboratories. A peak antibody concentration of 100 mIU/mL can be expected to fall significantly, even below 10 mIU/mL in about 5 years, which has been the basis for scheduling the booster dose of hepatitis B vaccine. There is

nothing very special about the threshold of 10 mIU/mL, except that this is a level that routine tests can reliably detect.

● A good response to the vaccine (see Table 32.4) is considered to be the achievement of anti-HBs level ⩾100 mIU/mL. This may give lifelong protection from symptomatic infection. An inadequate response is a level of <10 mIU/mL—these individuals make up 5–15% of those immunized (see Table 32.4 later in the chapter). The minimum protective level is 10 mIU/mL (WHO).

● There is some evidence that protective immunity can still be present with antibody levels <100 mIU/mL. It has also been suggested that immunity may persist for many years, even after antibody levels have fallen to below 10 mIU/mL or even to undetectable levels. In this case, it is suggested that one can rely on the memory cells reacting in the event of infection, that is, rely on the 'immunological memory' (cell mediated) to protect. In the USA it is accepted that the 'immunological memory' remains intact for at least 12 years and confers protection against chronic hepatitis B virus (HBV) infection, even though hepatitis B surface antibody (anti-HBs) levels may become low or decline below detectable levels. For children and adults whose immune status is normal, booster doses of vaccine are not recommended in the USA, nor is serological testing to assess antibody levels necessary. For haemodialysis patients in the USA a booster dose of vaccine is recommended when the anti-HBs level is less than 10 mIU/mL.

● The current advice in the UK is that individuals who remain at high risk of exposure to HBV should have their antibody level determined periodically. If the anti-HBs level falls below 100 mIU/mL, the need for a booster dose should be considered (unless they are HBsAg-positive, i.e. carriers).

● The administration of the vaccine to individuals known to be hepatitis B surface antigen-, or antibody-positive is unnecessary as they are carriers and immune. Inadvertent vaccination would merely boost antibody levels.

● The vaccine is ineffective when given to patients with acute hepatitis B during the incubation period.

● The vaccine may be given to HIV-positive individuals.

- The recombinant yeast hepatitis B vaccine may be given simultaneously with all other vaccines and immunoglobulins, but a different syringe and site should be used.
- This vaccine cannot cause liver cancer as it contains only purified surface antigen.
- Recipients of this vaccine can donate blood starting 48 h but best 1 week after a dose. A weak positive HBsAg reaction in blood donors has been reported 1–3 days after vaccination.
- Hepatitis B vaccine protects also against hepatitis delta (δ) as the latter only occurs in individuals infected with hepatitis B virus (see p. 337). This defective virus is unable to replicate without the simultaneous replication of HBV. Over 15 million chronic carriers of HBV are thought to be super-infected with the hepatitis δ virus, leading to a more severe form of hepatitis.
- *Nonimmunized contacts* of patients with acute hepatitis B should be passively immunized with hepatitis B immunoglobulin (HBIG) (see p. 161) and vaccinated simultaneously and at a different site.
- *Acute exposure* to infected blood should be treated by passive immunization with HBIG and active immunization with hepatitis B vaccine or a booster dose if previously immunized, unless known to have adequate protection level (>100 mIU/mL) of antibodies to the HBs antigen.
- The DoH recommends that all patients who are on dialysis, or who are approaching the need for dialysis, should be immunized against the hepatitis B virus (I would recommend that we also immunize them against Hepatitis A). Historically, it has been difficult effectively to immunize these patients against HB because there is a high non-response rate to vaccine in patients with renal impairment. Larger doses of the vaccine are necessary—at least double the normal dose (2 × 20 μg of Engerix B). A special formulation of the Aventis Pasteur MSD vaccine (HB-Vax II 40) has been licensed for this purpose and for immuno-suppressed patients (four times the normal dose).
- *Perinatal transmission* occurs when a mother who is positive for hepatitis B surface antigen infects her infant at birth. These babies have a 95% chance of becoming chronic HB carriers by the age of

6 months. Around 85% of infants born to mothers positive also to hepatitis B e antigen (HBeAg) become infected; such babies are more likely to become persistently infected than babies born to HbeAg-negative carriers. The most likely explanation is that HBeAg can cross the human placenta from mother to fetus.

The aim of immunoprophylaxis shortly after birth is to prevent perinatal transmission. The efficacy of HBIG is put at 50–90%, and that of the vaccine at 75–90%, while combined passive and active prophylaxis is well over 90%. The proposed action to be taken is as follows:

1 Infants born to mothers who are HbsAg-positive (carriers) are at greatest risk and best protected by being vaccinated (10 μg, SmithKline Beecham Pharmaceuticals; 5 μg, Aventis Pasteur MSD) at birth or as soon as possible thereafter, preferably within 12 h or a maximum of 48 h. At the same time, HBIG (200 IU) should be given in a different syringe and at a different site, if the mother is HBeAg-positive or the e markers are not known. HBIG need not be given if the mother is known to be anti-HBe-positive. The course of vaccination should be continued according to the accelerated schedule 0, 1, 2 and 12 months. One to three months after completion of vaccination, these infants should be serotested for HBsAg (identifies those infants that become clinically infected carriers) and anti-HBs (indicates response to the vaccine—see serological markers, Table 32.9 on p. 165). If the anti-HBs titre is less than 10 mIU/mL and the infant is HBsAg-negative, give three additional doses of vaccine at 0, 1 and 6 months and test for anti-HBs 1 month after the third dose. Alternatively, serotest 1 month after each of these three additional doses to determine whether subsequent doses are needed. If the anti-HBs titre after the initial course is between 10 and 99 mIU/mL give a booster 6 months later.

2 Infants born to mothers who had acute hepatitis B in pregnancy should receive four paediatric doses of hepatitis B vaccine at birth, 1, 2 and 12 months of age (the accelerated course), and seroconversion should be checked 1–3 months after completion of the administration of the fourth dose of the vaccine. This will indicate

response to the vaccine (there is a failure rate of 5–10%), and will also allow identification of those infants that are infected so that they can be referred for assessment and further management. HBIG (200 IU) should be given at the same time as the first dose of the vaccine, in a different syringe and at a different site, as above.

3 Infants born to mothers not tested during pregnancy: the DoH recommends that mothers are serotested for hepatitis B in the antenatal clinic. If a pregnant mother is in labour, having had no hepatitis B-tests during her pregnancy, blood should be taken as soon as possible for tests and the infant should receive the hepatitis B vaccine within 12 h of birth. If the mother is found to be HBsAg-positive (carrier), the infant should receive HBIG and vaccine as soon as possible and in any case within 7 days from birth. Subsequent vaccination should continue as for infants of HBsAg-positive mothers (see above).

• Antenatal screening for hepatitis B is strongly recommended. By April 2000, all health authorities should have introduced universal antenatal screening and immunization of babies at risk (Health Service Circular *HSC* 1998/127 and http:// www.open.gov.uk/doh/coinh.htm).

• There is no contraindication to breast-feeding if a baby starts immunization at birth and receives the full course.

• In the USA, two-thirds of the HBV-infected children do not have HBV-infected mothers. These infections result from close contact with HBsAg-positive people living in the child's household or other households [H. Mergolis in Needle Tips, Volume 10, No 1 Spring/summer 2000, p. 3].

• Hepatitis B, as a sexually transmitted disease, is the only such disease currently preventable by immunization. A complication of hepatitis B infection is hepatocellular carcinoma—this malignant complication can also be prevented by immunization.

Nonresponders to hepatitis B vaccine

The minimal protective titre of anti-HBs has been assumed almost universally to be 10 mIU/mL and immunological memory (see above) is thought to ensure protection even after circulating antibodies drop below this level or become undetectable. This is possible by the establishment of a pool of memory B lymphocytes to hepatitis B surface antigens following vaccination.

Studies of antibody response to hepatitis B vaccines (both plasma-derived and recombinant DNA) have shown that 5–15% of healthy immunocompetent subjects (about 5% of healthy infants, children and young adults) do not mount an antibody response to the surface antigen component present in these preparations (nonresponders = anti-HBs undetectable) or that they respond poorly (hypo-responders = anti-HBs <10 mIU/mL).

There is no universal agreement on how we should deal with nonresponders to hepatitis B vaccine. Here are some options.

• *USA*: Rely on immunological memory for long-term protection. There are follow-up studies extending for up to 10 years which show that protection persists even after anti-HBs responses have declined to undetectable levels and that vaccinees develop a rapid anti-HBs response when exposed to the virus or when given a reinforcing dose [Margolis (1993) *J. Infect. Dis.* 168, 9–14 and Wainwright *et al.* (1989) *J. Am. Med. Assoc.* 261, 2362–6]. Healthy vaccinees who develop levels of anti-HBs >10 mIU/mL have long-lived immunological memory for HBsAg. Many American researches support not giving boosters simply because levels of anti-HBs drop below 100 and over 10 mIU/mL. The American Academy of Paediatrics (*Red Book* 2000, p. 295) recommends reimmunization when the anti-HBs level is or drops below 10 mIU/mL. In such cases 1 to 3 doses of vaccine is recommeded but no further doses are recommended if the person remains anti-HBs-negative after revaccination.

• *UK*: The DoH recommends a repeat course if vaccine for nonresponders (anti-HBs less than 10 mIU/mL or not detectable), and a booster for those whose antibody level is 10–99 mIU/mL.

Give nonresponders up to three additional doses of the same vaccine, at 1–2-month intervals, with serological assessment of immunological response after each dose. Twenty per cent of non-responders usually seroconvert after the first additional dose and up to 50% after the third additional dose. For nonresponders who fail to produce any antibodies after one or two courses of one hepatitis B vaccine, a different hepatitis B vaccine may be tried, although there is no clinical evidence this will work.

Nonresponders (anti-HBs ⩽ 10 mIU/mL) can also be offered passive immunization with hepatitis B immunoglobulin (HBIG) after suspect exposure or injury. They should have their antibody to the core antigen (anti-HBc) determined in order to ascertain whether they have had hepatitis B infection in the past. If this antibody is negative, they have not had the infection in the past and they do need to receive HBIG.

● *Europe*: Professor Robert Steffen (Zurich, Switzerland) recommends that those with no or low response will require additional doses every 6–12 months. Some individuals are known to have seroconverted after more than 10 doses (personal communication).

● *In my practice* I have used an unlicensed method with considerable success. I use double the dose of the same or a different vaccine and serotest 2 months later. I repeat if necessary. Another method is to use the special formulation HB-Vax II 40 for patients on renal dialysis or the immuno-suppressed, in this case, for nonresponders (outside its license).

● In 1997, Dr Jane Zuckerman and coworkers [Zuckerman J. *et al.* (1997) *Br. Med. J.* 314, 329–33] showed that 69% of nonresponders to at least four doses of a licensed hepatitis B vaccine containing the S component, responded to a new hepatitis B vaccine (Hepagene) manufactured by Medeva Pharma Ltd, as yet unlicensed and not available in the UK. This vaccine is a third-generation vaccine containing pre-S_1, pre-S_2 and S antigenic components of both viral surface antigen subtypes *adw* and *ayw*. In a prelicensing study, Hepagene was used to treat carriers rather than to prevent infection. The study showed that the vaccine induces an immune response in carriers but it is presently unclear whether viral eradication can be achieved. Further studies are under way to provide more definitive evidence. This vaccine is awaiting EU approval for prophylaxis against hepatitis B infection.

● Seventy per cent of infant nonresponders to a repeat course of hepatitis B vaccine showed a good response and protective titres when they were reimmunized at 4 years of age [Tan *et al.* (1994) *J. Am. Med. Assoc.* 271, 859–61].

● In the general population, 5–15% will respond to hepatitis B vaccine with anti-HBs <10 mIU/mL or no detectable antibodies with the currently available methods of testing. Table 32.3 lists factors

Table 32.3 Factors negatively affecting response to hepatitis B vaccine.

● Increasing age (20% males, 3% females aged 15–20 years. 40% males, 18% females over 50 years)
● Male sex—females respond significantly better than males
● Male homosexuals—heterosexual males show a better response
● Chronic renal failure, renal dialysis (the immune response appears to be T-cell-dependent and therefore may be reduced by renal failure)
● Diabetes (70–80% seroconversion)
● Alcoholic liver disease, cirrhosis
● Malnutrition
● Obese individuals
● Cigarette smokers (50% lower antibody titres)
● Infection with HIV (seroconversion in 50–70% of cases)
● Immunosuppression by disease or treatment
● Genetic predisposition (e.g. HLA-B8, SCO1, DR3 homozygotes)
● Presence of hepatitis B infection (incubation time 45–180 days) at the time of vaccination—the vaccine may be ineffective
● Vaccine administered by route other than IM, and at a site other than the deltoid in adults and the anterolateral thigh in infants
● Incorrect vaccine storage, e.g. frozen
● Vaccine out-of-date

Table 32.4 Type of response to hepatitis B vaccine and the need for a booster dose—UK recommendations.

Type of response	Anti-HBs level (mIU/mL)	Booster dose recommendations
No response	Negative	Repeat vaccine course
Inadequate response	< 10	Repeat vaccine course
Low response	10 to < 99	6 months
Good response	⩾ 100	5 years single booster if still at risk. For those at very high risk, or immunosuppressed—check anti-HBs titre periodically

that may affect a response to hepatitis B vaccine. Table 32.4 indicates the action necessary according to response to the vaccine.

Individuals at high risk who persistently fail to respond to hepatitis B vaccination should be considered for passive immunization with HBIG in postexposure settings. They should be counselled about be-havioural and occupational risks.

Vaccine availability

• Engerix B (SmithKline Beecham Pharmaceuticals) is available in adult prefilled syringe (1 mL) each containing 20 µg of HBsAg protein, in packs of one and 10 (1 mL); adult vial (1 mL) containing each 20 µg , in packs of one and three (1 mL) and 10 (1 mL). Paediatric vial (0.5 mL) each containing 10 µg in packs of one.

• HB-Vax II (Aventis Pasteur MSD), available in prefilled syringe (1 mL) and vial (1 mL) for adults and adolescents, each containing 10 µg of HBsAg protein, in single packs.

HB-Vax II Paediatric (Aventis Pasteur MSD), available in prefilled syringe (0.5 mL), each containing 5 µg of HBsAg protein, in single packs.

HB-Vax II 40 (Aventis Pasteur MSD), available in suspension in vial (1 mL), each containing 40 µg of HBsAg protein, in single packs.

Storage. Between 2 and 8 °C. *Do not freeze.* Protect from light. Do not dilute. Shelf-life of 3 years. All vaccines should be well shaken to obtain a slightly opaque preparation.

Human hepatitis B immunoglobulin (HBIG)

• Human hepatitis B immunoglobulin (HBIG) is

prepared from the plasma of donors who have been found to have suitably high titres of hepatitis B antibodies. Each plasma donation and the final product are tested by validated procedures and found nonreactive for antibodies to HIV. Screening of blood donations is routine in the UK. The plasma used by BPL (Bio Products Laboratory, Elstree, Herts, UK) to manufacture their product is obtained from the USA where stringent screening processes are also in place.

• In the case of accidental exposure, allow the wound or cut to bleed and wash with soap and water. If the skin is contaminated, wash with soap and water. Rinse any eye splashes with water or sterile saline solution.

• Where immediate protection is required, such as after exposure to hepatitis B virus, HBIG and hepatitis B vaccine should be administered simultaneously, in separate syringes and into separate injection sites. Individuals who are known to have received hepatitis B vaccination in the past should be given a booster dose of vaccine unless they are known to have adequate protective levels of antibody, i.e. anti-HBs 100 mIU/mL.

• HBIG should be administered as soon as possible after exposure, preferably within 48 h and not later than 1 week. A second dose of HBIG should be given 4 weeks later unless:

(a) there is evidence of past hepatitis B infection in the recipient's pre-HBIG blood sample;

(b) tests show that the HBsAg-positive inoculum is anti-HBe-positive (low risk of infectiousness);

(c) hepatitis B vaccine was given at or about the time the first dose of HBIG was given.

• Babies born to mothers who had acute hepatitis B during pregnancy or early puerperium, or mothers who are HBeAg-positive, carriers or who

Table 32.5 Hepatitis B immunoglobulin is recommended in these circumstances.

- Accidental exposure to hepatitis B virus such as occurs when blood or other material containing surface antigen is inoculated, ingested or splashed onto mucous membranes or the conjunctivae. This is important for practice staff who perform invasive procedures and themselves fail to seroconvert
- Family contacts judged to be at high risk, and sexual contacts as well as carers of patients with acute hepatitis B
- Newborn of mothers with acute hepatitis B in pregnancy or early in the puerperium
- Newborn of mothers who are hepatitis B surface-antigen-positive, particularly if 'e' antigen is detectable. Such infants rarely display any symptoms but have a 95% chance of becoming chronic carriers

Table 32.6 Dosage of human hepatitis B immunoglobulin.

Age	Dose (IU)
Newborn	
IM soon after birth, within first 12 h	200 (DoH) or
Give simultaneously hepatitis B vaccine in a separate syringe and at a different site	40 IU/kg BW (BPL)
Children	
Age 0–4 years	200
Age 5–9 years	300
Age > 10 years	500
Adults	500

are HBsAg-positive should receive active/passive immunization. HBIG should be given as soon as possible after birth, preferably within 12 h. Efficacy of HBIG given at 12–48 h is presumed, but unproven. Hepatitis B vaccine should be given at the same time in a different syringe and at a different site. The second and third doses are given at 1 and 6 months after the first, or the accelerated schedule of 0, 1, 2 and 12 months is used. If vaccine is not given in the first 12 h after birth, the first dose should be given within the first 7 days. If vaccine admini-stration is delayed for as long as 3 months, a second dose of HBIG should be given.

- In up to 2% of cases, the passive/active immunization (HBIG/hepatitis B vaccine) is not effective. Infants should be serotested at 9 months of age or later (at least 1 month after the third vaccine dose), for surface antigen and antibody. If an infant is found to be surface-antigen- and -antibody-negative, he or she should receive a fourth dose of vaccine and be re-tested 1 month later for anti-HBs. If this fails, repeat the vaccine course later, definitely by the age of 4 years when 70% of infant nonresponders will produce detectable antibodies.

Table 32.5 shows circumstances where hepatitis

B immunoglobulin is recommended, while Table 32.6 shows dosage.

- HBIG should be used as a single dose IM and must never be given IV.
- Within 1 week from the onset of jaundice for sexual contacts and at-risk family members of an individual with acute hepatitis B.
- HBIG is not appropriate for travellers to high-risk areas. Hepatitis B vaccination is more appropriate under these circumstances.

HBIG availability

Human Hepatitis B Immunoglobulin intra-muscular (Bio Products Laboratory) is available in 2-mL ampoules (200 IU) and 5-mL ampoules (500 IU).

It is also available from the following sources:
- PHLS—Communicable Disease Surveillance Centres;
- local Public Health Laboratory Services;
- Blood Transfusion Service, Scotland;
- Public Health Laboratory, Belfast.

Storage. Between 2 and 8 °C in its carton. *Do not freeze.* Stored at 25 °C (in the dark): 1 week.

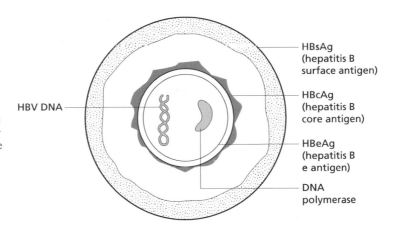

Fig. 32.1 The hepatitis B virus contains DNA surrounded by a core antigen envelope and is coated with an outside lipoprotein coat, the surface antigen (the major component of hepatitis B vaccine—initially known as Australia antigen), which is antigenically heterogeneous; it has four major subtypes: adw, ayw, adr and ayr. The 'e' antigen is a soluble protein of the core antigen, an indirect marker of infectivity contributing to the persistence of chronic infection.

HBV DNA

HBsAg (hepatitis B surface antigen)

HBcAg (hepatitis B core antigen)

HBeAg (hepatitis B e antigen)

DNA polymerase

Hepatitis B infection

Hepatitis B virus (HBV) (see Fig. 32.1) is a double-stranded deoxyribonucleic acid- (DNA) containing virus belonging to the class Hepadnaviridae. It replicates through an RNA intermediate, or 'pregenome'. The hepatitis core antigen is important in incorporating the pregenomic RNA. The virus replicates primarily in hepatocytes, releasing into the circulation hepatitis B surface antigen, 'e' antigen and HBV DNA. It remains potentially infectious for months when stored at approximately 32 °C and for years at –20 °C. Heat (100 °C for 30 min) can inactivate the virus.

HBV causes a spectrum of infection ranging from asymptomatic seroconversion to fulminant (0.1–1.0% of cases), fatal hepatitis. Its chronic complications include hepatic cirrhosis, necrosis, chronic active hepatitis and hepatocellular carcinoma, leading to a case fatality of 2%.

Lürman probably described the first hepatitis epidemic, which was related to a medical act (during a vaccination campaign against smallpox) in Bremen in 1885. However, it was not until the 1950s, with the development of hospital institutions and medical techniques, that cases of serum hepatitis in medical laboratory and ward staff, particularly in haemodialysis departments, were reported. By 1947 the terms hepatitis A and hepatitis B were introduced.

● The major modes of HBV transmission are by contact with blood or blood-derived fluids and through sexual activity. Apart from blood, it can be found in wound exudate, breast milk, semen, cervical secretions, vaginal fluid, tears and saliva, although the latter is not an effective vehicle for transmission. The virus has been shown to survive in dried blood, outside the body, for at least 1 week in ambient conditions.

● The routes of infection for children and adults are different. A woman infected with the HBV can pass it on to her baby at the time of childbirth (*perinatal—vertical transmission*) and almost all (up to 95%) these infants will themselves become HBV carriers. They will grow up to infect other children (*horizontal transmission*) through physical contact, skin conditions such as impetigo and scabies, or through cuts, grazes, bites. In adulthood, they in turn will infect their own children and others. Babies of HBeAg-positive mothers are at particular risk, with 70–90% of these infants becoming infected.

The most common modes of transmission in adults are *sexual contact*, both heterosexual and homosexual, parenteral and percutaneous inoculation *through blood and blood products*. This can take place through contaminated needles and syringes used by drug abusers and by some overseas medical establishments where disposable equipment is not always used or may not be available. Persons travelling abroad should be reminded about the dangers of being involved in road traffic, boat, mountain or ski accidents, sustaining contaminated wounds or other skin injuries. They should also avoid tattooing, ear-piercing, and sharing toothbrushes or razors. At greatest risk are

- Inappropriate sexual behaviour or personal contact
- Medical/dental interventions
- Accidents and casualty treatment
- Blood transfusion
- Intravenous drug use, sharing needles and syringes
- Adventure sports
- Acupuncture, tattooing and body piercing
- Autohaemotherapy (1–2 mL of blood from the patient, mixed with equal volume of saline and reinjected into the buttock or acupuncture points)
- Sharing razors and toothbrushes
- Haircut
- Massage (skin breaks)
- Administering or receiving first aid

Table 32.7 The main travel-related hepatitis B risk factors.

	HBV	HIV
Number of people estimated by the WHO to have been infected worldwide	2 billion	34 million
Number of hepatitis B carriers and AIDS cases	350 million	13 million
Minimum volume of blood required to transmit infection	0.00004 mL	0.1 mL
Risk of infection following a needle-stick injury with positive patient	27–43%	0.33%
Hepato-oncogenic	Yes	No
Kaposi's sarcoma	No	Yes
Vaccine preventable	Yes	No

Table 32.8 Comparison of hepatitis B and HIV—1999.

nonimmune healthcare workers for whom hepatitis B is a serious occupational hazard. Table 32.7 summarizes the main travel-related risk factors.

Permucosal route, e.g. splash of infected material onto the conjunctiva, can take place in the laboratory, the hospital ward, the treatment room, etc.

- Concentration of HBV in body fluids varies. It is *high* in blood, serum and wound exudate, *moderate* in saliva, vaginal fluid and semen, and *low or not detectable* in breast milk, tears, sweat, urine and faeces.

- Hepatitis B is extremely infectious. The minimum volume of blood required to transmit infection is minute: 0.00004 mL. It is estimated to be 100 times more infectious than the human immunodeficiency virus (HIV) (Table 32.8).

- Overall, over 50% of hepatitis B infection in

adults and the large majority (90%) of infection acquired in childhood is asymptomatic. Those who experience symptoms do so between 2 and 6 months after infection. These may include malaise, fever and headaches. Later on anorexia, nausea, vomiting and abdominal discomfort over the right hypochondrium. Jaundice may then follow, with pale stools and dark urine. The prognosis deteriorates with increasing age.

- Fulminant hepatitis B occurs in under 1% of cases. A person who becomes infected may die, although death is rare. Others (90%) recover and develop lifelong immunity. The serological loss of HBsAg and the presence of anti-HBs demonstrates resolution. About 2–10% of older children and adults, 25–50% of children aged 1–5 years old, 90% of children under 1 year of age, and 95% of

Table 32.9 Serological markers for hepatitis B infection and immunity.

Hepatitis B surface antigen (HBsAg)	The first screening test—detection of acutely infected patients, or carriers
Antibody to hepatitis B surface antigen (anti-HBs)	Indicates past infection or immunization and immunity
Hepatitis B e antigen (HBeAg)	Indicates active viral replication in acute infection and some carriers. The chronic carrier is at high risk of transmitting HBV infection
Antibody to hepatitis B e antigen (anti-HBe)	Present during and after recovery from hepatitis B, and in some chronic carriers. The chronic carrier is at low risk of transmitting HBV infection
Antibody to hepatitis B core antigen (anti-HBc)	Identifies persons who have had hepatitis B infection in the past (anti-HBc IgG), or have acute or very recent infection (anti-HBc IgM). It is not induced by immunization therefore it is negative in vaccinees who have never contracted hepatitis B infection
Hepatitis B virus DNA	Indicates viral replication at higher level. In chronic carriers it assesses infectivity and risk of transmission, disease activity and liver damage. Used in monitoring antiviral therapy

neonates infected at birth from their mothers (average among the under 5 year olds: 30–90%) progress to develop the chronic *carrier* state—a persistent infection, which can last for life.

● *The HBV chronic carrier* is defined as a person who is positive for surface antigen (HBsAg) for 6 months or more. Only 1–2% of these individuals will subsequently convert from HBsAg to anti-HBs-positive each year. Those with e-antigen (HBeAg) are highly infectious, while the presence of antibody to e-antigen (anti-HBe) indicates low infectivity (see Table 32.9). Approximately 5–10% will seroconvert from HBeAg to anti-HBe-positive each year. There is little correlation between the severity of the illness, and the amount or level of viral replication or viral antigen production. Male patients are more likely to remain chronically infected than female patients.

● Only a small percentage of carriers will have a history of infection—10% of children and 30–50% of adults. One of the reasons is because only a fraction of acute hepatitis B infections, approximately 2%, are reported among children younger than 5 years of age, even though this cohort accounts for nearly a third of all individuals with chronic infection [Margolis, H.S., Alter, M.J., Hadler, S.C., *et al.* (1991) Hepatitis B: evolving epidemiology and implications for control. *Semin Liver Dis* 11, 84–92].

● It is estimated that there are 350 million chronic carriers of hepatitis B virus worldwide. Many are lifelong carriers, although not all are infectious, and some clear the virus after varying intervals.

● *HBV carriers* most commonly (70–75%) display chronic, persistent hepatitis, which is generally asymptomatic and rarely progresses to serious liver disease, while a number of them have normal liver function tests. On the other hand, 25–30% of carriers (more likely the e-antigen carriers) go on to develop chronic active hepatitis, cirrhosis and, eventually, over an average of 20 years, primary liver carcinoma.

The rate of progression from chronic hepatitis B to liver cancer ranges from 0.2 to 0.7% per year, and from compensated cirrhosis to liver cancer from 0.2 to 8.0% per year [Fattovich G. *et al.* (1995) Occurrence of hepatocellular carcinoma and decompensation in Western European patients with cirrhosis type B. *Hepatology* 21, 77–82; Liaw Y. *et al.* (1989) Natural course after the development of cirrhosis in patients with chronic type B hepatitis: a prospective study. *Liver* 9, 235–41]. Over a quarter of all patients with chronic HBV (carriers) will die prematurely of liver cancer or cirrhosis [Alter M. (1996) Epidemiology and disease burden of hepatitis B and C. *Antiviral Therapy* 1(suppl. 1), 9–14].

Eighty per cent of all liver cancers are a consequence of infection with the hepatitis B virus, which is second only to tobacco as the most prolific carcinogen known to man. An estimated 850 000

Table 32.10 Hepatitis B notifications and deaths in England and Wales.

	1984	1987	1988	1989	1990	1991	1992	1993	1994	1995	1996	1997	1998	1999*
Notifications	2000	444	390	432	435	488	489	581	528	623	613	730	886	864
Deaths	69	69	59	58	53	53	79	35	29	61	62	64	54	63

Source: ONS, PHLS—Communicable Disease Surveillance Centre (CDSC).   *1999 figures provisional

deaths occur annually as a result of hepatitis B-related liver cancer. Infection by this oncogenic virus can be prevented by hepatitis B immunization. HB infection is responsible for 60 million cases of liver cirrhosis worldwide, more than the number of cases caused by alcohol.

• Overall, less than 0.5% of the UK population are chronic carriers of hepatitis B, although this may be considerably higher in certain ethnic subgroups and in long-stay institutions for the mentally handicapped [Bannister B., Begg, N. & Gillespie, S. (2000) In *Infectious Disease* 2nd Edn Blackwell Science, Oxford]. The overall prevalence of carriage in a study of 3781 sera of anonymous individuals aged 15–44 years submitted to 16 microbiology laboratories in England and Wales in 1996 was 0.37% [Gay N. *et al.* (1999) The prevalence of hepatitis B infection in adults in England and Wales. *Epidemiol. Infect.* 122, 133–8].

• The Scandinavian countries have the lowest carriage rates (0.05%). By contrast, in Southern Europe prevalence rates range from 0.5 to 2%, and the incidence rates of notified cases is about 6/100 000. In Central and Eastern Europe, as well as in the newly independent states, HBV is highly endemic. Carrier rates reach over 8% in the Central Asian Republics and in some countries in Eastern Europe, with reported incidence rates varying from 27/100 000 in Kazakhstan to 400/100 000 in Turkmenistan.

• In the UK, the prevalence is higher in certain inner-city areas where antenatal clinics report hepatitis B carriage in up to 1% of women tested. Carriage in antenatal women in the West Midlands ranged from 2% in those born outside the UK to 0.1% in those born in the UK [Boxall E. *et al.* (1994) *Epidemiol. Infect.* 113, 523–8]. The prevalence of anti-HBc was between 15 and 30% in injecting drug users attending specialist services (DoH 1997), and 17% in homosexual men attending genitourinary medicine clinics in London [Hart G. *et al.* (1993) *AIDS* 7, 863–9]. In a seroprevalence study in children aged 13–14 years (collected between 1986 and 1995), only 15/2025 (0.7%) were anti-HBc-positive [Hesketh L. *et al.* (1997) *Commun. Dis. Rep.* 4, R60–3].

• The average urban GP will have between five and 10 patients who are carriers on their list and will see a new symptomatic infection every 2 years. Over two-thirds of the carriers are not known to their GP, hence the importance of antenatal screening.

• The numbers of reports of acute hepatitis B to the Public Health Laboratory Service in 1984 for England and Wales were about 2000, while in 1995 they were about 623 (Table 32.10), with an estimated 25% of child cases proving fatal. The most common risk for exposure to acute symptomatic hepatitis B, based on laboratory reports in England and Wales in 1997, was identified as injecting drugs, followed by sex between men and women, and then sex between men.

• In the USA, it is estimated that 200 000–300 000 cases occur each year, while the number of hepatitis B carriers has reached 1.25 million. The incidence of hepatocellular carcinoma is increasing (by 71% from 1976 to 1995), and the increase is expected to continue until the rate of the major cause—infection with hepatitis B or C—is brought under control.

• About 8–13% of HB infection cases in the UK are thought to have been acquired abroad (Table 32.11) and the most common risk factor is sexual contact (56%), followed by medical treatment (15%), and intravenous drug use (5%)—the most common risk factor in those remaining in the UK (around 45% in 1998). It has been estimated that 18% of travellers over 65 years who became ill were admitted to hospital while abroad and therefore exposed potentially to infection.

A study of 16- to 40-year-old UK holiday-makers showed that 17 out of 354 travellers abroad had sex with a new partner (5%). Despite 12 of these (71%) carrying condoms, the same number of people had sex without a condom at least once [Gillies P. *et al.* (1992) HIV-related risk behaviour in UK holiday-makers. *AIDS* 6(3), 339–41]. This is mirrored by another UK study, which reported that only 41% of holiday-makers who had sex while abroad always used condoms [Ford N. & Eiser J.R. (1995) Risk and liminality. In: *Health and the International Tourist. The HIV-Related Socio–Sexual Interaction of Young Tourists*, pp. 153–75. Routledge Press, London]. The use of condom showed some relation to age: 17- to 18-year-olds were more likely to use condoms than 23- to 26-year-olds.

Serological markers
(see Table 32.9)

• Infection with HBV results in the appearance of core antibody in the serum, and in most people this antibody will persist for many years, indicating past infection. Those who become carriers of the HBV will persistently test positive for surface antigen. Those who become immune will test positive for antibody to the surface antigen.
• Immunization with hepatitis B vaccine results in seropositivity for surface antibody alone (anti-HBs-positive).
• If the previously immunized person is found to be positive for core antibody, it indicates that this person has previously acquired hepatitis B infection or it may coincide with acute clinical hepatitis. If, in addition, this person has persistent surface antigenaemia, he or she is at high risk (one in four) of chronic hepatitis, which can lead to cirrhosis and hepatocellular carcinoma.
• A successfully immunized person with persistent

protective antibody to HBsAg (anti-HBs >100 mIU/mL), when exposed to infection, may become infected, as shown by anticore sero-onversion, but this is rarely associated with acute hepatitis.
• A typical serological profile in a chronic carrier includes the presence of the HBsAg, with high replicative state and infectivity suggested by HBeAg, lack of anti-HBe and detectable HBV DNA. About 10–15% of HBeAg-positive patients undergo spontaneous remission in disease activity each year. When this happens there is loss of HBV DNA, followed by loss of HBeAg and the appearance of anti-HBe.

For an interpretation of hepatitis B serological markers please refer to Table 32.12.
• *Transmission of hepatitis B by blood transfusion*: the most significant and cost-effective advances in reducing the risk of post-transfusion hepatitis have resulted from the selection of safer blood donors (acceptance of volunteer rather than paid donors, banning of blood collections from prisoners) and the screening of blood for HBsAg that was introduced in the 1970s, and hepatitis C antibody that was introduced in the early 1990s.

A review by Soldan and coworkers [Soldan *et al.* (1999) *Br. Med. J.* 318, 95] showed 24 cases associated with transfusion (out of 4185 infections reported in 1991–97) in England and Wales. In 10 cases investigation was not possible or inconclusive (donors could not be identified or retested). Of the 14 probably infectious donations, three were from HBsAg-negative donors during acute hepatitis B infection and 11 were from negative donors during late carriage of the virus. The authors concluded that most of these infectious donations could have been detected by testing for antibodies to core antigen (anti-HBc).

It has been known since the 1970s that, infre-

	History of travel			Number	
	Yes	No	No information	Notified	Laboratory-confirmed
1996	79	92	397	613	568
1997	82	129	441	730	652
1998	89	140	614	886	843

Table 32.11 Laboratory-confirmed cases and notifications of hepatitis B infection in England and Wales (1996–98).

Source: ONS, PHLS Communicable Disease Surveillance Centre.

Serological markers	Result	Interpretation
HBsAg Anti-HBs Anti-HBc	All negative	Susceptible
HBsAg Anti-HBs Anti-HBc	Negative Positive Positive or Negative	Immune
HBsAg Anti-HBs Anti-HBc IgM anti-HBc	Positive Negative Positive Positive	Acutely infected
HBsAg Anti-HBs Anti-HBc IgM anti-HBc	Positive Negative Positive Negative	Chronically infected

Table 32.12 Interpretation of the hepatitis B serological markers.

quently, HBV is transmitted by transfusion from chronic HBV carriers with subdetectable concentrations of HBsAg. Such infectious units can be detected by testing for anti-HBc. The problem lies more with the specificity of anti-HBc assays and new techniques for donor screening are being developed, such as the nucleic-acid-testing (NAT). Calculations based on reasonable but unverifiable assumptions indicate that the frequency of HBV transmission by chronic carriers negative for HBsAg is 1 in 52 000 [Sacher R. *et al.* (2000) Prevention of transfusion-transmitted hepatitis. *Lancet* 355, 331–2].

In the largest study so far in the UK, Regan and coworkers followed up recipients of 20 000 units of blood and tested them 9 months later to identify transmission of hepatitis B or C, HIV, or human T-cell leukaemia/lymphoma virus. No transfusion-transmitted infections were identified. Three patients acquired hepatitis B during or after hospital admission but not through transfusion. The researchers concluded that the current risk of transmission of these infections through transfusion in the UK is very small, although hospital-acquired infections may arise from sources other than transfusion [Regan F. *et al.* (2000) Prospective investigation of transfusion transmitted infection in recipients of over 20 000 units of blood. *Br. Med. J.* 320, 403–6].

Seven transfusion-transmitted infections were

identified in the UK from October 1998 to September 1999. Of these, one case was hepatitis B and another case hepatitis C. These were detected in asymptomatic recipients who were tested after donors had received positive test results. The donation infectious for hepatitis B was collected from a donor with an HBsAg-negative, acute infection; that for hepatitis C was released into the blood supply after an error in the testing process yielded a false negative result [Serious Hazards of Transfusion Scheme. *Annual Report 1998–99* (2000) SHOT, Manchester—for a copy of the report Tel.: 0161 251 4208].

Management of hepatitis B

● *Fulminant infection*: liver transplantation if it is clear that the patient will not survive otherwise. α-interferon has not been found to be beneficial in these cases.

● *Acute infection*: most cases resolve spontaneously. No treatment in the form of α-interferon or other antiviral agent is indicated in the absence of complications.

● *Chronic infection*: α-interferon is effective in 35–40% of patients. It is indicated in patients HBeAg and/or HB DNA and raised at least twice the upper limit of normal of aminotransferases (the aspartate is the more important). Permanent loss of HB DNA and HBeAg is considered a response to antiviral treatment. Eradication of the infection is possible in only a minority of patients. α-interferon has little effect in immunosuppressed patients, including patients on renal dialysis, patients with malignancies receiving chemotherapy, and patients with liver, heart or kidney transplant.

Famciclovir has been used to treat severe recurrence of hepatitis B infection after transplantation. Lamivudine is a potent inhibitor of human HBV as well as HIV.

The global problem

HBV has infected about 2 billion people according to a WHO estimate. There are an estimated 20 million new infections per year worldwide. Worldwide, it causes an estimated 4 million acute infections every year. Chronic HBV infection is responsible for about 60 million cases of liver cirrhosis, more than the number caused by alcohol [Kane M. (2000) *Action on hepatitis B as an occupational hazard.* No.1 Viral Hepatitis Prevention Board, 4]. Globally, it is the ninth most common cause of death Between 1 and 2 million people die each year from acute or chronic sequelae of HBV infection, 850 000 deaths each year are estimated to be a result of hepatocellular carcinoma as a consequence of past HBV infection.

The WHO estimates that medical treatment with blood-infected needles results in 8–16 million cases of hepatitis B infection a year worldwide.

About 350 million people are carriers of HBV. Many are lifelong carriers, although not all are infectious, and about 25% of carriers develop serious liver disease, such as cirrhosis and hepatocellular carcinoma. Of these carriers, the WHO estimates that 60 million will die from liver cancer and 45 million from liver cirrhosis.

It has been estimated that in Europe there are between 900 000 and 1 million new HB cases every year, of which 90 000 will become chronic carriers and 20 000 will die from cirrhosis or liver cancer. This magnitude of disease burden makes it one of the most significant health problems worldwide.

● The prevalence of hepatitis B infection, that is the percentage of the population who have serological evidence of prior HBV infection, varies markedly in different parts of the world (see Table 32.13 and Fig. 32.2).

● Natives of China, Hong Kong, Malaysia, Vietnam and Singapore have a particularly high carriage rate of HBV.

● The risk of HB is low in tourists who stay in endemic areas for a short time, provided they are not involved in any kind of accident, do not require dental or medical intervention, such as blood transfusion, and do not break fundamental rules about personal hygiene and contact. Travellers are at increased risk of accidents while abroad. In fact, trauma is the most common travel-related illness and road traffic accidents and falls on land are common causes of injury. Young males are particularly at risk of accidents. Trauma is the most common cause of death in those under 50 years of age.

● When assessing risk for travellers consider the following:

the likelihood of direct contact with infected blood or other body secretions, for example through accidents, or of intimate sexual contact with potentially infected persons;

Table 32.13 Prevalence of hepatitis B carrier state and serological evidence of prior HBV infection.

High endemicity	8–20% chronic carriers. 70–95% prevalence Central and Southern Africa, South-East Asia, Central Asia, China, Amazon Basin, Alaska, Pacific Islands, the Caribbean
Intermediate endemicity	2–7% chronic carriers. 30–50% prevalence North Africa, Southern and Eastern Europe, Middle East, Russian Federation, Indian Subcontinent, Japan, Central America and around the Amazon Basin
Low endemicity	< 2% chronic carriers. 4–6% prevalence North and Western Europe, North America, Southern South America, Australia, New Zealand

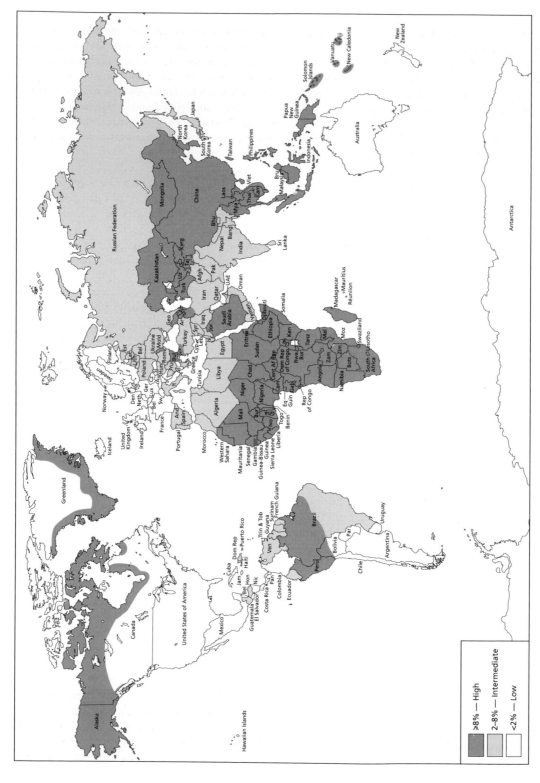

Fig. 32.2 Worldwide distribution of hepatitis B carrier state prevalence (this map generalizes available data.)

the prevalence of HBV carriers in the destination population;

the duration of the planned trip;

the traveller's activities when at destination;

the traveller's fitness and level of health.

- The objectives of hepatitis B immunization are to:
  - (a) prevent chronic HBV infection;
  - (b) prevent chronic liver disease;
  - (c) prevent primary hepatocellular carcinoma;
  - (d) prevent acute symptomatic hepatitis B infection.

The WHO aims to control rather than eliminate hepatitis B (because of the 350 million carriers). In 1991, the Global Advisory Group of the WHO's Expanded Programme for Immunization (EPI) called for all countries to introduce hepatitis B vaccine into their national immunization programmes by 1997. The implementation of this policy throughout the world will lead, in due course, to a marked reduction of the reservoir of HBV carriers and ultimately it could lead to the eradication of HBV infection.

The WHO's objective is to reduce the incidence of new carriers, especially children, by 80% by the year 2001, and eventually to eliminate both the million plus deaths that occur annually from HBV and the resulting liver complications—cirrhosis and primary liver cancer.

More than 90 countries, including most European countries and the USA, have already met this call. European countries that have not are the UK, Sweden, Norway, Finland, the Netherlands, Slovakia and the Czech Republic. The last two countries are interested in implementing programmes of universal hepatitis B immunization of infants and and/or adolescents.

The correct control strategies for HB infection control are:

- safe, effective vaccines;
- high-risk-groups immunization;
- universal immunization.

The current UK policy

The DoH's current policy is to target the high-risk hepatitis B groups, but even in well-defined, well-motivated and well-educated risk groups, such as healthcare workers, vaccine coverage is not high enough. As for much larger high-risk groups, such as male homosexuals, intravenous drug users or sexually promiscuous individuals, no country has been successful in reaching them. This failure is one of the reasons why most industrialized countries in Western Europe, North America and Asia now recommend routine immunization of infants and/or adolescents.

Low endemicity is not a valid reason to ignore the WHO advice. The UK has substantial populations of ethnic minorities, refugees and immigrants from areas of high endemicity who continue to maintain transmission. Injecting illegal drugs is an ever-increasing problem. In addition, the continuous increase in foreign travel means that more and more British people are now at risk of contracting the disease.

In order to reduce the burden of chronic hepatitis B in the UK and the other developed countries, a global effort to immunize children in the highest prevalence countries is necessary, as per WHO recommendations. This is a huge financial burden on the developing countries, one that must be shouldered partly by the industrialized countries.

Is hepatitis B immunization cost-effective?

The DoH thinks not. This was also a common attitude in the USA (also an area of low endemicity) until the CDC (Centres for Disease Control) showed that hepatitis B immunization was cost-effective, and even more so than *Haemophilus influenzae* b. Once infant immunization was introduced in the USA, bulk purchasing of the vaccines made them much cheaper (66 pence per shot). Further, research has shown that, assuming a not overly ambitious coverage of 68%, vaccinating infants against HBV would result in a net saving of approximately US$19.7 million per year; targeting adolescents would save US$3.5 million per year. H. Margolis at the CDC [Margolis H.S. *et al.* (1995) Prevention of Hepatitis B virus transmission by immunization: an economic analysis of current recommendations. *J. Am. Med. Assoc.* 274, 1201–8] has calculated that the cost per year of a life saved by HB infant immunization ($1852) was lower than that of antepartum administration of anti-Rh immune globulin to prevent rhesus isoimmunization ($2329), and considerably lower than those of neonatal intensive care ($7987) and coronary artery bypass surgery ($10 595).

Cost-effectiveness studies performed in countries with low endemicity, such as Belgium [Van Damme P. *et al.* (1995) Hepatitis B prevention in Europe: a preliminary economic evaluation. *Vaccine* 13 (suppl. 1), S54–7], Canada [Wrahn M. & Detsky A.S. (1993) Should Canada and the United States universally vaccinate infants against hepatitis B? *Med. Decis. Mak.* 13, 4200], USA [Margolis H.S. *et al.* (1995) Prevention of Hepatitis B virus transmission by immunization: an economic analysis of current recommendations. *J. Am. Med. Assoc.* 274, 1201–8], and even here in the UK [Mangtani P., Hall A.J. & Normand C. (1995) Hepatitis B vaccination: the cost-effectiveness of alternative strategies in England and Wales. *J. Epidemiol. Comm. Health* 49, 238–44] consistently find that universal HB immunization is economically attractive. Economic arguments can no longer be used to delay the implementation of universal hepatitis B immunization in countries with low endemicity such as the UK.

At a presentation during the 1999 ISTM meeting in Montreal, it was pointed out that if the whole population of Germany (80 million) was to receive hepatitis B vaccine, it would still cost less than the total cost to the health services of liver transplantation, chronic hepatitis B, cirrhosis and liver carcinoma.

Are countries that have introduced universal hepatitis B immunization seeing the benefits?

The *New England Journal of Medicine* [(1997) 336, 1855–9] published a Taiwanese study showing that universal hepatitis B immunization of children over a 10-year period, reduced the incidence of liver cancer in children. The average annual incidence of liver cancer in children of 6–14 years of age in Taiwan declined from 0.7 per 100 000 children between 1981 and 1986, to 0.36 between 1990 and 1994 ($P < 0.01$), following the introduction of

the mass vaccination of neonates in 1986 and preschool children in 1987.

In Italy, the average morbidity rates for hepatitis B in the period 1988–91 was 6.7 cases per 100 000 population. In 1991 mandatory immunization of infants and adolescents against hepatitis B was introduced. By 1995, vaccine coverage rate was over 90% and morbidity 5.3 cases per 100 000. By 1994, there was a dramatic decline in HBV infection rates of the order of a 50% reduction of acute hepatitis B in subjects aged 15–24 years compared with 1988 [Mele E. *et al.* (1997) Control of hepatitis B in Italy. In: *Viral Hepatitis and Liver Disease*, (Hollinger F., Lemaon S. & Margolis H. eds), pp. 675–7. Edizioni Minerva Medica, Turin]. The combination of nationwide vaccination of infants and adolescents, as well as prevention programmes targeted at high-risk groups have contributed to the control of hepatitis B that was once one of the major health concerns in Italy.

Since the introduction of routine hepatitis B immunization in the Alaska native population in 1983, the incidence of acute hepatitis B has fallen by over 98% and no new carriers have been detected among those who have been immunized [Wainwright R. *et al.* (1991) Duration of immunogenicity and efficacy of HB vaccine in a Yupik Eskimo population. Preliminary results of an 8-year study. In: *Viral Hepatitis and Liver Disease* (Hollinger F., Lemaon S. & Margolis H. eds), pp. 762–6. Williams and Wilkins, Baltimore].

In an area of The Gambia, the prevalence of chronic HBV infection in children declined from 12% to just 0.5% within 6 years of the introduction of routine infant immunization [Whittle H. *et al.* (1991) Vaccination against HB and protection against chronic viral carriage in The Gambia. *Lancet* 337, 747–50].

The World Bank's 1993 World Development Report stated that the addition of hepatitis B vaccine into national immunization programmes (along with the yellow fever vaccine) was among the most cost-effective health interventions in most developing countries.

The way forward in the UK

Hepatitis B is a preventable disease. Every child

born with hepatitis B who becomes a chronic carrier, and every adult that suffers from chronic liver disease or liver cancer as a result of HBV infection is, in my view, a case of national negligence.

In about 30% of patients with hepatitis B the mode of infection is not known. This in itself is a powerful argument for universal immunization.

The right way forward is universal infant HB immunization because infected children are more likely to become chronic carriers and it is easy to reach them through our primary care-based effective immunization target programmes. In addition, we should introduce catch-up immunization of adolescents (the group that 'spreads' the infection more than others), and continue targeting high-risk groups.

Combined vaccines are in advanced stages of licensing. Such polyvalent vaccines will include the common childhood vaccines and, in addition, hepatitis B. Such a development should certainly encourage the DoH to introduce hepatitis B immunization into the UK schedule. Hepatitis B is a serious and highly infectious disease, and it is preventable. Universal infant, adolescent and at-risk groups immunization would largely eradicate the disease and its sequelae.

The United Kingdom Advisory Group on Hepatitis—guidelines for protecting healthcare workers and patients from hepatitis B

All UK practices have been circulated with the Health Service Circular (HSC) 2000/020 on this subject. This new HSC supplements previous guidance (1993 and 1996) on hepatitis B-infected health care workers (see below). Its aim is to reduce further the risk of transmission of hepatitis B virus (HBV) infection to patients. It has implications across primary and secondary care.

Summary

Previous guidelines did not allow doctors and nurses to perform 'exposure prone procedures' if they were HBeAg positive. This still applies.

They allowed those who were anti-HBe positive but HBeAg negative to perform such procedures. The new guidance excludes those with increased viral load and specifies procedures to be followed in such cases.

Date for completion of testing in practices: 1st June 2001

Exposure prone procedures

Exposure prone procedures are defined by the DoH [UK Health Departments (December 1998), *AIDS/HIV Infected Health Care Workers: Guidance on the management of infected health care workers and patient notification*] as 'those invasive procedures where there is a risk that injury to the worker may result in the exposure of the patient's open tissues to the blood of the worker. These include procedures where the worker's gloved hands may be in contact with sharp instruments, needle tips or sharp tissues (e.g. spicules of bone or teeth), inside a patient's open cavity, wound or confined anatomical space where the hands or fingertips may not be completely visible at all times'.

For primary care it is important to note that procedures where hands and fingertips of the worker are visible and outside the patient's body at all times, and internal examinations or procedures do not involve possible injury to the worker's gloved hands from sharp instruments and/or tissues, are not considered to be exposure prone procedures. Such procedures include:

- taking blood (venepuncture);
- routine vaginal examinations;
- fitting intrauterine contraceptive devices (coils) and surgical insertion of depot contraceptive devices—provided fingers remain visible at all times when sharp instruments are in use;
- minor surface suturing (NB. Excision of lipomata and sebaceous cysts are considered exposure prone procedures);
- the incision of abscesses;
- simple endoscopic procedures (including gastroscopy) but not where there is a significant risk of biting of the worker's fingers as in dealing with a violent or fitting patient;
- setting up and maintaining IV lines. Central lines are included provided any skin tunnelling procedure used for setting them up is performed in a nonexposure prone manner;

• simple vaginal delivery and the use of scissors to make an episiotomy cut (NB. Infiltration of local anaesthetic prior to an episiotomy, and suturing of an episiotomy are considered exposure prone procedures); and

• general nursing procedures;
  If in doubt, check with the Occupational Health Physician.

The United Kingdom Advisory Group on Hepatitis—guidelines for protecting health-care workers and patients from hepatitis B

These guidelines (Health Service Guidelines (93) 40) were issued to UK healthcare workers in August 1993. A supplementary letter (NHS EL(96) (77)) was issued in September 1996. Their purpose was:

• to ensure that healthcare workers who may be at risk of acquiring HBV from patients are protected by immunization;

• to protect patients against the risk of acquiring HBV from an HBeAg-positive (highly infectious) healthcare worker.

They recommended that:

• healthcare workers who are HBeAg positive (highly infectious) must not carry out 'exposure prone procedures' in which there is a risk that injury to themselves could result in their blood contaminating a patient's open tissues;

• all healthcare workers who perform 'exposure prone procedures' should be given the hepatitis B vaccine. Their level of seroconversion should be checked 2–4 months after the third dose. Those found to have antibody to surface antigen level (anti-HBs) <10 mIU/mL, with their consent, should be tested for serological markers of past or current HBV infection.

(a) Those without markers of previous infection (anti-HBc negative, anti-HBs negative) may be at risk of hepatitis B infection. Their practice need not be restricted provided that occupational exposures are promptly reported and managed appropriately. Consider another course of vaccine and/or regular testing.

(b) Those found to have naturally acquired im-

munity (anti-HBc positive, HBsAg-negative) are not at risk of infection.

(c) Those found to have a current infection/be carriers (HBsAg positive, anti-HBe positive) should have markers of infectivity checked. If e antigen positive, exclude from all 'exposure prone procedures' and refer for treatment and occupational advice. HBeAg and HBsAg carriers should not undertake invasive procedures. If e antigen negative, or anti-HBe positive or negative, there is no need to change work practices (this is the main point that has changed with the new guidelines—see below).

These guidelines apply to all healthcare workers, e.g. doctors, nurses, midwives, dentists, dental workers, medical and dental students, etc. Employers should make compliance with the guidance a condition of service for new staff appointed to posts that will involve 'exposure prone procedures', and should also ensure that locum or agency staff have complied with the guidance.

The new guidance (HSC 2000/020) aims to protect against transmission from hepatitis B infected but e antigen negative healthcare workers. This is because several incidents in recent years have shown that some health care workers with HBV infection/carriers who are negative for HBeAg may still infect patients during exposure prone procedures.

The new guidance recommends that the healthcare workers who are hepatitis B surface antigen (HBsAg) positive (HBV infected/carriers) and HBeAg negative and currently performing exposure prone procedures should have their viral load measured.

• If the healthcare worker's HBV DNA concentration in blood (viral load) exceeds 1000 genome equivalent per millilitre they will not be allowed to perform exposure prone procedures.

• If the viral load does not exceed 1000 /mL they will not be restricted but should be advised by the occupational health physician on minimizing the risk of transmission to patients and should be retested every 12 months. They should cease performing exposure prone procedures if the viral load subsequently exceeds 1000 /mL or they are suspected or shown to have transmitted HBV to a patient.

Blood samples from healthcare workers who

perform exposure prone procedures for the purpose of testing for current hepatitis B infection or response to vaccine should be taken directly by the occupational health service or by a person commissioned to do so by the occupational health service. Occupational Health Physicians are ethically and professionally obliged not to release information without the consent of the individual that has been tested. On the other hand there are occasions when an employer may need to be advised that a change of duties should take place, but hepatitis B status itself will not normally be disclosed without the healthcare worker's consent (Fig. 32.3).

In any investigation of possible transmission of blood-borne virus infection from a healthcare worker to a patient, blood samples should be obtained directly by a member of the incident Investigation Team or a person commissioned to do so on their behalf.

An e-antigen positive healthcare worker, who is successfully treated with α-interferon, and whose e-antigen negative status is sustained for 12 months after cessation of treatment, may be able to resume exposure prone procedures provided they satisfies the criterion of viral load contained in the new guidance.

The Primary Care Organizations are required to ensure that initial assessments on viral load in HBeAg negative HBV infected/carrier (HBsAg positive) healthcare workers who perform exposure prone procedures are completed by 1 June 2001 (this guidance applies also to Secondary Care and Community Trusts).

The practice may not have performed any tests on doctors and staff performing exposure prone procedures. Liaise with the Occupational Health Physician for hepatitis B screening.

The individual has been immunized but has not sero-converted (no anti-HBs detected). Liaise with the microbiologist as there is a need for carrier state in

Fig. 32.3

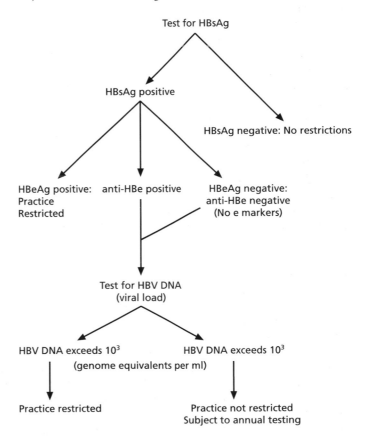

the individual to be excluded (is the person HBsAg-positive and anti-HBc positive?). You will also receive advice about re-vaccination.

Need to check viral load. Liaise with the Occupational Health Physician and microbiologist—the blood sample will need to be sent to a special laboratory.

The cost of testing is borne by the employer.

You can find information on: www.doh.gov.uk/coinh.htm and http://www.doh.gov.uk/nhsexec/hepatitisb.htm

At the Department of Health you can contact: Dr Hugh Nicholas, Room 635, Skipton House, 80 London Road, London SE1 6LH. Telephone: 020 79721533. E-mail: hugh.nicholas@doh.gsi.gov.uk.

HBsAg mutants, our future concern

HBV vaccination programmes have reduced carrier rates and acute morbidity in endemic regions of the world, and have an excellent safety track record. However, now viruses with mutations in the a determinant of the HBsAg are being found in vaccines, carrier populations after nucleoside drug therapy, and liver transplant recipients treated with hepatitis B immunoglobulin. Worryingly, the neut-ralizing antibodies raised by vaccination may not be effective against these mutants.

The Gly145Arg mutant is the most frequent and stable postvaccination HBsAg mutation seen. A large study of 345 infants in Singapore born to mothers with HBsAg and HBeAg who received HBIG at birth and plasma-derived hepatitis B vaccine at a dose of 5 or 10 µg within 24 h of birth and then 1 month and 2 months later revealed 41 breakthrough infections with HBV, despite the presence of anti-HBs [Oon C. *et al.* (1995) Molecular epidemiology of hepatitis B virus vaccine variants in Singapore. *Vaccine* 13, 699–702]. This mutant is increasingly being detected in vaccines in several other countries. It can be transmitted vertically or horizontally to immune individuals and to carriers of wild-type HBV.

Viruses carrying these mutants may not be detected with standard immunobased assays for HBV. This can lead to HBV being undetected in blood supplies. It is to be hoped that this problem will be solved by improving existing detection kits and by implementing new technology such as DNA chips.

● Ante-natal hepatitis B tests are explained in two leaflets produced by the Children's Liver Disease Foundation. Copies can be obtained by calling the Foundation on 0121 2123839 or via their website at http://www.childliverdisease.org

Information

For doctors:
● The CDC (USA) website: http://www.cdc.gov/ncidod/diseases/hepatitis
● Disease and vaccine information from the CDC: http://www.cdc.gov/nip/publications/acip-list.htm
● The American Digestive Health Foundation's website: http://mars.gastro.org/adhf/viral/hep.html
● The John Hopkins University's website: http://www.hopkins-id.edu/diseases/hepatitis/index.hep.html
● Hepatitis Information Network (Hepnet), Canada: http://www.hepnet.com

For patients:
● The Hepatitis Foundation international website: http://www.hepfi.org/infomenu.htm

Hepatitis B is a notifiable disease.

Chapter 33

Hepatitis A and B combined vaccine

Contraindications to the vaccine

- Acute febrile illness.
- Severe reaction to a previously administered combined hepatitis A and B vaccine, or monovalent hepatitis A or hepatitis B vaccines.
- Severe hypersensitivity to any component of the vaccine—aluminium, phenoxyethanol.
- Children under 1 year of age—the hepatitis A component is not licensed for this age. Children under 1 year can receive the hepatitis B monovalent vaccine.
- Pregnancy and lactation are relative contraindications and vaccination should be considered only if a mother is at risk of both viruses.

Possible side- and adverse effects

Local reactions

Local reactions include mild, transient soreness, redness and swelling.

General reactions

General reactions are similar to those experienced with the monovalent hepatitis A (see p. 141) and hepatitis B (see p. 153) vaccines.

Flu-like illness, fatigue, dizziness, nausea, vomiting, abdominal cramps, rash pruritus are rare. Neurological complications are very rare indeed.

The vaccine

The vaccine combines the existing monovalent hepatitis A and hepatitis B vaccines of the manufacturer (Table 33.1).

Administration

- The dose is 1.0 mL for adults and 0.5 mL for children age 1–15 years, given IM to the deltoid muscle in adults and anterolateral thigh or deltoid in children under 6 years.
- Patients with thrombocytopenia or bleeding disorders may receive the vaccine subcutaneously,

Table 33.1 Administration specifications for the combined hepatitis A and B vaccine (Twinrix).

	Adults (16 years and over)	Children (1–15 years)
Hepatitis A antigen	720 EL.U	360 EL.U
Hepatitis Bs antigen	20 µg	10 (g
Aluminium salts	0.45 mg	0.25 mg
2-phenoxyethanol	5.0 mg	2.5 mg
Isotonic solution	1.0 mL	0.5 mL

Schedule: 0, 1, 6 months

Route: IM (deltoid, anterolateral thigh in very young children)

Boosters: with monovalent vaccines
  Hepatitis A—every 10 + years
  Hepatitis B—single booster at 5 years for those who continue to be at high risk

Table 33.2 Who should receive the combined hepatitis A and B vaccine?

Short-term travellers staying for 1 month or more
Long-term travellers
Frequent travellers
Expatriate workers
Travellers coming into contact with locals, e.g. immigrant, especially children visiting homeland
Occupational groups such as aid workers, missionaries, healthcare workers, military, diplomatic personnel
With risky lifestyles: IV drug users, adventurous risking injury, homosexuals, men and women with multiple sexual partners or whose sexual behaviour is likely to place them at risk
Chronically ill travellers with underlying health problems that may necessitate seeking medical care abroad

Table 33.3 Hepatitis A and hepatitis B transmission.

Hepatitis A predominantly	Hepatitis B predominantly	Both A and B
Impure water	Medical/dental procedures	Accidents
Unhygienic food	Acupuncture, tattoos, ear-piercing	Contact with locals
		Sexual contact
		Blood transfusion

Table 33.4 Risk areas for hepatitis A and hepatitis B.

Hepatitis A	Hepatitis B
Low endemicity	
70–90% by age 50 years	4–6%. Chronic carriers < 2%
North America	North America
Australasia	Australasia
North and West Europe	North and West Europe
Japan	
Intermediate endemicity	
90% by age 25 years	30–50%. Chronic carriers 2–7%
Southern and Eastern Europe	Southern and Eastern Europe
Russian Federation	Russia Federation
Middle East (parts)	Middle East, North Africa
	Indian subcontinent
	Central America and around the Amazon
	Japan
High endemicity	
90% by age 10 years	50–95%. Chronic carriers 8–20%
Africa	Central and South Africa
South-East Asia	South-East Asia
China	China
Central and South America	Amazon basin
Middle East (parts)	Pacific Islands
Eastern Europe	

although this route of administration could result in suboptimal immune response to the vaccine.
- Patients with impaired immunity or on haemodialysis programmes may require additional doses of the vaccine in order to achieve adequate protective antibody titres.
- Serotesting for adequate antibody is necessary for the hepatitis B component 2–4 months after completion of the primary course for patients at increased risk (see p. 157).
- The vaccine will not prevent infection by the hepatitis C or E viruses. It will protect infection by the hepatitis δ (delta) virus—a defective virus that is too small to replicate unless it can attach itself to the surface antigen of the hepatitis B virus.
- Protection against hepatitis A and hepatitis B develops within 2–4 weeks. Table 33.2 gives advice on who should receive the vaccine.
- An accelerated schedule is not as yet licensed in the UK. Work undertaken by J. Zuckerman and coworkers at the Royal Free Hospital in London shows that a 0, 7, 21 days with a booster dose at 12 months schedule provides adequate protection for both infections.

Vaccine availability

Twinrix Adult (1.0 mL) and Twinrix Paediatric (0.5 mL) (SmithKline Beecham) are available in packs of one and 10 prefilled syringes.
Storage. Between 2 and 8 °C. *Do not freeze.* Do not dilute. Shelf-life 24 months.

Combined hepatitis A and B immunization

The introduction of the combined hepatitis A and B vaccine heralds the beginning of a future trend in travel vaccinations—the combination vaccines. Among the advantages are the following:
- reduction in the number of medical visits, injections, time necessary;
- increase in compliance, acceptance, coverage;
- dual protection against two infections that share similar characteristics in transmission (Table 33.3) and endemicity (Table 33.4). There is a considerable overlap of high-endemicity areas of hepatitis A and B so that travellers are often considered to be at risk from both viruses.

Chapter 34

Influenza

Contraindications to vaccination

- Acute febrile illness.
- Severe reaction to a previously administered influenza vaccine.
- Severe hypersensitivity to hens' eggs, chicken embryo (the virus used to produce the vaccine is grown in allantoic fluid) or any other constituents of the vaccine.
- Severe hypersensitivity to thiomersal or antibiotics used during the manufacture of the vaccines (Table 34.1).
- Pregnancy, unless a pregnant woman has other medical conditions that place her at increased risk of complications from influenza, in which case immunization should be considered. Lactation is not a contraindication to vaccination.

Possible side- and adverse effects

Local reactions

Transient swelling, redness, pain and induration may occur.

General reactions

General reactions include myalgia, malaise, headaches, arthralgia and fever for 1–2 days, beginning 6–12 h after vaccination. Neurological and anaphylactic reactions are very rare.

The incidence of Guillain–Barré syndrome is estimated to be one episode in every one million doses given. During a vaccination programme against swine influenza in the USA it was 1 in 100 000—the cause was not established. Anecdotal cases of asthma attacks after vaccination have been reported, but their significance and true relation to the vaccine are uncertain.

Often, vaccinees, especially the elderly, claim that influenza vaccine 'causes them flu'. They should be assured that the vaccine does not cause influenza but, in common with all other vaccines, it may cause 'flu-like' symptoms usually for 1–3 days after vaccination. In addition, many other respiratory viruses circulate during the cold months of the year.

The vaccine

The vaccine is made from egg-grown viruses, which are inactivated and highly purified. The

Vaccine	Antibiotics	Thiomersal
Fluvirin	Neomycin Polymyxin	Yes
Influvac	Gentamycin	Yes
Inactivated influenza vaccine (split virion) BP Pasteur	Neomycin	Yes
Begrivac	Polymyxin	No
Fluarix	Gentamycin	Yes

Table 34.1 Influenza vaccines where antibiotics or thiomersal are used in the manufacturing process.

vaccine is trivalent and contains two type A strains (H1N1 and H3N2) and one type B strain, representing the most recent influenza viruses circulating in the world. The types are recommended annually (in February for the northern hemisphere) by the WHO and the UK Joint Committee on Vaccinations and Immunizations Advisory Group. Their recommendations are based on the prevailing isolates received by the WHO from the four international reference centres (London, Atlanta, Tokyo and Melbourne) and approximately 110 national laboratories in more than 80 countries. The manufacturers then have until September to grow the chosen strains in eggs and prepare vaccine stocks—hence the importance of practices ordering their influenza vaccine supplies early (in spring). The need for annual production of vaccine with different virus strains results mainly from the ability of the influenza virus to undergo antigenic 'shift' and 'drift' (see p. 83). The WHO recommendations for the southern hemisphere (May to October) are issued in the preceding September.

For the *northern hemisphere* 2000/2001 season the WHO recommended the following strains to be incorporated in the influenza vaccines: A/Moscow/ 10/99 (H3N2)-like virus, A/New Caledonia/20/99 (H1N1)-like virus, and B/Beijing/184/93-like virus. The *southern hemisphere* influenza vaccines for the May to October 2000 season should contain: A/ Moscow/10/99(H3N2)-like virus, A/New Caledonia/20/99(H1N1)-like virus, and B/Beijing/184/ 93-like or B/Shangdong/7/97-like virus.

Salk first described a killed influenza vaccine in 1945. Early whole virus vaccines contained intact, formalin-inactivated virus and were associated with many adverse effects. Many of our elderly patients still remember the pre-1966 live attenuated vaccines, when 'having the vaccine was virtually as bad as having the disease'. The modern subunit vaccines we use today are very well tolerated and evoke a good serological response.

Two forms of subunit vaccine are available: split virus vaccines (Begrivac, Inactivated influenza vaccine BP Pasteur, Fluarix) contain fragmented virus particles that have been partially purified by extraction with organic solvents, and sub-unit surface antigen vaccine (Fluvirin, Influvac), which is composed of highly purified haemagglutinin and neuraminidase antigens. The vaccines are equivalent in efficacy and adverse reactions.

Administration

- Children aged 6 months to 12 years, who may not have been previously infected or who have not received the flu vaccine (unprimed), require two doses of the vaccine. The second dose should be given after an interval of at least 4 weeks (Table 34.2).
- When a 0.25-mL dose is indicated, the prefilled syringe should be held in an upright position and half the volume should be eliminated, the remaining volume should be injected.
- Influenza vaccine should be given by IM or deep SC injection. The deltoid muscle is the recommended site for adults and older children, the anterolateral thigh for children under 1 year of age. In adults, and especially elderly patients, as a precaution the left arm should be avoided because of the possibility that left upper limb pain experienced may be attributed to the influenza vaccine when, in fact, this may be a symptom of myocardial ischaemia/ infarction (I have had such a case). Patients with bleeding disorders should have the vaccine by the SC route and in consultation with their physician.
- Allow the vaccine to reach room temperature before injection.

Table 34.2 Administration specifications for all available influenza vaccines.

Age	Dose (ml)	Route	Reinforcing dose 'Unprimed child'* aged 6 months to 12 years	Booster
6–35 months	0.25–0.50	IM or deep SC	4–6 weeks	None
Children from 36 months	0.50	IM or deep SC	4–6 weeks	None
Adults	0.50	IM or deep SC		None

*An 'Unprimed child' is not previously infected or immunized.

- The vaccine is effective if given 1 month (but at least 10 days) before exposure to the virus is anticipated. The UK influenza vaccination programme starts in October.
- Clinical effectiveness in adults is about 70–80%. In patients over the age of 65 effectiveness in preventing clinical illness is 30–40%. More importantly, influenza vaccination in the elderly is associated with a significant reduction in the severity of disease, incidence of bronchopneumonia, rate of admission to hospital by as much as 60% and mortality by around 40% compared with matched controls (CMO's letter of 1 August 2000, available on the Internet at: http://www.open.gov/doh/cmo/cmoh.htm). High immunization coverage (over 80%) of the elderly in residential or nursing homes appears to generate sufficient herd immunity that limits the spread of the disease.
- Seroprotection is generally obtained within 2–3 weeks. Postvaccination immunity lasts for 6–12 months.
- Antibody response in patients immunosuppressed by disease or treatment may be insufficient.
- Immunize HIV patients annually and particularly before travel.
- The antibody titres induced by influenza vaccine decline over a period of 3–6 months. Avoid administering the vaccine too far in advance of the influenza season. As the antibody level may take up to 10–14 days to rise, the ideal time to vaccinate is in October in anticipation of influenza activity by mid-November. For continuous protection, vaccinate annually.
- Revaccination each year should take place with the currently recommended vaccine and any unused vaccines from the previous year should be discarded.
- Ensure that the practice has a yearly influenza immunization programme in place, which includes the recall of high-risk patients for revaccination.
- Flu vaccine can alter the hepatic clearance of several commonly used drugs, among them warfarin, phenytoin and theophylline. These changes do not seem to be clinically significant. None the less, the GP and nurse should be alert to this possibility.

- Inactivated (killed) influenza vaccine does not cause influenza, neither does it protect from other influenza viruses not contained in the vaccine, nor from other organisms that may cause respiratory and generalized infections during the influenza season. The expectations of patients therefore may differ from what the vaccine can deliver and should be warned about this.
- As the 'at-risk groups' for influenza and pneumococcal infection are similar, consider combining influenza with pneumococcal immunization—the pneumococcal vaccine is given once only. Asplenic patients require yearly influenza vaccination.

Who should receive the vaccine?

The DoH's Chief Medical Officer writes to GPs yearly giving advice on the recommendations for influenza immunization for all those in whom the disease is more likely to be a serious illness. These are individuals with:

(a) chronic respiratory disease, including asthma;
(b) chronic heart disease;
(c) chronic renal disease;
(d) diabetes mellitus and other endocrine disorders;
(e) immunosuppression as a result of disease or treatment, including patients with anatomical or functional asplenia;
(f) those living in long-stay residential accommodation (residents of nursing homes, residential homes and other chronic care facilities);
(g) all those aged 65 years and over.

The DoH does not recommend routine immunization of fit children and adults, including healthcare and other key workers such as home-care staff, district nurses, carers and household members of high-risk persons, but leaves the final decision as to who should be offered immunization to the patient's medical practitioner. The extension of the DoH's recommendations to include all people aged 75 years and over (1998) was welcome, because many elderly people will have some conditions that put them at special risk of complications resulting from influenza. A further extension to 65 years and over was announced in 2000. Patients 65 years and over make up about 20% of a GP's list, although this depends greatly on the area; some coastal towns are favoured by people who have retired. Elderly people without high-risk con-ditions do have an increased morbidity resulting from influenza, although to a lesser degree than do those with underlying medical conditions.

In the USA, vaccination is recommended for the following groups of people who are at increased risk for complications from influenza or who have a higher prevalence of chronic medical conditions that place them at risk for influenza-related complications:

● people aged 50 years and over;
● residents of nursing homes and other chronic-care facilities that house people of any age who have chronic medical conditions;
● adults and children who have chronic disorders of the pulmonary or cardiovascular systems, including asthma;
● adults and children who have required regular medical follow-up or hospitalization during the preceding year because of chronic metabolic diseases (including diabetes mellitus), renal dysfunction, haemoglobinopathies or immunosuppression (because of disease or treatment);
● children and teenagers (aged 6 months to 18 years) who are receiving long-term aspirin therapy (at risk of developing Reye's syndrome after influenza infection);
● women who will be in the second or third trimester of pregnancy during the influenza season; and
● all health care workers, including night and weekend staff, are recommended for vaccination.

Vaccine availability

All influenza vaccines are available in a prefilled single-dose (0.5 mL) syringe. Shake the syringe well to distribute the suspension uniformly before injecting.
● Begrivac (Wyeth Laboratories).
● Fluarix (SmithKline Beecham Pharmaceuticals).
● Fluvirin (Medeva Pharma).
● Inactivated Influenza Vaccine (split virion) BP (Aventis Pasteur MSD).
● Influvac (Solvay Healthcare).

Storage. Between 2 and 8 °C. *Do not freeze*. Protect from light. Allow the vaccine to reach room temperature before use.

Influenza infection

This infection is caused by an orthomyxovirus, of which there are three antigenically distinct types: A, B and C. In fifteenth century Florence, the influence (influenza) of the stars on the planets was thought to be the cause of this short, febrile illness. In 1931, influenza virus type A was isolated from pigs and 2 years later from humans; type B was isolated in 1940 and type C in 1947. The first description of influenza we have comes from Hippocrates in 412 BC. The first documented influenza pandemic occurred in 1580.

Influenza A is the most important influenza virus in humans but can also infect many different animal species including horses, pigs, whales, seals and a large variety of birds. It has been the cause of many epidemics and pandemics such as the Spanish flu in 1918, Asian flu in 1957, Hong Kong flu in 1968 and Red flu in 1977. An extraordinary mutation may have been the reason why the 1918 influenza A virus (H1N1) proved so lethal, causing the death of 30 million people, many of whom were healthy and young (compare this to the 8.5 million people that lost their lives in World War I, 1914–18). In the UK, between September and November 1918 at the peak of the outbreak, 225 000 people died. There is evidence that the viruses that caused these epidemics originated from animals: 1918, swine; 1957 and 1968, avian strains.

The 1989/90 influenza epidemic was the worst to have hit England and Wales since 1976 and was most probably caused by type A. During the epidemic, there were almost 29 000 more deaths than would be expected for that time of the year. Of these excess deaths, 60% were in women and more than 85% were in people aged over 65 years. In 1993, there were more than 13 000 excess deaths attributed to influenza in Britain. Every year we expect to see 3000–4000 deaths in the UK as a result of influenza, with incidence rising during epidemics.

Influenza A viruses are classified into subtypes on the basis of their two surface glycoprotein

Fig. 34.1 The influenza virus.

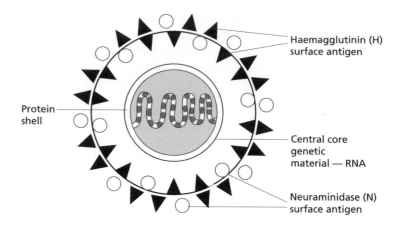

Haemagglutinin (H) surface antigen

Protein shell

Central core genetic material — RNA

Neuraminidase (N) surface antigen

antigens, haemagglutinin (H) and neuraminidase (N) or sialidase (Fig. 34.1). The human disease is caused by three H (H1, H2, H3) and two N (N1, N2) antigenic subtypes. Each human virus contains a combination of one type of H and one of N. A series of minor changes in the gene that encodes H can occur ('antigenic drift'), so that antibodies no longer recognize this antigenic site and previous infection or immunization becomes ineffective. These 'drifts' result from a high number of mutations that affect the H surface glycoprotein. Occasionally there is a major change in the H surface antigen ('antigenic shift'). This requires a double infection, that is infection of the same cell by two viruses. This is thought to occur when whole segments of RNA from animal viruses are incorporated into human viruses. A virus with an entirely new H emerges and can result in a pandemic. A cell that is infected simultaneously by two strains of type A virus with haemagglutinins or neuraminidases of different serotypes produces hybrid viruses. All combinations are theoretically possible and lead to more radical changes than those associated with antigenic drift. Such recombinations also take place in nature and have been responsible for pandemics.

Influenza B viruses also undergo mutations and change exclusively through antigenic drift, although less frequently as they are more stable. Influenza B viruses only have one subtype of H and one of N—they do not divide into subtypes. They are found exclusively in humans but an extension to animals was recently found with the identifica-

tion of influenza B virus in seals by a Dutch team (oral presentation at the Good Vaccination Practice Conference, Monaco, April 2000).

Influenza virus infection does not stimulate permanent immunity to reinfection with the same subtype of virus because of the new emerging variants. The same will apply to immunity acquired by vaccines, which is even less effective. Protection from vaccination lasts for about 6 months to 1 year. There is therefore a need for annual vaccination in order to provide continuing protection.

Presentation

Influenza is a highly contagious acute viral disease of the respiratory tract affecting all ages and about 20% of the population annually, although only a small number consult a doctor. It occurs worldwide in the winter or early spring. The highest transmission period in the northern hemisphere is from November to March while in the southern hemisphere this is April to September. In the tropics, it occurs throughout the year.

Transmission is airborne by droplets, particularly in enclosed spaces, when an infected person talks, coughs or sneezes. The virus can persist for hours particularly in cold and low-humidity environments. The incubation time is 1–3 days. The patient excretes the virus in respiratory secretions already a day or two before the symptoms develop and until about 5–7 days after. They therefore remain infectious for others from a day or two before and for 3–5 days after the onset of clinical symptoms in adults, and an average of 7 days (up to 13 days) in children. Because of the symptoms, it is often assumed that influenza is a systemic infection. In fact, the influenza virus stays in the respiratory tract and has not been found beyond this site. Unlike some other viruses, such as varicella, influenza is not blood borne; the primary site of viral replication is the respiratory tract.

It presents with sudden onset pyrexia (38–40 °C, peaks within 24 h of onset and lasts 1–5 days), headaches, coryza, anorexia, chills, arthralgia and myalgia. A dry cough can follow with a sore throat and malaise. Vomiting and, more rarely, diarrhoea can also occur, especially in children. In mild-to-moderate cases, it is a self-limiting disease lasting about 72 h, with recovery within 7 days. In more severe cases, the virus can invade the lungs (primary viral pneumonia) or contribute to a secondary bacterial lung infection.

A distinction should be made between a cold and influenza according to the symptoms. The cold presents gradually, over days, with milder symptoms and only sometimes with a mild fever while the patient with influenza looks ill, the fever is marked, headaches are severe and symptoms develop rapidly. Malaise and muscular aches and pains in the case of a cold are mild, while in influenza these are profound and severe, to the point that the patient finds it extremely difficult to get out of bed. Nasal congestion in the case of a cold is usually prominent and the appetite is often unaffected. In influenza, nasal congestion can be minimal and the appetite is very limited if any. Sore throat and cough may occur in both cold and influenza.

Influenza can be complicated by acute exacerbations of chronic respiratory disease: viral (influenza) pneumonitis; secondary bacterial pneumonia; otitis media; croup and bronchiolitis in infants and young children; febrile convulsions; Reye's syndrome; myositis; myocarditis; Guillain–Barré syndrome; transverse myelitis; and encephalitis. Most at risk are patients who, because of their age or underlying health problems, are unlikely to cope with the disease.

There is some evidence that influenza A infection may be associated with fetal or perinatal mortality. Large epidemiological studies are necessary to confirm this association. None the less, GPs and nurses should be aware of the possibility of influenza A infection adversely influencing fetal survival. Increased rates of miscarriage, stillbirth and premature birth have been observed during the 1918 and 1957 pandemics.

According to the DoH and the Royal College of General Practitioners (RCGP), a weekly consultation rate of 50–200 per 100 000 patient population reflects normal winter activity. A rate of 200–400 reflects above-average winter activity. The official definition of an influenza epidemic is 400 cases per 100 000 population in 1 week.

Management

Physical rest, fluids and paracetamol are important. Within about 72 h the patient is starting to feel better. Signs that should alert the physician to a bacterial respiratory infection complicating influenza are breathlessness, purulent sputum, pleuritic pain, with the illness extending to well over 72 h without signs of improvement. Provided the patient does not exhibit cyanosis, hypotension (diastolic blood pressure dropping below 70 mmHg), tachypnoea over 25 breaths per minute, diffuse fine crepitations, or vomits, dehydrates or appears confused, they can be looked after in the community (at home). Antibiotics need to target the causative agents of bacterial lung infection which are mainly *Streptococcus pneumoniae* (38%), *Staphylococcus aureus* alone (19%) or in combination with other agents (7%), *Haemophilus influenzae* (11%) and other Gram-negative bacteria including group A β-haemolytic streptococci. Amoxycillin, cephalosporins or erythromycin are a good choice. Reserve ciprofloxacin for unresolving or complicated chest infections.

The first specific therapy to be available for influenza A virus is amantadine hydrochloride; it is ineffective against type B virus. It prevents viral penetration of the cell membrane and has no direct viricidal action. It does not interfere with antibody production, whether from the vaccine or an actual infection, and best results are achieved when it is given within 48 h of onset of symptoms.

Although it is as effective (60–80%) as influenza vaccine in preventing influenza A virus, it is not a substitute for annual immunization of groups 'at risk'.

The DoH recommends amantadine during an outbreak of influenza A in the following circumstances, although it warns that indiscriminate use of amantadine could lead to viral resistance:
• for nonimmunized patients 'at risk' for 2 weeks while the vaccine takes effect;
• for patients 'at risk', in whom immunization is contraindicated (I would personally add, also for those at risk who refuse immunization), for the duration of the outbreak;
• for healthcare workers and other key personnel to prevent disruption of services during an epidemic.
In addition, consider amantadine in the following:
• immunodeficient persons who may have poor antibody response to the vaccine;
• nonimmunized carers at home;
• persons with influenza A, to decrease the duration of fever and other systemic symptoms provided it can be started within 48 h of their onset.

The recommended dose is 100 mg daily. Adverse reactions occur in 5–20% of patients and include nausea, anorexia, light-headedness, insomnia, headaches, restlessness, anxiety, difficulty in concentrating and even depression. Epileptic fits may occasionally occur, mainly in elderly patients taking more than 100 mg/day. Exercise care in patients with renal impairment as amantadine is excreted renally and can cause neurological side-effects.

Neuraminidase promotes influenza virus release from infected host cells (which are turned into 'flu factories' by the invading influenza virus) and facilitates virus spread within the respiratory tract. Several potent and specific inhibitors of this enzyme have been developed. The sialic acid analogues specifically inhibit both influenza A and B virus neuraminidase, thus viral growth and spread to other cells. Unlike amantadine, which targets the M2 protein ion channels of influenza A viruses (B viruses lack M2 protein), these neuraminidase inhibitors inhibit replication of both influenza A and B viruses. Zanamavir, administered by inhalation, has been licensed in the UK. Oseltamivir, administered orally, was expected to have been available for the winter season of 2000/01 but did

not file for a license. Zanamavir is administered by inhalation from a dry powder inhaler (diskhaler), two (5-mg) doses twice daily for 5 days starting as soon as possible, within 48 h of the onset of symptoms. It is licensed for the treatment (not prevention) of influenza in people aged 12 years and over.

Zanamavir was the subject of a rapid appraisal by the National Institute of Clinical Excellence (NICE) in 1999. The Institute concluded that, on the basis of clinical trial evidence, the use of Zanamivir within 48 h of the onset of symptoms of influenza reduces the duration of the symptoms by 1 day (1.2 days in at-risk persons). In 2000, NICE revised its guidance. The use of zanamivir is recommended only when 'flu is circulating in the community, for the treatment of at-risk adults able to commence treatment within 48 hours of the start of their symptoms and suffering from diabetes, cardiovascular disease (not hypertension), chronic respiratory disease (asthma, COPD) or immunosuppression, or are aged over 65.

The manufacturer of Zanamavir (Glaxo-Wellcome) has issued a warning to doctors that it could cause bronchospasm and serious respiratory deterioration. Caution should be exercised when prescribing this drug for influenza to patients with asthma or chronic obstructive pulmonary disease.

Seasonal variations in heart disease and influenza immunization

Numerous studies in the past have suggested that infection may promote atherosclerosis, myocardial infarction (MI), stroke, restenosis, aortic aneurysm and peripheral vascular disease. A possible relationship between influenza and MI was first suggested after epidemics of influenza struck Europe and the USA in the early 1990s. In those epidemics, about half of the excess mortality was attributed to causes other than influenza, including heart disease. As influenza immunization reduces the risk of acquiring influenza, and of hospitalization and death, particularly among the elderly, would influenza vaccination reduce the incidence of MI in patients with established coronary atherosclerosis?

This was the hypothesis researchers from the

University of Texas, Houston, School of Medicine, under Dr Ward Casscells set out to examine with a retrospective case–control study. This they performed on patients with a previous history of MI, who were seen in the hospital outpatients department during the influenza season of October 1997 to March 1998. They presented their results at the 49th Annual Scientific Session of the American College of Cardiology in Anaheim in March 2000.

After adjustment of other predictive variables, such as smoking, hypertension, hyperlipidaemia, medication, previous influenza immunization and vitamin intake, influenza vaccination was found to be associated with a 67% reduction in the risk of subsequent MI. Such a case–control study is not definitive, but can generate new hypotheses. Would the use of amantadine or a neuraminidase inhibitor prevent further MI in these patients? What is the role of chest infections (the researchers did not examine this parameter)? Does pneumococcal vaccination also protect against MI? Does influenza vaccination protect those under 65 years of age with no coronary heart disease (CHD) risk factors?

Practice immunization programme

In the UK in the 1989 epidemic, only 10–20% of those people considered to be 'at risk' did in fact receive the vaccine. Following this epidemic, in 1991/92 the uptake was raised to 41%. In 1996/97 less than 44% of elderly patients within the 'at risk' groups received the vaccine according to the PHLS. A much greater effort to target these people is therefore needed by the members of the primary healthcare team. All patients classified by the DoH as 'at risk' (these include all individuals over 65 years of age) should be immunized if they agree. Do not forget the practice staff.

The practice morbidity data, the age–sex register and the computerized repeat prescription system will be necessary. The practice can post invitations or attach them to the repeat prescriptions, and put posters up in the waiting room. As influenza activity is rarely significant before the end of November, the best time to start the immunization campaign is in August and vaccinations in October. Experience from previous years and practice data should give an idea of the number of doses of influenza vaccine needed.

A practice influenza immunization programme needs to have the following elements:
- identified target group held on a database;
- effective call and recall system;
- an effective mechanism for dealing with defaulters;
- year-on-year patient education and vaccine promotion programme;
- a healthcare team committed to prevention.

Practices in England and Wales can recover their vaccine purchasing expenses and even make a profit by buying and dispensing the vaccine under paragraph 44.5 of the *Statement of Fees and Allowances*—Red Book (SFA) (see p. 243). The practice profit depends to a great extent on the discount obtainable when buying directly from the manufacturers or wholesalers. In addition, an item-of-service fee is payable by the DoH for vaccinating patients aged 65 or over. Vaccination of patients under this age with chronic disease does not qualify for this IOS.

Influenza is a highly infectious disease that spreads rapidly in the community, especially in institutions. Epidemics occur in an unpredictable manner. Quite a number of patients tend to think of influenza as a relatively mild disease because it is confused with the common cold and other types of respiratory tract infections. In fact, influenza is a potentially lethal condition, especially in at-risk and elderly patients, and preventing it is an important community task for the GP and the primary healthcare team.

The case for influenza immunization

An estimated 10% of the population worldwide or about 500 million people 'catch' influenza each year [Ghendon Y. (1992) Influenza—its impact and control. *World Health Stat. Q.* 45, 306–10]. This could translate into about 5 million people in the UK each year.

Each year influenza is associated with substantial morbidity, increased absenteeism from work and school and considerable misery for many thousands of individuals and families. The infection exerts a considerable drain on both human and economic resources. Employees not only report absent from work but also reduced effectiveness on return to work. Hospital resources become overburdened owing to increased acute admissions, particularly among the elderly and patients at risk of complications. Even in a non-epidemic year, influenza has been shown to have a considerable impact on productivity, and lead to substantial consumption of healthcare resources [Keech M. *et al.* (1998) The impact of influenza and influenza-like illness on productivity and healthcare resource utilization in a working population. *Occup. Med.* 48, 85–90].

Influenza in the young and healthy causes a significant increase in absenteeism, but is rarely life-threatening. In older people, it is a major cause of hospitalization and mortality during winter months. Even in a nonepidemic year, it is estimated that as many as 3000–4000 deaths in the UK are attributed to influenza. Over 80% of deaths occur among people over 65 years of age [Nicholson K.G. (1990) Influenza vaccination and the elderly. *Br. Med. J.* 301, 617–18].

The present UK national policy set by the DoH continues to be for annual selective immunization of all people over the age of 65, and 'high-risk' patients for whom influenza is more likely to be a serious or complicated illness, regardless of age. A similar policy is followed by the Netherlands, Denmark, Sweden and Finland. Canada, Australia, New Zealand and France have extended their recommendations to include all elderly people (usually aged 65 years and over) and others outside this age group whose underlying chronic illness places them at high risk of influenza and its complications. With the adoption of this policy in the UK, it has made targeting of high-risk groups more straightforward, much easier to achieve and it will not discriminate against people who have led healthier lifestyles—they, too, need protection. Even better, would be an extension to age 60 and over.

In 2000, the US Advisory Committee on Immunization Practices (ACIP) recommended the lowering of the age for routine influenza vaccination from 65 to 50, in order to increase vaccination levels in the 50–60-year-old age group. Between 24–32% of persons in this age group have a chronic medical condition that places them at high risk for influenza-related hospitalization and death. Vaccination levels of high-risk persons aged 50–60 have been low, and aged-based strategies are usually more successful than risk-based vaccination strategies.

Studies have shown that influenza immunization produced a reduction of more than 50% of cases of respiratory illness, pneumonia, hospitalization and mortality. A UK study has shown that immunizing patients against influenza can reduce mortality by about 40%, and repeated annual vaccinations can reduce mortality by 75% [(1995) *Lancet* 346, 591–5].

An American study [Nichol, K.L., Lind, A., Margolis, K.L. *et al.* (1995) The effectiveness of vaccination against influenza in healthy working adults. *New Engl. J. Med.* 333, 889–93] looked into the effectiveness of vaccination against influenza in healthy, working adults aged 18–64 years. Those receiving the vaccine reported 25% fewer episodes of upper respiratory illness, had 43% fewer days off work and made 44% fewer visits for medical consultation regarding upper respiratory illness than those injected with placebo—results that will be greatly welcomed by the UK medical practices and industry.

Another American study [Nichol, K.L., Margolis, K.L., Wuorenma, J. & Von Sternberg, T. (1994) The efficacy and cost effectiveness of vaccination among elderly persons living in the community. *New Engl. J. Med.* 331, 778–85] showed that for each season there was a reduced rate of hospitalization for pneumonia and influenza (by 48–57%) and for all acute and chronic respiratory conditions (by 27–39%) in those receiving the vaccine. Mortality from all causes was also reduced by 39–54%. The direct cost savings attributable to influenza vaccination in this study averaged $117 per patient for each of the 41 418 people immunized during the 3 years of the study.

In October 2000, an American study that ran between 1997 and 1999 concluded that influenza vaccination of healthy working adults aged 18 to 64 years can reduce the rates of influenza-like illness (by 34%), lost workdays (by 32%) and physician visits (by 42%) during years when the vaccine and circulating viruses are similar. The vaccine efficacy was 86%. However, they also found that vaccination may not provide overall economic benefits (net cost $11.17) in those years when the vaccine does not match circulating viruses [Bridges, C.B., Thompson, W.W., Meltzer, M.I., *et al.* (2000) Effectiveness and cost-benefit of influenza vaccination of healthy working adults: a randomised controlled trial. *J. Am. Med. Assoc.* **284**, 1655–1663].

Another study evaluated the effect of influenza vaccination in day-care children on reducing influenza morbidity among their household contacts. They found that unvaccinated household contacts of influenza-vaccinated day-care children had 42% fewer febrile respiratory illnesses compared with unvaccinated household contacts of control children. Among school-aged household contacts (aged 5–17 years), there was an 80% reduction among contacts of vaccinated children vs. contacts of unvaccinated children in febrile respiratory illnesses [Hurwitz, E.S., Haber, M., Chang ,A. *et al.* (2000) Effectiveness of influenza vaccination of day care children in reducing influenza-related morbidity among household contacts. *J. Am. Med. Assoc.* **284**, 1677–1682].

Influenza vaccine is effective in preventing infections in healthcare professionals and may reduce the number of days lost as a result of illness, according to a US study [Wilde J. *et al.* (1999) Effectiveness of influenza vaccine in health care professionals, a randomised trial. *J. Am. Med. Assoc.* **281**, 908–13]. The trial was carried out between 1992 and 1995 in two teaching hospitals in Baltimore. A total of 264 subjects without chronic medical problems were recruited. Researchers found that immunization achieved an 88% reduction in influenza A infections ($P = 0.001$) and 89% for influenza B ($P = 0.03$). Among the influenza vaccinees, cumulative days of reported febrile respiratory illness were 28.7 per 100 subjects compared with 40.6 per 100 subjects in controls ($P = 0.57$), and days of absence were 9.9 per 100 subjects against 21.1 per 100 subjects in controls ($P = 0.41$). The authors concluded that these data support a policy of annual influenza vaccination of healthcare professionals.

Nosocomial infection with influenza poses an important risk for elderly patients in long-term care. A Glasgow team investigated whether voluntary vaccination of healthcare staff in long-term geriatric hospitals would lower the rates of virologically proven influenza and mortality among patients compared with current practice of no routine vaccination. They found that in the hospitals where the healthcare workers were offered vaccination (50.9% uptake), there was a significant decrease in mortality among patients from 22.4% in 'nonvaccine' hospitals to 13.6% in the 'vaccine' hospitals. There was no decrease in the frequency of nonfatal influenza infection [Carman W. *et al.* (2000) Effects of influenza vaccination of healthcare workers on mortality of elderly people in long-term care: a randomised controlled trial. *Lancet* **355**, 93–7]. The research team has also found serological evidence of influenza infection in 23% of hospital staff in a winter season, and warns that there is a significant potential for staff to infect patients. Protecting staff may therefore be a useful additional strategy to lower transmission among frail, elderly patients for whom vaccination offers incomplete protection.

In the October 1996 issue of *Effectiveness Matters*, the NHS Centre for Reviews and Dissemination recommended annual influenza immunization of everyone aged over 65 years. They based this recommendation on a systematic review of research showing that vaccinating elderly people against influenza is an effective, safe and cost-effective way of reducing influenza-related deaths and illness.

Another British review published in 1998 [McColl A. *et al.* (1998) Performance indicators for primary care groups: an evidence based approach. *Br. Med. J.* **317**, 1354–60] pointed out that influenza immunization for those aged 65 and over was likely to be cost effective. They calculated that 108 people aged over 65 need to receive influenza vaccination each year to prevent one death. In a population of 100 000 this intervention could prevent 146 deaths each year.

I would support influenza vaccination being extended to all those over 60 years of age in the UK. At the time of concerns with escalating NHS costs and shortages of hospital facilities and rising acute admissions to hospitals, it would be prudent for the DoH to extend its influenza vaccination recommendations to all above 60 years of age. We will not just increase the chances of survival in our patients who have retired, but we will also improve their quality of life by a simple annual jab in the arm.

Why can we not recommend annual influenza immunization to anyone, of any age, who wants to decrease his/her likelihood of catching influenza? Employers and DoH should seek to have a common policy.

Numbers needed to treat (NNT)

Using UK mortality data and the effectiveness figures from UK studies, it has been estimated that in 1989 the number of older people who have needed to be vaccinated to prevent one death would have been 40 in high-risk groups and 240 in other groups. In the nonepidemic year of 1993, these figures were 80 and 500, respectively.

Taking into consideration the fact that we expect two cases of influenza in every 23 people aged over 60 years, and using the numbers-needed-to-treat (NNT) method, one case in every 23 can be prevented by influenza immunization, thus immunization prevents half the cases of influenza in people over 60 years of age. The NNT in healthy adults is 9.2 (7.8–11.1). This means that for every nine healthy adults given influenza vaccine, one will avoid having influenza that would have had it if they had not been vaccinated [(2000) *Bandolier 73*, 7(3), 8]. Infected healthy adults can spread the infection to individuals in the 'at risk' groups.

A new flu virus—a new pandemic?

In 1994 Shortridge isolated avian H1N1 influenza virus from pigs and found evidence of pig-to-pig spread. The fear now is that a bird–pig–man triangle can become a potential source of a viral shift that could start a pandemic of human influenza [(1997) *Lancet* 349, 36].

The outbreak of avian flu in Hong Kong began in May 1997, when a 3-year-old Chinese boy died from respiratory failure secondary to viral pneumonia and Reye's syndrome (recognized influenza complications). The strain of the virus that struck the boy was identified in August as H5N1, a typically avian influenza virus that infects predominantly chickens. The boy and his family had not come into contact with these birds and none of the boy's family tested positive for antibodies to H5N1. On the other hand, one of the doctors that treated the boy at Queen Mary Hospital did test positive raising the possibility of human-to-human transmission. By December, antibodies to H5N1 virus were found in another eight out of a total of 502 contacts of further cases that had occurred in Hong Kong, none of whom had serious symptoms.

Until the middle of January 1998 there had been 18 confirmed cases with six deaths reported to the WHO. The Hong Kong administration took the precaution of destroying over a million chickens and banning imports of live poultry from China.

The influenza virus strain H5N1 is not new. It was first isolated in South Africa in 1961 and has since caused epidemics in poultry. In late March and early May 1997 there was an outbreak in three farms in Hong Kong with a mortality rate coming close to 100%.

The puzzle of viral transmission

New strains of human flu emerge after the influenza virus genes have intermingled in pig cells with genes from strains of human or avian flu, or both. This is possible in pigs as they possess human and avian flu receptors. The question now is how did this exclusively avian H5N1 virus managed to infect humans? Is this through a chance contact between human and bird, or bird faeces, or direct human-to-human transmission? If this avian virus acquires the ability to be transmitted from human to human then the entire world is vulnerable as a pandemic could follow.

The virus characteristics

Scientists from the USA and Hong Kong have found that the H5 protein contains multiple basic amino acids adjacent to the cleavage site of the viral haemag-glutinin (H). This feature is characteristic of highly pathogenic viruses such as the one that resulted in the pandemic of 1918. Most flu viruses infect the respiratory and alimentary tracts. These extra amino acids may permit the H5N1 flu virus spread beyond these tracts, e.g. to the heart and brain.

Person-to-person transmission has not been confirmed so far in any of the reported cases. The doctor that treated the young boy had antibodies to the virus but did not become ill. The worry is that the currently circulating H5N1 strain could mix with another strain more adept at passing on to humans. This could trigger a pandemic. China is the hypothetical epicentre from where a pandemic virus will emerge next, but it is reasonable to assert that it could do this anywhere in the world, where there are concentrations of birds, perhaps pigs, and human beings.

Logistic and ethical dilemmas in case of a pandemic

From the time the Hong Kong problem was identified to the point when the laboratories were possibly able to produce a vaccine for that strain, a year had passed. New techniques for massive production of influenza vaccines are necessary so that they can be produced with speed, and so that we do not have to rely on the availability of hens' eggs in cases of unforeseen increased requirements.

A further problem is the number of vaccines that we could produce with the present production capabilities we have. In case of pandemic, the vaccine-producing countries will be able to produce only a relatively limited number of vaccines. The question is who will get the available vaccines? How are we going to prioritize? What about supplying vaccines, if any, to the developing world? France is a vaccine-producing country. It now needs 6 million doses per year. In case of a pandemic it will need for itself 60 million doses of vaccine.

The WHO published its pandemic planning document (http://www.who.int/emc and search under influenza) in April 1999. It outlines the need for adequate planning by countries to deal with an influenza pandemic. Many developed countries, including the UK, France, Belgium and Switzerland, have a plan in place, while a number do not (Germany, Netherlands, Japan, China).

An influenza pandemic would have particular impact in developing countries, where influenza vaccine, antiviral drugs and health professionals are in short supply. These countries need to develop a pandemic plan around available resources. New data from the 1918 pandemic has showed the appalling impact in areas such as sub-Saharan Africa and India. Of the estimated 30 million deaths, 17 million occurred in India, where there was a death rate of 30 per 100 000 population, compared with 5 per 100 000 in Europe and North America.

Risk of influenza to travellers

Influenza viruses circulate throughout the world. Travellers are exposed to these viruses outside their country's influenza season. The risk of exposure to influenza during travel depends on the time of the year, destination, type of travel, e.g. large organized tourist groups containing people from different areas in the world, the mode of travel, e.g. ship, aeroplane.

Persons at increased risk for complications of influenza should consider immunization before travel, if they were not vaccinated during the preceding winter. Summer outbreaks have frequently been reported on cruises in North America and in the Mediterranean. In 1998, an estimated 850 000 travellers, many elderly, from at least 45 countries, visited Alaska during the May–September summer travel season. An estimated 40 000–50 000 cases of influenza-like illness occurred during the summer outbreaks and several elderly travellers died from complicating pneumonia. Influenza-like symptoms were reported by 72% of the passengers aboard an aircraft that happened to encounter a 3-h delay on the ground and with inoperative ventilation.

More recent approaches to influenza vaccination

DNA vaccines are a long way from being made available (see p. 15). Live attenuated, cold-adapted, reassortant influenza virus vaccines have already been tried in children. They can be given intranasally, are well tolerated and produce good antibody response. They have not as yet come up for licensing in the UK but they are used in Russia.

Several live virus influenza vaccines have been develped in the past 25 years or so. One major concern has dogged live virus influenza vaccine development from the beginning: the possibility that the attenuated vaccine virus could reassort with virulent wild-type virus and produce a new agent to which the population is susceptible. The result, some scientists hold, could well be an influenza pandemic paralleling that of 1918–1919.

Information (websites)

• Updates on influenza activity in the UK can be found on the PHLS website: http://www.phls.co.uk/facts/influenza/Activity9900/fluact02.htm

• WHO influenza global network of centres, information for the public: http://oms.b3e.jussieu.fr/flunet

• The WHO's geographical information system to monitor influenza activity: http://www.who.int/emc/diseases/flu/index.html

• Information from national laboratories in WHO Weekly Epidemiological Report: http://www.who.int

• Influenza surveillance data collected weekly by CDC: http://www.cdc.gov/ncidod/diseases/flu/weekly.htm. Influenza activity updates on http://www.phls.co.uk/facts/influenza/fluactivity0001.htm

• Surveillance for Influenza—USA: http://www.cdc.gov/epo/mmwr/preview/mmwrhtml/ss4903a2.htm

• Information on influenza pandemic (FluAid): http://www.cdc.gov/od/nvpo/pandemics/

• CDC vaccination information: http://www.cdc.gov/nip/publications/mmwr/rr/rr4903.pdf

• The over-65s national coverage of influenza immunization was 61% at the end of November 2000—a remarkable achievement of co-operation between the DoH and primary care.

Chapter 35

Japanese B encephalitis

Contraindications to vaccination

- Acute febrile illness.
- Severe sensitivity to a previously administered Japanese B encephalitis vaccine.
- Severe sensitivity to the preservative thiomersal.
- Cardiac, hepatic and renal conditions, especially during acute exacerbations, unstable neurological conditions, immunodeficiency, and malignancy—lack of data on efficacy and adverse reactions of vaccine.
- Persons with history of allergies (including allergy to drugs), urticaria, especially to hymenoptera (bee stings) and history of angio-oedema have a greater risk of allergic reactions to the vaccine.
- Pregnancy, unless the pregnant woman is travelling to an endemic area with very high risk of infection.
- No data are available on the safety and efficacy of the vaccine among children under 1 year of age. Whenever possible, vaccination should be deferred until after the first year of life.

Possible side- and adverse effects

Local reactions

Swelling, redness and pain developing within hours to several days after vaccination occur in about 20% of vaccinees.

General reactions

Up to 10% of vaccinees suffer malaise, headaches, rigors, fever, nausea, vomiting, abdominal pain, myalgia. Urticaria, angio-oedema, dyspnoea and anaphylaxis within minutes and as long as two weeks after vaccination occur in approximately 0.3% of vaccinees. Encephalitis, encephalopathy, seizures and peripheral neuropathy are estimated to occur in 1–2.3 vaccinees per million.

Observe all persons receiving the vaccine for at least 30 min in the clinic and warn them about the possibility of delayed urticaria and angio-oedema. Advise them to defer international travel and remain in an area with ready access to medical care for at least 10 days after receiving the last dose—most reactions occur after the first dose within 10 days, with the majority (88%) occurring within 72 h. Instruct them to seek immediate medical care and take an over-the-counter antihistamine, if available, at the outset of any allergic reaction, particularly oedema of the extremities, face, lips and oropharynx. Consider supplying adrenaline injection to patients with a history of strong allergic reactions to insect stings or history of urticaria. If travel is soon or imminent, assess the risk of exposure to the virus against the risk of having a delayed allergic reaction and advise the traveller accordingly.

The vaccine

Both viral inactivated vaccines available in the UK are derived from infected mouse brain. They are prepared with the Nakayama strain, produced by the Research Foundation for Microbial Diseases of Osaka University (Biken).

Administration (Table 35.1)

- The two doses of the primary course can be given 1–2 weeks apart and induce seroconversion of approximately 80%. The third dose (at 30 days) increases seroconversion to 90–99%.

Table 35.1 Administration specifications for Japanese B encephalitis vaccine.

Age (years)	Dose (ml)	Route	Schedule			Reinforcing dose	Boosters
			Routine	Emergency	Extreme emergency		
JE-Vax (Aventis Pasteur MSD)							
1–3	0.5	SC	0, 7, 30 (3 doses)	0, 7, 14 (3 doses)	0, 14 (2 doses)	—	2 + years
> 3 and adults	1.0	SC					
Japanese B encephalitis vaccine (Korea Green Cross Corporation)							
1–3	0.5	SC	0, 7–14 (2 doses)	—	—	1 year (1 dose)	3 years (annually if at high risk)
> 3 and adults	1.0	SC					

● Both available vaccines are unlicensed and not available on the NHS. They can be purchased privately on a 'named-patient' basis only.

Vaccine availability

● JE-Vax—lyophilized Japanese B encephalitis vaccine Biken (Aventis Pasteur MSD) available in 1-mL vials.
● Japanese B encephalitis vaccine (Korea Green Cross Corporation) distributed in the UK by MASTA, available in 1-mL vials.

Storage: Between 2 and 8 °C. *Do not freeze.* Use within 8 h of reconstitution.

Japanese B encephalitis infection

Japanese B encephalitis is a mosquito-borne flavivirus infection that is endemic throughout most of the Far East and South-East Asia.

The hosts are mainly pigs, migrating birds and ducks. Transmission to humans is by the bite of infected rice field-breeding mosquitoes of the genus *Culex* that feed on pigs and birds (*Culex tritaeniorhynchus*). Fewer than 1–3% of mosquitoes are infected with the virus. The incubation period is 4–14 days. One in 200 infections becomes clinically apparent (99.5% asymptomatic) and the case fatality rate is estimated at 20–30%, with up to 50% of the survivors being left with neurological damage. Only 0.1–0.2% of infection is encephalitic. Most disease is reported in young children. Japan and China are now undertaking immunization of children. The peak season is the summer monsoon months (June–September), but sporadic cases occur throughout the year.

The disease occurs mainly in children under 15 years of age (85% of reported cases) in endemic areas. The development of symptomatic disease and neuroinvasive disease, as well as case fatality, may be more likely with advancing age (> 55 years of age). About 30 000–50 000 cases are reported annually from the affected areas of Asia, with an incidence rate of about 10 per 10 000. It is thought that the incidence of the disease is grossly underreported as in most cases infection causes a very mild disease. In India, only 1 in 500 infected children are symptomatic. The risk for contracting the disease has been estimated at one case per month per 5000 exposed travellers. The disease kills around 11 000 inhabitants and leaves another 9000 disabled every year.

Japanese B encephalitis is found exclusively in Asia, particularly in Bangladesh, India (in the East and South), Sri Lanka (north), Nepal, Burma, Thailand, Laos, Cambodia, Vietnam, Indonesia, Brunei, Borneo, Papua New Guinea, Philippines, Hong Kong, Korea, China and Japan (see Fig. 35.1).

Bali is a popular destination and there have been suggestions that the vaccine should be adminis-

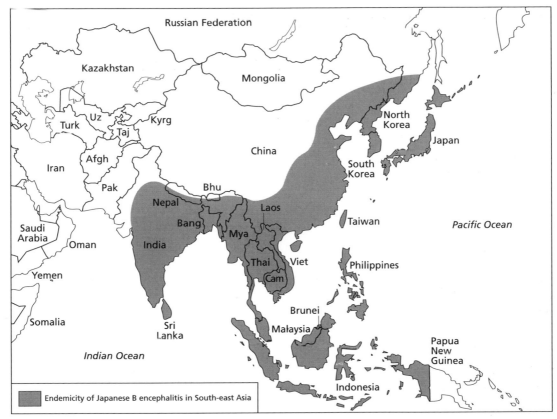

Fig. 35.1 Endemicity of Japanese B encephalitis in South-East Asia.

tered to short-term travellers to Bali because of reports of the death of a 51-year-old Danish man, who contracted Japanese B encephalitis after a 12-day stay in Bali, as well as the acquisition of the disease by a Swedish 60-year-old woman who stayed on the island for 10 days (both cases in 1995) and an Australian girl in 1989 after a 2-week holiday. There is no agreement on this recommendation.

No effective or specific treatment is available for Japanese B encephalitis.

● Disease and vaccine information from the CDC: www.cdc.gov/nip/publications/acip-list.htm.

The future

There is a need to identify the inactivated vaccine components that produce hypersensitivity, and study the appropriate interval for boosters as this issue requires clarification.

The Chinese have developed a live attenuated vaccine from Japanese encephalitis virus strain SA 14–14–2 which was passed through weaning mice and is produced in primary baby hamster kidney cells. This vaccine has been shown to be safe and immunogenic with an effectiveness rate of 98%. Further controlled studies on the safety are necessary. It requires two injections, none the less its cost is low ($0.03 per dose), which suggests it might be useful in the WHO Expanded Programme on Immunization.

Prevention

Prevention is by avoiding mosquito bites and by immunization. Precautions against insects should be taken, especially at dusk and dawn. Prevent mosquito bites by keeping arms and legs covered after sunset, and using insect repellents.

Vaccination is recommended for travellers to

endemic areas of South-East Asia and the Far East if one of the following conditions applies:
• short-term visitors to rural endemic areas if they undertake extensive outdoor activities;
• visitors staying more than 1 month in endemic areas, especially if they visit rural areas;
• consideration should be given to frequent visitors (e.g. those engaged in trade or commerce) to cities surrounded by endemic areas;
• expatriates living in endemic areas.

Chapter 36

Plague

Contraindications to vaccination

- Acute febrile illness.
- Severe reaction to a previously administered dose of the vaccine.
- Severe hypersensitivity (anaphylactic reaction) to phenol, beef protein and soya casein.
- Pregnancy, unless the mother is at high risk.

Possible side- and adverse effects

Local reactions

Swelling, redness and pain occur in approximately 10% of vaccinees.

General reactions

General reactions include headaches, fever, malaise and lymphadenopathy. Rarely urticaria and nausea, vomiting, myalgia, arthralgia and leucocytosis may occur.

The vaccine

Formalin-inactivated whole-cell *Yersinia pestis* vaccine has been grown in artificial media and preserved in phenol.

Administration (Table 36.1)

- The vaccine is administered by IM injection into the deltoid region.
- Seroconversion is estimated at 92% within 2 weeks of the second dose. Duration: 6–12 months.
- No safety or effectiveness data exist to support vaccination of individuals under 18 and over 61 years of age.
- Recommended generally for persons who will have direct contact with wild or commensal rodents or other animals in plague-epizootic areas, and for persons who will reside or work in plague-endemic rural areas where avoidance of rodents and fleas is difficult. In particular for:

  (a) veterinary surgeons, laboratory workers, geologists or biologists working directly with *Yersinia pestis*-infected animals;

  (b) long-stay travellers to endemic areas where the risk of contracting the disease is high;

  (c) workers travelling to disaster endemic areas;

  (d) military personnel deployed in endemic areas.
- It is not recommended for routine immunization of travellers.

Vaccine availability

The vaccine is not available in the UK and has to

Table 36.1 Immunization with plague vaccine.

First dose	Second dose	Third dose	Early booster	Further boosters
1 mL	0.2 mL 1–3 months after first	0.2 mL 5–6 months after second	Three booster doses 0.2 mL each, every 6 months if still at risk	0.2 mL every 1–2 years if risk of exposure persists

be imported from the USA on a 'named-patient' basis only. Contact Greer Laboratories Inc. (see p. 402). Readers in the UK should note that Bayer is not able to supply the vaccine. Store the vaccine at 2 to 8 °C. Discard if frozen.

Plague infection

The name plague is derived from the Greek plaga/ plege, which means a 'blow' or 'wound'. It is known in the West as the Black Death.

It is caused by *Yersinia pestis*, a bipolar strain, Gram-negative rod. It infects rodents and other animals. About 30 different kinds of fleas can transport the bacterium from one animal host to another (humans are a host, too).

Bubonic plague is transmitted by the bite of an infected flea or rodent, while pneumonic plague is transmitted by aerosols during direct contact with an infected patient or an infected animal.

The incubation time is 2–6 days for the bubonic plague and slightly shorter for the pneumonic variety. Symptoms include fever, headaches, myalgia, rigors and pain in the groin because of the lymphadenopathy. The condition can progress to septicaemia. The onset of symptoms is usually sudden, appearing 2–7 days after the infected flea bite. The organism can be isolated in blood cultures, cerebrospinal fluid or in sputum. It is sensitive to tetracycline and streptomycin.

Plague can be found in the western USA, parts of South America, Asia and Africa. In 1990, there were 7631 cases reported in 19 countries and 570 deaths but generally, an average of 1200 cases and 180 deaths were reported to the WHO between 1980 and 1994. Among countries reporting cases are the USA (10–30 cases/year), Kenya, Equator and Peru.

The control of fleas and suppression of the rodent population are important epidemic measures in countries that face the problem of plague. Appropriate short-term chemoprophylaxis is with tetracycline/doxycycline during periods of exposure. Trimethoprim-sulfamethoxazole is an acceptable substitute for use in children.

Plague is a notifiable disease.

● Disease and vaccine information from the CDC: www.cdc.gov/nip/publications/acip-list.htm.

Chapter 37

Pneumococcal infection

The polysaccharide pneumococcal vaccine

Contraindications to vaccination

- Acute febrile illness.
- Severe reaction to a previously administered dose of the vaccine.
- Severe hypersensitivity to thiomersal (Pnu-Imune).
- Children under 2 years of age—the vaccine has limited immunogenicity in these children (poor response, safety and efficacy not established).
- Pregnancy—it is not known whether the vaccine can cause fetal harm. The vaccine should not be used in pregnancy. If it is decided to immunize a pregnant woman with high-risk conditions such as cardiopulmonary or sickle cell disease, and it is not possible to vaccinate before pregnancy, it is advisable to wait until after the first trimester—the hospital consultant must be consulted.
- Breast-feeding is normally a contraindication.
- Revaccination within 3 years—high risk of adverse reactions.
- Revaccination of children under 10 years of age.
- Patients on immunosuppressive therapy or who have received it within the past 10 days.
- The vaccine should be avoided during chemotherapy or radiotherapy and less than 10 days prior to commencement of such therapy because the antibody response is poor. Vaccination could be considered 6 months after completion of chemotherapy and/or radiotherapy.
- Patients with Hodgkin's disease who have received extensive chemotherapy and/or nodal irradiation.

Possible side- and adverse effects

Local reactions

Redness and pain occur in up to 50% of vaccinees, also swelling and occasionally induration.

General reactions

Fever, headaches, malaise and myalgia are seen in less than 1% of vaccinees. Rash, urticaria, arthralgia rarely occur. Very rarely neurological disorders, including Guillain–Barré syndrome, glomerulonephritis, relapse of thrombocytopenia in patients with idiopathic thrombocytopenic purpura within 2 weeks of vaccination and lasting up to 2 weeks, and anaphylactic reaction.

Revaccination within 3–5 years or vaccination of individuals who have previously received the 14-valent pneumococcal vaccine was associated with increased risk of reactions (because of high levels of circulating antibodies). The same applies to the present 23-valent vaccine.

The vaccine

The 23-valent pneumococcal vaccine contains puri-fied, capsular polysaccharide antigens of 23 pneumococcal serotypes responsible for 85–90% of bacteraemic infections. It has replaced the 14-valent vaccine.

The 23-valent vaccine contains 25 µg of each capsular polysaccharide antigen (the 14-valent vaccine contained 50 µg of each antigen). In common with other polysaccharide vaccines, it does not induce T-cell-dependent responses associated with immunological memory. Following vaccination, well over 80% of healthy adults will develop a good antibody response for 5 years that will

Table 37.1 Administration specifications for polysaccharide pneumococcal vaccine.

Age	Dose (ml)	Route*	Boosters
Adults	0.5	Deltoid SC/IM	5–10 years (not < 3 years) for high-risk persons (check antibody titres first)
Children 2 to 10 years	0.5	Anterolateral thigh or deltoid SC/IM	No booster

*The IV and ID routes must be avoided.

decline over the next few years (average protective level 7–10 years). Among the elderly, children with nephrotic syndrome or asplenic patients, this decline starts earlier so that protective antibody levels may not be present 6 years or more after vaccination. Immunosuppressed patients and young children respond less well to the vaccine.

Children under 2 years of age do not mount a good antibody response to the currently available polysaccharide vaccines.

Administration (Table 37.1)

● Protective antibody levels usually develop by the third week following vaccination. The protective efficacy of the vaccine in preventing pneumococcal pneumonia is 65–70%, and for bacteraemia 64%. It is less effective in those who are immunocompromised, chronic alcoholics, and in patients with multiple myeloma and Hodgkin's lymphoma.

● Boosters are not normally recommended other than for high-risk patients (see below) after 4–10 years. The presence of high pneumococcal antibody levels at the time of administration of a booster is associated with higher risk of local and general reactions. If in doubt, measure the specific antibody level (undertaken in only a few centres). Revaccination with 23-valent vaccine is recommended for high-risk individuals who have received the 14-valent pneumococcal vaccine (available in the UK before 1983) more than 6 years previously.

● Clearly mark the notes of patients immunized to avoid accidental revaccination.

● When elective splenectomy or chemotherapy/radiotherapy is planned, the vaccine should be given, at the latest, 2 weeks before the procedure.

Ideally, enough time should be available before the procedure for measurement of specific antibody levels after immunization that will show whether the patient has responded to the vaccination. In post-traumatic splenectomy, give the vaccine immediately after recovery and before leaving the hospital.

● Patients who require penicillin or other antibiotics for prophylaxis against pneumococcal infection should not discontinue their treatment after vaccination.

● The vaccine is effective in preventing severe pneumococcal infections such as pneumonia or meningitis, but it gives no protection against more common infections where the *Pneumococcus* can be implicated, such as otitis media or exacerbations of chronic bronchitis. There are 84 known capsular pneumococcal serotypes (not all equally pathogenic) and only 23 serotypes are contained in the vaccine.

Indications

In the UK the DoH recommends pneumococcal vaccination for anybody over 2 years of age in whom pneumococcal infection is likely to be more common and/or dangerous. In particular, the DoH recommends the vaccine for those with:

● asplenia or severe dysfunction of the spleen, including homozygous sickle-cell disease and coeliac syndrome;

● chronic renal disease or nephrotic syndrome;

● immunodeficiency or immunosuppression resulting from disease or treatment, including HIV infection at all stages (the earlier the HIV patient is vaccinated, the better the response);

● chronic heart (e.g. heart failure), lung (e.g. chronic obstructive pulmonary disease (COPD)) and liver disease, including cirrhosis;

● diabetes mellitus.

Advanced age is not included in the DoH recommendations, contrary to the advice of the WHO [Fedson, D. *et al* (1989) WHO recommendations on pneumococcal vaccination: immunization of elderly people with polyvalent pneumococcal vaccine. *Infection* 17, 437–41] and recommendations in the USA [CDC MMWR. Prevention of Pneumococcal Disease. Recommendations of the Advisory Committee on Immunization Practices. ACIP. April 4, 1997/Vol. 46/No. RR-8] where all adults aged 65 years and over are recommended for immunization. In one study [Steven, N. & Wright, P. (1992) Pneumococcal immunization and the healthy elderly. *Lancet* 340, 1036–7], only one in three patients over 65 years of age with pneumococcal infection had risk factors that would have made them eligible for immunization under the UK recommendations. Several case–control studies have shown the efficacy of pneumococcal vaccine for selected elderly populations, both healthy and with coexisting disease.

Another group of patients that should be vaccinated, but not included in the DoH's recommendations, are patients with chronic alcoholism [American College of Physicians, reference given above; Obaro, S. *et al* (1996) The pneumococcal problem. *Br. Med. J.* 312, 1521–5].

● The DoH advises performing opportunistic pneumococcal immunization on at-risk non-immunized patients at routine GP or hospital consultations, at discharge after hospital admission, or when immunizing next time against influenza (pneumococcal vaccine is given once only). The aim is to curb rising infection in the UK caused by growing antibiotic resistance.

● A USA study [Nichol K.L. (1999) The additive benefits of influenza and pneumococcal vaccinations during influenza seasons among elderly persons with chronic lung disease. *Vaccine* 17, S91–S93] found that pneumococcal vaccination alone caused a 27% reduction in hospitalization from pneumonia, although this was not statistically significant (that of influenza vaccine was 52%). However, the effects were additive when given with influenza vaccine. Both vaccines were associated with significant reductions in deaths and, again, the protective effects were additive.

● Further data on pneumococcal and influenza vaccination is now available [Nichol K.L. *et al.* (1999) The health and economic benefits associated with pneumococcal vaccination of elderly persons with chronic lung disease. *Arch. Intern. Med.* 159, 2437–42]. A cohort study of 1898 patients over 65 years old with chronic lung disease was followed over a 2-year period. Pneumococcal vaccination was associated with significantly lower risks for pneumonia/influenza leading to hospitalization (43% decrease in hospitalization, $P = 0005$) and for all cause mortality (29% decrease in deaths, $P = 0.008$). These effects were additive to those of influenza vaccination: hospital admissions for pneumonia and all cause mortality decreased by 72 and 82%, respectively, in those given both vaccines. Economic analyses based on USA costs estimated a remarkable 2-year healthcare cost saving of almost $300 per person vaccinated for this particular high-risk group.

● Most patients who are candidates for pneumococcal immunization are also candidates for annual influenza immunization.

Vaccine availability

● Pneumovax II (Aventis Pasteur MSD), available in a 0.5-mL single-dose pre-filled syringe. Inspect before injection (clear, colourless liquid without suspended particles).
● Pnu-Immune (Wyeth Laboratories), available in a 0.5-mL single-dose vial.

Storage: Between 2 and 8 °C. *Do not freeze.* No dilution or reconstitution is necessary.

Future pneumococcal vaccines

In the UK, pneumococcal infections are more common in children under 2 years and adults over 50 years; those over 65 years are 2–5 times more likely to develop pneumococcal infection than the general population. The introduction of a childhood conjugate pneumococcal vaccine is a priority. This is expected to have an impact on invasive pneumococcal infection such as pneumonia, otitis media, and the need for tympanostomy tubes. The present polysaccharide pneumococcal vaccine does not induce immunological memory. Polysaccharide conjugate vaccines covering 7, 9 and 11 serotypes are now undergoing trials before application to be licensed. Starting in April 2000, the PHLS is carrying out a trial, on behalf of the DoH, of three unlicensed conjugate pneumococcal vaccines involving 600 infants.

T. Lieu and coworkers have calculated that the introduction of a conjugate pneumococcal vaccine for healthy infants in the USA will prevent 116 deaths, 12 000 cases of bacteraemia and meningitis, 53 000 cases of pneumonia, and 1 million episodes of otitis media [Lieu T. *et al.* (2000) Projected cost-effectiveness of pneumococcal conjugate vaccination of healthy infants and young children. *J. Am. Med. Assoc.* 283, 1460–8]. Before accounting for vaccine costs, the vaccination programme would save $342 million medical and $415 million in work-loss and other costs from averted pneumococcal disease. Vaccination of healthy individuals would result in net savings for society if the vaccine cost is less than $46 per dose, and net savings for the healthcare payer if the vaccine cost is less than $18 per dose. The manufacturer's list price in the USA is $58 per dose (2000). With present calculations this is cost-effective but not cost-saving. On a league table for cost-effectiveness of health interventions, the cost per life saved is $80 000 (in comparison, for influenza vaccination of people aged 65 years and over the cost per life saved is $1300 and $2800 for cervical smears every 3 years in women in this age group), $160 per otitis media episode, $3200 per pneumonia case, $15 000 for bacteraemia, and $280 000 for meningitis prevented.

Wyeth Laboratories is seeking a European licence for its conjugate pneumococcal vaccine, Prevenar. A UK licence is expected in the first quarter of the year 2001. In trials, this vaccine has shown dramatic efficacy for invasive disease, excellent efficacy for pneumonia and good efficacy for otitis media at 57% as regards to vaccine serotypes; this equates to 34% of pneumococcal otitis media, and 6% of general otitis media infections.

Pneumococcal conjugate vaccines are produced by coupling the saccharide to one of the following protein carriers: tetanus toxoid, diphtheria toxoid, CRM_{197} protein, and meningococcal outer membrane complex. Such vaccines are immunogenic in infants and other at-risk groups. They are able to induce immunological memory, and mucosal antibodies as demonstrated in phase II studies. This means the conjugate vaccine may prevent mucosal infections, thus reducing the spread of pneumococcal disease. This will be especially important if it reduces the spread of antibody-resistant pneumococcus.

In the USA the pneumococcus causes 16 000 cases of bacteraemia, 1400 cases of meningitis and 7 million cases of otitis media in children under 5 years of age. In February 2000, the US Food and Drug Administration (FDA) approved Prevnar (Wyeth-Lederle Vaccines), a 7-valent pneumococcal conjugate vaccine. In a large-scale clinical trial in the USA, this vaccine was shown to have 100% efficacy (95% CI 75.4–100%) in preventing invasive pneumococcal disease, caused by the seven serotypes included in the vaccine, after immunization at 2, 4, 6 and 12–15 months of age. It is hoped that widespread use of this vaccine could possibly reduce the spread of drug-resistant pneumococci in the future. The US Advisory Committee on Immunization Practices (ACIP) recommends the use of Prevnar for all infants up to the age of 23 months, and in certain older children aged 24–59 months belonging to high-risk groups.

Pneumococcal infection

Streptococcus pneumoniae (the pneumococcus) is a lancet-shaped, Gram-positive diplococcus and was first isolated in 1881 by Pasteur in France and Sternberg in the USA. Eighty-five pneumococcal serotypes have been identified. Certain serotypes are prevalent in adults and others in children.

Pneumococcal infections are most common during the winter months. Many people (up to 30% of healthy adults and up to 60% of healthy children) carry the organism in their nasopharynx without symptoms. Transmission is via droplets of respiratory tract secretions, from person-to-person in close contact (i.e. within 1–2 m). The incubation period is 1–3 days. Most cases of pneumococcal infection occur in individuals who are already asymptomatic carriers of the disease. Clinical illness develops when the pneumococci spread to tissues outside the nasopharynx [Fedson D.S. & Musherr D.M. (1994) Pneumococcal vaccine. In: *Vaccines* (Plotkin S.A. & Mortimer E.A. eds), pp. 517–64. W.B. Saunders, Philadelphia]. Patients described as 'at risk' above (see Vaccine) are at increased risk of pneumococcal infection.

Surveillance reports of invasive pneumococcal disease in elderly people 65 years of age show an annual incidence of 31 per 100 000 population in England and Wales (1996 data), and 34 per 100 000 in Scotland (1997 data). The true incidence in most developed countries is about 50 per 100 000 among the elderly.

Pneumonia is the third biggest killer in the UK (Office of Health Economics, 1997) and the pneumococcus accounts for up to 30–60% of community-acquired pneumonia. In one study it was put at 76% [Noah, N. (1988) Vaccination against pneumococcal infection. *Br. Med. J.* 297, 1352]. It is common in elderly people among whom it causes severe illness and up to 10–20% mortality [Salisbury, D. & Begg, N. (1996) *Immun-ization Against Infectious Disease*. HMSO, London], especially in patients who develop bacteraemia or meningitis. In one study [Steven, N. & Wright, P. (1992) Pneumococcal immunisation in the healthy elderly. *Lancet* 340, 1036–7], the case : fatality ratio for patients over 65 years of age was 40%. In another study, out of 5837 cases of pneumococcal pneumonia, 12% were fatal [Daniel, R. *et al.* (2000) Mortality from invasive pneumococcal pneumonia in the era of antibiotic resistance. *Am. J. Pub. Health* 90, 223–9].

Patients at risk of severe pneumococcal infection are patients with absent or non functioning spleen, renal and cardiac failure, chronic pulmonary or liver disease, chronic alcoholics and diabetes mellitus. Also children under 2 years of age, elderly people, smokers, patients with skull fractures, with blocked Eustachian tube, influenza, anaemia, primary and secondary antibody deficiency, e.g. hypogammaglobulinaemia, immunodeficiency including HIV and malignancy. Smoking is an independent risk factor for pneumococcal (influenza and meningococcal) disease by a factor of 4, and in passive smokers by a factor of 2.5.

At particular risk are patients with impaired immunological response to the pneumococcus, that is, patients with splenic dysfunction or post-splenectomy, patients with sickle-cell anaemia, Hodgkin's disease, congenital or acquired immuno deficiency (including HIV), nephrotic syndrome and organ transplantation.

Symptoms depend on the site of infection, therefore they can be those of pneumonia, empyema, meningitis, pericarditis, endocarditis, peritonitis, otitis media or arthritis.

Over the past two decades, strains of the pneumococcus resistant to penicillin and other antibiotics have become widespread and have been increasing all over the world.

The most common manifestation of pneumococcal infection is *pneumonia*. The onset of illness is usually sudden with fever, rigors, myalgia, weakness, anorexia, chest pain (from involvement of the pleura) and cough, initially nonproductive, but later purulent. Pneumococcal pneumonia is estimated to affect 1 in 1000 adults each year—about 53 000 cases in the UK, 4500–9000 deaths in England and Wales every year. The incidence is higher among the elderly and patients with asplenia, Hodgkin's disease, myeloma, cirrhosis, heart disease and renal failure. The case-fatality rate is about 10–20%. In a British study in Nottingham [(1988) *Lancet* ii, 255–8], it accounted for 76% of primary pneumonias in adults admitted to hospital and for 89% of deaths from this cause. We admit to hospital one in five cases.

The annual incidence of *pneumococcal meningitis* in the UK is 1 per 200 000 of the population (mostly children aged under 1 year)—about 400 reported cases per annum. Mortality rate is 22%, increasing to 59% in patients over 75 years.

Pneumococcal bacteraemia occurs in all age groups with an incidence of 4.8–9.2 (average 7) per 100 000 population. Among persons over 65 years the incidence is 50 per 100 000, and in children under 2 years it is 160 per 100 000. It has been estimated to develop in up to 30% of cases of pneumococcal pneumonia. The estimated mortality rate is 20%, in the over-75-year-olds this rises to 28% but among high-risk patients, such as the immunosuppressed, it is estimated to be over 40%.

Household and intimate contacts of cases of meningococcal disease have a 500- to 1200-fold increase in risk of disease. The first 7 days of the illness is the most contagious period but may persist for several weeks and even months. The local consultant for communicable disease control may suggest prophylaxis with an antibiotic, usually rifampicin (for dosage see Table 26.6, p. 119, under meningococcal infection) for the index case as soon as they can take oral medication (unless on the effective ceftriaxone) and to household/intimate contacts.

McDonald and co-workers [McDonald, Friedman, E., Banks A. *et al* (1997) Pneumococcal vaccine campaign based in general practice. *Br. Med. J.* 314, 1094–8] have calculated that a Health Authority with a population of 500 000 can expect an annual incidence of:

• 400 cases of pneumococcal pneumonia in adults, with 40–80 deaths;
• 43 cases of pneumococcal bacteraemia, with 6–11 deaths;
• 3–4 cases of pneumococcal meningitis, with one death.

The average length of hospital stay of patients with community-acquired pneumonia is 11 days. One in 10 will require intensive care management [MacFarlane, J. (1995) The clinical impact of pneumococcal disease. In: *The Clinical Impact of Pneumococcal Disease and Strategies for its Prevention* (R. T. Mayon-White, ed) pp. 9–15 Royal Society of Medicine International Congress and symposium Series 210, London].

Globally, pneumococcal bacteria cause a massive burden of disease. Pneumonia is the most common cause of death among children. Every year, it kills over a million children under 5 years old in the developing world. There are 20 000 deaths a year in the USA, 90% of them at age 65 years and over. The main cause of pneumonia is *Streptococcus pneumoniae*. It accounts for 70% of all cases of pneumonia and is responsible for 20–25% of total mortality among children in developing countries. Travellers who should consider immunization are those travelling to sub-Saharan Africa, India and Nepal.

Information on community-acquired pneumonia can be found on the website of the University of Texas: www.utexas.edu/pharmacy/courses/phr385e/community_pneu/index.htm.

Asplenia

The spleen has an important role in removing bacteria and parasitized red cells from the circulation. It also produces proteins, such as properdin and tuftsin that have a role in complement activation and opsonization, respectively. Splenectomy has been estimated to carry a lifetime risk of overwhelming sepsis of up to 5%, although the risk is probably highest in the first 2 years after splenectomy and higher in children than in adults [O'Neal B.J. & McDonald J.C. (1981) The risk of sepsis in the asplenic adult. *Ann. Surg.* 194, 775–8].

Patients with surgical or functional asplenia (patients after bone marrow transplantation, with sickle-cell disease and some haemoglobinopathies) have reduced clearance of encapsulated bacteria, such as the pneumococcus, from their bloodstream. After splenectomy overwhelming infection can follow, caused most often by *Streptococcus pneumoniae* and *Haemophilus influenzae* type b. Before splenectomy, patients should receive pneumococcal and *H. influenzae* b vaccines (check that the child has not already received Hib) and seroconversion should be checked before the surgical procedure. If immunization was not performed before splenectomy, it should be carried out after the operation. Asplenic individuals respond poorly to polysaccharide vaccines. Antibody levels are lower than in normal hosts and wane more rapidly.

All patients with anatomical splenectomy or functional asplenia should be considered for the following vaccines.

• *Pneumococcal vaccine*—if not given before, it should be given as soon as possible after the operation and before discharge from hospital. Boosters are needed every 5–10 years as indicated by antibody titres. Asplenic patients with lymphoproliferative disorders or sickle-cell anaemia may require reimmunization earlier, after 3–5 years. The recommended pneumococcal antibody post splenectomy is > 40 u/mL.
• *H. influenzae* b vaccine—in the case of a child, check that the vaccine has not already been given. The need for boosters is still unclear.
• *Influenza vaccine*—should be given annually.
• *Meningococcal A + C vaccine*—its routine use is not recommended in the UK other than in cases of

contact or in outbreaks caused by group A and/or C. It is recommended for asplenic patients travelling to areas where there is an increased risk of group A or C infection. For boosters, see Table 26.2 on p. 114. Children in the UK receive the *meningococcal C conjugate vaccine* (since October 1999). If they are to travel abroad, they should, in addition, receive the plain polysaccharide meningococcal A + C before they are expected to travel in order to acquire protection against the A sero-group (see meningococcal vaccine on p. 113).

Because pneumococcal antibody levels may decline rapidly in some high-risk groups, GPs should consider monitoring these antibody responses, perhaps annually or biannually (the test can only be undertaken in a few centres). Some patients, in fact, may need reimmunization earlier than the recommended 5–10 years.

Antibiotic prophylaxis. In children, the risk of infection after splenectomy is high enough to justify a tablet of phenoxymethylpenicillin (penicillin V 125 mg up to age 6 years, 250 mg from 6 years onwards) twice daily, or amoxycillin (aged 0–5 years 10 mg/kg day, 5–14 years 125 mg/day—co-amoxiclav may be used), at least until their sixteenth birthday. Patients who are allergic to penicillin should take erythromycin.

Ideally, postsplenectomy patients should take prophylactic penicillin for life. On the other hand, not many patients are willing to comply. In adulthood, by 2 years after splenectomy, the risks of overwhelming infection are much reduced to the point that prophylaxis could then be reserved for only the most vulnerable (those with malignant haematological disease or immunosuppression). The adult prophylactic dose is: penicillin V 250–500 mg twice daily or amoxycillin (co-amoxiclav) 250–500 mg daily.

Patients who are unwilling to take regular penicillin should be made aware of the risks and supplied with penicillin to take immediately at the onset of suggestive symptoms.

Give the patient a splenectomy leaflet and a card to carry. Consider recommending a Medic-Alert bracelet.

Prophylactic antibiotics are taken irrespective of whether the patient has been fully immunized. If a patient is not taking antibiotic prophylaxis, he/she should do so during periods of travel and should keep a therapeutic course of antibiotics in reserve (penicillin V: children up to age 14 years 200–300 mg/kg day in six divided doses, maximum 6 g; adults, 1–2 g every 4–6 h; amoxycillin: under 1 year, 62.5 mg every 8 h; 1–5 years, 125 mg every 8 h; 5–14 years, 250 mg every 8 h; adults, 0.5–1.0 g every 8 h). A local doctor should be consulted immediately should infective symptoms of rigors, malaise or pyrexia occur. Local medical advice is very important because of a high incidence of penicillin-resistant pneumococci in Spain and some other European countries and, of course, malaria and other pyrexial disease in endemic countries.

Finally, asplenic patients should be warned that they should avoid animal bites, especially dog bites as these can transmit the bacteria *Capnocytophaga canimorsus*, which can lead to septicaemia and death if not treated early and appropriately with co-amoxiclav or erythromycin. They should avoid blood-borne protozoal infection such as babesiosis. *Babesia* species is a red cell parasite that occurs along the eastern seaboard of the USA and in some parts of northern Europe. It is transmitted by ticks. Asplenic patients should avoid travelling to malaria-endemic areas, especially areas where falciparum malaria predominates. They should consider avoiding travel to areas such as coastal West or East Africa, where transmission rates of malaria are high. Strict adherence to the appropriate prophylaxis for the area being visited and avoidance of mosquito bites are essential.

Information

Additional information is available from the following sources.

● *Information about splenectomy for patients*, which includes a card to carry, is available from: DoH, PO Box 410, Wetherby LS23 7LL. Fax: 0990 210 266.

● *Factsheet on splenectomy and infection*, available from Oxfordshire Health Authority, Manor House, Headley Way, Oxford OX3 9DZ.

● Medic-Alert Foundation International, 1 Bridge Wharf, 156 Caledonian Road, London N1 9UU. Tel.: 020 7833 3034, or Freephone 0800 220 386.

● CDC disease and vaccine information. Website: www.cdc.gov/nip/publications/mmwr/rr/rr4608.pdf.

Chapter 38

Rabies

Contraindications to vaccination

- Acute febrile illness.
- Severe general reaction to a previously administered rabies vaccine, except for postexposure treatment.
- Severe sensitivity to neomycin or β-propiolactone.
- Pregnancy, unless there is a significant risk of infection, in which case pre-exposure prophylaxis is indicated. Pregnancy is not a contraindication to postexposure prophylaxis.
- Rabies is almost always fatal therefore for postexposure treatment, all contraindications should be ignored.

Possible side- and adverse effects

Local reactions

Swelling, redness and pain may develop within 24–48 h from administration.

General reactions

There may be myalgia, headaches, fever, nausea or vomiting within 24 h of administration. Urticaria, pruritus, malaise may occur in 1–6% of vaccinees 2–21 days after vaccination. Very rarely Guillain–Barré syndrome and anaphylactic shock occur. Reactions can become more severe with repeated doses. Up to 6% of persons, 2 to 21 days after receiving booster doses of the human diploid cell vaccine, may experience an immune complex-like reaction characterized by urticaria, pruritus, malaise, nausea, vomiting, arthralgia, angio-oedema. It is rare in persons receiving primary immunization with human diploid cells vaccine.

The vaccine

The virus in Rabies Vaccine BP (Aventis Pasteur MSD) is inactivated with β-propiolactone. It is a freeze-dried suspension of Wistar rabies virus strain, cultured on human diploid cells (HDCV). It contains traces of neomycin.

Neither the purified chick embryo cell (PCEC) nor the rabies vaccine adsorbed (RVA) vaccines were available during the first half of the year 2000 in the UK. Rabipur (Chiron Behring), a PCEC vaccine, was licensed and expected to be made available at the end of 2000 (see p. 210).

Administration

The dose is the same for all ages. It should be given by IM or deep SC injection. It is free in the UK (on the NHS) for people at specified occupational risk (see below). It is not available on the NHS for routine immunization of travellers, who should be issued with a private prescription or given the vaccine privately.

- The three-dose course (0, 7, 28 days) is recommended in the UK (Table 38.1). For those people going on a one-off trip, the old two-dose regimen (0 and 28 days) may give adequate protection. If they remain at continued risk, they should receive a reinforcing dose 6–12 months later, with boosters at 2- to 3-year intervals.
- Antibodies appear 7–14 days after the first dose and peak within 30–60 days. For full protection the third dose is required. Adequate titres usually develop within 2 weeks after the third dose and they persist for at least 1 and usually 3 years. The three-dose course causes seroconversion virtually in all immunocompetent recipients (essentially 100%). It is therefore unnecessary to test seroconversion routinely, except in individuals who

Table 38.1 Pre-exposure immunization for rabies.

Immunization	Dose (ml)	Route*	Schedule (days)
First dose	1.0	IM or SC	0
Second dose	1.0	IM or SC	7
Third dose	1.0	IM or SC	28 (Rabipur 21–28)
Booster	1.0	IM or SC	Every 2–3 years (if at continued risk; Rabipur 2–5 years)

*The IM route is preferable. If the SC route is chosen in exceptional circumstances, the vaccine should be given by deep SC injection.

have experienced a severe reaction to a previous dose of anti-rabies vaccine to confirm the need for reinforcing dose. On the other hand, individuals exposed to or working with the virus should have regular 6-monthly antibody testing. The WHO recommended minimum protective rabies virus neutralizing antibodies titre is 0.5 IU/mL.

● Insufficient response may be achieved in patients immunosuppressed by treatment or disease.

● Exercise caution in patients with bleeding diathesis, i.e. patients on anticoagulants, when using the IM route.

● There is no licensed minimum age for the rabies vaccine—there are no data available for the under 1 year olds.

● Although the general teaching of not repeating interrupted courses applies, in the case of rabies an exception is made because it is such a fatal disease. The manufacturer Aventis Pasteur MSD suggests the following action in the case where the HDCV course is interrupted:

Three-dose course (0, 7, 28 days)

(a) If interruption after the first (day 0) dose is less than 3 months: restart course.

(b) If interruption after first and second (days 0 and 7) doses is over 6 months: restart course.

(c) If over 5 years have elapsed since the three-dose primary course: restart course.

Two-dose course (0, 28 days)

If more than 2 years have elapsed since the 6–12 month missed booster was due: restart course.

● The painful abdominal injections were abandoned in the mid-1970s. The HDCV is almost painless. It should be administered by IM injection, into the deltoid region (never use the gluteal region) and in very young children in the anterolateral aspect of the thigh.

● Other regimens/routes of administration not covered by the manufacturer's product licence in the UK and therefore on the doctor's own responsibility are the following:

Accelerated course allowing completion of the regimen within 1 week: three full-dose (1-mL each) IM injections at three sites on day 1, with a booster dose on day 7. The WHO no longer recommends this.

The Zagreb protocol consists of two 1.0-mL IM injections on two sites (right and left deltoid) on day 0, followed by a further two injections on days 7 and 21. This schedule induces an early antibody response.

Intradermal (ID) vaccine schedules utilize less vaccine and reduce the cost when many people need to be immunized. It should be noted that the lyophilized vaccine, once reconstituted, must be used within an hour. Thus, it is only of use in larger centres and when group exposure occurs. Children receiving ID vaccination may have lower rabies-neutralizing antibody levels than children receiving the vaccine IM. Immune protection is estimated to commence after 2 weeks from when the first ID dose was given. The intradermal route should only be used by experts in ID injections, otherwise consideration should be given to checking the antibody titre. It should not be used in patients concurrently taking chloroquine or mefloquine for malaria prophylaxis as they may interfere with antibody response to the intradermally administered HDCV. If the traveller will be taking chloroquine or mefloquine for malaria prophylaxis, the ID HDCV series must be completed well before (1–2 months) antimalarials are started. If this is not possible, the IM dose/route should be used.

The Thai Red Cross Intradermal Schedule (two-site intradermal regimen, 2-2-2-1-1) consists of 0.2 mL (0.1 mL if another vaccine is used with a diluent of 0.5 mL instead of 1 mL) of reconstituted vaccine given at two sites on days 0, 3, 7, and at one site on days 28 and 90 (five visits).

The Oxford Intradermal Schedule (eight-site ID regimen, 8-4-1-1) consists of 0.2 mL (or 0.1 mL depending on dilution—see above) vaccine given at eight sites on day 0, at four sites on day 7, and single sites on days 28 and 90 (four visits). It is used in some countries in Asia and Africa.

If rapid immunization is necessary, as in the case of staff caring for a patient with rabies, 0.1 mL of vaccine can be given ID into each of the four limbs (0.4 mL in all) on the first day the need arises.

● Pre-exposure immunization does not eliminate the need for additional therapy after a rabies exposure (see below) but simplifies postexposure treatment by decreasing the number of vaccine doses needed and eliminating the need for rabies-specific immunoglobulin.

● The vaccine is available free (from the PHLS) on the NHS for the following people at occupational risk (as suggested by the DoH in its publication *Memorandum on Rabies: Prevention and Control,* 2000):

(a) laboratory workers handling the virus;

(b) those who, in the course of their work, may be at risk of exposure to infection as a result of the regular handling of imported animals that either may not have completed quarantine or may not have fulfilled the requirements of the Pet Travel Scheme, e.g.

at animal quarantine centres;

at zoos;

at research and acclimatization centres where primates and other imported animals are housed;

at ports, e.g. certain Customs and Excise Officers;

agents authorized to carry imported animals;

(c) veterinary and technical staff in the State Veterinary Services;

(d) local authority inspectors appointed under the Animal Health Act 1981 (it only includes dog wardens who are also inspectors);

(e) workers in enzootic areas abroad, who, by the nature of their work, are at special risk of contact with rabid animals (e.g. veterinary staff, zoologists);

(f) health workers who are likely to come into close contact with a patient with rabies;

(g) licensed bat handlers.

● Rabies serum antibody titres should be determined at regular intervals, i.e. every 6 to 24 months depending on risk and degree of exposure, in those who are at risk in the course of their work (see above). The WHO recommended titre of antibody is $\geqslant 0.5$ IU/mL.

● The vaccine is not available on the NHS for all others, although it is recommended for travellers to areas where they may be exposed to high risk of infection or to remote areas where medical treatment may not be immediately available (more than a day). In such cases, travellers can obtain the vaccine by private arrangement from their GP or commercial travel clinics. Consider immunization of children and adults going to live in countries such as India or Thailand.

Post-exposure treatment

● The first dose of the vaccine should be given as soon as possible after the suspected contact (day 0). Human rabies immunoglobulin is only necessary if the person with the suspected contact has not previously been fully immunized (Table 38.2). Start treatment immediately and stop if it is subsequently proved the suspect animal is free of rabies.

● Immediately after exposure, wash lesions copiously and thoroughly with soap or a detergent and running water for at least 5 min. The aim of washing is to destroy the virus before it has time to multiply and penetrate the peripheral nerves. Apply 40–70% alcohol, tincture or aqueous solution of iodine. A good alternative is cetrimide solution 0.1% BPC. Cover with a simple dressing. Do not suture the wound for at least 24–48 h to prevent the virus from spreading into the nerve fibres. If suturing is necessary, rabies immunoglobulin should be infiltrated around the wound.

● If necessary, antitetanus prophylaxis and an antibiotic (co-amoxiclav) should be considered to avoid additional infections.

Table 38.2 Post exposure treatment for rabies—DoH recommendations.

Immunization status	Dose of vaccine (ml)	Route— deltoid	Schedule (days)	Rabies-specific immunoglobulin 20 IU/kg body weight on day 0*
Fully immunized	1	IM or SC	0, 3–7 days (two doses)	Not usually necessary
Nonimmunized	1	IM or SC	0, 3, 7, 14, 30 days (five doses). Stop if animal found conclusively to be free of rabies	Half infiltrated around the wound, the rest IM into the gluteal region
				Necessary for cases from 'high risk' countries (see Table 38.6)

*Immunoglobulin is not necessary for postexposure cases from 'low-risk' countries (see Table 38.6). It should be used for cases from 'high-risk' countries (see Table 38.7).

• Local medical advice should be sought regarding necessary action.

• In the case of domestic animals, advise the patient to ask to see the last vaccination certificate. The dog or cat should be observed for 15 days (the DoH in its 'Memorandum on Rabies Prevention and Control' does not give advice regarding other animals). Exchange address/telephone numbers so that the casualty can be notified should the animal begin to behave abnormally. Inform the local police and, in case of difficulty, the British Consular officer.

• On return to the UK, report to the Duty Port Medical Officer at the Health Control Unit before passing through customs/immigration controls. Otherwise, report to own GP.

• If the animal is wild or stray, inform the local police. The local doctor will advise whether postexposure treatment is necessary. It may be safer to consider such an animal as rabid.

• Animal bites and the need for postexposure treatment in countries of no or low risk should be judged separately. Local advice is very important.

• Returning travellers who report possible exposure to rabies should receive immediate treatment. For contact numbers see below under 'Information'.

Suggested action in some specific situations

• The patient previously received a brain-tissue-derived vaccine (as opposed to the HDCV or the PCEC culture vaccine): treat such patients as if they have never been immunized.

• The patient was severely exposed to rabies, the vaccine was started, no rabies-specific immunoglobulin was given, and the patient returns after day 7 from exposure: still give the immunoglobulin to the wound sites and complete the immunization course.

• The exposed person presents for treatment after a considerable delay: there are no firm guidelines, so it may be safer from the medicolegal point of view to give full postexposure treatment, including injection of the wound sites with rabies-specific immunoglobulin (the incubation period is from 5 days to over 1 year).

• The patient has multiple bites on the face and neck and the volume of the rabies-specific immunoglobulin is not sufficient to be infiltrated in all sites: dilute it to make up an adequate volume.

• The most common causes of treatment failures are a result of incomplete or delayed treatment, omission of rabies-specific immunoglobulin administration, surgical interference with bite wounds prior to infiltration with immunoglobulin, and improper use of immunoglobulin (e.g. failure to inject all wounds).

• Warn the travellers that in the case of a suspect bite, they need postexposure treatment even if they had previously received the vaccine—they must seek local medical advice without delay.

• Table 38.3 contains the WHO advice for postexposure treatment.

Table 38.3 WHO-Guide for postexposure treatment.

Category	Type of contact with a suspect or confirmed rabid domestic or wild animal, or animal unavailable for observation	Recommended treatment
I	Touching or feeding of animals. Licks on intact skin	None, if reliable case history is available
II	Nibbling of uncovered skin. Minor scratches or abrasions without bleeding. Licks on broken skin	Administer vaccine immediately according to the 0, 3, 7, 14, 30-day schedule*
III	Single or multiple transdermal bites or scratches. Contamination of mucous membrane with saliva (i.e. licks)	Administer vaccine* and rabies immunoglobulin immediately

*Stop treatment if animal remains healthy throughout an observation period of 10 days or if animal is killed humanely and found to be negative for rabies by appropriate laboratory techniques.

Vaccine and immunoglobulin availability

• Rabies vaccine BP (Aventis Pasteur MSD)—HDCV, available in single-dose vial with disposable syringe containing 1 mL of diluent (Water for Injections BP with no added preservatives). The Public Health Laboratory Services (Virus Reference Division) Tel.: 020 8200 4400 will supply the HDCV vaccine for pre-exposure immunization for those at occupational risk. In Scotland details of availability of vaccine from SCIEH, Tel.: 0141 300 1100.

• Rabipur (Chiron Behring—available from MASTA), powder in vial, diluent in ampoule with syringe and needle. This PCEC vaccine was recently made available. Pre-exposure course similar to the HDCV vaccine. Booster 2–5 years. Lower reaction to boosters expected—one application may be for individuals who have reacted to HDCV.

• Human Rabies Immunoglobulin intramuscular (Bio Products Laboratory) is available in single-dose vials of approximately 2-mL volume. For NHS use, it is supplied through the PHLS centres.

Storage. Between 2 and 8 °C. *Do not freeze.* Use within 1 h after reconstitution.

Rabies infection

Rabies is probably the oldest recorded infection of mankind. The word 'rabies' comes from the Sanskrit word 'rabbahs' which means 'to do violence'. It refers to the Vedic period of India (30th century BC), when the God of Death was depicted being attended by a dog, his constant companion and the emissary of death. The earliest known reference to rabies can be found in the Eshmuna code of Babylon from the 23rd century BC, which details a dog owner whose pet causes someone's death by rabies. In ancient Egypt, god Sirius was imagined in the form of a furious dog. The Greeks were familiar with the disease since Homer's time; in the *Iliad*, Hector is called a 'mad dog'. Aristotle thought that only animals were susceptible to rabies. The real breakthrough in the history of the disease came in 1885 when Pasteur developed the first rabies vaccine. According to the Spanish physician Dr Gomez-Alonso, Count Dracula was no vampire, but had rabies. The symptoms of the advanced form of disease, when the virus attacks the brain, matched the description of the ancient legend. They include a fondness for biting, blood and sex. Dr Gomez-Alonso believes the vampire legends were triggered by an eighteenth century epidemic of the rabies virus in Hungary.

The rabies virus belongs to the genus *Lyssavirus* and occurs primarily in animals. It is an acute encephalomyelitic virus infection that produces an acute febrile illness with rapidly progressive central nervous system symptoms. There can be agoraphobia, hypersexuality, persistent insomnia, aversion to mirrors (can suffer spasms at the sight of mirrors), later hydrophobia, dysphagia, hallucinations, convulsions, paralysis and almost always (untreated) ends in death as a result of respiratory paralysis. The annual mortality rate (deaths/million population) is 0.023 in the USA, 4.5 in Thailand, 11 in Indonesia, 18 in Bangladesh, and 35.5 in India.

The virus is a single-stranded RNA rhabdovirus and is transmitted to humans by the bite or scratch of an infected animal, rarely through mucous membranes. Most animals, when infected, become ill within 3 days, hence the 10-day standard period of observation of a suspect animal. Other modes of transmission are by transplantation (such as corneas) or airborne (migrating bats). After inoculation, the virus replicates locally and spreads through peripheral nerves to the central nervous system where it causes encephalitis. The nearer to the central nervous system the infected bite, the shorter the incubation time will be—it ranges between 4 days to well over 1 year (average 3–8 weeks) and even 7 years. Bites on the face therefore are most dangerous. Children are often bitten on the face or neck, causing a short incubation period.

In Europe, the red fox is predominantly infected, although during the last decade the incidence has fallen dramatically. This is largely a result of the success of coordinated wildlife vaccination programmes, together with effective vaccination of domestic animals. In Turkey dogs are predominantly infected. Apart from foxes and dogs, other animals that can become infected are cats, bats, deer, badgers, horses, cattle, skunks, racoons, coyotes, jackals, wolves, kangaroo, rats, cotton rats, common field voles, monkeys and others (Table 38.4).

Rabies is endemic in all continents except Antarctica and Australasia (Fig. 38.1). Table 38.5 shows the countries that are thought to be of 'no risk'. Travellers to these countries may not need postexposure prophylaxis. Table 38.6 shows the countries considered 'low risk'. Table 38.7 shows the countries considered 'high risk'. See 'Information' below for contact telephone numbers.

The last indigenous case in the UK was in 1902, and all subsequent nonindigenous cases have been imported, with the exception of a single rabid bat on the Sussex coast in 1996. The last person to die in the UK of rabies was a 19-year-old man who had been bitten by a stray dog while in Nigeria before his return to the UK. Between 1977 and 1987, six cases were reported in the UK, three of them in children bitten by dogs on the Indian subcontinent.

Table 38.4 Predominant global rabies animal reservoirs.

Animal	Area
Dogs	Throughout the world, particularly Asia, Africa and Latin America
Foxes	Europe, Arctic and North America
Raccoons	Eastern USA
Skunks	Midwestern USA, Western Canada
Coyotes	Asia, Africa, North America
Mongooses	Indian mongoose in the Caribbean islands; yellow mongoose in Asia and Africa
Bats	Insectivorous bats in North America and Europe; vampire bats from Northern Mexico to Argentina

Table 38.5 Countries of **no risk** according to the DoH February 2000—no postexposure prophylaxis needed.

Region	Countries
Europe	Cyprus, Faroe Islands, Finland, Gibraltar, Greece, Iceland, Ireland, Italy (except the northern and eastern borders), Malta, Norway (mainland), Portugal, Mainland Spain (except N. African Coast), Sweden, UK
Americas	Anguilla, Antigua and Barbuda, Bahamas, Barbados, Bermuda, Cayman Islands, Dominica, Guadaloupe, Jamaica, Martinique, Montserrat, Netherlands Antilles, St. Christopher & Nevis, St. Lucia, St. Martins, St. Pierre & Miquelon, St. Vincent & Grenadines, Turks & Caicos Islands, Virgin Islands
Asia	Japan, Singapore, Taiwan
Oceania	American Samoa, Australia, Belau, Cook Islands, Federated States of Micronesia, Fiji, French Polynesia, Guam, Kiribati, New Caledonia, New Zealand, Niue, Northern Mariana Islands, Papua New Guinea, Samoa, Solomon Islands, Tonga, Vanuatu, Western Samoa

Country
Belgium, Denmark, France, Germany, Luxembourg, Netherlands, Switzerland, Canada, USA
Note: For the risk of rabies in different parts of the USA, contact the Centre for Disease Control and Prevention, USA Department of Health and Human Services. National Centre for Infectious Diseases, Atlanta, Georgia 30333, USA. Website: http://www.cdc.gov

Table 38.6 Countries considered of **low risk**—DoH February 2000. In postexposure, vaccine only required.

Country
Colombia, Ecuador, El Salvador, Guatemala, Parts of Mexico, Peru Most other countries in South America
India, Nepal, Pakistan, Philippines, Sri Lanka, Thailand, Vietnam Most other countries in Asia
Turkey Africa

Table 38.7 Countries considered of **high risk**—DoH February 2000. In postexposure, vaccine is necessary. Previously nonimmunized individuals need vaccine and immunoglobulin.

In contrast, in 1992, 12 cases of human rabies were reported in Europe (11 in the former Soviet Union and one in France—imported from Algeria). During the same year, the number of animal rabies cases reported in Europe was 11 000 (66% in foxes). Between 1986 and 1996, 17 European countries reported human rabies (187 nonimported cases, mainly from Turkey, Romania and Russia). Nowadays, on average, every year in Europe there are about 20 000 animal cases. Thirteen human deaths were reported in Europe in 1997, 10 of which occurred in the Russian Federation.

The incubation period in animals varies greatly. In dogs, it is usually between 3 and 8 weeks. The saliva of animals may be infectious already before clinical signs appear, usually 3–5 days, exceptionally up to 2 weeks, or up to 29 days in foxes.

The current strategy for the elimination of rabies in Europe is by vaccinating domestic animals parenterally and by oral vaccination of foxes. Distribution of attenuated live vaccine was via impregnated chicken heads acting as bait. A new bait consisting of fat and fish meal has improved the seroconversion rate and facilitated mass production.

Countries free from rabies impose strict control in animal traffic across borders. Animals that are brought in legally are isolated and placed under observation—for 6 months in the UK. In the summer of 1999, the Government signalled the end of the UK's 100-year-old quarantine laws, which are the world's toughest antirabies regulations, by announcing a pilot scheme for pet passports. Under the new rules, as from April 2000, travelling dogs and cats are able to enter Britain without going into quarantine if they have not been to a nonqualifying country in the 6 months before entry to the UK, they are fitted with a microchip under their skin, and have full antirabies vaccination history. Vaccination should have been followed up by blood test showing satisfactory level of protection against rabies, and 6 months should have elapsed since that blood test was performed. Veterinary checks will be recorded and the microchip number written on a certificate which will be signed by a vet, who has treated the animal before embarkation for the UK, to prevent the spread of certain tapeworms and ticks, carried by cats and dogs. Only pets (dogs and cats) from specified Western European countries and assistance dogs from Australia will be allowed to enter Britain under the pilot, which if successful, will be followed by the Pet Travel Scheme (PETS)—to be introduced by April 2001. In the future, consideration will be given to extending the scheme to additional species and further qualifying countries. Animals landed from small boats and yachts are not eligible for the 'Pet Travel Scheme'.

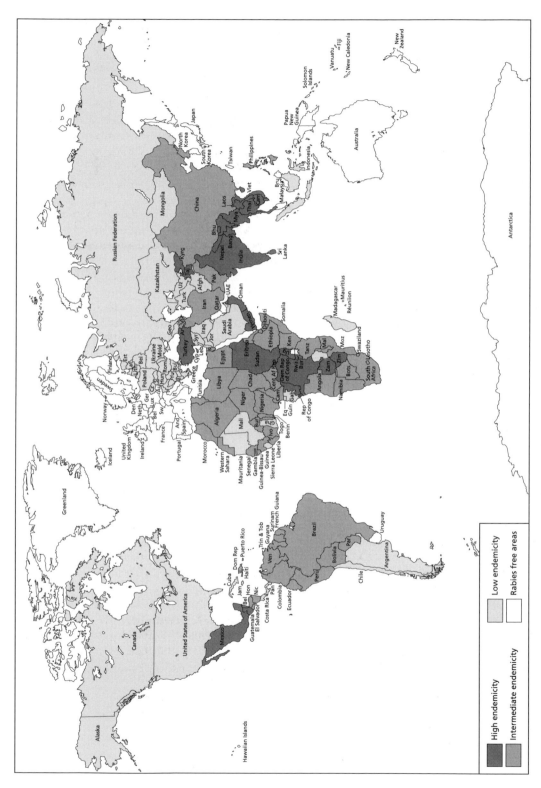

Fig. 38.1 Worldwide distribution of rabies infection. (This map generalizes available data.)

High endemicity
Intermediate endemicity
Low endemicity
Rabies free areas

213

Pet animals travelling within the United Kingdom and the Republic of Ireland will continue to be able to do so without restriction.

One of the problems doctors may face is that individuals bitten by animals that are accompanying their owners on a holiday here in the UK or animals that have just returned from Europe will see a doctor for advice. Where there is clinical suspicion of rabies, the doctor should proceed to 'postexposure' treatment as per available guidelines (see above). All emergency treatment in the UK is free at the point of delivery.

The majority (82%) of the estimated 35 000–50 000 annual human deaths (WHO 1997) worldwide occur in canine endemic regions with a large stray dog population. In about 10% of cases, the scratch or bite of an infected cat is responsible. India accounts for the majority of the 33 000 human deaths in Asia (WHO 1997). The risk to travellers is unknown but the annual incidence of rabies in expatriates is about 2%.

An estimated 10–12 million people receive treatment (one or more doses of postexposure rabies vaccine) each year after being exposed to animals suspected of having rabies. An estimated 5 million are treated in China, over 1 million in India, and 51 000 in Europe (1997).

Rabies control

Rabies control consists of:
- avoiding contact with animals (domestic and wild) in endemic areas;
- never handling bats, especially if they look sick or are injured;
- immunization of domestic animals;
- vaccination programmes for wild animals;
- prompt treatment of suspected exposure to rabies;
- pre-exposure immunization of people at risk because of their occupation and of travellers to endemic areas;
- immunization programmes for the population of high-risk area countries;
- quarantine of imported animals.

Information (websites)

- 'Pet Travel Scheme': For up-to-date government information telephone 'The Pet Line' on 0870 2411 710, or E-mail: pets@ahvg.maff.gov.uk Alternatively, use the website: http://www.maff.gov.uk/animalh/quarantine/default.htm
- The DoH's *Memorandum on rabies: prevention and control* can be found on http://www.doh.gov.uk/memorandumonrabies/
- The WHO report on Rabies: request by E-mail: on cdsdoc@who-int or on the website: http://www.who.int/emc-documents/rabies/whocdscraph994c.html
- *Pre-exposure*: Telephone advice for health professionals on pre-exposure rabies vaccination can be obtained from the Travel Unit, Communicable Disease Surveillance Centre on 020 8200 6868. In Scotland, contact SCIEH on 0141 300 1100.
- *Post-exposure*: Advice from the PHLS Virus Reference Division in London (Tel.: 020 8200 4400), in Scotland (Tel.: 0141 531 5900 or SCIEH 0141 300 1100), and in Northern Ireland (Tel.: 01232 329 241). Enquiries of foreign health authorities regarding the health of the animal involved in an incident, telephone the Communicable Diseases Office of the DoH on 020 7972 1522. USA: http://www.cdc.gov/epo/mmwr/preview/mmwrhtml/00056176.htm
- Country-by-country rabies risk: The Virus Reference Division, Central Public Health Laboratory, Colindale, London, NW9 5HT, Tel.: 020 8200 4400. In Scotland, SCIEH, Clifton House, Clifton Place, Glasgow, G3 7LN, Tel.: 0141 300 1100.
- Rabies vaccine for those at occupational risk: PHLS Virus Division, Tel.: 020 8200 4400. In Scotland details of availability of vaccine from SCIEH, Tel.: 0141 300 1100.

Rabies is a notifiable disease.

Chapter 39

Tick-borne encephalitis

Contraindications to vaccination

- Acute febrile illness.
- Severe hypersensitivity to egg protein.
- Severe hypersensitivity to a previously administered tick-borne encephalitis vaccine.
- Pregnant or lactating mothers should only received the vaccine after careful consideration, if they are going to be at high risk.

Possible side- and adverse effects

Local reactions

There may be swelling, redness and pain around the injection site and swelling of the regional lymphatic glands.

General reactions

Pyrexia may occur, especially in children, not usually over 38 °C and lasting up to 24 h following mainly the first dose of the vaccine, also headaches, myalgia, arthralgia, neck pain. These symptoms subside within a few days. Rarely neuritis may occur. In some patients the vaccine may cause aggravation of autoimmune diseases, such as multiple sclerosis, iridocyclitis.

The vaccine

Viral-inactivated whole-cell vaccine is used. It is not licensed in the UK and not available on the NHS—available on a 'named-patient' basis, privately only.

Administration

There is no age limit for vaccination, but children under 1 year of age should only be vaccinated if there is an actual risk of infection. The dose is the same for all ages and the primary course consists of three doses of the vaccine (Table 39.1).

- In vaccinees up to the age of 30 years, seroconversion may reach 100%, and in the over 60 year olds 93% can be achieved after the third dose. The length of protection after the second dose is 1 year, and after the third dose, 3 years.
- If rapid immunization is required, three doses of *Encepur* (Chiron Behring, Germany) can be administered according to the following schedule: 0, 7, 21 days. Seroconversion can be expected, at the earliest, 14 days after the second dose. A booster dose should be given 12–18 months later.
- Immunization should preferably be given in the winter months. If it is started in late spring or early summer (during seasonal tick activity), it is recommended that the second dose is given 2 weeks after the first in order to seroconvert as soon as possible.

Table 39.1 Administration specifications for tick-borne encephalitis vaccine.

Immunization	Dose (ml)	Route	Schedule
First dose	0.5	IM	0 months
Second dose	0.5	IM	1–3 months after 1st dose
Third dose	0.5	IM	9–12 months after 2nd dose
Booster	0.5	IM	Every 3 years

- Immunosuppressed patients and patients aged 60 and over, should have their antibody titre checked 4–8 weeks after the second dose of the vaccine (or after the third dose if the rapid immunization schedule was used). Repeat the second dose if at this stage seroconversion is unsatisfactory and give the third dose according to the immunization schedule.
- After administration of tick-borne immunoglobulin, allow at least 4 weeks before vaccinating.
- Patients with bleeding diathesis can receive the vaccine subcutaneously.

Vaccine availability

- Fsme-Immun Inject Vaccine (Hyland Immuno Baxter Healthcare Ltd; manufactured by Immuno AG/Austria) is available in individual prefilled syringe containing 0.5 mL suspension. Available on a 'named-patient' basis. Shelf-life: 12 months.
- Encepur (Chiron Behring, Germany) is available in a prefilled syringe, single dose. Available on a 'named-patient' basis, from MASTA. Shelf-life: 18 months.

Storage. Between 2 and 8 °C. *Do not freeze.*

Tick-borne encephalitis immunoglobulin

Tick-borne encephalitis-specific immunoglobulin is available for postexposure prophylaxis of non-immunized (whether by choice, or when the vaccine is contraindicated, or the first injection was given 1–4 days before infection) and immunosuppressed persons. It can be administered before exposure and up to 96 h (4 days) after exposure, i.e. after a tick bite in a tick-borne encephalitis endemic area.

Dosage

The immunoglobulin should be warmed to body temperature and administered slowly by deep IM injection. If large doses are required (›5 mL), administer them in divided doses at different injection sites. The gluteal muscle (buttock) is a good site for injection.
- *Pre-exposure prophylaxis.* Before a possible

exposure, the dose is 0.05 mL/kg BW. The protection commences within 24 h and lasts for approximately 4 weeks. If the risk continues, another dose should be administered.
- *Postexposure prophylaxis.* 0.2 mL/kg BW, administered up to 4 days after a tick bite.

In the case of a tick bite before or within 2 weeks after the first dose of the vaccine, the specific immunoglobulin should be given as follows.

Tick bite before or up to 4 days after the first dose of the vaccine:

0.1 mL/kg BW (days 1 and 2 after tick bite);
0.2 mL/kg BW (days 3 and 4 after tick bite).

Tick bite more than 4 days after first dose. Give only the second dose of the vaccine immediately and continue vaccination schedule as normally.

Tick bite before the administration of the third dose. Adhere to the vaccination schedule and perform the third dose when it is due.

If more than 4 days (96 h) have elapsed since an established or suspected tick bite, do not administer the immunoglobulin for 28 days (the maximum incubation period for the infection) as it could adversely affect the course of the tick-borne encephalitis infection.

Immunoglobulin availability

FSME-Bulin specific immunoglobulin (Baxter Hyland Immuno—manufactured by Immuno AG/Austria) is available in vials containing 1, 2, or 5 mL, on a 'named-patient' basis.

Storage: Between 2 and 8 °C. Protect from light. Shelf-life: 3 years.

Tick-borne encephalitis infection

Tick-borne encephalitis is one of the arbovirus infections (others are yellow fever, dengue fevers and Japanese B encephalitis). It is transmitted by the bite of blood-sucking infected *Ixodes* ticks, which feed on a wide range of birds and forest mammals. Less commonly it is transmitted through drinking unpasteurized milk from infected animals such as cows and goats. Humans mainly pick up the ticks through contact with infested undergrowth and grasses, especially during April through to August or in September to October after long, hot, humid summers. It is not transmitted from person-to-person.

The incubation period ranges from 2 to 28 days and the effects vary from subclinical infection through a febrile illness to frank meningo-encephalitis (in 6–10% of patients). Recovery without sequelae is the general rule. The case fatality is around 1% with worse prognosis among the elderly. Very few ticks (1–2%) are infected except in central Europe and Asia where up to 5% of ticks are infected. The disease rarely occurs at altitudes above 1000 m or in urban areas.

Distribution of the European subtype is mainly in low, warm, forested areas, especially with heavy undergrowth, in parts of Slovenia, Croatia, Czech Republic, Slovakia, Germany, Austria, Switzerland, Poland, Denmark, Latvia, Russia, Ukraine, Scandinavia, Belarus, Romania and Bulgaria. The risk per week in Austria, according to Du Pont and Steffen is 1 per 77 500 [Manual of Travel Medicine and Health, 1999. B.C. Decker Inc., Ontario, Canada]. In Central Europe the *Ixodes vicinus* ticks are the main vectors of tick-borne encephalitis (Fig. 39.1).

Ixodes persulcatus ticks are the vectors of Russian spring-summer encephalitis, a Far Eastern subtype of tick-borne encephalitis virus that occurs predominantly in sections of Russia, China and Korea (Fig. 39.2).

At-risk groups

- Travellers at particular risk are campers, hikers and ramblers in Alpine meadowland in late spring and summer.
- Collectors of mushrooms and berries in the woods and forests.
- People working in agriculture and forestry.
- Armed forces in Central Europe.

Prevention

- Advise travellers to avoid tick-infested areas.
- Dress appropriately. Ticks travel upwards, so cover ankles, legs and arms, as much skin as possible. Tuck trousers into socks.
- Avoid crouching without the protection of trousers in endemic areas (the disease is more common in women).
- Use insect repellents containing diethyl toluamide (DEET) or permethrin on clothes, especially socks, and camping gear.
- Remove ticks immediately by pulling them directly out of the skin with a slight jolt using either forceps, tweezers or with fingers, but without rotation. Grip the tick as far as possible towards the front of its head and remove the whole tick. If parts of the tick remain stuck in the skin, do remove them as soon as possible. Suffocating the tick with oil, cream or any other substances is not recommended as this may induce injection into the body of more infectious material.
- Avoid unpasteurized dairy products.
- Consider immunization for individuals with a high-risk exposure.

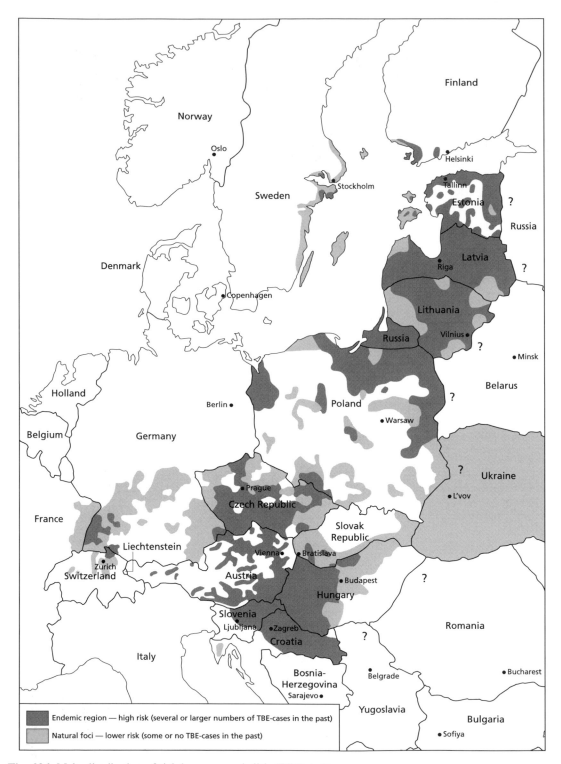

Fig. 39.1 Main distribution of tick–borne encephalitis (TBE) in Europe.

218

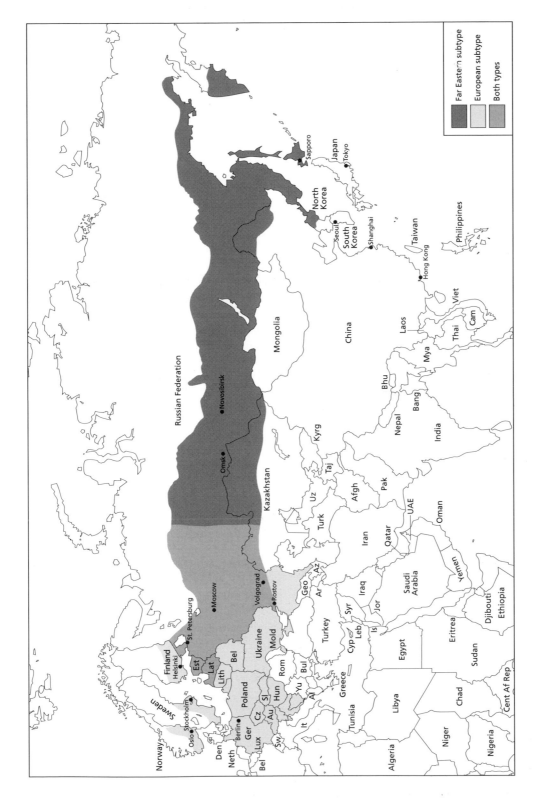

Fig. 39.2 Distribution of Western and Eastern subtype of tick-borne encephalitis virus.

219

Chapter 40

Typhoid

Vi antigen vaccines

Contraindications to vaccination

- Acute febrile illness.
- Severe reaction to a previously administered dose of the vaccine.
- Children under 2 years of age (Typherix, SmithKline Beecham) and 18 months (Typhim Vi, Aventis Pasteur MSD). Children under 18 months of age may show a suboptimal response to the vaccine and typhoid is rare in this group. The decision to vaccinate children under 18 months should be based upon the risk of exposure to typhoid.
- Pregnancy and lactation are a relative contra-indication (lack of data) and the vaccine should only be given if there is a clear risk of infection.

Possible side- and adverse effects

Local reactions

Swelling, redness and pain may occur in two-thirds of vaccinees (Typhim Vi data). Soreness was the most common reaction and has been reported in approximately 7% of recipients of Typherix. These occur in the first 48 h after vaccination.

General reactions

Myalgia, malaise, nausea, headaches and pyrexia are seen in up to 9% of recipients.

The vaccine

The two parenteral vaccines available in the UK contain purified Vi polysaccharide antigen extracted from the bacterial capsule of *Salmonella typhi* strain Ty2. Vi antigen is important in inducing protective antibodies against typhoid. It does not protect against paratyphoid fevers A and B because the causative agents, *S. typhi* A and B, do not have a Vi antigen. Each 0.5-mL dose of vaccine contains 25 µg of the Vi capsular polysaccharide antigen.

Administration (Table 40.1)

- The vaccine should be given by IM (Typherix), and deep SC or IM (Typhim Vi) injection. Exercise caution in patients with bleeding diathesis; following IM injection firm pressure should be applied to the site of injection for at least 2 minutes (Typherix).
- Antibody seroconversion is seen in over 95% of vaccinees at 2 weeks post vaccination.
- It confers over 55–75% protection against typhoid in recipients. Optimal protection is achieved within 14 days from vaccination and lasts for at least 3 years.

Table 40.1 Vaccination specifications for the Vi antigen vaccines.

Age	Primary course	Revaccination
Typhim Vi Adults and children over 18 months	0.5 mL SC/IM (single dose)	0.5 mL SC/IM every 3 years
Typherix Adults and children over 2 years	0.5 mL IM (single dose)	0.5 mL IM every 3 years

- In the UK, it is not recommended during an outbreak of typhoid fever as it does not give immediate protection and may even temporarily increase susceptibility to infection.

Vaccine availability

- Typhim Vi vaccine (Aventis Pasteur MSD) is available as a single-dose, prefilled syringe in packs of one and 10. Shake before use.
- Typherix vaccine (SmithKline Beecham) is available as a single-dose, prefilled syringe in packs of one and 10. Shake before use. It is supplied with a choice of two needles; a 1-inch (25 mm, 23G) blue and a 5/8-inch (16 mm, 25G) orange needle (see Choice of needle length on p. 17–18). Both vaccines have detachable labels, which can be peeled off the prefilled syringe and placed directly onto patient records.

Storage. Between 2 and 8 °C. *Do not freeze.*

Oral typhoid vaccine

Contraindications to vaccination

- Acute febrile illness.
- Acute gastrointestinal illness. Do not vaccinate while diarrhoea and vomiting persist.
- Severe reaction to a previously administered dose of the oral vaccine.
- Immunodeficiency and malignancy.
- HIV-positive individuals, whether asymptomatic or symptomatic.
- Pregnancy and lactation, unless the mother is at great risk of infection (it is not known whether the vaccine can cause fetal harm or whether it is passed in human milk).
- Children under 6 years of age—safety and efficacy have not as yet been established.
- Interactions include:
  (a) sulphonamides and antibiotics (delay vaccination for > 24 h after their administration), as they may be active against the vaccine strain causing inhibition of the protective immune response;
  (b) mefloquine for malarial chemoprophylaxis should not be taken on the same day—separate by at least 12 h (> 24 h in the USA);
  (c) oral polio vaccine (OPV) should be separated from the oral typhoid vaccine by 3 weeks because of possible interference of the immune response in the gut (UK DoH). The USA CDC advises that available data do not suggest that simultaneous administration of OPV or yellow fever vaccine decreases the immunogenicity of the Ty21a oral typhoid vaccine. Furthermore, they advise that if typhoid vaccination is warranted, it should not be delayed because of the administration of viral vaccines, and that simultaneous administration of Ty21a and immunoglobulin does not appear to pose a problem.

Possible side- and adverse effects

Transient mild nausea, vomiting, abdominal cramps and urticarial rash occur in less than 1% of vaccinees. There may be diarrhoea in 0.1–20% (usually mild) and fever in 1–5% of vaccinees.

The vaccine

Each oral vaccine capsule contains 2×10^9 organisms of the attenuated *S. typhi* strain Ty21a in a lyophilized form.

Administration

- The vaccine capsule should be swallowed whole (do not chew) immediately after placing it in the mouth, with a cool liquid (no warmer than 37 °C), approximately 1 h before a meal (Table 40.2).
- The capsules must be kept refrigerated and all three doses must be taken to achieve maximum efficacy.
- Protection against typhoid commences approximately 7–10 days after completion of the three-dose course and is optimum at 14 days. Duration of protection is about 1 year in European [DoH] and 5 years in US/Canadian travellers.
- A three-dose alternate-day schedule of the oral typhoid vaccine achieves protection of 70% (range 33–94%). In a study among previously unexposed subjects with a multidose schedule (five to eight doses), 87% protection was achieved.

Table 40.2 Administration specifications for oral Ty21a typhoid vaccine.

Age	Primary course		Booster for travel to endemic areas
	Dose	Frequency	
Adults and children > 6 years	1 capsule every other day	3 doses*	3-dose course annually

*In the USA, four doses are used, with a booster every 5 years under conditions of continued or repeated exposure.

- There is no need to separate the administration of the oral typhoid vaccine from other parenteral live vaccines or HNIG.
- The US Public Health Service Recommendations advise that it is necessary to restart an interrupted course of oral typhoid vaccine.
- The liquid formulation of the vaccine is not yet available in the UK.

Vaccine availability

Vivotif typhoid live oral vaccine (MASTA). One pack comprises three enteric-coated capsules, each representing one dose. The blister containing the vaccine capsules should have an intact foil seal.

Storage. Between 2 and 8 °C in a dry place, protected from light. It is important to stress to the patients who will self-administer the vaccine that it must be refrigerated at these temperatures.

Whole-cell typhoid vaccine

This vaccine is no longer available in the UK.

Which vaccine?

No vaccine is a substitute for close attention to personal, food and water hygiene. Both parenteral and oral vaccines confer comparable protection against the disease so the only differences between them are the routes of administration, dose schedules and contraindications. It is therefore reasonable to advise the following:
- when the primary course is to be given parenterally, the Vi antigen vaccine is preferable (it involves only a single injection);
- if the patient prefers the oral route for vaccination, or if he/she has a phobia of needles, the oral typhoid vaccine can be used.

Note: No item of service fee is payable for the oral typhoid vaccine (self-administered by the patient) and most Health Authorities in England and Wales do not reimburse to nondispensing practices the cost of the vaccine under SFA paragraph 44, 1–5. This scheme does not apply to Scotland and Northern Ireland.

Typhoid fever infection

'Typhos' in Greek means mist or fog, indicating the confusion many pyrexial illnesses caused bacteriologists. Typhoid fever is a potentially lethal infection that follows ingestion of the bacterium *Salmonella* serotype *typhi*. The incubation period is 1–3 weeks. It can affect any age, but is more often found in children and less often in adults. Unlike most other gastrointestinal infections, which predominantly affect children aged 6 months to 3 years, the incidence of typhoid peaks between 5 and 12 years. In a study from India published in 1999 [Sinha A. *et al.* (1999) Typhoid fever in children aged less than 5 years. *Lancet* 354, 734–7] the researchers found 25% of cases were in children under 3 years of age, 44% in those under 5 years.

The onset is insidious with headaches and lethargy being the usual presenting symptoms. It then progresses to myalgia, abdominal discomfort, cough malaise, constipation and later bloody diarrhoea with rigors. A characteristic pink papular rash 2–4 mm in diameter ('rose spots') may appear on the trunk of white patients in 25–50% of cases—they disappear on pressure. There is bradycardia relative to the high fever in less then half the patients and often splenomegaly with a distended abdomen. Hepatomegaly occurs in one-third of cases, and in one-third of these jaundice is also present. By the third week in untreated cases the patient is still pyrexial, toxic and confused. The abdomen is distended and the diarrhoea can resemble 'pea soup'. Bowel perforation occurs in 2% and haemorrhage in 4% of cases. Bacteraemia, myocarditis and pneumonia can lead to death.

Typhoid is not a diarrhoeal but a systemic disease. The infective agent is shed in faeces, typically as long as 6 weeks to 3 months after infection. Take blood cultures (especially in the first 10 days of illness) and stool cultures (or rectal swabs) if there is difficulty of diagnosis. Culture of bone marrow is the most sensitive method and can be used to establish a definite diagnosis. The Widal test can confuse the picture as it can be positive because of previous typhoid immunization, or earlier infection with salmonellae or other Gram-negative bacteria that share similar antigens (serological evidence alone is not enough to make a diagnosis).

The level of mortality in developed countries is 1.3–8.4% (highest among the elderly, lowest with treatment) and in developing countries 12–32%.

Endemic or epidemic multiresistance to antibiotics (ampicillin, trimethoprim, chloramphenicol) is reported in several countries. The management of typhoid fever centres on rehydration. If antibiotics are used, ciprofloxacin and chloramphenicol are the agents of choice. Repeated negative stool cultures are necessary to ensure eradication is complete. Twenty per cent of patients continue to excrete the organism for 2 months after the onset of illness.

About 3% (range 2–5%) of patients will continue to harbour the organism in their gallbladder for many years after infection; they become chronic carriers and excrete it periodically in their stools. High Vi capsular antibody is suggestive of a carrier state. Options for treatment include prolonged antibiotic courses and cholecystectomy.

Typhoid fever is acquired through contaminated food and drink in 90% of cases and by direct contact with a patient or a chronic carrier in 10%. Spread is usually faecal–oral. *Salmonella typhi* thrives on cold meats and shellfish. Excreta of a human case of typhoid or a chronic carrier can contaminate food and water. Sewage and water supplies can be important sources of infection. It is therefore predominantly a disease of countries economically underdeveloped, with poor sanitation, while it is uncommon in affluent parts of the world.

Eradication of typhoid in the community involves the provision of pure, clean water, proper sewage disposal systems, identification and treatment of chronic carriers and immunization. The reservoir of bacteria is strictly in humans. They can, however, survive several months in soil or water. Heating water to 57 °C destroys *S. typhi* by removing the Vi antigen. Iodination and chlorination are also effective ways of killing typhoid bacilli.

In England and Wales in 1999 150 cases of typhoid fever were reported, 122 in 1998 and 140 in 1997. The majority (about 88%) are travellers returning from abroad, especially from the Indian subcontinent (84% of those that have stated the country of infection in 1998). A few cases (16 in 1997, 13 in 1998 and 18 in 1999) are contracted in the UK from carriers who were exposed to the disease previously, usually abroad.

Typhoid immunization is recommended for travel to all countries except northern and western Europe, North America, Japan, Australia and New Zealand. It is also recommended for laboratory workers handling specimens, which may contain typhoid organisms.

● The seroprotective level of the typhoid antibody following vaccination is ≥ 1 µg/mL.

● According to WHO estimates, the global incidence of this disease is around 16 million cases each year and 600 000 deaths. The highest incidence occurs across the tropical belt, with the Indian subcontinent and Asia having approximately 80% of the world's cases (Fig. 40.1). Some low endemicity remains in southern and eastern Europe.

● The risk to travellers is estimated by Du Pont and Steffen [Manual of Travel Medicine and Health, 1999. B.C. Decker Inc., Ontario, Canada] to be over 10 cases per 100 000 visitors in the Indian subcontinent, parts of South America (mainly Peru) and West Africa (Senegal), while for North Africa (Egypt, Morocco) and Haiti it is 4–10 per 100 000 visitors. Most at risk are persons visiting relatives in their native country.

● Travellers should be advised that the most effective prevention of typhoid fever is by strict adherence to the rules on food, water and beverages. Immunization provides a good second line of protection.

● In exceptional cases where chemoprophylaxis is necessary, the quinolones can be used.

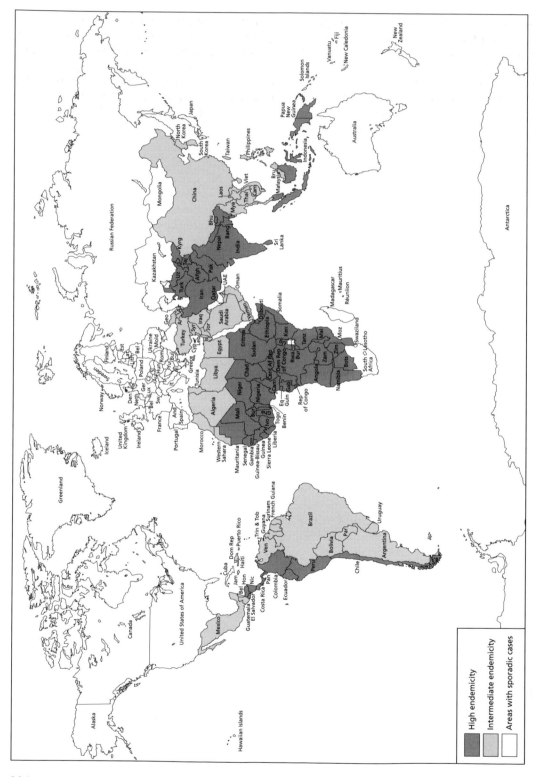

Fig. 40.1 Worldwide distribution of typhoid fever infection. (This map generalizes available data.)

High endemicity

Intermediate endemicity

Areas with sporadic cases

● Staying in the best hotels does not always guarantee a trouble-free stay. An employee or even the orange juice (as in the case of a New York resort hotel) can be the source.

● Queen Victoria's husband Prince Albert died from typhoid at Windsor Castle in December 1861. Thirty-seven years later, in 1898, vaccination against typhoid was introduced. 'Typhoid Mary', an immigrant cook from Europe who was a carrier, spread typhoid fever among upper-class families in New York, causing illness in 54 people and three deaths.

● Disease and vaccine information from the CDC: www.cdc.gov/nip/publications/acip-list.htm

Typhoid fever is a notifiable disease.

Chapter 41

Varicella

Contraindications to varicella vaccine

- Acute febrile illness.
- Severe hypersensitivity to a previously administered dose of the vaccine.
- Severe sensitivity (anaphylactic reaction) to neomycin, traces of which are contained in the vaccine.
- Immunosuppressed patients during intense immunosuppressive therapy, including radiotherapy.
- HIV patients.
- Children with aplastic anaemia.
- With low lymphocyte count of less than 1200/mm^3.
- Within 3 months from administration of varicella-zoster immunoglobulin (VZIG)—it can negatively interfere with antibody production after vaccination.
- Within 3 weeks of administration of another live virus vaccine but may be administered simultaneously and at different sites. In the case of measles vaccine, if not given simultaneously, allow 1 month between two vaccines as measles vaccination may lead to short-lived suppression of the cell-mediated response and therefore reduce the efficacy of the varicella vaccine.
- Pregnancy and for 3 months before—adequate contraception should be used for 3 months after vaccination of women of child-bearing age.
- Aspirin should be avoided for 6 weeks after vaccination because of the possible risk of developing Reye's syndrome.

Possible side- and adverse effects

Local reactions

Pain, induration and redness sometimes occur for a short time.

General reactions

Papulovesicular eruptions, sometimes accompanied by fever, may appear a few days or weeks after vaccination. The vaccine can produce an attenuated subclinical varicella infection in susceptible persons.

The vaccine

A live attenuated varicella vaccine is available in the UK on a 'named-patient' basis (unlicensed), for immunocompromised patients such as children with leukaemia, or about to have kidney transplants, etc.

The OKA strain of live attenuated varicella vaccine was developed in the early 1970s in Japan for use in immunocompromised children at risk of varicella.

Administration

A single dose of the vaccine is given for children aged 9 months to 12 years, while older children and adults receive two doses of vaccine, 6 weeks apart by SC injection. It is reserved in the UK for immunocompromised patients. Maintenance chemotherapy is withheld for 1 week before and 1 week after the first dose of the vaccine, while steroids are withheld for an additional week. Efficacy of the vaccine is estimated at 85%.

Revaccination is not necessary unless so indicated following titration of varicella antibodies.

About 90% of healthy children are protected after one dose of the vaccine (a suggestion is to consider incorporating varicella immunization at 15 months of age for all children), while in healthy young adults protection is about 70% after two doses. A vaccinee who is not completely protected from chickenpox usually has a modified illness after exposure to infection.

Postexposure vaccination within 3 days of contact may prevent development of varicella in 90–100% of healthy children.

Varicella vaccine induces both humoral and cellular immunity. Vaccine-induced immunity is maintained after two decades of follow-up [Kamiya H. & Ito M. Update on varizella vaccine. Curr Opin Pediatr 1999; 11 : 3–8]. The vaccine may also be effective as post-exposure prophylaxis [Watson B. *et al.* Post-exposure effectiveness of varicella vaccine. Pediatrics 2000; 105 : 84–88], but its role in the prevention of Zoster and the question of booster doses is unresolved.

Some individuals show increases of antibodies against varicella-zoster virus (VZV) some time after vaccination; it is suggested that this finding is a result of immunological boosting caused by exposure to wild-type VZV in the community. About 25% of adults, and immunocompromised children and adults, will lose detectable antibodies within 1 year from vaccination. It is of concern that these individuals might then become exposed to wild-type virus and contract severe varicella. High-risk patients should have measurements of their varicella antibodies taken periodically after immunization, so that the need for a booster dose can be identified.

Breast-feeding is not a contraindication to vaccination.

Vaccine availability

Varilrix (SmithKline Beecham). The lyophilized vaccine is available in single-dose vials with a diluent in ampoules and prefilled syringes. Ensure the vaccine dissolves completely. Available on a 'named-patient' basis from the manufacturer.

Storage. Between 2 and 8 °C. *Do not freeze diluent.* Use immediately after reconstitution.

Human varicella-zoster immunoglobulin

Contraindications to immunoglobulin

- Patients with thrombocytopenia.

- Previous anaphylactic reaction following administration of human varicella-zoster immunoglobulin.

Possible side- and adverse effects

Local reactions

There may be short-term discomfort at the site of injection.

General reactions

Very rarely anaphylaxis may occur, especially in patients who have had an atypical reaction to blood transfusion or treatment with plasma derivatives and in patients who are already seropositive if determined by a sensitive assay (e.g. latex agglutination) or enzyme immunoassay.

The immunoglobulin

Human varicella-zoster immunoglobulin (HVZIG) is manufactured from the pooled plasma of donors with high titres of varicella-zoster antibody.

Each plasma donation and the final product are tested by validated procedures and found non-reactive for hepatitis B surface antigen and also antibodies to HIV-1, HIV-2 and hepatitis C virus.

Administration (Table 41.1)

Table 41.1 Human varicella-zoster immunoglobulin dosage.

Age (years)	Dose (mg)	Route
0–5	250	IM
6–10	500	IM
11–14	750	IM
⩾15	1000	IM

- HVZIG is available in a single-dose vial of 250 mg strictly for IM use.
- It does not prevent infection if given within 72 h of exposure but may attenuate an attack if given within 10 days after exposure.
- Of all adults in the UK over the age of 20 years, 90% show evidence of previous infection with

VZV. Contacts of immunosuppressed patients without a definite history of chickenpox should be screened for antibody to the virus.

Human varicella–zoster immunoglobulin is recommended for individuals in contact with chicken-pox or shingles in the following groups:

• immunocompromised patients (see definition on p. 45) by disease or treatment and pregnant women who are seronegative for VZV antibody;

• recent (within 6 months) bone marrow transplant recipients regardless of history of chickenpox;

• symptomatic HIV-positive individuals unless known to have VZV antibodies (asymptomatic HIV-positive individuals in contact with chickenpox or shingles do not require the immunoglobulin);

• infants up to 4 weeks after birth whose mothers develop chickenpox (not shingles) in the period 7 days before to 1 month after delivery;

• infants in contact with chickenpox or shingles in the first 28 days whose mothers have no history of chickenpox or who, on testing, have no antibody;

• premature infants in contact with chickenpox or shingles born before 28 weeks of gestation or with a birthweight of less than 1 kg—even if the mother gives a positive history of chickenpox, they may not possess maternal antibody;

• pregnant women exposed at any stage, but especially during the first 20 or the last 3 weeks, without a history of chickenpox who are found not to possess antibody to the virus. About two-thirds of pregnant women in the UK have antibody despite a negative history. This immunoglobulin does not prevent infection but it may attenuate maternal disease.

The following infants, aged less than 1 month, will possess antibody to the virus, therefore they do not require the immunoglobulin:

(a) those born more than 7 days after the onset of maternal chickenpox;

(b) whose mothers have a positive history of chickenpox and/or a positive antibody result (with the exception of premature infants as described above);

(c) whose mothers develop zoster before or after delivery.

• Particular attention should be paid to patients receiving high doses of corticosteroids (children on $\geqslant 2$ mg/kg/day of prednisolone, or an adult on > 40 mg/day). Do not stop the corticosteroid. Administer the immunoglobulin (unless shown to have antibody to the virus) and seek prompt specialist care and urgent treatment (e.g. systemic aciclovir).

Immunoglobulin availability

Human Varicella–Zoster Immunoglobulin intramuscular (Bio Products Laboratory) available in 250-mg single-dose vial.

For NHS use only, it can be obtained from all Public Health Laboratory Services, from The Laboratories, Belfast City Hospital, or from the Blood Transfusion Services in Scotland.

Storage. Between 2 and 8 °C. *Do not freeze.*

Varicella and zoster infection

Varicella (chickenpox) is a highly infectious disease with humans being the only reservoir of the virus. It is caused by the varicella zoster virus. Primary infection results in chickenpox. It persists in a latent form and reactivation results in herpes zoster (shingles). Chickenpox is endemic throughout the Western world.

The virus is transmitted directly by personal contact with chickenpox or shingles lesions or by air-borne droplet infection. Most cases of chickenpox occur in children between 5 and 10 years of age. In children, it is usually a mild disease, much less severe than in adults. The infection can be severe in immunocompromised patients, in neonates and in pregnant women, particularly in the first trimester (fetal varicella syndrome).

Nearly everyone (90%) in the UK has had the infection by the age of 40 years. Most adults with negative or unknown history of chickenpox are likely to be immune.

The incubation period is usually 2–3 weeks. Patients are contagious 1–2 days before the characteristic vesicles appear and until they dry. The disease is seasonal, in winter and spring, with a peak between March and May.

The complications of primary varicella disease

include scarring, pneumonia, haemorrhagic problems, meningoencephalitis, acute transverse myelitis, hemiparesis, osteomyelitis, acute epiglottitis, thrombocytopenia, leukopenia, myocarditis, pyogenic sepsis, and fetal varicella syndrome when infection occurs in the first trimester (microcephaly, cataracts, limb hypoplasia, growth retardation).

Reactivated varicella (shingles) can cause blindness, postherpetic neuralgia and encephalitis. Approximately one in five people develop shingles at some time in their lives. Patients with active shingles can transmit chickenpox. Reactivation has been associated with increasing age, HIV infection and cancer.

Primary infection or vaccination provides longterm immunity. Exogenous infection in individuals who have had chickenpox has been demonstrated by a rise in antibody titre but this does not lead to clinical manifestations (the child 'does not get chickenpox twice'). Exogenous infection boosts the immunity.

Chickenpox in children does not require specific treatment unless severe and/or in immunocompromised patients who should receive human varicella-zoster immunoglobulin IM and oral aciclovir (20 mg/kg BW to a maximum of 800 mg, started within 24 h of onset of rash and repeated at 6-hourly intervals for 5 days). If a patient is on corticosteroids, they should not be stopped—seek specialist advice. Adults with severe chickenpox or shingles could also receive aciclovir. Famciclovir and valaciclovir are licensed also for the treatment of herpes zoster in adults. For indications of varicella-zoster immunoglobulin, see p. 228.

Figures for the UK show that chickenpox causes an average of 30 deaths each year, and one-third of these are associated with immunosuppression. In 1996, 39 people died from chickenpox, most of them were adults.

Chickenpox in pregnancy

During the first two trimesters of pregnancy, it may result in chickenpox embryopathy, which may include microcephaly, hydrocephalus, limb hypoplasia, microphthalmia, cataracts, uveitis, skin scarring and growth retardation. The overall risk to the fetus is estimated at less than 1% in the first 12 weeks. The critical period is 13–20 weeks of pregnancy when the risk to the fetus is thought to be around 2%. In the last trimester, it may result in neonatal chickenpox, which, if severe, may be associated with a mortality as high as 30%.

If a pregnant mother comes into contact with a case of chickenpox and there is a definite history of chickenpox, she can be reassured. If there is no such clear history, blood must be sent to the local PHLS microbiology department for same-day assay of antivaricella-zoster antibodies. Such antibodies are usually present in two-thirds of mothers and they can be reassured. If antibodies are absent, the PHLS will advise on the administration of HVZIG.

Children with chickenpox

Children with chickenpox should not be given aspirin as the combination may lead to Reye's syndrome, which can be fatal.

In the USA, before January 1996 when the varicella vaccine became available for routine immunization, about 4 million cases occurred each year (mostly in children under 15 years), 400 000 cases of zoster, 9300 hospitalizations and 50–100 deaths. Now that the vaccine is in routine use for children, it is estimated that for every dollar the US spends on the vaccine, they save $5 (the study assumed a preschool vaccine uptake of 97%). Immunization against varicella protects not only against chickenpox but also against developing later shingles. On the other hand, frequent contact with chickenpox is associated with a lower risk than average of contracting shingles [Solomon B.A. *et al.* (1998) Lasting immunity to varicella in doctors study (LIVID) study. *J. Am. Acad. Dermatol.* 38, 763–5].

Here in the UK, we can only hope future combined vaccines will have the varicella vaccine incorporated so that it will be easier to obtain approval from the DoH to add varicella to our childhood immunization programme. Work at the PHLS has calculated that we would need to vaccinate a child for less than £9 for this immunization to be cost-saving. Another worry is that of longterm immunity: will the vaccine protection wane with time such that varicella infection is merely postponed to later in life? With our present knowledge it is unclear when booster doses should be given, or indeed whether they will be needed at all.

In the meantime, chickenpox is increasingly affecting pre-school children in the UK. Between 1983 and 1998, age-specific incidence of chickenpox derived from consultations with GPs taking part in the Royal College of General Practitioners Weekly Returns Service doubled in children aged 0 to 4 years, halved in children aged 5 to 14 years, and fell by almost a third in adults aged 15 to 44 years. This downward shift in age of contracting chickenpox may be a result of increased social contact between preschool children [Ross A, Fleming D. (2000) Chickenpox increasingly affects preschool children. *Commun. Dis. Public Health* 3, 213–215].

Information

● Disease and vaccine inforamtion from the CDC: www.cdc.gov/nip/publications/acip-list.htm.
● Information on shingles for patients: http://www.medinfo.co.uk/conditions/shingles.html

Chapter 42

Yellow fever

Contraindications to vaccination

- Acute febrile illness.
- Infants below the age of 9 months—infants under 4 months of age are more susceptible to adverse reactions of the vaccine (encephalitis) than older children and this risk is age-related. Consider vaccination of infants aged between 4 and 9 months only if travelling to an infected area and at increased risk.
- Previous severe reaction to the vaccine.
- Anaphylactic hypersensitivity to hens' eggs. As a result of changes in the manufacturing process the vaccine available in the UK no longer contains neomycin and polymyxin.
- Pregnancy, although if a pregnant woman must travel to an area of high yellow fever risk, vaccination should be considered as the risk of infection may outweigh the small theoretical risk to the fetus from vaccination. It is best to postpone travelling. The WHO advises that vaccination against yellow fever is permitted after the sixth month of pregnancy when justified epidemiologically [*International Travel and Health*, WHO (1999) 88]. It is not known whether the yellow fever virus or the antibodies cross the placenta during pregnancy, or are excreted in breast milk during lactation. An unreferenced entry in the *US Pharmacopeia Drug Information* 1998, 18th edition, confirms that 'yellow fever vaccine is not distributed into milk following vaccination and therefore, may be given to nursing mothers'. A breast-feeding mother may receive the vaccine if travelling to a highly endemic area.
- Immunodeficiency and malignancy.
- HIV-positive individuals whether asymptomatic or symptomatic—insufficient evidence as to the safety of its use (DoH advice). Consider sup-plying the traveller with a letter of exemption. Travellers with asymptomatic HIV infection who cannot avoid potential exposure to yellow fever could be offered the choice of immunization. The WHO recommends yellow fever vaccination in asymptomatic HIV infection, and states that there is insufficient evidence to permit a definitive statement on whether administration of this vaccine poses a risk for symptomatic HIV-infected persons [*International Travel and Health*, WHO (1999) 66]. Most physicians caring for people with HIV would be reluctant to give yellow fever vaccine to patients with CD4 lymphocyte counts below $500/mm^3$ and would offer waiver letters for travel purposes.
- Within 3 weeks of administration of another live virus vaccine (ignore in the case of OPV and immediate travel), but may be administered simultaneously and at a different site. Within 3 weeks of administration of the live bacterial BCG.
- Give the cholera vaccine (not available in the UK) simultaneously or, better still, separate by 3 weeks as it may inhibit antibody response to both vaccines.
- Concurrent vaccination against hepatitis B may reduce antibody titres expected from yellow fever vaccine, and probably of that from hepatitis B vaccine. Where possible, separate theses two vaccines by 3–4 weeks.

Yellow fever vaccine may, if necessary, be given simultaneously with human normal immuno-globulin (HNIG), which in the UK is unlikely to contain antibody to the yellow fever virus. Ideally, the HNIG should be administered 3 weeks after the vaccine. If the HNIG was given first, 3 months or at least 6 weeks should elapse before the vaccine is given.

Possible side- and adverse effects

Local reactions

Local reactions include swelling, redness and pain lasting 2–5 days (5%).

General reactions

These are generally mild. Headaches, myalgia and low-grade fever occur in 2–5% of vaccinees, lasting 5–10 days after vaccination. Less than 0.2% will need to limit their activities. Rash, urticaria and jaundice are extremely rare (less than 1 in a million) and occur primarily in vaccinees allergic to eggs. Encephalitis associated with vaccination was reported worldwide in 18 cases out of more than 200 million doses of the vaccine and mainly occurs in infants.

The vaccine

It is a live, attenuated, virus vaccine prepared from the 17D strain of yellow fever virus grown in chick embryos. It contains traces of neomycin and polymyxin.

Administration (Table 42.1)

• The reconstituted vaccine should be given within 1 h by deep SC injection. The dose is the same for all ages and induces seroconversion in nearly 100% of recipients.
• It is recommended that, apart from travellers, laboratory workers handling infected material should be immunized.
• The immunity, which probably lasts for life, is officially accepted for travel for 10 years starting from 10 days after primary immunization and immediately after a booster.

• For the purposes of international travel, the vaccine is administered only at Yellow Fever Vaccination Centres approved by the DoH. These centres meet stringent conditions regarding transportation, handling, storage, administration and documentation. They issue the International Certificate of Vaccination for Yellow Fever, which is required for entry into or exit from some countries.
• The GP should supply an official letter of exemption to a patient who cannot, for medical reasons, receive the vaccine. However, certain countries may not accept this letter, so it may be necessary to use this letter to obtain an official waiver stamped by the embassy of the countries to be travelled through or to. Otherwise, the traveller may risk quarantine or sometimes vaccination at the border using needles of sometimes questionable sterility.
• The international Certificate of Yellow Fever Vaccination is the only certificate that represents a vaccination internationally regulated. The WHO recommends this immunization for all travellers to countries situated in the endemic areas (see Fig. 42.1), especially for travel outside the urban areas, even if these countries have not officially reported cases and do not require evidence of immunization upon entry. In the 'endemic' areas, the potential for transmission exists, while 'infected' areas are countries whose officials have reported human cases to the WHO.
• The requirement for immunization is not only to protect the individual but to prevent the disease spreading further in that country or transferring it to another country where the *Aedes aegypti* mosquitoes are present and therefore transmission is possible. South-east Asia and the Indian subcontinent have the mosquito but not the disease. They require a Certificate of Yellow Fever Immunization from travellers coming from an endemic area.

Table 42.1 Administration specifications for yellow fever vaccine.

Dose (ml) > 9 months of age and adults	Route	Schedule	Booster
0.5	SC	Once only	Every 10 years (for travellers)

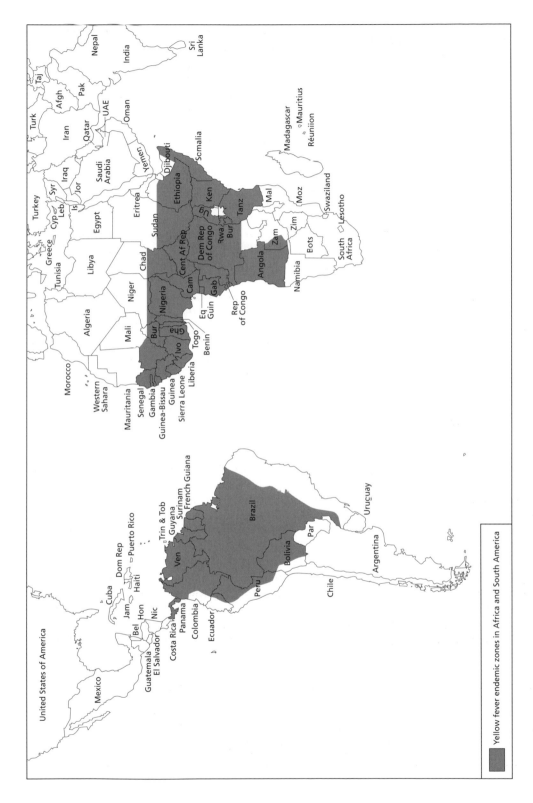

Fig. 42.1 Yellow fever endemic zones in Africa and South America.

Yellow fever endemic zones in Africa and South America

233

Vaccine availability

Yellow fever vaccine live BP (Medeva Pharma) is available as freeze-dried vaccine supplied to designated centres in packs of five single-dose and five-dose vials with diluent. Vaccination is available from DoH-approved Yellow Fever Vaccination Centres only.

In order to assist vaccine shortages, Aventis Pasteur MSD imported their vaccine from France in 2000. This yellow fever vaccine is unlicensed, in multidose vials (10 doses).

Storage. Between 2 and 8 °C. *Do not freeze diluent.* Protect from light. Reconstituted vaccine should be used within 1 h.

Yellow fever infection

The virus is believed to have originated in Africa and to have crossed the Atlantic by trading and slaving ships, which may have introduced one of its important vectors, the mosquito *Aedes aegypti*. The first reported outbreak was in Barbados in 1647. It is today endemic in equatorial Africa and in parts of South America (Fig. 42.1).

Yellow fever is a tropical, urban and rural arbovirus infection (of the *Flavivirus* genus) transmitted by mosquitoes. It occurs: in the tropics of Africa between 15N and 10S parallels (especially western Africa including Ghana, Nigeria and adjacent countries) and is worst during late rainy and early dry season; in South America (especially Peru, Bolivia, Brazil and the neighbouring countries) and the southern part of Central America (that includes Panama with extension to Trinidad and Tobago) and is worst between January and March. It is totally absent from Asia despite the presence there of its vector and animal reservoir.

The main vector is the (female) mosquito *A. aegypti* in Africa, while in South America are the forest-dwelling *Haemagogus* and *Sabethes* mosquitoes. The mosquito acts also as a reservoir, as once infected it remains so throughout its life.

In jungle yellow fever, the mosquitoes transmit the disease among nonhuman primates (monkeys are the main hosts) but also humans when the opportunity arises. In urban/rural yellow fever, the disease is transmitted in a cycle from human to mosquito to human—the mosquitoes live permanently or seasonally in shelters such as discarded coconut shells, water pools and reservoirs close to human dwellings.

After an incubation period of 3–6 days, the disease may be completely asymptomatic or it appears in a mild form with nonspecific flu-like symptoms, or it may cause fever, vomiting, red tongue, swollen bleeding gums, congested conjunctivae, haemorrhage and jaundice. The death rate ranges from less than 5% (in the indigenous population) to more than 60% in nonimmune adults. Death occurs within 10 days from the onset of symptoms. The WHO estimates that there are probably 300 000 cases and 20 000 deaths a year from the disease, although only 1439 cases and 491 deaths were notified to the WHO in 1993–97.

There is no specific treatment except for the relief of symptoms. On the other hand, vaccination has almost total efficacy. Recovery from yellow fever results in lasting immunity. Immune mothers may pass on passive immunity to their infants that can last up to 6 months.

During the past decade, we have witnessed a 'dramatic resurgence' of the disease in Africa, according to the WHO. Some 200 000 cases of yellow fever occur every year in 33 endemic countries on the continent (the vast majority of them in sub-Saharan Africa), with a combined population of 468 million. Of great concern is the fact that the *A. aegypti* mosquito is now widespread in many African cities.

The incorporation of yellow fever vaccine into the routine Expanded Programme on Immunization (EPI) was recommended in 1998 by a joint WHO/UNICEF Technical Group on Immunization in Africa. In order to avoid the need for a return visit it was suggested to immunize against yellow fever at 9–12 months of age when the children will normally receive the measles vaccine. Unfortunately, many of the African countries worst hit by the resurgence of yellow fever are also among the poorest on the continent and are unable to afford the vaccines with their own resources.

Control of yellow fever is by:
• eradication of the vector in rural and urban areas;

- avoidance of mosquito bites. Mosquitoes that transmit urban yellow fever generally feed indoors and outdoors during the early morning and late afternoon. Covering up, using insect repellents containing DEET, or similar, and the use of mosquito nets are very important measures;
- immunization (mass and routine) against yellow fever is most important, especially of the jungle type;
- community clean-up campaigns to eliminate the mosquitoes breeding sites;
- wearing clothes that cover most of the body, staying in well-screened areas;
- sleeping under bed nets treated with permethrin;
- isolation of yellow fever patients in mosquito-proof rooms to prevent further spread of the virus into the mosquito population;
- epidemic control;
- continuous surveillance.

The risk to travellers is considered to be low as most are immunized.

Some countries require vaccination only if a traveller arrives from an infected area. Check the current US biweekly Blue Sheet to determine whether any country on the itinerary is currently infected with yellow fever by accessing the Blue Sheet on the CDC website: http://www.cdc.gov/travel

Disease and vaccine information from the CDC: www.cdc.gov/nip/publications/acip-list.htm

Yellow fever is a notifiable disease.

Part 4

The Practice and Immunization

Chapter 43

Immunization fees and the UK GP

A UK GP is an independent contractor, not a health service employee. Most of the income of British GPs derives from providing services to NHS patients and this is funded centrally by the Department of Health (DoH).

GP earnings from immunizations are derived from:
- immunization target payments;
- item-of-service fees for immunization;
- direct payment by patients;
- personal dispensing of vaccines by GPs in England and Wales.

Target payments

The target payments for immunization were imposed on GPs as part of the 1990 contract. The fees payable to GPs depend on the percentage of the target population who receive the vaccinations and whether this percentage is above the targets set by the Government, currently 70% vaccination uptake for the lower, and 90% for the higher target fee. Furthermore, these fees vary according to how much of the work is undertaken by the GP and how much by other agencies, such as immunization clinics run by health authorities or hospitals.

For target payments purposes, childhood immunizations are divided into two sections. The first is the percentage of children on the practice list who, by the age of 2 years, have achieved full Group 1 (diphtheria, tetanus, polio—three doses), Group 2 (pertussis—three doses), Group 3 (measles/mumps/rubella (MMR)—one dose), and Group 4 (*Haemophilus influenzae* b—three doses or the over-13-months single dose) immunization on the first day of the quarter. The meningococcal C conjugate vaccine attracts an item-of-service fee.

The second target payment is the percentage of those who have received boosters for diphtheria, tetanus and polio by the age of 5 years. The second MMR was expected to have entered this target in 1999 but this did not happen and GPs continue to receive an item-of-service fee instead.

The target population includes all children on the practice list who are 2 years (or 5 years for the second target population) on the first day of a quarter.

It has been calculated that the average GP list (1884 patients) will include 22 children aged 2 or under. A doctor achieves the 90% target if 90% or more of the children aged 2 or under are immunized, in which case the higher target rate is payable (£2685 p.a. in April 2000). If they do not achieve this target, but nevertheless achieve 70% or more (but under 90%), the lower target fee is payable (£895). Proportionate target payments for the preschool boosters (children age 5 or under) are £795 and £265, respectively.

The children could have been immunized in their present or previous practice. If there are more than 22 children on a doctor's list, the target payment is proportionately higher. However, any immunization courses completed outside general practice (e.g. in a health authority-run clinic) will lead to a proportionately reduced payment (but they do count towards achieving the percentage target).

Item-of-service (IOS) fees

These are paid to GPs by the Government only when a particular vaccination is given as a matter of public policy, either for persons remaining in this country or those travelling abroad that qualify. Fees are paid at two levels. Level B fee (£6.45 in April 2000) is paid for the last in a course of two or more vaccinations or a reinforcing dose, or for vaccinations that are in a single dose. Level A fee

(£4.45) is paid for all other vaccinations. Level B is higher than A. Claims should be made on the Items-of-Service Multi-Claims GMS4 form (England and Wales).

Health Authorities have discretion to pay an item-of-service fee to GPs for vaccinations they administer in the case of local outbreaks of a disease, or any emergency programmes provided:

● the GP is not employed by the Health Authority for a session during which the vaccinations are performed;

● the Health Authority's public health physician recommends the vaccinations, or subsequently approves the vaccination—as in the case of close contacts of a person suffering from a specific infectious disease.

This scheme is covered by the Statement of Fees and Allowances, paragraph 27.4. Item 13 of paragraph 27/Schedule 1 specifies that this only applies to diphtheria, tetanus, poliomyelitis, anthrax, typhoid, rabies, infectious hepatitis and *Haemophilus influenzae* b.

The DoH agreed in 1999 to give GPs an IOS fee for meningococcal C vaccination, and in 2000 for influenza vaccination of any patient aged 65 and over.

Immunizations attracting an item-of-service fee

Persons not travelling abroad

● *Diphtheria and tetanus either separately or combined*: for children aged 6 years and over who have not had the basic course of immunization or a reinforcing dose. Also for staff in hospitals considered at risk of infection.

● *Tetanus*: for children not previously immunized aged 15–19 years, and nonimmunized persons. For previously immunized persons having a booster on leaving school, entering higher education or starting work; thereafter, for those who have not had a booster during the previous 5 years or more.

● *Poliomyelitis*: for nonimmunized 6–40-year-olds; parents or guardians of children receiving oral polio. Groups at risk such as GPs, dentists, ambulance staff, GP practice staff in contact with patients, etc. For a reinforcing dose for persons

aged 6 years and over, and previously immunized: at school, school leaving, entering higher education or starting work, and groups at risk as above.

● *MMR*: children given the second MMR dose at or near the routine preschool immunizations; children not previously immunized with MMR aged 6–15 years;

● *Measles*: children who have not previously been immunized against measles and who have not had measles, aged 6–15 years. They should receive the MMR.

● *Rubella*: girls aged 10–14 years who have not previously had and are not currently receiving the MMR vaccine. Seronegative nonpregnant women of child-bearing age. Seronegative male staff working in antenatal clinics.

● *Haemophilus influenzae b*: no IOS fee is payable for persons aged 2 years and over. Under 2 years, children are covered by the target payments.

● *Meningococcal C conjugate (MenC)*: an IOS fee is payable for infants aged 2, 3 and 4 months and schoolchildren that have not received the vaccine at school. *Meningococcal A + C polysaccharide*: there is no provision for an IOS fee—other than for immunizing students during the 1999 campaign when the MenC was in short supply.

● *Infectious hepatitis*: the DoH in its Statement of Fees and Allowances (SFA—'Red Book') does not clarify which hepatitis the term 'infectious hepatitis' covers. It is presumed to cover all types, and a fee is payable for vaccinating those at risk in institutions, through work, and others recommended through health officers, i.e. the Public Health Department of the Local Health Authority.

● *Anthrax*: for workers exposed to special risks of contracting anthrax, such as those working in establishments such as tanneries, glue, gelatine, soap and bonemeal factories and woollen mills.

● *Typhoid*: staff in hospitals considered to be at risk of infection.

● *Rabies*: vaccination of individuals considered by the DoH (*Memorandum on Rabies: Prevention and Control*—February 2000—www.doh.gov.uk/memoradumonrabies/ to be at special risk because of their employment:

(a) laboratory workers handling the virus;

(b) those who in the course of their work may be

at risk of exposure to infection as a result of the regular handling of imported animals that either may not have completed quarantine or may not have fulfilled the requirements of the Pet Travel Scheme, e.g.

> at animal quarantine centres;
> at zoos;
> at research and acclimatization centres where primates and other imported animals are housed;
> at ports, e.g. certain Customs and Excise Officers;
> agents authorized to carry imported animals.

(c) veterinary and technical staff in the State Veterinary Services;

(d) local authority inspectors appointed under the Animal Health Act 1981 (it only includes dog wardens who are also inspectors);

(e) workers in enzootic areas abroad, who by the nature of their work are at special risk of contact with rabid animals (e.g. veterinary staff, zoologists);

(f) health workers who are likely to come into

(g) licensed bat handlers.

● *Influenza*: for all patients aged 65 and over.

Persons travelling abroad

In certain circumstances, the DoH will pay an IOS fee:

● *Tetanus, diphtheria*: no special provisions are made for these two vaccines as regards travellers, so regulations for 'Persons not travelling abroad' will apply.

● *Typhoid*: travellers to an infected area or where typhoid immunization is a condition of entry. Travellers to all countries except Canada, the USA, Australia, New Zealand and northern Europe. The DoH will not pay a fee for the oral typhoid vaccine (self-administered by the patient) despite the fact that the patient is counselled by the GP or nurse before the vaccine is prescribed. Level B payment is payable for the parenteral typhoid vaccine (single injection).

● *Cholera*: travellers to an infected area or where cholera immunization is a condition of entry. All travellers to Africa and Asia. The parenteral vaccine is not available in the UK. The oral cholera vaccines are anticipated to become available in the future.

● *Poliomyelitis*: travellers to an infected area or where polio immunization is a condition of entry. Travellers to all countries except Canada, the USA, Australia, New Zealand and Europe (includes Cyprus and Turkey).

● *Infectious hepatitis*: this is assumed to refer to all types of hepatitis, although the Local Health Authorities usually pay an item-of-service fee for the administration of hepatitis A vaccine or immunoglobulin. Health Authorities differ in their interpretation of payments for hepatitis A vaccine. For persons travelling outside northern Europe, Australia and New Zealand, particularly those who are going to reside for 3 months or longer or who, if infected, might be less resistant because of a pre-existing disease, or who are travelling to areas of poor sanitation (degree of exposure to infection likely to be high). The DoH advises Health Authorities to make a level B payment for the concluding dose of hepatitis A vaccine, whether the present two-, or the previous, three-dose type is used [Health Circular FHSL (94)49 of 24 October 1994]. This could apply to the combined hepatitis A and B vaccine (Twinrix) where three doses are given. None the less, some Health Authorities are known to have paid fee A for the first dose, too. If the combined hepatitis A and B vaccine is used, an IOS fee, when appropriate, is paid for the A component of the vaccine.

The DoH does not pay an IOS fee for travel immunizations such as hepatitis B, tetanus, diphtheria, meningococcal, yellow fever, rabies, Japanese B and tick-borne encephalitis. The GP may be able to claim an IOS fee if the traveller requires the vaccine because he or she lives in the UK and an IOS fee is payable for patients not travelling abroad, e.g. tetanus and/or diphtheria.

Where the GP does not receive an IOS fee, he or she is allowed to charge the traveller a fee (but see below for other conditions that need to apply in such a case). The relevant paragraph in the 'Terms of Service for Doctors', which is contained in the NHS (General Medical Services, GMS) Regulations 1992, as amended, is number 38, sub-paragraph (h), which deals with immunizations for travel abroad. It states that GPs can charge for treatment consisting of immunization for which no remuneration is payable by the Health Authority through the Red Book and which is requested in connection with travel abroad.

In the case of the combined hepatitis A and B vaccine, and in the absence of clear guidance from the DoH with regard to hepatitis B, the GP should claim an IOS fee, if applicable, for hepatitis A. For the combined hepatitis A and typhoid vaccine, claim for typhoid first, and for hepatitis A when you give the hepatitis A reinforcing dose. Some health authorities pay for both hepatitis A and typhoid when the combined vaccine is used. For tetanus, the GP could claim an IOS fee whether the person is travelling or not, as long as the previous dose of the vaccine was given 5 or more years previously.

Not all Local Health Authorities interpret 'The Red Book' as it is written, so you may find that in one area GPs receive a fee that may not be available to fellow GPs in another area.

In the absence of a specific IOS fee, local primary care organizations can purchase vaccine directly from the manufacturer and pay GPs an incentive to vaccinate patients using a section 36 Local Development Scheme. This scheme gives Health Authorities and Primary Care Organizations flexibility to improve the development and responsiveness of General Medical Services, by giving local GPs financial incentives beyond those set out in the SFA. Incentives can be paid for enhancing GMS service to certain specified standards, or providing it in a particular way, which is negotiated locally. Payments must not duplicate existing arrangements provided for in the SFA. Further information about Local Development Schemes is available in the Health Service Circular HCS 1999/107.

Direct payments

Direct payments are only allowed from non-NHS (private) patients; also from NHS patients travelling abroad where their immunization is not covered by the SFA. Examples are hepatitis B, meningococcal, pneumococcal, influenza, oral typhoid, yellow fever, rabies, and tick-borne and Japanese B encephalitis. GPs are also allowed to charge NHS patients requesting international vaccination certificates, whether the vaccine was given on the NHS or privately.

GPs in the UK are allowed to charge a fee for prescribing or providing (not for both) drugs that a patient requires to have in his or her possession *solely in anticipation of the onset of an ailment while the traveller is outside the UK*, but for which he or she is not requiring treatment in the UK when the drug is prescribed. An example is loperamide for possible diarrhoea while abroad.

If a patient with the intention to travel abroad requests a drug he or she *requires intermittently*, e.g. for the relief of migrainous headaches, this should be prescribed on the National Health on an FP10—the drug may be necessary and be taken while still in the UK.

If a patient is travelling abroad for an *extended period (over 3 months)*, all regular and intermittent medication to be used abroad should be issued on a private prescription, but at least 1 month's grace (on FP10) should be considered.

When issuing a private prescription for *malaria prophylaxis* or if they provide the medication, GPs are allowed to charge a fee for one but not for both.

The position on selling travel kits to travelling patients is not clear as it can be seen to be breaching the GPs' Terms of Service.

GPs or practice nurses cannot charge their registered patients a fee for seeing them in the practice travel clinic and giving them advice. The GP could be found in breach of their Terms of Service if they were to do so.

A GP is allowed to charge a patient for administering the vaccine, for which the Health Authority does not pay an IOS fee, only if the patient is travelling abroad, e.g. hepatitis B or typhoid for travel to Australia. In addition, the GP can charge the patient the cost of the vaccine—he cannot issue an FP10 or claim reimbursement of this vaccine.

One of the common problems in travel clinics is the patient who has the first dose of the vaccine, but fails to return for the subsequent doses/boosters. In order to minimize the chance of default, consider:
• giving the vaccinee a card with the date and time of the next appointment;

Table 43.1 List of vaccines that can be purchased and dispensed by non-dispensing GPs in England and Wales under SFA paragraph 44.1–5.

- Cholera (vaccine currently not available)
- Hepatitis A
- Hepatitis B
- Hepatitis A & B
- Hepatitis A & typhoid
- Low-dose diphtheria and tetanus vaccine for adults and adolescents (in prefilled syringe)
- Meningococcal A & C
- Tetanus
- Typhoid
- Influenza
- Pneumococcal

NB: The oral typhoid vaccine may be prescribed on the NHS but it is not reimbursable, by all Health Authorities, to non-dispensing GPs in England and Wales under SFA 44.1–5. This does not apply to dispensing GPs.

- keeping a record of the vaccinee's name and address so that a reminder card can be sent by post in case of default;
- use a computer prompt (see Electronic Recall Systems for completion of immunization, Chapter 45).

Personal dispensing of vaccines/availability of vaccines on the NHS

Nondispensing GPs in England and Wales (does not apply to Scotland or Northern Ireland) can claim a fee for purchasing and dispensing certain vaccines under paragraph 44.1–5 of the SFA. The vaccines may be administered by the doctor or the nurse and they are generally vaccines that are not supplied free to GPs (see Table 43.1 for a list). They are bought in bulk directly from the manufacturer, local pharmacy or other supplier and administered to NHS patients of the practice.

Almost all vaccine suppliers operate discount schemes for GPs. The greater the discount, the greater the (additional) practice profit. The largest discounts tend to be in the most competitive areas or when a large number of vaccines are purchased.

Overall, the government reimburses the GP the following:

- the drug tariff (trade) basic price;
- an on-cost allowance of 10.5% of the basic price before deduction (reduction—see below) of any Government discount under paragraph 44/Schedule 1;

- a container allowance of 3.8 pence per prescription;
- a dispensing fee of 113.1 pence (in year 2000)—reduced further when over 400 scripts per GP are submitted, according to a sliding scale;
- an allowance in respect of VAT, calculated as a percentage (17.5%) both of the basic price less any Government discount (reduction—see below), and of the container allowance.

Since April 1995, the Government has been applying its own discount (reduction) in the reimbursement fee payable to GPs, according to a scale contained in paragraph 44/Schedule 1. The reduction applies to the total basic price of all prescriptions submitted for pricing by the GP. If the total basic price is up to £2000, a reduction of 3.17% applies. For between £2001 and £3000, a 5.93% reduction applies, and so on.

Note: the patient does not (and should not be asked to) pay a prescription charge. The GP should raise a prescription for each item administered except for the eight vaccines (Table 43.2), which are claimed as a bulk entry using Form FP34D (Appendix).

All prescriptions should be noted, counted and sent under cover of Form FP34D to the Prescription Pricing Authority (PPA) by the fifth day of the month following that to which the prescriptions relate. There is a different address for England and Wales (see p. 407).

Table 43.2 Vaccines claimed in bulk and not individually, under SFA paragraph 44.1–5.

Cholera (vaccine not available in the UK)
Hepatitis A
Hepatitis B
Influenza
Meningococcal A + C
Pneumococcal
Tetanus
Typhoid

An FP10 (a prescription) is not accepted by the Prescription Pricing Authority (PPA) for reimbursement for these vaccines.

Charging the NHS patient

Paragraph 38(h) of the 'Terms of Service' allows GPs to charge patients a fee 'for treatment consisting of an immunization for which no remuneration is payable by the Health Authority in pursuance of the Statement made under regulation 34 and which is requested in connection with travel abroad'.

Paragraph 43(1) specifies that 'a doctor shall order any drugs or appliances which are needed for the treatment of any patients to whom he is providing treatment under these terms of service by issuing to that patient a prescription form, and such a form shall not be used in any other circumstances'.

As paragraph 38(h) of the 'Terms of Service' allows GPs to charge patients for the provision of the vaccines in Table 43.3, these vaccines cannot be prescribed on an FP10 under paragraph 43(1).

The Health Authorities receive the individual practices' prescribing analysis and cost (PACT) data. They, in turn, have the right to demand from practices repayment of any vaccine that, in their opinion, was given to a person not entitled to receive that vaccine on the NHS.

Where the GP cannot claim remuneration from the Local Health Authority for administering a vaccine to a traveller, and the vaccine was purchased by the practice privately, he or she may charge the patient certain fees. The British Medical Association (BMA) used to recommend fees up to February 2000, and these fees are mentioned here. In effect, the practice may charge whatever sum it considers reasonable. Below are the last issued BMA fees:

Table 43.3 Vaccines not available on the NHS for travellers (they cannot be issued on the NHS where the sole purpose of immunization is travel).

- Japanese B encephalitis
- Rabies for travellers*
- Influenza†
- Tetanus‡
- Tick-borne encephalitis
- Pneumococcal†
- Yellow fever
- Diphtheria‡
- Meningococcal A + C†
- Hepatitis B†

*See p. 240 for special groups for whom this vaccine is available on the NHS.
†It may be decided that the patient would need this immunization even if they were not travelling abroad, e.g. for an asplenic patient, a male homosexual, etc. In this case, the vaccine is available on the NHS (no IOS fee from the Health Authority and no fee from patient).
‡May qualify for IOS fee. Therefore, prescribable/reimbursable on the NHS, if it satisfies criteria for 'persons not travelling abroad' (see p. 240).

Table 43.4 Vaccines not reimbursed under SFA paragraph 441–5.

- Yellow fever
- Tick-borne encephalitis
- Japanese B encephalitis

- fee per course of immunization: £23—usually charged at the first visit;
- the cost of the vaccine purchased privately.

Tables 43.3 and 43.5 indicate the vaccines that are not available on the NHS where the sole purpose of obtaining the vaccine is travel, and the vaccines that are centrally supplied by the DoH's official distributors are therefore not prescribable on FP10 and not attracting a reimbursement of vaccines fee.

Where the GP receives an item-of-service fee, he or she cannot charge the patient and it is fraudulent to do so. However, a GP may charge for a vaccination certificate (£8 or any other amount) in all cases if the patient requests it.

Other certificates that relate to travel, and for which the GP is entitled to charge a fee are shown in Table 43.6. The BMA last recommended a specific fee for each category in February 2000.

Tough new competition laws in the UK have forced the BMA to suspend the annual update of

Table 43.5 Vaccines centrally supplied—excluded from reimbursement under SFA paragraph 44.1–5.

Diphtheria vaccine adsorbed for children (no longer available in the UK as from summer 2000)
Diphtheria (low-dose) vaccine adsorbed for adults
DT—diphtheria/tetanus
DTwP—diphtheria/tetanus/whole-cell pertussis
DTaP—diphtheria/tetanus/acellular pertussis
DTaP–IPV—diphtheria/tetanus/acellular pertussis and inactivated polio
Hib—*Haemophilus influenzae* b
DTwP–Hib—diphtheria/tetanus/whole-cell pertussis and *Haemophilus influenzae* b combined products for administration as one injection
MR—measles/rubella
MMR—measles/mumps/rubella
Meningococcal C conjugate
Pertussis acellular—on a 'named-patient' basis (not available as from September 2000)
Poliomyelitis—oral
Poliomyelitis—inactivated (injectable)
Rubella (for children and adult women)
Td—tetanus and low-dose diphtheria for adults and adolescents in ampoule presentation (for children aged 10 years and over)
Tuberculin purified protein derivative
BCG

Table 43.6 Certificates relating to travel for which the GP is entitled to charge a fee (BMA recommended—February 2000).

- Travel cancellation insurance certificate £13.50–£29; examination and report £58.50
- Fitness to travel certificate £8–£23
- Fitness to travel examination with report £58.50
- Fitness to travel—extract from records £31
- Freedom from infection certificate £8–£23
- Certificate of negative HIV result for travel (patient) £46
- Passport countersignature £20
- Private prescription (e.g. for antibiotic) £8
- International certificate of vaccination (issued by nurse or doctor) £8
- Administration of a course of vaccine £23

suggested category D and medicolegal fees for GPs. Regulators at the Office of Fair Trading believe these fees may now be in breach of the 1998 Competition Act, which came into force on 1 March 2000. Practices should set their own fee structure.

Summary points for travel vaccines

- The NHS practice-registered patient traveller cannot be charged for administration and/or cost of the vaccine if one the conditions below exists:
    (a) GP is able to claim an IOS fee from the Health Authority;
    (b) GP claims reimbursement of the cost of the vaccine;
    (c) GP prescribes the vaccine on FP10 (NHS prescription);

(d) GP uses a vaccine centrally supplied (free).
- If the GP is unable to claim from the Health Authority an IOS fee for administering a travel immunization to an NHS practice-registered patient traveller, and the patient does not medically need the vaccine here in the UK (does not belong to a group at risk—see individual vaccine chapters), he or she can charge the patient a fee for administration and/or cost of the vaccine provided the vaccine is purchased privately.
- If an NHS practice-registered patient traveller is charged a fee for travel immunization, the GP cannot:
    (a) prescribe the vaccine on an FP10;
    (b) recover the cost of the vaccine by claiming reimbursement from the NHS;
    (c) use a (free) centrally supplied vaccine;
    (d) charge the patient for the vaccine if it is allowed free to the patient on the NHS (he or

she has a 'right' to it), e.g. a nonimmunized practice patient travelling to India has a right to hepatitis A immunization, as long as the practice makes it available to its patients, but has no right to such vaccine on the NHS if he or she is travelling to Germany.

● Vaccines supplied free to GPs by agents of the DoH, e.g. Farillon Ltd (see Table 43.5) are for NHS use only and can be used as per SFA recommendations for patients 'travelling' and 'not travelling abroad'. In this case the patient is charged nothing.

● If the GP has reason to believe a particular NHS patient traveller needs to be immunized against a particular disease not covered by the Statement of Fees and Allowances, he or she has two options:

(a) either to purchase the vaccine privately and charge the patient the vaccine cost and/or for administration of the vaccine (a traveller to Mecca for the Hajj, a traveller to Thailand);

(b) to prescribe the vaccine (except those in Table 43.4) on an FP10 or claim reimbursement of the cost of the vaccine from the NHS, in which case the patient is charged nothing (an asplenic traveller to Mecca for the Hajj, a male homosexual traveller to Thailand).

● A patient that is not registered in any way with the practice, for immunization purposes is considered to be a private patient and should be charged fully. The GP should take care not to use a NHS vaccine. He should purchase the vaccine privately. This could apply to a patient registered with another practice in the town, attending your travel clinic.

For a comprehensive table on charging the NHS patient traveller for immunizations see Table 43.7.

Table 43.7 Charging the NHS practice-registered patient traveller for immunizations.

Vaccine	NHS			Private	
	Centrally supplied	FP10 or reimbursed†	IOS fee claimable‡	Charge patient	Charge patient vaccine cost and administration
Diphtheria	Yes	No	Child over 6 years for primary course and reinforcing dose	No	No—vaccine centrally supplied
Tetanus	No	Yes	Every 5 years or more	No	If non-traveller fee not payable, e.g. booster under 5 years and vaccine purchased privately
Diphtheria/Tetanus combined (Td)	Yes (ampoule)	No (ampoule) Yes (prefilled syringe)	As for diphtheria and/or tetanus School leavers (use the ampoule)	No	If IOS fee is not claimable and vaccine (prefilled syringe) purchased privately
Hepatitis A	No	Yes	Outside Australia, New Zealand, and Northern Europe	No	If IOS fee not claimable and vaccine purchased privately
Hepatitis A & B	No	Yes	Hepatitis A & B: claim for hepatitis A	No	
Hepatitis A and Typhoid	No	Yes	Yes, for both. If not consider 1st claim for typhoid, and 2nd for Hepatitis A at reinforcing dose	No	If IOS fee not claimable and vaccine purchased privately

continued

Table 43.7 *cont.*

Vaccine	NHS				Private
	Centrally supplied	FP10 or reimbursed†	IOS fee claimable‡	Charge patient	Charge patient vaccine cost and administration
Hepatitis B	No	Yes	No	No	If vaccine purchased privately
Japanese B encephalitis	No	No	No	No	Yes
Meningococcal A + C	No	Yes	No	No	If vaccine purchased privately
Pneumococcal	No	Yes	No	No	If vaccine purchased privately
Poliomyelitis	Yes	No	Outside Europe (includes Turkey and Cyprus), Canada, USA, Australia and New Zealand. Infected area. Immunization is a condition of entry	No	No—vaccine centrally supplied
Rabies	No Yes, from PHLS for the special groups at risk	No	No Yes, for the special groups at risk (see p. 240)	No	Yes No, for the special groups at risk
Tick-borne encephalitis	No	No	No	No	Yes
Typhoid Vi antigen (inj.)	No	Yes	Outside N. Europe, USA, Canada, Australasia. Infected area Immunization is a condition of entry	No	If IOS fee is not claimable and vaccine purchased privately
Live (oral)	No	Yes (some Health Authorities have reimbursed)	No for oral (patient self-administers the vaccine)		
Yellow fever	No	No	No	No	Yes (from approved centres)

† Reimbursed under SFA paragraph 44.1–5 for non-dispensing GPs in England and Wales.
‡ IOS, item of service fee.

Chapter 44

Immunization and audit

Medical audit is a systematic way of looking critically at the work healthcare workers are involved in to see whether a change could lead to an improvement. It is a useful tool by which we can check that what *we are* doing is what we think *we ought to* be doing, and what improvements can be made.

Audit can be very well applied to immunization. You may, for example, want to see whether all patients for whom annual influenza vaccination is recommended do indeed receive the vaccine. Audit will measure the practice performance with regard to the influenza campaign. Such an audit will not only show how well (or badly) the practice is doing, but will also stimulate discussion among the members of the primary healthcare team, encourage change (if it is required) and allow for reassessment of changes by being repeated every year.

Here are two examples of audit that the practice could adopt or modify with regard to influenza immunization and hepatitis B practice staff immunization status. They can be modified to cover any other immunization.

Audit of influenza immunization

The audit method

● *The rationale*: patients at risk of complications from contracting influenza because of their medical condition or age could benefit from annual influenza immunization.
● *The aim*: to examine whether all patients for whom the DoH recommends annual influenza immunization have received the vaccine this year.

Criteria

The proposed criteria relate to patients for whom the DoH recommends annual influenza immunization. Patients with the following conditions/situations should have received the vaccine during the previous 12 months:
● chronic heart disease;
● chronic respiratory disease, including asthma;
● chronic renal disease;
● diabetes mellitus and other endocrine disorders;
● immunosuppression as a result of disease or treatment, including asplenia or splenic dysfunction;
● all patients aged 65 years and over;
● people living in residential homes.

Standard

That 80% of these patients should have received the influenza vaccine this year (choose another standard if you wish). The ideal but, probably, nonachievable standard would have been 100%.

Method of data collection

● Nominate members of staff to carry out the audit data collection, meet with them and explain the aims and proceedings.
● Identify patients with various conditions by the practice disease register or repeat prescriptions, opportunistic surgery attendance, health promotion or specific disease clinics, over-75s checks and personal memory (doctor, nurse and staff). Patients in residential nursing homes can be identified by their address.
● Ideally, you will wish to include in this audit all your patients in the target group, but this will probably not be possible because of the numbers. Select an appropriate size for a representative sample (Fig. 44.1).
● Scrutinize each set of notes to determine the

Fig. 44.1 Sample size for 95% confidence level of results (± 5%). [**From Derry J. (1993)** *Managing Audit in General Practice* 1, 17–20, by kind permission of the publishers, Hayward Medical Communications Ltd.]

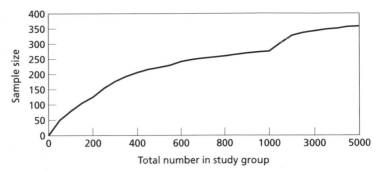

Table 44.1 Example of a data evaluation sheet.

No.	Name*	Date of birth*	Sex	Flu vaccine (Y/N)	Date (month/year)
1	Smith, PA	2/5/25	M	Y	Oct. 1999
2	Taylor, JA	2/8/13	F	N	—
3	Patel, P	11/3/19	F	N	—
4	Wallace, AN	19/11/03	M	Y	Nov. 1999
5	Ryan, T	6/3/15	F	Y	Oct. 1998
6	Roberts, NY	4/11/05	M	Y	Jan. 2000
7	Alexander, JN	6/8/09	M	N	—
8	Morris, AC	30/9/14	F	N	—
9	Marsh, TS	26/2/26	F	Y	Dec. 1999

*Computerized practices may wish to use the patient's computer number instead.

presence or absence of flu vaccine administration this year (October–April) and transfer information on spreadsheets or a specially written computer program.

● Interrogate the computer if all flu vaccinations are normally recorded on it.

● Agree on a reasonable time scale for completion of data collection.

● Prepare the data for analysis by collating the information on computer or data evaluation sheets (Table 44.1). You may find it easier to compile a separate data collection sheet for patients in each of the DoH at-risk groups.

Compare performance with standards

Have at least 80% of patients with chronic conditions, people over 65 years of age, and all living in residential accommodation, as recommended by the DoH received the influenza vaccine this year?

If you have not achieved your set standards, decide on a course of action. You may decide that you will plan your next influenza campaign early,

order your vaccines early, organize nurse-run influenza vaccination clinics or increase the number of such clinics, write to your target patients, attach to the repeat prescriptions a letter of invitation to an influenza vaccination clinic, put posters in the waiting room, personally (and all members of the primary healthcare team) promote immunization against influenza, and so on.

Remeasure performance

Once all changes have been introduced and complied with, the practice will wish to evaluate the changes and ensure it now reaches, as near as possible, 100% standard. A repeat audit will show exactly that.

Remeasure your performance annually by repeating this audit.

Audit protocol for practice staff hepatitis B immunization status

Practices require the GPs and nurses to produce

evidence of hepatitis B immunity. Quite a number of practices extend this requirement to all staff. This is to comply with the United Kingdom Advisory Group on Hepatitis—Guidelines for protecting healthcare workers and patients from hepatitis 8 [(93)40]. It recommends that practices ensure that staff who may be at risk of acquiring hepatitis B virus from patients are protected by immunization.

A member of staff need not be involved in 'exposure-prone procedures' to put themselves in danger of contracting the hepatitis B virus from a patient. If a patient is brought in bleeding or collapses in the waiting room, the receptionist may be the first person to attend/give first aid.

As the employer, the GP has responsibility for protecting his or her staff from contracting hepatitis B. Do you know how many (and which members) of your staff are susceptible to the virus (i.e. unprotected?) If you do not, this simple audit may give you the answer.

The audit method

The rationale: to ensure that all practice members of staff are protected against hepatitis B virus infection.

Target group

All members of the primary healthcare team (PHCT) employed by the practice. You will do well if you include the doctors in the target as not only is it vital that they are immune, but they can be a good example to staff and lead from the front.

Criterion

Members of the PHCT should have adequate levels ($\geqslant 100$ mIU/mL) of antibody to hepatitis B surface antigen (anti-HBs).

Standard

100%, i.e. all in the target group should comply with the criterion.

Method of data collection

All members of the PHCT employed by the practice will be required to produce written evidence from the laboratory of their anti-HBs status. The Practice Manager will collect all written evidence submitted and will present the results.

Members of staff and GPs will have their blood samples taken after prior arrangement with the local occupational health service. Once the reports are available, they will be entered into a spreadsheet (Table 44.2).

It is important to explain to the staff the purpose of this audit and the benefits to themselves and patients. Answer all their questions and give them time to consider this request.

Decide in advance what you will do in the case

Table 44.2 Audit of PHCT members' (employed by the practice) hepatitis B immunity—data entry sheet.

			Level of immunity		
No.	Name	Actual anti-HBs (mIU/mL)	Good ($\geqslant 100$	Low 10–99	Inadequate < 10 or 0
1					
2					
3					
4					
5					
6					
7					
8					
etc.					
Total					

where staff refuse to provide evidence of hepatitis B immunity or a blood sample. Consider obtaining legal/BMA advice if needed.

Agree necessary change

Consider each member of the PHCT separately and, if any action is necessary, discuss this privately and confidentially with the member of staff concerned and obtain their agreement to the proposed action.

Implement change

Among the changes you will wish to introduce may be the following:
- those with low immunity (anti-HBs = 10–99 mIU/mL) should consider having a booster;
- those with inadequate immunity (anti-HBs <10 mIU/mL) should consider a repeat course of hepatitis B vaccine;
- those with no antibodies present should consider a repeat course of hepatitis B vaccine, with the same or a different vaccine;
- all staff who receive a booster or a full course should be advised to have their antibody level checked by a blood test 8 weeks after the booster or completion of the course.

Specific problems of interpretation

This refers to staff involved in 'exposure-prone procedures' whose anti-HBs level remains inadequate, i.e. 'nonresponders' (see chapter on hepatitis B on p. 153).

Additional information on audit

Sampling your practice list

If your practice has relatively few people who require a particular vaccine, you may be able to search all the notes or access the information from the practice computer. However, in some cases you may have to take a representative sample of case notes if, for example, you need to review more than 100 patients and the information is not on computer.

If you audit only a proportion of your notes, you need to review a representative sample. This does not require a great deal of statistical sophistication. Simply use Fig. 44.1 to determine the sample size with 95% confidence of result $\pm 5\%$.

Assume, for example, your audit reveals that only 50% of your high-risk target group have been vaccinated. Provided you used the right sample size, then you are 95% confident that $50 \pm 5\%$ (i.e. 45–55%) have been vaccinated.

After selecting the sample size, you need to decide which of the following methods you will use to sample patients' notes:
- *Random sampling*. Allocate all patients in the target group a successive number. Draw random numbers using tables or the random number generator on a scientific calculator or a bingo-style counter. Clearly, each patient is equally likely to be selected for the audit.
- *Systematic sampling*. Suppose, for example, that your practice identifies 400 patients at high risk of needing a particular vaccine. Figure 44.1 shows that to be confident that your results apply to the remaining patients, you need to audit 200 records. Using systematic sampling, you should audit every second set of notes $(400/200 = 2)$.
- *Stratified sample*. Split the target patients into groups (strata), e.g. males and females. This may be the best method to sample patients' notes for a hepatitis B vaccination audit. Divide patients into groups: homosexual men, high-risk occupations, intravenous drug abusers, for example. Then select them using either random or systematic sampling from within the group. If the group is small, audit them all.
- *Cluster sampling*. This method audits a 'group' or 'cluster' of patients and extrapolates the results to a larger population. So, for example, results from one or two GPs could be extrapolated to others in the practice. However, cluster sampling may be difficult to perform without someone feeling that they have been 'singled out'.

Chapter 45

Electronic recall systems for completion of immunization

This section provides general advice, which readers should modify according to their requirements.

Instructions for vaccine booster trawl using EMIS computer system

(With kind permission from Egton Medical Information Systems Ltd.)

To construct a search you must know the following information:

● How, for example, the first Havrix injection is recorded in the immunization notes for a patient (e.g. 1st Hepatitis A Vaccination or 1st Havrix Mono).

● How the second Havrix (booster) is recorded in the immunization notes for a patient (e.g. 2nd Hepatitis A Vaccination or Booster Hepatitis A or 2nd Havrix Mono).

This can vary from practice to practice.

In addition to this you must know how far back you want to search. You need to specify date ranges for each search. Search as far back as you wish for the initial injection, but remember that the date range for the booster should be 6 months later, e.g.

1st Hepatitis A Vaccination
Earliest date: 1/1/98; Latest date: 1/1/99
Booster Hepatitis A Vaccination
Earliest date: 1/7/98; Latest date: 1/7/99

Common problems

Q *I'm not sure what the immunizations have been recorded under.*

A Look up a patient who you know has received the vaccinations and note down what has been recorded under their immunization history. If several different things have been recorded (i.e. multinurse practice using different terminology) then you can search for all of these by

adding a feature, but selecting for this feature to be EITHER/OR instead of SHARED; e.g. search for:
EITHER: 1st Hepatitis A Vaccination
OR: 1st Havrix Monodose

Q *The search doesn't bring up anyone.*

A Do each search separately:

● First, look for everyone who has received the first injection. Print this search out.

● Secondly, look for everyone who has received the reinforcing dose. Print this out.

● Put the two sheets side by side and tick off on the reinforcing dose sheet everyone who appears on the first injection sheet. This will give you a list of people who have had the first but not the second.

To construct the search

From the main menu select ST SEARCH & STATISTICS
B PATIENT SEARCHES
A BUILD/PERFORM NEW SEARCH
A PERFORM SEARCH ON TODAY'S PRACTICE POPULATION

Search Construction screen
A ADD FEATURE

Select Type screen
2 CLASSIFICATION CODES

Instead of typing I for immunization type in:
1st Hep A

This brings you to all the hepatitis injections recorded. Whatever the nurse records the first hepatitis A injection as, select this now by pressing the relevant letter,

e.g. A 1ST HEPATITIS A VACCINATION
B ENTRIES BETWEEN 2 SPECIFIED DATES
WILL BE SEARCHED
Enter the earliest and latest dates you want to search, e.g.

Earliest 1/1/98
Latest 1/1/99

The system asks you if you want to include current active problems—N

This feature is A SHARED. You have instructed the computer to search the database for everyone who has received an initial injection of Havrix.

We now need to add to this to search for those who have not had the Havrix booster.
You should be at the search construction screen.
A ADD FEATURE
2 CLASSIFICATION CODES
Type in HEPA
Again this brings you to all the hepatitis injections recorded.
Whatever the nurse records the booster hepatitis A injection as, select this now by pressing the relevant letter, e.g.
B 2ND HEPATITIS A VACCINATION
B ENTRIES BETWEEN 2 SPECIFIED DATES
This should be 6 months later from the earliest and latest dates you selected for the initial, e.g.

Earliest: 1/7/98
Latest: 1/7/99

+ Problem Questionnaire

As we want to pull up a list of those who have NOT had the booster this feature is B EXCLUDED

Check details, press return to complete.
If these features are correct press Y
Give the search a title, e.g. HAVRIX BOOSTER RECALL

Run the search now, it should take a few seconds.

Go into:
S SEARCH RESULTS
2 ONE OFF SEARCH

Find your search title, e.g. HAVRIX BOOSTER

RECALL
B NAMES AND ADDRESSES
2 ALPHABETICAL
1 NO DIVISION
F FHSA FORMAT

Either 8 View to screen or 7 to print out

Instructions for Hepatyrix booster trawl using EMIS computer system

The aim of this document is to help you construct a search for patients requiring a hepatitis A booster and exclude those who have current typhoid protection.

To construct a search you must know the following information:
● how the first Havrix injection is recorded in the immunization notes for a patient (e.g. 1st Hepatitis A Vaccination or 1st Havrix Mono);
● how the second Havrix (booster) is recorded in the immunization notes for a patient (e.g. 2nd Hepatitis A Vaccination or Booster Hepatitis A or 2nd Havrix Mono);
● how typhoid vaccinations have been recorded.

The first part of the search uses the same criteria as the Havrix booster trawl. Follow STEP 1 and STEP 2

Search Construction screen
A ADD FEATURE

Select Type screen
B CLASSIFICATION CODES

Type I for immunization type:
This brings you to all the injections recorded.
Whatever the nurse records the typhoid injection as, select this now by pressing the relevant letter; e.g.
Read code for typhoid vaccination
B ENTRIES BETWEEN 2 SPECIFIED DATES
WILL BE SEARCHED
We need to search back 3 years ago from today's date. Anyone who has received a typhoid vaccination in this time will not be eligible for a Hepatyrix

vaccination, as they will still be covered for typhoid; e.g.

Earliest: 3 years ago from today's date
Latest: Press RETURN for today's date
This feature is B EXCLUDED

You have instructed the computer to search the database for everyone who has:
● received an initial injection of Havrix;
● not returned for a booster dose within a certain time;
● no typhoid protection.

Check details, press RETURN to complete
If these features are correct press Y

Give the search a title, e.g. PATIENTS ELIGIBLE FOR HEPATYRIX
Run the search now, it should take a few seconds.
Go into
S   SEARCH RESULTS
3   ONE OFF SEARCH

Find your search title, e.g. PATIENTS ELIGIBLE FOR HEPATYRIX
B NAMES AND ADDRESSES
ALPHABETICAL
NO DIVISION
F FHSA FORMAT

Either 8 View to screen or 7 to print out

Instructions for printing labels using EMIS computer system

CSV files

When using EMIS it does not always give you the option of printing out the labels that you want.

There is a way around this if you are confident with Excel and Mail Merge in Microsoft Office.
1   When you have completed the search on EMIS it gives you the option to print or save. Select **Save**.
2   In the save file, it gives you a few options to where you would like to save the file and you want to choose **Save as Comma Separated Version**—(CSV) on A:/drive.
3   Put a clean floppy disk in the A:/drive and press enter.
4   Move the disk to another computer, which has MS Office, and open up the file in an Excel Spreadsheet. (This will now act as a database.) Save as a .XLS file.
5   Open up a Word document and select Tools and Mail Merge. (This is where your knowledge of Mail Merge kicks in.) Choose labels and use the .XLS file as your data source (**Open Data Source**). Insert the fields and merge the document. Save this and print labels.

Booster audit using VAMP system

The example below takes you through the stages needed to produce a list using VAMP of patients who have had their first dose of Havrix but have not presented for their second. It may look complicated but by following the process below the whole thing takes about 10 min.
1   From main menu choose TRANSACTION: ENTER
2   Type 'SR' (search): ENTER
3   Choose PREVENTION OPTIONS: ENTER
4   Choose IMMUNIZATION/VACCINATIONS: ENTER
5   This will present a screen requiring fields such as name/age/sex, etc. Pressing ENTER 9 times will fill in with defaults, e.g. age range 0–110. Use the defaults as this captures everyone.
6   Choose IMMUNIZATION RECORDS: ENTER
7   The period of search should be completed as required. Suggest 'from' date should go back 2 years and 'to' date should be 6 months prior to current date. ENTER
8   Against vaccination type. Type 'HEPATITIS A': ENTER × 3
9   A box should appear asking for stage of vaccination: choose 1ST STAGE: ENTER × 4
10 The report should now run. (If it does not, press ENTER again!)
11 Once completed press ENTER
12 Choose SAVE/PRODUCE GROUPS: ENTER

13 Enter Name (I suggest HEP1): ENTER × 2
14 Report is now saved as HEP1: ESC
15 You are now returned to position (3) above. Proceed from (3) as before. However, when you get to position (5) fill in all the defaults with the ENTER key **except**: 'SEARCH ON GROUP OF PATIENTS'. Here you should type 'HEP1'
16 Proceed as before until (9) where you should choose: 2ND STAGE: ENTER
17 Proceed as before until (12). This time call it HEP2: ENTER × 2
18 Report is now saved as HEP2: ESC
19 From search menu choose PROCESS GROUPS: ENTER
20 Choose COMBINE GROUPS: ENTER
21 Enter Name of 1st Group (HEP1): ENTER
22 Enter Name of 2nd Group (HEP2): ENTER
23 Enter Name of 3rd Group (I suggest HEP3): ENTER
24 Select EXCLUDING PATIENTS COMMON TO BOTH GROUPS: ENTER
25 Choose SAVE PRINT LAST REPORT: ENTER
26 Choose REPORT HEADINGS: ENTER
27 Select the fields you want in your report, i.e. name, address, post code, telephone number by typing the field number and pressing ENTER each time.
28 Now persuade the practice to set their printer up with labels and print report!

Note

If you wish to do a sanity check, select one of the patients from the hard copy report, return to the main menu. Select Transaction and type 'N'. This will then prompt you for forename and surname, enter these. Once it has brought the patient up press ENTER again and this will take the details to the top of the screen. Now type 'PD' against the transaction prompt and this will bring up the patient record where the date for the initial dose will be recorded (if the report is correct there will be no recorded date for the booster).

Any problems call the VAMP helpdesk on 020 7501 7010.

Instructions for printing labels using VAMP computer system

1 Click on the icon for PRINT LABELS.
2 *Single patient or group*—First select whether you are printing a single patient label (Single patient), the default, or multiple labels (check the Group Box).

If selecting a single patient, click on the SELECT PATIENT button to display the SELECT A PATIENT screen. Select the patient you want.

If selecting a group, click to highlight the group listed in the group window. Once selected the group is shown in the SELECTED GROUP window, together with the number of patients in the group in PATIENT COUNT.
3 *Single/Multiple labels*—the default is to print one label per patient. Amend this for more labels for each patient.
4 *Label format*—Select the size of the label stationery, which is loaded in the printer. (It gives you quite a few options but you want the Laser—L7163 or L7160 as you can order the labels from SB).
5 Do you wish to check Label alignment? If it is selected, this will give a preview of the labels against gridlines.
6 *Print Options*—click on PRINT OPTIONS (see *Printer and Print options*) to select PRINTER, then OK
7 Check that your label stationery is correctly loaded into the label printer before finally clicking on PRINT. EXIT will close the screen.
8 All directions for the booster trawl are in the help file on all VAMP computers and they are worth printing out and using each time.

Immunization audit using AAH Meditel

(With kind permission of Topex Health Ltd.)

Using reports and formats for medication searches system 5

Predefined Letter Editor

The Predefined Letter editor (PDL) is an option on page 21 of the System 5 menu configuration. To edit or add a predefined letter within System 5, you will need some knowledge of Lyrix word processing. Please refer to the Lyrix reference guide.
● At the System 5 Main Menu type RP or 21 and press ENTER.
● Type PDL and press ENTER to access the Predefined Letter Editor.
● At the screen prompt type in a predefined letter code, or select F3 codes for a picking list of predefined letters already created. To create a new letter type a unique four-character code at the prompt, i.e. MDLT and press ENTER.
● Type a title for this letter on the first line of the blank document and press ENTER.
● Type the body of the letter as required. The practice header details and the salutation are not required when composing the letter as these will be merged when the report is run.
● Press ESC followed by e to exit and save the Lyrix document.

Your predefined letter can now be used from within the RR option. The use of format LETP allows the creation of a predefined letter for each of the patients selected from the report.

Basic Filter Report for Medication

In this example the practice requires a report to find all patients on a particular drug and requires a letter sent to each of these patients. The letter required will first have been set up using the Predefined Letter example. It is important to decide what medication or medication range is required for the search and what period of time an issue has been made for it to be deemed current. In this example any medication issued during the last

3 months (91 days) will be classed as current.
● From the System 5 Main Menu type RR and press ENTER
● The Report processing screen is displayed with the cursor active in the From Index field
● Type 2 for Read Code Quick report. Alternatively select from the codes available using F3
● At Selected By type in the required read code or type a synonym and select from the picking list as required, e.g. type, cl3. and press ENTER to include all patients on any Salbutamol Inhalation Preparations.

A filter will need to be created to find all patients that have had a current issue of this medication. The medication search that has just been created will search for all patients issued with the medication ever. The filter will allow the identification of only those patients having an issue in the last 3 months (91 days).
● With the cursor active on the Filter Group field select F4 Filters
● The Filter Group Editor is displayed. This allows the linking of the required criteria set up as individual filters. Filters that have been set previously are displayed at the bottom of the screen and can be used within the filter group as required. To create a new filter select F6 Filters
● The Filter screen is displayed. Select F4 add to create new filter
● Type a filter code name of four characters to identify this filter, e.g. **01 where ** are your initials
● Type a meaningful title for the filter, e.g. 'Issues Salbutamol Last 3 months' and press ENTER
● Three filter types are displayed, each allowing for the searching of specific information. At filter type select M for Medication information.

The criteria that are available within the medication filter allow the searching of five medication criteria.
● a—Prescribed and authorized:
  a range of drug read codes may be specified which are authorized for issue, i.e. medication that has outstanding issues 1/2, 5/6. The doctor who authorized this medication may also be supplied.
● f—authorized date:
  a range of dates that a medication has been

authorized can be specified either relatively or absolutely. The doctor who authorized the medication can also be specified. The medication is included within authorization date regardless as to the authorization status, i.e. includes medication that is 1/1, 0/1 and 3/4, etc.

- i—issue date:

  the date that the medication was issued can be specified either relatively or absolutely. The doctor who authorized the medication can also be specified.

- p—prescribed ever:

  searches for any item of medication that has been prescribed at any time. The doctor who authorized the medication can also be specified.

- u—unused medication:

  the period in which medication is unissued can be specified either relatively or absolutely. The doctor who authorized the medication can also be specified.

- Select F3 Codes at according to (this is not displayed on screen) and select the required criteria to search for the information. Select Line 2—i issue date and press ENTER.

- The date at which that medication has been issued can be specified either relatively or absolutely. Type L (last) *followed by* 3 *followed by* M (months). (In this example we have used 3 months as an indication that the patient is currently on this medication).

- The system requires the medication code to be analysed. Type in the start medication code, cl3. *Salbutamol inhalation preparations.*

- We require the full range of medication within this hierarchy. Press ENTER to include the full range.

- A doctor that authorized the medication can be specified if required. Press ENTER to include all doctors' authorizations.

- Further filters can be entered at this point. Select F8 end to complete the filters.

- The Filter Group screen is redisplayed. Select F4 add to create new filter group.

- Enter a four character code that will be used to identify this Filter Group, e.g. **01 (where ** are your initials) and press ENTER.

- Type a meaningful title for this filter group, e.g.

'Issue Salbutamol Last 3 months' and press ENTER.

- Type in the code of the filter that has been created, e.g. **01 (where ** are your initials).

- The title of the filter is completed. The cursor becomes active in the 'If True' field. As this group only contains one filter Continue or Select can be used to include those that match the filter. Type in C and Continue appears in the 'if true' field.

- The cursor moves to the 'if false' field. This specifies what happens to the patients that have not had an issue in the last 3 months. Type E and Exclude appears in the 'is false' field. The remainder of the records, i.e. those that have had an issue in the last 3 months will be selected.

- Select F8 to End and F8 to return to the RR screen.

- Type the four-character code used to identify the Filter Group., e.g. **01 and press ENTER.

- Select a suitable sort order for this report. Type S for Surname and Initial or alternatively select a required sort order by selecting F3 codes and choosing from the list available.

We require a letter to be printed for each of the patients found by the report. It is always a good idea to run the report to screen using the default SHRT—Short Patient Data first to check the quantity and accuracy of the search criteria.

- For Format type LETP. Alternatively select the format by selecting F3 and choosing from the list available.

- The file/printer defaults to S—Screen Pause. Press ENTER to accept default or select F3 codes for a picking list of other available outputs.

Three additional fields are displayed at the bottom of the report. These fields allow the specification of the required letter and letter options.

- The 'text file to include' is the four-character code given to the letter that has been created using PDL. A list of letters is available by selecting F3 codes. Type in the four character code, e.g. MDLT.

- The 'Mark notes with code' is an optional field that can be used automatically to mark the selected patient's notes with a Read code selected at the report run time. To enter a code, either type a Read code directly or search using a Synonym. In this example no code is required so press ENTER to leave blank.

● The 'Address to Patient if aged under (years)' is also optional and allows the entering of a minimum age that letters will be addressed to the patient. Any patients that are under the specified age will have letters addressed to the parent or guardian. We require no minimum age in this example so press ENTER to leave blank.

● Select F7 Run and the report will display to the requested output.

● Select F8 exit to return to the System 5 Main Menu.

Patient Lists

Patient Lists can be created within the menu option SL. A Patient List consists of patient numbers and is used as the input within the report-processing screen. Patient Lists can be created either manually or by using the report-processing screen to create a list of patients selected within the report criteria.

● From the System 5 Main Menu type SL and press ENTER

The system prompts for a list name to create or edit.

Type a four character filename and press ENTER.

● A skeleton Patient List is displayed within a Lyrix file, together with information to assist in creating a Patient List.

● Using the down and right arrow keys position the cursor to the right of the !!T. Type a title for this Patient List and press ESC followed by B

● The cursor will become active in the bottom left corner of the file.

● Press ENTER to create a blank line at the end of the file.

● Type in the first patient number to be included within the Patient List and press ENTER

● Repeat the process ensuring that each patient number is on a separate line and contains no blank lines.

● After the last patient number press ESC followed by E to save the file.

Note: It is important that the document contains no blank lines and that the text contained at the top of the file is not altered or the list will not work correctly.

Editing a Patient List

● From the System 5 Main Menu type SL and press ENTER

● Type the four character filename of the list to be edited and press ENTER

● Edit the Patient List as necessary.

● Press ESC followed by E to save the changes to the file.

Letter to Patient (LETP)

One format that can be used with the Patient Lists option is Letter to Patient. A predefined letter will be created for each of the selected patient groups.

From the System 5 Main Menu type RR and press ENTER

● At 'From Index' type 0 (Sorted File).

● For 'Selected By' type the four character filename of the patient list to be used in the report and press ENTER

● If the correct filename has been used, the system will display that the input file is present.

● No filters are required press ENTER to accept default 0 (no filters).

● No sort order is required press ENTER to accept the default 0 (no sort order).

● At 'Format' type LETP (Letter to Patient) and press ENTER

Three additional fields are displayed to specify the criteria for the selected format.

● At File/Printer press ENTER to accept the default S (screen pause) or select a suitable printer or file for the report output.

● The 'text file to include' is the four-character code given to the letter that has been created using PDL. A list of letters is available by selecting F3 codes. Type in the four character code, e.g. MDLT

● The 'Mark notes with code' is an optional field that can be used automatically to mark the selected patient's notes with a Read code selected at the report run time. To enter a code, either type a Read code directly or search using a Synonym. In this example no code is required so press ENTER to leave blank.

● The 'Address to Patient if aged over (years)' is also optional and allows the entering of a minimum age that letters will be addressed to the patient. Any patients that are under the specified age will have letters addressed to the parent or guardian. We require no minimum age in this example so press ENTER to leave blank.

- Select F7 Run and the report will display to the requested output.
- Select F8 exit to return to the System 5 Main Menu.

COST—Prescribing cost

The COST format can be used to not only provide detailed information about the prescribing of medication but to create a list of the selected group for use with other formats or as a means of identifying patients on a particular medication.

This format is used to report on the prescriptions issued to patients in the chosen group. The format looks at each issue given to patients in the chosen date range and considers the cost of that issue (at the time of issue), calculated by the system. The report prints the number of items and their total cost at the end of the report. The report also prints the number of items and their total cost at the end of each patient.

The format also allows you the following choices, that is, whether to:
- display every item or only those over a certain cost;
- limit the date range chosen;
- restrict to a certain Read code or Read code chapter;
- display patients with no scripts in a certain range;
- display total cost only, or every item;
- specify just NHS or just Private scripts (or both);
- display only patients whose total drug cost exceeds the chosen amount.

Prescribing cost report

In this example we will look at the prescribing cost to all our Asthmatics (.H43.) during the last 12 months.

From the System 5 main menu select RR and press ENTER

- At From Index type 2 (Read code quick) and press ENTER
- At selected by: type .H43. and press ENTER
- No filters are required press ENTER to accept default 0 (no filters).
- At Sort Order type G (Registered GP/Surname) and press ENTER
- At Format type COST (Prescribing cost output) and press ENTER
- Press ENTER to accept default output of Screen Pause.

Four additional fields are displayed to specify the criteria for the selected format.
- At display each item type Y and press ENTER to display all drug issues.
- At lower cost level type 0.00 and press ENTER to display all items regardless of cost.
- At start date range type L12M and press ENTER to look at prescribing cost over the last 12 months only.
- At end date range press ENTER to look back 12 months from today.
- Select F7 run.

The report will run and the prescribing cost for each of the practice asthmatics will be displayed along with the total prescribing cost for the whole practice.

Prescribing budget report

In this example we wish to find those asthmatics who have a total prescribing cost of over £800.00 during the 12-month period 1/4/97–31/3/98.
- Find all asthmatics as per previous example.
- At display each item type X and press ENTER to only display if the total cost exceeds a set level.
- At lower cost level type 800.00S and press ENTER to display only those whose cost exceeds £800.00 with the S suppressing those patients who do not qualify therefore omitting them from the report output.
- At start date range type L12M and press ENTER to look back 12 months.
- At end date range type 31/03/98 so the system will look back 12 months from 31 March 1998.
- Select F7 run.

Using Patient List within report processing

The report will run with the output only displaying those patients who match the criteria. The output will display a list of patient numbers who match the criteria. To display the full patient information this can be done as follows.

● At from index type 0 (sorted file) and press ENTER
● At selected by: type COST and press ENTER (Input file is present will be displayed).
● No filters are required press ENTER to accept default 0 (no filters).
● At Sort Order type G (Registered GP/Surname) and press ENTER
● Select a suitable format or press ENTER to accept SHRT (Short patient data).
● Press ENTER to accept default output of Screen Pause
● Select F7 run

The report will produce a list of patient details included within the report for asthmatics with a prescribing cost over £800.00

Specific medication searches

In this example we wish to find all patients who have had an issue of Zovirax shingles packs in the last 6 months.

● At from index type 2 (Read code Quick) and press ENTER
● At selected by: type ,ei19 and press ENTER
● No filters are required press ENTER to accept default 0 (no filters).

● At Sort Order type G (Registered GP/Surname) and press ENTER
● At format type COST (prescribing cost output) and press ENTER
● Press ENTER to accept default output of Screen Pause

Four additional fields are displayed to specify the criteria for the selected format.

● At display each item type N,EI19 and press ENTER to display only the total cost for Zovirax shingles packs.
● At lower cost level type 0.00S and press ENTER to include all issues and suppress those patients with no issue of Zovirax.
● At start date range type L6M and press ENTER to look back over the last 6 months.
● At end date range press ENTER to look back 6 months from today.
● Select F7 run

The report will now run and produce an output of only those patients issued with the medication over the specified time period.

Other COST format options

The read code search can include any level of the read code hierarchy. To display only respiratory drugs you can use Y,C or to display inhalation preparations Y,C12 can be used.

Other options available from within lower cost level field include:

● S, Suppress details
● N, NHS issues only
● P, Private scripts only

Chapter 46

The practice nurse and immunization

Part of the work of the practice nurse is to promote the benefits of and to carry out immunization. In most circumstances, immunization is an elective procedure, particularly for young children. The vaccines used to immunize children against infectious diseases are among the safest drugs available, provided their contraindications are observed.

It is important to understand the difference between immunization and vaccination, as these two terms are often used interchangeably in practice. To immunize is to make immune, especially by inoculation but also by injection of human immunoglobulin, whereas to vaccinate is to inoculate (a person) with vaccine so as to produce immunity against a specific disease. Immunity is an intrinsic or acquired state of resistance to an infectious agent. Natural immunity is acquired following infection and the subsequent production of antibodies, whereas immunization is achieved following the administration of antigens to stimulate the production of antibodies and induce immunity artificially. Therefore, vaccination is the act of vaccinating against a disease, with immunization being the acquisition of immunity to the disease. Vaccination does not always result in immunization; it may not lead to seroconversion and seroprotection—see p. 29 for factors that can adversely influence seroconversion.

Although the immediate goal is the prevention of infectious disease in the individual and the community, the ultimate objective is eradication. In countries with successful immunization programmes, virtual elimination of tetanus, diphtheria, poliomyelitis, pertussis, measles, mumps and rubella is being observed. We have already seen the eradication of smallpox from the world and poliomyelitis from the Americas.

An essential part of the role of the practice nurse is to understand fully the reasons for immunization, contraindications, adverse reactions and special precautions indicated for each infectious disease vaccine. Most of the necessary descriptive and factual background is contained within this book; it is important that this information is used, coupled with the nurse's teaching and counselling abilities, to promote health in the practice population.

The GP, practice nurse and other team members must agree protocols for immunization to ensure both safety and high standards of practice. While the practice nurse should encourage immunization at all times, there must be respect for individual choice, and patients or parents should not be cajoled into vaccination against their wishes. A better approach would be to explain and discuss the risks of refusal of immunization. We advise. It is the patients or parents who decide.

The GP contract (April 1990) introduced target payments for childhood immunizations, with 70% achievement as the lower target and 90% as the higher target. Practice nurses should familiarize themselves with the statutory changes, which take place from time to time in immunization programmes.

Most importantly, the practice nurse should be able to promote immunization in the community and carry out successful immunization campaigns. No child should be denied immunization. To deny a child immunization may be to deny that child good health, sometimes life.

Medicolegal aspects of immunization and the nurse

The practice nurse has two main responsibilities in the administration of vaccines to a patient. The first of these responsibilities is to ensure his or her own competence in undertaking the activity, and the second is to ensure that the correct vaccine is given to the right patient and in the correct way and circumstances.

Following through the guiding principles associated with any activity, the nurse giving a vaccine must have had specific and adequate training to carry out the procedure; his or her employer must be satisfied with the competence of the nurse and the nurse must feel that she or he is equipped and competent to undertake this exercise.

The nurse who gives any vaccine must have a thorough knowledge of that vaccine, its correct dosage, route of administration, adverse effects, contraindications and compatibility. He or she has to ensure that the prescribed vaccine by the GP is the right one, the patient is fit to receive it and that he or she administers the vaccine correctly. The nurse must also be able to recognize and treat any postvaccination reactions, including anaphylactic shock. Only when these criteria have been met should the nurse be involved in immunization procedures.

Having established the appropriate knowledge base, the nurse needs to give due regard to the 'legal' processes which govern the administration of medicines. It is recommended that nurses refer to the Standards for the Administration of Medicines' (UKCC 1992—update expected later in year 2000).

The most obvious point is that, at present, nurses are not in a position to prescribe vaccinations themselves; as such, the nurse will have to establish that a 'prescription' originated by the GP is in existence. This prescription can be in any form of an instruction in an individual's notes or record card, or may take the form of a 'patient group direction'. This latter form of prescription is probably the most common means by which a practice nurse will operate an immunization clinic and the Medicines Act has recently been amended to reflect this in English Law (Health Service Circular NHSE 200 Patient Group Directions, HSC 2000/026—it applies to the NHS in England).

One further step, which should be followed through before giving any vaccine, is to ascertain the informed consent of the patient receiving the dose or, in the case of a child, the consent of the responsible adult.

In summary, a doctor may delegate the responsibility for immunization to a nurse if that nurse:

● has received adequate training in the recognition and management of anaphylaxis with appropriate resuscitation equipment and drugs (e.g. adrenaline) being available at the place of work where the vaccinations will normally take place;

● has received appropriate training and is competent in all aspects of immunization. These should include identification of the need and contraindications to vaccination, appropriate information for patients on significant risks or side-effects, use of correct injection site and technique, recognition and treatment of postvaccination reactions;

● is willing to undertake immunizations and, if so, is professionally accountable for this work as defined in the UKCC advisory document *The Scope of Professional Practice and Standards for the Administration of Medicine*;

● has the consent of his or her employer such as agreed, signed and dated patient group directions which outline the responsibility of the team involved.

A doctor can prescribe unlicensed drugs, or licensed drugs for an unlicensed indication if, in his or her clinical judgement, there is a need to do so. However, the patient must be fully informed.

Not infrequently, the nurse may be in a situation where the vaccine to be given is unlicensed. A nurse can accept responsibility to administer an unlicensed vaccine provided:

● the unlicensed vaccine has been prescribed by the doctor on a 'named-patient' basis;

● the nurse fully informs the patient that:

(a) the vaccine is unlicensed and that means this vaccine has not been through the normal regulatory procedures of the UK government;

(b) this vaccine may have as yet unknown side-effects;

(c) the known side-effects are explained to the patient.

● the nurse is certain that the action he or she is about to take will be that of which a responsible body of medical opinion would approve [the 'Bolam Test' (1957)];

● the doctor who is delegating the administration

of this vaccine has done so to a nurse who is reasonably competent, and trained to standards expected for administrating vaccines (as outlined above);

● the patient consents to having this vaccine.

It is to be hoped that quite a number of the practice nurses' issues on supply and administration of medicines will be improved if we see the implementation and further extension of nurse prescribing.

Patient Group Directions for prescription only medicines

Up to August 2000, these were called 'group protocols'. *The Oxford Dictionary* defines protocol as 'terms agreed in conference and signed by the parties'. The Medical Defence Union (MDU) in London has, in the past, issued the following advice.'Protocols are documentary evidence of the agreement by a team of healthcare professionals on the care that they intend to offer to patients and how this is to be delivered. Protocols are not procedures. They describe the WHO, WHERE and WHY rather than detail the precise HOW.'

Members of the primary health care team use protocols to promote a more consistent approach to patient care. Protocols also ensure the requirements of accountability have been met in that they described the agreed normal practice in an area of care, e.g. pretravel health education advice. In the event of a complaint the practice protocol in use at the time of the incident is useful as evidence of normal practice; also that the care provided was at the standard required by the 'Bolam Test' (see page 262). For examples of protocols, access http://www.groupprotocols.org.uk.

The Medicines Act of 1968 allows only doctors, dentists and vets to prescribe prescription only medicines (POMs). The Act allows others to administer POMs in accordance with the written or verbal direction of the medical practitioner.

The Government set up the *Review of Prescribing, Supply & Administration on Medicines* in March 1997. Dr June Crown, President of the Faculty of Public Health Medicine, led the review. The interim report focused on providing a report to Ministers on supply and administration of medi-

cines under group protocols and was published in April 1998. It recommended that group protocols can be used as direction to administer POMs, and provided clear guidance on the development of protocols for the administration of POMs.

Health Service Circular 2000/026 [DoH (1999) *Review of Prescribing Supply and Administration of Medicines. The Final Report*. DoH London] sets out amendments to section 5(1)(b) of the Medicines Act 1968 and the POMs Order 1997. This Act applies to the NHS and covers treatment provided by NHS Trusts, Primary Care Trusts, Health Authorities, GPs, dentists, Walk-in Centres and NHS funded Family Planning Clinics.

At the same time the legal term for 'group protocols' for POMs has been changed to '*Patient Group Directions*'. These apply to nurses, midwives, health visitors, optometrists, pharmacists, chiropodists, radiographers, orthoptists, physiotherapists and ambulance paramedics. They can supply and/or administer medicines as named individuals. The Medicines Control Agency (MCA) will monitor compliance with amended legislation and failure to comply could result in a criminal prosecution under the Medicines Act [NHSE (2000) *Patient Group Directions (England Only)* HSC 2000/026].

Newer drugs, indicated by a black triangle in the British National Formulary (BNF), could not have normally been administered under 'group protocols' in the past. HSC 2000/026 allows for black triangle vaccines to be included in 'patient group directions' provided they are used in accordance with the schedules recommended by the Joint Committee on Vaccination and Immunization. Patient group directions will not cover unlicensed medicines.

From 9 August 2000, patient group direction must include the following:

● name of the business to which the direction applies;

● date the direction comes into force and expiry date;

● description of the medicine to which the direction applies;

● class of health professional who may supply or administer the medicine;

● signature of doctor or dentist as appropriate, and pharmacist;

- signature by appropriate health organization;
- clinical condition or situation to which the direction applies;
- clinical criteria under which the patient is eligible for treatment;
- exclusions from treatment under the direction;
- circumstances in which further advice should be sought from a doctor or dentist;
- arrangements for referral for medical advice;
- details of dosage, maximum dosage, quantity, strength, route, frequency and duration of administration;
- relevant warnings including potential adverse reactions;
- details of necessary follow up action;
- record keeping arrangements; and
- date for review (generally two years) after which the direction will not be valid.

The Primary Care Organizations' Clinical Governance leads will probably be responsible for facilitating the establishment of patient group directions in the practices.

Influenza vaccine Patient Group Direction

The example given below has been designed by JB Medical and is presented here with kind permission of Dr Jonathan Belsey, Managing Director. Readers can find a broad range of medical and surgical conditions, in each case addressing issues of needs assessment, clinical evidence, audit, guidelines and Patient Group Directions by accessing the http://www.jbmedical.com. A Primary Care Organization (PCO) subscription will allow open access to *Primary Care Toolkit* for all practices and individuals within the PCO.

Situations covered by the Patient Group Direction

The direction covers the administration of influenza vaccine by the health professionals named above to patients registered with the practice.

Groups eligible for vaccination

The target group for vaccination is as follows.
- All patients aged 65 or over.
- All patients with chronic heart disease.
- All patients with chronic respiratory disease including asthma.
- All patients with chronic renal disease.
- All patients with diabetes mellitus.
- All patients with immunosuppression due to disease or treatment.
- All patients in long-term residential care.
- Insert other groups to be included for routine vaccination—consider: pregnancy after the first trimester, children, health care workers or employees who deal with children, e.g. teachers, other occupational groups.

This Patient Group Direction applies to *Insert practice name* and covers the administration of influenza vaccine by the practice nurses/nurse practitioners employed to work on these premises, namely *insert names of staff*

It was developed by *insert GP name*

In conjunction with *insert senior pharmacist name insert Clinical Governance lead or appropriate alternative name insert health professional representative name*
It comes into effect on *insert date* and expires on *insert date*

Signed
. . . . GP
. . . . Pharmacist
. . . . PCG/T representative
. . . . Health professional representative
Date *insert date*

Groups excluded from vaccination

All patients with severe sensitivity to hens' egg who have experienced any of the following symptoms after eating egg:
● hives/urticaria;
● swelling of the lips or tongue;
● acute respiratory distress or collapse;
● known IgE sensitivity to egg;
● all patients who experienced severe reaction to the vaccine in the past; and
● any patient who has a fever at the time of vaccination (minor illness otherwise does not contraindicate receiving the vaccine).

Class of medication included

Approved split virion or surface antigen influenza vaccines which comply with the World Health Organization recommended viral strains for the year in question.

Dosage details

Storage

The vaccine will be stored as prefilled syringes in a designated refrigerator between 2 and 8°C. The temperature will be checked and recorded at the start and end of every vaccination clinic or every day if more stringent criteria are desired by the staff member running the clinic.

Dose

Adults. 0.5 mL By deep subcutaneous or intramuscular injection in the deltoid muscle of the nondominant arm
Children. 3–12 years: 0.5 mL. 6–35 months: 0.25 mL to 0.5 mL. All ages to be repeated after 4–6 weeks if not previously vaccinated and given by deep subcutaneous or intramuscular injection into the anterolateral aspect of the thigh or deltoid from one-year-old.
Maximum dose. Adults should receive only one dose each year. Children receiving the influenza vaccine for the first time should receive no more than two doses the first year and only one dose in subsequent years.

Checklist before administering vaccine

There should be a doctor or another nurse who has up to date training in the administration of vaccines and the treatment of anaphylaxis on the premises for the duration of the vaccination clinic.
● Suitable resuscitation equipment should be readily available in the room.
Pre-filled syringe of adrenaline 1/1000 (1 mg/mL) suitable for subcutaneous or intramuscular injection.
Airway.
Nebuliser and beta-agonist solution.
Injectable hydrocortisone and antihistamines.
Intravenous giving set with colloid solutions.
● Check the vaccine is not out of date and has not been frozen or stored above 8C.
● Check that the patient (or his or her parent/guardian if a child) consents to receiving the vaccine and has been given adequate information on the vaccine and potential problems.

When to seek further advice

● The patient reports other symptoms in response to egg
● *Insert other conditions which you wish to prompt referral to the doctor*

Possible adverse reactions

● Discomfort and swelling at the injection site lasting up to 2 days in up to two-thirds of patients. Treat with self-administration of paracetamol if required.
● Fever, aching muscles and joint pains beginning a few hours after injection and lasting up to two days, occurs rarely in children and no increased risk in healthy adults or the elderly. Treat with paracetamol suspension: Child up to 1 year 60–120 mg; 1–5 years 120–250 mg; 6–12 years 250–500 mg; over 12 years 500 mg–1 g; all doses up to 4 times daily
● Guillain–Barré syndrome has been reported in one vaccination campaign, occurring in 1 per million vaccinations. A patient who develops any of the following symptoms over the few days after the

Table 46.1 To distinguish fainting from anaphylaxis

	Fain/panic attack	Anaphylaxis
Age	Adult and older child (young children rarely faint)	Any age
Central pulse (carotid, femoral)	Present and strong, but heart rate may be slow	Weak or absent, heart rate fast
Breathing	May be fast and gasping, voice normal	Stridor and wheeze, hoarse voice, may stop breathing
Blood pressure	Normal or low but returning to normal in 1–2 min	Very low with fast heart rate
Skin	May be pale and sweating	Pale or widespread flushing, may have urticarial weals or swelling round the mouth, the tongue, or face
Other symptoms	May feel nauseous, dizzy, tingling in fingers or round mouth from hyperventilation	
What to do	Lie on left lateral side until regain consciousness, then lie down with feet raised for 10–15 min. If in doubt of diagnosis treat as anaphylaxis.	Lie on left lateral side with airway if needed. Call for help. Administer adrenaline subcutaneously, or intramuscularly if loss of consciousness, repeating up to 3 times if no response within 5 min each time. Intramuscular hydrocortisone or antihistamine; nebulized salbutamol if bronchospasm, transfer to hospital urgently.

vaccine should be referred for medical assessment urgently:

persistent tingling in the fingers or feet;
weakness in the limbs, trunk, chest wall or face muscles;
unsteadiness and clumsiness;
urinary incontinence or retention;
difficulty with breathing;
fainting or panic attack; or
anaphylaxis. This may be mild, with slowly increasing peripheral oedema and urticaria, or more severe with circulatory and breathing problems (Table 46.1).

When to follow up patients

Insert details of when you think this is appropriate: after any adverse reaction or from a list of more severe reactions?

Records

The following information must be recorded in the patients' notes:

- Vaccine given
- Batch number
- Name of person who performed the vaccination
- Any adverse events experienced by the patient

Anaphylaxis or other significant adverse reactions should be notified to the CMS using the yellow card system by *insert name of person responsible for notifying CSM.*

Computer records

These should be updated with the relevant Read Code *insert Read code favoured for the practice.*

Claiming reimbursement

The GMS 4 forms should be filled in after every vaccination clinic by *insert name of person responsible for this* and sent to the Health Authority without undue delay, to enable the Health Authority to collect data on how many of the target population have been immunized.

Chapter 47

Practice nurse: pre-vaccination checklist

- Has the GP (the prescriber) issued a prescription or given written instructions in the patient's notes, or have you got a patient-specific protocol or a patient group direction?
- Check the patient's details are correct and confirm them with the patient: name, address and date of birth. Do these details match the prescription already written?
- Has the patient had this vaccine before? If yes, is this vaccine appropriate now?
- Has the patient had any reaction, especially severe, to a previous dose of this vaccine? If yes, do not vaccinate and consult with the prescriber.
- If indicated, has the patient had antibodies to the disease tested? Does the patient need the vaccine (e.g. a patient with a past history of jaundice requesting hepatitis A immunization)?
- Is the patient feeling well? Have they a fever?
- Is the patient immunosuppressed by disease or treatment? If yes, consult with the prescriber.
- Has the patient receiving a live vaccine had an injection of immunoglobulin less than 3 months ago? If yes, consult with the prescriber.
- Has the patient receiving a live vaccine received another live vaccine (viral or bacterial) during the past 3 weeks? If yes, do not vaccinate and consult with the prescriber.
- Has the patient ever had an anaphylactic reaction to this or another vaccine, an antibiotic or hens' eggs? If yes, consult with the prescriber, as the vaccine may be contraindicated or special precautions may need to be taken.
- Is the patient now pregnant or planning to become pregnant soon? You may need to discuss vaccination with the prescriber. For advice on immunization and pregnancy, see p. 327.
- Advise the patient to avoid pregnancy and for how long, if appropriate.

- Check that no other contraindications to the vaccine exist.
- In the case where for travel a vaccine is 'sometimes recommended': inform the patient of this and ask them to take the decision whether to have the vaccine.
- Discuss with the patient vaccine side-effects. You may need to put in context severe side-effects and compare them with similar complications from the disease. Reassure the patient about mild reactions and what action, if any, they should take.
- Advise on the length of the vaccine course, number of doses needed, set dates for further doses to be given if it is appropriate.
- Arrange for postvaccination antibody level check if appropriate (e.g. in the case of hepatitis B immunization and high-risk patients).
- As no vaccine is 100% effective, discuss with the patient the importance of scrupulous personal, food and water hygiene and personal contact if this is appropriate.
- Advise the patient what the vaccine does not protect from (e.g. the influenza vaccine does not protect from all influenza viruses).
- Discuss the degree of protection the vaccine you are about to administer affords.
- Identify the right vaccine: check the outer packaging of the vaccine (no matter how familiar you are with it):
  (a) check the expiry date;
  (b) check name and expiry date on the vaccine vial/syringe;
  (c) note the name and batch number and record both in the patient's notes;
  (d) in addition: record the date the vaccine is given, the name of the vaccine and whether it is part of the primary (which dose) course or a booster;

(e) sign the entry in the notes.

• Are you satisfied the correct storage conditions have been observed?

• Reconstitute freeze-dried vaccines only with the diluent supplied and use within the manufacturer's recommended period after reconstitution.

• Add diluent slowly to avoid frothing.

• Check that the colour of the reconstituted vaccine is that stated by the manufacturer in the package insert.

• Ask the patient preferably to sit or lie down, especially if they have vaccination/needle phobia.

• Although not necessary, if you choose to clean the skin with alcohol or other disinfecting agent, allow it to evaporate before administering the vaccine.

• Ensure you have the patient's permission to administer the vaccine before giving it. You advise; they decide.

• Choose the appropriate site for injection (some vaccines, such as hepatitis B, should not be given in the buttock) and route (e.g. subcutaneous for yellow fever vaccine).

• Check that the dose of vaccine is appropriate to the age of the person to be vaccinated.

• If you are satisfied you have taken all precautions and there are no contraindications, with the patient's consent, administer the correct vaccine with the correct technique at the correct site, via the correct route and in the correct amount.

• If two or more vaccines are given simultaneously, record the relevant sites in the patient's notes.

• Observe the patient after immunization for 20 min. This may mean the patient will remain at the surgery, in the waiting room, where they can be seen by a member of staff, for example the receptionist. Only release them if they look and feel well.

• Ensure the patient is in good health and not experiencing any immediate adverse reactions before you ask them to wait in the waiting room.

• If possible, speak to the patient once more before they leave the surgery.

• Ensure correct disposal of the vaccine vial/syringe.

• Return all unused/unopened vaccines to the practice pharmacy fridge immediately after administering the vaccine or at the end of the immunization clinic.

• If in doubt, do not vaccinate, but consult with the prescriber.

Part 5

Travel Health

Chapter 48

Introduction to travel health

International travel

Over the last few years there has been a revolution in the travel industry, with great reductions in the cost of flights, enabling more people to travel not only more often but also further afield. The speed and ease of air flights as well as the comfort of sea cruises today have also greatly encouraged travel. The World Tourism Organization recorded 561 million visits in 1995, the majority in the developed countries. This figure rose to 613 million in 1997. Europe was the most popular destination with 333 million tourist arrivals. During the same year, over 21 million Europeans travelled to Asia, the Pacific, Africa and the Middle East. Another 16 million visited the Americas while the majority of Europeans took their holidays within Europe (275 million visits), although long haul visits increased by 11.8% in 1995.

The number of travellers from a developed country visiting a developing country is about 50 million every year and rising. They are exposed to different climatic, environmental and cultural circumstances, as well as to a range of infections not normally encountered in the Western World. The vast majority of travellers visit Europe. Table 48.1 shows the percentage of visitors worldwide in 1976 and 1997.

Table 48.1 Worldwide travel trends in 1976 and 1997.

Area	1976 (%)	1997 (%)
Europe	69.2	59.0
East Asia/Pacific	3.9	14.7
Americas	22.5	19.4
Africa	2.1	3.8
South Asia	0.7	0.7
Middle East	1.6	2.4

According to DuPont and Steffen [Manual of Travel Medicine and Health. 1999. B.C. Decker Inc., Ontario, Canada], the international tourist receipts amount annually to 380 billion US dollars. The world's top spenders were Germany (48 billion), USA (46 billion), Japan (36 billion), United Kingdom, France, Italy, Austria, the Netherlands (all spending over 10 billion each). The top earners of these leisure funds were the USA (61 billion), France, Italy, Spain, United Kingdom, Austria, and Germany (all earning over 10 billion each).

International migration

It is estimated that between two to four million people migrate permanently every year. Mass migration may be forced as well as voluntary. Migration may be induced by wars, land and economic pressures, the perceived need to improve the quality of life.

The world-wide flow of migration is from:

- east to west
- south to north
- developing to developed countries
- villages and country areas to metropolitan areas

Historically, immigration has been to a number of traditional recipient countries such as Australia, USA, and Canada. Now, however, Europe has become a common destination for many migrants. These migrants have challenging physical and mental problems. Nearly all refugees have higher incidence of nutritional deficiencies, depression, hepatitis B, tuberculosis, and intestinal parasites.

UK residents and travel

UK residents are travelling abroad more frequently than ever before. According to the 1998 report of the Office for National Statistics (ONS) in 1994, UK residents made 39.6 million visits abroad. This figure rose to 42 million in 1996 and 50.9 million in 1998—the highest growth rates in visit numbers since the mid-1980s. At the same time spending by UK residents abroad increased from £14.4 billion in 1994 to £16.2 billion in 1996 and £19.5 billion in 1998 (ONS, Travel Trends 1998).

In comparison, visits to the UK by overseas visitors are showing signs of slowing down. In 1998, the ONS estimates that 25.7 million such visits were made, more than double the visits made in 1978. However, the growth of overseas residents' visits to the UK between 1997 and 1998 was the lowest since 1991 when the Gulf war led to a fall in the number of visits to the UK (ONS, Travel Trends 1998).

In 1998, spending by overseas residents during their stay in the UK was £12.7 billion. Compare this to the £19.5 billion spent by UK residents travelling abroad and the UK is left a record £6.8 billion deficit—£2.1 billion more (worse) than in 1997. Exchange rate movements have had a significant effect on both overseas and UK residents' travel. In contrast, the balance of payments for travel in 1978 was showing a surplus of £1 billion (ONS, Travel Trends 1998).

The main reason for travel abroad by UK residents is holidays. In 1998, holidays (including tours) accounted for 32.3 million visits abroad, while business accounted for 8 million, visiting relatives and friends 6.5 million and miscellaneous

4 million (Fig. 48.1). In total, 50.9 million visits abroad were made by UK residents in 1998 (ONS, Travel Trends 1998).

The most popular destinations for the UK traveller in 1998 were France (11.5 million visits), followed by Spain (9.6 million), the Irish Republic (3.9 million), USA (3.5 million) and Germany (2 million). The total number of UK residents' visits to EU Europe in 1998 was 37.2 million, to non-EU Europe (includes Turkey, Central and Eastern Europe, and former Soviet Union Countries) 4.3 million, North America 4.2 million, while the rest of the world (Central and South America, Caribbean, Africa, Middle East, Asia, Australasia, etc.) attracted 5.2 million UK visitors (Fig. 48.2; ONS Travel Trends 1998).

If we were to deduct the number of visits UK residents made outside North America, Australia, New Zealand, Japan, and EU Europe we find that about 8.84 million visits were made in predominantly developing countries in 1998. The largest increase in visits was recorded for Central and South America—42% more visits in 1998 than in 1997. The bulk of this growth was in holidays to Mexico (ONS, Travel Trends 1998).

The most popular mode of travel for visits abroad is still by aeroplane. In 1998, airlines transported abroad 34.3 million UK residents, while 10.5 million travelled by sea and 6 million through the Channel tunnel (ONS, Travel Trends 1998).

About 75 000 medical insurance claims are made every year. Of the UK residents that fall ill

Fig. 48.1 Reasons UK residents travel abroad and number of visits (1998)

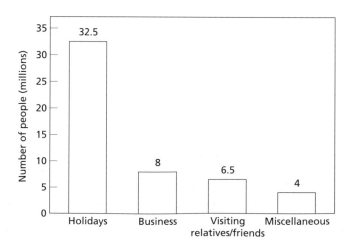

Fig. 48.2 Number of UK residents' visits abroad and destinations (1998).

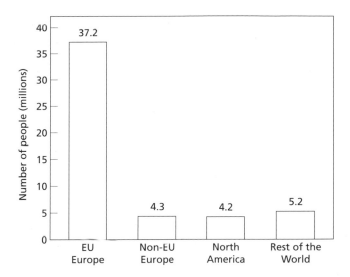

abroad, 69% require minimal intervention, 10% require to see a doctor or a nurse in the host country, 20% are repatriated and 1% require air ambulance. Trauma is still the most common cause of falling ill abroad, followed by gastrointestinal disease, cardiovascular diseases and general infections.

Infectious disease and travel

The greatest morbidity risk in travellers is pre-existing disease such as cardiovascular, respiratory, rheumatic, gastrointestinal, etc. In American travellers this amounts to about 27% of all deaths abroad. The western traveller dies abroad most commonly from cardiovascular disease (50–69%), followed by injury or accidents (20–25%). Infection accounts for only 1–4% of deaths abroad. For the 'locals', it is a different story.

Infectious disease is the world's leading cause of death, accounting for over 17 million (one in three) of the 52 million deaths occurring every year among the 5.75 billion people on this earth. The majority of those killed by infectious disease (about 9 million) are young children. Among the biggest killers are acute lower respiratory infections (4 million children), tuberculosis (3 million people), diarrhoeal disease (3 million children), malaria (2 million people), hepatitis B and its liver sequelae (1–2 million people). Table 48.2 shows

the 10 most common causes of death in 1996 as estimated by the WHO.

Emerging infectious disease—climate changes

It has been estimated that 1 billion people in the world today lack access to adequate sanitation services and safe water. Such poverty in the developing world has obvious global implications such as political instability, overpopulation, disease harbouring and spreading, difficulties in instituting preventive measures, etc. In the developing world, the chance of dying is almost 30 times greater for an infant, 40 times greater for a child, and more than 1000 times greater for a pregnant woman compared to their counterparts living in an industrialized nation.

While the world is battling with existing infectious disease, new diseases emerge. In fact, during the past 20 years at least 30 new diseases have emerged to threaten the health of hundreds of millions of people. The second major problem is the emerging resistance by disease-causing organisms to antimicrobial drugs and other agents, posing a major public health problem worldwide.

Global warming is not new. Present global temperatures have been in a warming phase that began 200–300 years ago. Average temperatures

Cause of death	Number (millions)	Percentage of total
Infectious and parasitic disease	17.3	33
Diseases of circulation (stroke, heart attack, etc.)	15.3	29
Cancer	6.3	12
Death at birth or shortly afterwards (prematurity, asphyxia, trauma, infection)	3.7	7
Chronic lung disease (bronchitis, emphysema)	2.9	6
External causes (accidents, suicides)	1.0	2
Malnutrition, diabetes and related conditions	0.9	2
Death of mother as a result of pregnancy, childbirth	0.6	1
Mental disorders such as dementia, alcohol dependence	0.3	< 1
Miscellaneous or unknown	3.7	7
Total	52.0	100%

Table 48.2 The 10 most common causes of death in 1996 worldwide estimated by the WHO.

are now approaching those at the height of the Medieval Warm Period, near the end of the twelfth century. The intervening centuries included a much colder period, the Little Ice Age, by far the most important climatic fluctuation in recent history. Our concern now is that human activities may be modifying the natural climate. A decline in temperatures from the 1940s to the late 1970s gave rise to worries that industrial pollutants were causing global cooling. Subsequent warming has been attributed to increased concentrations of atmospheric carbon dioxide produced by burning fossil fuels, and other greenhouse gases.

The average global temperature rose steadily from 13.5 °C in 1860 to 14.4 °C in 1998. This has an effect on weather (extreme weather conditions), infectious disease, animal and reservoir hosts, as well as population density and movement. Warmer temperatures are causing:
- lengthening of mosquito seasons;
- rapid mosquito development;
- rapid pathogen development;
- northward extension of species' ranges.

Three-quarters of the world's population live in developing countries. More than one-fifth of the world's population lives in extreme poverty. Almost one-third of all children are undernourished. Half the people in the world lack regular access to the most needed essential drugs. More than 90% of the expected population growth in the coming decades will be in the developing regions of Asia, Africa and Latin America. Two-thirds of people living in sub-Saharan Africa are desperately poor. More money is spent on debt servicing than on health and education, standards of which continue to deteriorate. Within Africa, corruption, wars and lack of commitment to health (especially women's health) have contributed towards the appalling health indices we see today.

The increase in international travel, trade and tourism means we have the means of transporting fast disease-producing organisms from one continent to another and from one country to another. Air travel in particular has increased by almost 7% a year in the last 20 years and further increases of over 5% a year during the next 20 years are predicted.

The social and economic cost of infectious diseases on countries as well as communities, families and individuals can be enormous. An epidemic or the endemicity of an infectious disease in a country can deprive it of foreign currency income from food trade and tourism. The affected communities and individuals quickly feel the knock-on effect.

Infectious diseases cause almost 60% of death and disability in the world's poorest 20% of population.

Controlling infectious diseases is in everybody's interest and is a global challenge. Most important is the introduction of environmental sanitation measures, coupled with better understanding of infectious disease epidemiology. This is followed in importance by the discovery of new antibiotics to replace those to which the disease-producing organisms are developing resistance, and the development of vaccines.

Better technology and mass production of vaccines have helped to reduce their cost. Despite this, many developing countries are unable to purchase them. The WHO, as well as many charitable organizations, makes vaccines available to these countries. In addition, a differential price for vaccines is operated by some vaccine manufacturers, whereby the same vaccine is offered at a higher price to western countries so that it can be offered at a much lower price to developing countries.

Our task is to make the world a safer and healthier place in which to live.

Chapter 49

Travel clinics

We are now witnessing a boom in international travel. In 1948 world airlines transported 4 million international passengers—in 1990 that figure rose to 1160 million, of which 31 million were UK residents. Air travel is predicted to increase by $> 5\%$ a year during the first 20 years of this century.

In 1998, UK residents made 50.9 million visits abroad. Of these, 32.3 million were for holidays and 6.5 million for visiting friends and relatives, giving a total of 38.8 million visits for pleasure. Most of these were in Europe (see previous chapter). UK residents make about 8.84 million visits to predominantly developing countries (ONS, Travel Trends 1998).

The Travellers' Omnibus Survey 1999 explored the attitudes and behaviour of travellers towards travel health. It found that:
- 67% of travellers visiting at-risk destinations did not seek travel health advice before travel;
- 51% of them travelled unprotected against hepatitis A, hepatitis B and typhoid, the three most common vaccine-preventable travel-related diseases;
- of those travelling unprotected, 24% were unaware of the risk to their health, 31% considered the risk too low to justify vaccination, and 30% were given incorrect travel health advice;
- of those travellers failing to seek travel health advice, 81% proceeded to travel unprotected to an at-risk destination.

The main function of the Travel Clinic is to provide a travel service that suits the needs of the population it serves. GPs and practice nurses have an important role in giving people both general and specific advice about travel abroad. Such advice may be generic but it should also be tailor-made for that particular trip of the traveller. Furthermore, they have the responsibility to recognize any disease 'imported' from abroad and to treat

those returning unwell. Travel medicine has therefore become established as a speciality area within the general practice setting. The contribution of practice nurses has become invaluable, as many of them run the travel clinics under the guidance of the GP.

It is important to note that fewer than 5% of travel-related illnesses are currently preventable by vaccines and that the most common illnesses acquired abroad are preventable by measures other than immunization.

In general, 'low-risk' travellers are holiday-makers or business people staying in high standard hotels or major cities. 'High-risk' travellers are:
- pregnant women;
- young children;
- the elderly, especially those with coexisting disease;
- patients with dental problems needing attention while abroad;
- individuals who, for any reason (e.g. accident) require blood transfusion while abroad;
- patients who have anatomical or functional asplenia;
- those immunosuppressed by disease or treatment, including HIV patients;
- healthcare personnel and others going to work or stay for a considerable time or to live in developing countries;
- 'sex travellers';
- travellers who participate in casual sex;
- adventure travellers who put themselves at risk of trauma, etc.;
- backpackers;
- those who undertake tattooing and body piercing while abroad;
- individuals who have migrated away from endemic areas and their children who are brought up in the new country when they return home after a

long absence, especially when staying with relatives.

It should be emphasized to travellers that immunization against infectious diseases does not give complete protection. It is not a substitute for adherence to recommended preventive hygiene measures and proper personal contact. The importance of good personal precautions should be stressed, such as care over eating and drinking, avoiding excess exposure to sun, insect and animal bites and sensible personal contact and hygiene.

Before providing prospective travellers with advice, immunization or prophylaxis, the medical adviser needs to take into consideration the following:

- the individual's age, sex, physical and mental condition;
- family medical history, such as epilepsy in first-degree relatives;
- whether the individual is intending to become or is now pregnant or breast-feeding;
- any pre-existing medical or dental disease and any important operations such as splenectomy;
- their current medication and any known allergies;
- are they known to have glucose-6-phosphate dehydrogenase (G-6-PD) deficiency—this may become essential with future antimalarials expected on the market;
- any previous travel (in)tolerance of prophylactic antimalarial drugs;
- the type of travel (e.g. tourism, visiting relatives, adventures, work abroad);
- mode of travel to and at destination (e.g. aeroplane, train, road vehicle, ship, hired car/moped/bicycle, etc.);
- the parts of the country the traveller plans to visit;
- the kind of activities the traveller intends to undertake (beach, safari, jungle exploration, climbing, backpacking, trekking, bungee jumping, etc.);
- type of accommodation during travel and hygiene standards expected (hotel, guesthouse, relatives);
- degree of contact with locals;
- any specific health risks that may arise in that country;

- the traveller's habits and expectations, any special activities planned (at altitude, diving, trekking);
- the date of departure;
- the length of time to be spent abroad and in particular areas;
- the areas or countries that will be involved in the travel and their requirements;
- the risk of exposure to infectious disease in relation to the traveller's immunity;
- the latest advice available (must have access to it).

Good travel advice is that which has a chance to be followed by the traveller—sensible and practical which does not hinder the individual's enjoyment of travel and at the same time helps to reduce the risk of disease or health problems. This may involve:

- providing advice on management of pre-existing disease while abroad;
- providing advice on self-medication and the management of risk factors and illness abroad;
- education to influence the traveller's behaviour;
- prophylaxis using vaccines, medication or devices.

The most common cause of death abroad is cardiovascular disease (most deaths in the over-50s) followed by accidents and injuries (most deaths in the 20–29 years age group). Trauma is the most common cause of death in travellers under 50 years of age. The most common affliction travellers are likely to experience is diarrhoea. Malaria and hepatitis A are the next most common infectious diseases travellers acquire. About 18% of travellers over the age of 65 who become ill while abroad have to be hospitalized.

One particular group of travellers that may fail to seek advice are individuals living in Western countries whose families originate from the tropics or the Indian subcontinent. They perceive themselves as immune when in reality they face the same health risk as any other traveller, and even higher as they tend to stay with relatives.

Table 49.1 gives an example of a traveller's questionnaire/assessment that can be used in the Travel Clinic, supplemented with information on particular immunizations in Table 49.2. Table 49.3 shows my practice travel clinic questionnaire.

Table 49.1 The table shows the basic questions a travel questionnaire should contain.

Traveller's questionnaire/assessment

Personal details: Name:
Date of birth: Telephone No:
Address:
Practice computer number:

Medical/dental disease history relevant to travel (active and relevant past conditions):
Physical health (good, moderate, poor health):
Medication taken:
Functional disability, any physical disability (incontinence, predisposition to motion sickness):
Mental health and psychological problems (phobias, anxiety, depression, dementia):
Allergies:
Previous tolerance of travel medication, i.e. specific malaria prophylaxis:
Contraception: Pregnant: Breast-feeding:
Sexual health needs:
Smoking:
Vaccination history (including reactions):
Departure date:
Duration of travel:
Country/ies and particular areas to be visited:
If only staying in major city/ies, any possibility of travel outside the city:
Type and style of travel (package, city tours, safari, backpacking, visit to relatives, etc.):
Mode of travel to and at destination (air, sea, land and what kind of vehicle):
Accommodation (hotel, staying with relatives, etc.):
Reason for travel (holiday, business, voluntary work):
Length of stay in particular areas:
Special activities (diving, camping, bungee jumping, altitude, etc.):
Insurance (adequate, need to contact British Heart Foundation, British Diabetic Association, etc.):
Special considerations (terminal illness, condition needing attention during travel):
Contraindications to flying (any present):

Advised malaria chemoprophylaxis:
Advised immunizations:

Table 49.2 Traveller's questionnaire—immunizations.

Vaccine	Primary course	Last booster	Vaccine	Primary course	Booster
Diphtheria			Hepatitis A		
Tetanus			Hepatitis B		
Pertussis			Influenza		
Haemophilus influenzae b			Japanese B encephalitis		
Meningococcal			Tick-borne encephalitis		
conj. C, A + C					
Poliomyelitis			Rabies		
MMR			Typhoid Vi Typhoid oral		
BCG			Yellow fever		
Pneumococcal					

Table 49.3 The author's practice travel clinic questionnaire.

The Ringmead Medical Practice

TRAVEL QUESTIONNAIRE

To be completed by patient

Name: _____   Date of birth: _____

Departure date: _____   Length of stay/holiday: _____

Countries to be visited, including 'stop-overs':

_____

_____

Type of holiday: Staying Within Resort ☐ Back packing ☐ Trekking ☐ Safari ☐ Other ☐

Current medication (including steroids, chemotherapy,   _____
                    contraception):

_____

Important past medical history: _____

Allergies: _____

Previous vaccines: _____

Females: I am not pregnant ☐   I have no reason to suspect I am pregnant ☐

. . . .

To be completed by nurse

	Recommended	Given		Recommended	Given
Tetanus	☐	☐	Comb. Diphth/Tetanus	☐	☐
Polio	☐	☐	Low Dose Diphtheria	☐	☐
Typhoid	☐	☐	Comb. Typhoid/Hep. A	☐	☐
Hepatitis A	☐	☐	Combined Hep. A + B	☐	☐
Hepatitis B	☐	☐	Meningococcal A + C	☐	☐
Rabies	☐	☐	Influenza	☐	☐
Yellow fever	☐	☐	Tick-borne encephalitis	☐	☐
Pneumoccocal	☐	☐	Japanese B encephalitis	☐	☐

Advice has been given regarding:
Food/water (Diarrhoea) Management   ☐
Sun protection   ☐
Care re: sexual behaviour   ☐
Mosquito bite protection   ☐
Malaria medication: 6. Other   ☐
   1. Chloroquine & Proguanil   ☐   7. Stand-by treatment   ☐
   2. Chloroquine   ☐   Malaria management:
   3. Mefloquine   ☐   8. Recognition of symptoms   ☐
   4. Doxycycline   ☐   9. Length of prophylaxis   ☐
   5. Malarone   ☐   10. Malaria advice sheet given   ☐

I have discussed all the above with the Practice Nurse and have had the opportunity to ask questions.

Signature: _____   Date: _____

Chapter 50

Advice to travellers

Eating and drinking

Gastrointestinal problems, predominantly diarrhoea and vomiting, are the major cause of illness for travellers abroad. Give advice on how to avoid these problems as well as what to do with some medications in the case of diarrhoea and vomiting (this applies particularly to patients on diuretics and angiotensin-converting enzyme inhibitors where diarrhoea can lead to dehydration and kidney failure). The traveller could avoid a considerable number of problems if they could remember nine words and adhere to the advice: *boil it, cook it, peel it, or forget it.*

Practical advice could include the following .

Water

- Wash hands after using the toilet and before handling or eating food. Use paper towels or hot air to dry hands. Avoid used, damp, cloth towels—better to drip dry hands.
- Drink plenty, avoid tap water. Adequately chlorinated water will afford significant protection against viral and bacterial water-borne diseases but chlorine alone may not kill some enteric viruses and the parasitic organisms that cause amoebiasis, and cryptosporidiosis. Uncontaminated rain, spring or deep well water is usually safe.
- Unless one is sure about the safety of the local water do not use it. To prepare water for drinking, cleaning teeth, washing salads or making ice there are a number of methods that can be employed.

Boil the water

This is by far the most reliable method to make water of uncertain purity safe for drinking. Boiling water at 100 °C for 10 min kills all known enteric pathogens. This may not be a problem if fuel is available in good supplies. Practically, water should be brought to a rolling boil for 5 but no less than 1 min and then allowed to cool to room temperature. Cover the container while cooling. In order to improve the taste, add a pinch of salt, or pour the water several times from one container to another, or shake it in a clean, sterilized container, not plastic. Because the decrease in atmospheric pressure at high altitudes changes the temperature at which water boils, add 1 extra minute of boil for every 1000 m (3000 feet) above sea level.

Chemically disinfect water

To disinfect water chemically, (if very unsafe filter it first—see below) add 2% tincture of iodine; five drops per litre for clear water or 10 drops per litre for cloudy water. Allow it to stand for 20–30 min and add orange or soluble vitamin C if you need to disguise the iodine taste. Iodine is available in tablets, crystals and aqueous solution too. This method cannot be relied upon to kill *Cryptosporidium* unless the treated water is allowed to stand for 15 h before drinking. Exercise care in pregnant women, young children under 6 years old, sufferers of thyroid disease, and generally avoid using iodine for longer than 6 weeks. Chlorine can also be used for chemical disinfecting of water but it does so in a much slower way than iodine by a factor of 2–3. Its germicidal activity varies greatly with the pH, temperature and organic content of the water to be purified, and it is generally less reliable than iodine. It does not kill amoebic cysts. Household bleach is a source of chlorine and is sometimes used as a water disinfectant—1–2 drops per litre of water, allow to stand for 20 min. Such a solution should smell and taste slightly of chlorine. Its agitation during transport accelerates chlorine loss and this is a distinct disadvantage.

Water filtration

It may be necessary to filter water when there is a need to remove suspended material in cloudy water before (not after) boiling or chemically disinfecting. It is also a convenient alternative to boiling, especially when boiling is not practical or possible. Water is forced through filters either by gravity or through an attached pump or direct pressure from tap water through a special attachment. A large variety of filters exist on the market ranging from small units for the use of individuals, such as backpackers, to large units for a group of travellers, as in expeditions. Reverse-osmosis filters provide protection against viruses, bacteria and protozoa, but they are larger and more expensive. Microstrainer filters with pore sizes of between 0.1 and 0.3 μ can remove bacteria and protozoa but not viruses. If such filters are used the water should, after filtration, be treated with iodine or chlorine in order to kill viruses. Ceramic filters have small pore sizes and the best are those with pores of 0.5 μ, impregnated with silver (in which case do not boil the filter as part of filter maintenance) which kills microorganisms. Filters with iodine-impregnated resins are most effective against bacteria and viruses but the contact time with iodine in the filter is too short to kill *Giardia* in cold water and it will not kill *Cryptosporidia*. Proper maintenance of water filters according to the manufacturer's instructions is essential for optimum function.

Further advice on safe water

- Use bottled water from a reputable commercial producer. The seal must be intact and opened in your presence. Carbonated water is preferable—it is unlikely to have been filled from the tap.
- As a last resort, tap water that is uncomfortably hot to touch and is allowed to cool may be safer than cold tap water.
- Avoid ice in drinks or in contact with food; it could have been made with tap water.
- It is usually safe to drink wine, beer and minerals in cans or bottles as long as the seal is intact. However, water on the outside of cans or bottles might be contaminated. Wipe clean the surface that will come into contact with the mouth. Better to use a sterile, individually wrapped straw.
- Hot coffee or tea is generally safe but the water should be boiled for 5 min (in the case of an electric kettle that switches off automatically remove the lid while boiling).
- Use safe or preboiled water for cleaning teeth.
- Drink only pasteurized milk, otherwise boil it at 55 °C for 30 min or at 65 °C for 1 min.
- Avoid drinking from straws (they might have been washed in contaminated water) unless individually wrapped.
- Always carry a safe drink with you. This can be in a vacuum flask or other clean containers.
- Avoid excessive alcohol as, among other actions, it can lead to dehydration.
- Do not open your mouth while taking a shower or swimming (recreational water is often contaminated). Prepare a very hot bath and allow it to cool before getting in. Chlorine-smelling pools are safer. Swimming in rivers and ponds may result in skin and/or generalized infections such as bilharzia. Sea water near towns may be sewage-polluted.

In case of diarrhoea substitute solid food and milk with clear fluids or a carbohydrate-containing proprietary salt and sugar solution. If none is available, make one by mixing 1 level teaspoon of salt and 8 level teaspoonfuls of sugar in 1 litre of safe water.

Food

- Eat freshly cooked food that is roasting hot, thoroughly cooked—especially meat and seafood. Pink meat should be avoided.
- All raw food is subject to contamination.
- Avoid cooked food that has been kept at room temperature.
- Avoid leftovers or reheated food.
- Soft cheeses may be a source of listeriosis or brucellosis.
- Ensure the yolk in the egg to be eaten is cooked until solid.
- Avoid food, sauces and relishes left out and exposed to flies.
- Spicy foods do not lessen the risk of contamination.
- Avoid shellfish (clams, mussels, oysters, prawns, etc.) and raw fish.

- Avoid cold cuts, salads, raw vegetables, water-melons (sometimes they are injected with water to increase their weight).
- Avoid dairy products such as puddings or any-thing else unless you are sure pasteurized milk was used.
- Avoid ice-cream from unreliable sources, espe-cially kiosks and street vendors. Do not eat it if melted and refrozen.
- Only eat fruit you can peel personally. Peel tomatoes too.
- Eat food from sealed packs or cans—but not if the can appears 'swollen'.
- Avoid food from street vendors. Beware of kebabs where the meat is packed tightly and therefore may not be cooked through.
- Eat in busy, clean restaurants.
- Spare a thought about the plates and cutlery you are going to use—they should have been washed with detergent, clean water should have been used and they should have been protected from flies. Ask to see the kitchen if necessary.
- Wash your hands in clean water before you eat and only eat food that you have personally handled.
- Thoroughly wash hands with (preferably the liquid) soap, in warm running water and dry under air dryers or use disposable towels.
- At the bar, give the bowl of salty nuts a miss— you do not know the level of personal hygiene of other users or the barman.
- Never forget the rule: '*Boil it, cook it, peel it—or forget it*'.
- Breast-feeding confers best protection in very young children. If the child is on formula milk, ensure safe or preboiled water is used.

Road traffic and other accidents, sea and alcohol

Warn travellers that more Britons die abroad in road traffic accidents or by drowning than from all immunizable diseases added together. Accidents are the second most common cause of death (after cardiovascular disease), and the premier cause of death in young people.

- Remember roads in many developing countries can be unmade, narrow, unlit at night, badly engin-eered, poorly maintained, unsafe. Drivers do not always observe speed limits, pedestrian crossings or traffic signals.
- Being involved in an accident may mean having a blood transfusion or operation.
- Cars, coaches, buses and scooters can be unroadworthy and badly maintained, uninsured drivers may be poorly trained, working long hours or even on illegal drugs. Do not get on overloaded buses.
- If you rent a vehicle, check that it is in good condition, the brakes are working, it has seatbelts, inspect to ensure that tyres, windscreen wipers and lights are in good working order, and the vehicle is covered by adequate insurance.
- Avoid night driving.
- Do not drink (any amount of) alcohol and drive.
- Always wear seatbelts.
- Avoid motorbikes and scooters. If you must ride them, insist on a good quality crash helmet or take your own.
- Avoid overcrowded public vehicles.
- Ensure you are familiar with local traffic sys-tems, road conditions and regulations.
- Do not take nonprescribed drugs—your risk for accidents increases, and prison sentences can be very severe.
- Do not drink alcohol and swim.
- Do not dive into unfamiliar swimming pools— check the depth of water before diving.
- Never swim alone. Do not swim far out to sea. Watch for strong sea currents. Do not take inflat-able air-beds or toys into the sea.
- Do not swim for at least an hour after a meal or alcohol.
- Supervise children by water very closely, espe-cially those on airbeds.
- Look out for jelly fish and sea urchins.
- Ask for information about local safe beaches.
- Do not swim in freshwater streams, canals and lakes in Central Africa, South America (some parts only) or South-East Asia because they are liable to be infested with snail hosts of schistosomiasis (bilharzia), or in water with algae, or infested with rats or urine from animals (risk of Weil's disease— leptospirosis).
- Ensure watersports are properly supervised and the equipment is in good order.
- Keep away (and supervise children) from bal-

cony barriers—quite often they are low enough for people to lose their balance and fall.

● Avoid coming into contact with domesticated animals and their bites.

● Minimize the risk of assault by being with others, not going out at night, choosing streets that are well lit and not deserted, not wearing expensive watches or jewellery or carrying expensive cameras or other equipment.

● Get to know about the 'no go' areas and avoid them.

● Remember the local hospitals may not be what you are accustomed to at home and the danger of using blood contaminated with hepatitis B, hepatitis C and/or HIV is real.

● If water-skiing, wear wetsuits (protects women from high-speed douching of infected water).

● Always wear appropriate protective footwear (sandals, flip-flops)—foot injuries on the beach are common.

● Beware of electrical and/or gas heating/cooking equipment; fires, electrocution and carbon monoxide poisoning are possible.

● Avoid smoking in bed. Check there are smoke detectors in your hotel and room.

● If you are using a tent, think of possible floods, avalanches, robbery attacks, entry of dangerous animals, snakes and insects. Take time to survey the area.

● Be fit enough for the sport you are undertaking, e.g. skiing and climbing.

● Do not undertake bungee jumping as it is very dangerous and may result in fractures, ocular haemorrhage, lens subluxation, retinal detachment, hearing loss, quadriplegia, foot drop and death. In addition, it may invalidate the traveller's insurance (some policies have an exclusion).

Sun warnings

Solar ultraviolet radiation is approximately 200–400 nm in wavelength. The long wavelengths (315–400 nm) UVA do not cause sunburn but are responsible for many photosensitivity reactions, photodermatoses, and are implicated in long-term skin damage and pathogenesis of skin cancer. Their long-term effects can take 10–20 years to become apparent. The medium wavelengths (280–315 nm) UVB cause sunburn and contribute to the long-term effects of solar ultraviolet radiation, namely premature skin ageing (photoageing—wrinkled, mottled, leathery skin) and skin cancer.

Current sunscreens block both UVA and UVB to varying degrees. The sun protection factor (SPF) is defined as the ratio of the least amount of ultraviolet energy required to produce a minimal erythema on skin protected by sunscreen to the amount of energy required to produce the same erythema on unprotected skin. The SPF indicated on the preparation with a number provides guidance on the degree of protection offered against UVB. For example, a correctly applied sunscreen with an SPF of 15, reduces the ultraviolet radiation exposure to the skin to 1/15th of its original value. In other words, it enables the person to remain 15 times longer in the sun without burning.

The ability to protect against UVA is indicated by a star rating system graded 1–4. This system indicates the protection against UVA relative to protection against UVB for the same product. A product with 4 stars protects equally against UVA and UVB, 1 star indicates the poorest level of protection against UVA compared with UVB. Still, we must remember that such preparations do not prevent long-term damage to skin associated with UVA, which may not be apparent for years later (10–20 years). In order to achieve the best protection against UVA, preparations that contain titanium dioxide should be used as they reflect ultraviolet radiation (e.g. RoC Total Sunblock, Spectraban Ultra lotion, Sun E45). Sunscreens that contain cinnamates, benzophenones or dibenzoylmethanes absorb ultraviolet radiation.

Sunscreen preparations with SPF 15 and above are available on NHS prescription for patients with abnormal cutaneous photosensitivity resulting from genetic disorders or photodermatoses, including vitiligo and those resulting from radiotherapy. Also, for chronic or recurrent herpes simplex labialis. Such prescriptions should be endorsed with 'ACBS' (Advisory Committee on Borderline Substances).

The primary function of sunscreens is to prevent sunburn. This is phototested *in vivo* at an internationally agreed application thickness of 2 mg/cm^2. Several studies have shown that users of sunscreens apply much less than this, usually between 0.5 and 1.3 mg/cm^2. It follows therefore that in view of the application thickness most users will achieve only a quarter to half of the value expected from these products. This is one of the reasons sunbathers suffer sunburns despite using high factor sunscreens. The others are over-exposure to sun in the belief that they are protected, and missing parts of the body, e.g. behind the ears.

A convenient way of classifying correctly applied sunscreens, for travellers with no special skin problems is the following:
• SPF 25 and above: suitable for travellers exposed to strong sunshine, especially children;
• SPF 15–24: for travellers who burn easily or who are in the sun for several hours;
• SPF 8–14: for travellers already tanned who stay in the sun for short periods;
• SPF 4–7: for travellers with darker skin, and for those who stay in the shade;
• SPF under 4: do not have any practical application as sunscreens.

If the traveller suffers from sunburn, they should stay out of the sun until the skin has healed. Taking cool showers, applying calamine, aloe vera lotion, or yoghurt may help to ease soreness, itching and redness.

A heatstroke may occur when the function of the sweat glands begin to deteriorate and the body overheats. This may come on gradually but also suddenly, causing the individual to feel weak, exhausted, thirsty, possibly with headaches and muscle cramps. The traveller's condition can then deteriorate, the body temperature rises to $> 39\ °C$, they may vomit, become drowsy, confused, irrational, and may soon collapse. Such a person must be placed in the shade, gently fanned or sponged with a cool, wet cloth, and fluids should be given by mouth if conscious and parenterally if in coma.

Advice for travellers should include the following.
• Gradual exposure to the sun, wearing a hat and sunglasses, sunscreen creams, and avoidance of direct sun between 11.00 and 15.00 h are essential.
• Overexposure to sunlight causes sunburn, premature skin ageing and an increased risk of skin cancer. In the UK, the incidence of newly diagnosed skin cancer appears to be doubling every 10 years. There were over 40 000 cases in 1997.
• Remember, ultraviolet radiation is most powerful on the equator.
• You are still exposed to the sun's effects under a cloud.
• Overheating of the body may lead to sunstroke or heat stroke.
• Avoid strenuous activity at midday.
• Drink plenty of fluids and avoid alcohol.
• Avoid excess coffee, especially during the hot parts of the day.
• If sweating a lot, consider adding some salt to your food, provided you drink plenty of fluids and you do not suffer from a cardiac condition that involves fluid overload.
• Limit exposure to sun at the start of the holiday—grade exposure to sun in half-hour intervals.
• Use appropriate sunscreen agents liberally and at regular intervals (every 2–3 hours). Use water-resistant sunscreen for children playing in water or if you are undertaking water activities. The higher the SPF, the greater the protection, the longer you can stay in the sun. Take special care of ears, eyelids, nose, lips, shoulders and upper legs. Cover well the areas of the skin not used to sun exposure (topless bathing).
• Wear a hat and protect eyes with good quality sunglasses—still apply sunscreen to face and neck. Wear long-sleeved shirts.
• The face is exposed to sun from reflective surfaces such as water and sand. Protect with sunscreens, especially under the eyes.
• Certain drugs (e.g. doxycycline, thiazides) can make the skin more sensitive to sun. Consult your doctor or pharmacist before travelling.
• For tanning, use a high SPF lotion to start with and reduce slowly, so that at the end of the day you do not feel sunburned.
• Use a moisturizing 'aftersun' cream/lotion regularly and frequently.
• Always carry a sufficient number of sunscreen lotions, of varying SPF (the higher the factor, the higher the protection).
• Remember, babies (best keep them out of direct sunlight, especially if under 9 months of age), children and the elderly are particularly at risk. Also, fair-skinned people, especially with blue eyes

and/or red hair, patients with previous skin cancer and those with skin pigment conditions such as albinism.

- Dress children in long-sleeved shirts and hats.
- Wear sunglasses, which filter UV to protect the eyes.
- High humidity and increased perspiration favour the growth of fungi and bacteria on the skin. Taking frequent showers (three or more) helps to keep the body cool. After showering, dry between folds of skin and apply a light dusting powder.
- If you notice any unusual skin changes or if your pigmented moles change in size, shape or colour, become itchy or bleed, show them to your doctor.
- Bursting blisters resulting from sunburns should be avoided as this may lead to infection.

Blood-borne and sexually transmitted diseases

Inappropriate sexual behaviour abroad increases the risk of contracting HIV 300-fold. Apart from HIV, travellers could contract hepatitis B, hepatitis C, herpes, syphilis, chancroid, gonorrhoea, gardenerella vaginalis, chlamydia, trichomonas vaginalis, candida, human papillomavirus, cytomegalovirus, pubic lice and scabies. A common assumption is that people are more likely to engage in high-risk sexual behaviour when travelling than when they are at home. HIV-1 seems to be more readily transmitted from men to women than from women to men, so women are at increased risk of heterosexual HIV-1 transmission. Men's risk behaviour abroad reflects their behaviour at home, whereas women's risk behaviour is frequently shaped by the background of their sexual partners [Bloor M. *et al.* (1998) Differences in sexual risk behaviour between young men and women travelling abroad from the UK. *Lancet* 352, 1664–8].

Casual encounters are frequent. A study at a London clinic [Daniels *et al.* (1992) *Int. J. STD AIDS* 3, 427–8] found that 51% of heterosexual men, 36% of homosexual men and 20% of women had had sex with a previously unknown contact while on holiday during the 6 months before the study. The long-stay traveller is more likely to have a 'local' sexual liaison. In the *Communicable Diseases Scotland Weekly Report A* (1993,

286/3) it was reported that 80% of the total cases of heterosexually contracted AIDS reported in the UK were acquired abroad. Women are two to four times more susceptible than men to contracting AIDS from unprotected intercourse (hepatitis B is 100 times more infectious than HIV).

Bloor *et al.* (see above) examined the sexual behaviour of young people aged 18–34 years who had travelled abroad from the UK without a partner during the previous 2 years (summer of 1994 and 1996). They found that one in 10 reported sexual intercourse with a new partner. Travellers who reported a new sexual relationship abroad were also likely to report large numbers of sexual partners at home. Of the 400 people who had a new sexual partner abroad, 300 (75%) used condoms on all occasions with the new partner.

- Avoid having casual relationships but if you have sex with someone new, always use a condom. Pack an adequate supply of good quality condoms, do not rely on the availability and quality of local condoms (buy condoms in the UK with the British Standard Kitemark or an EN600 mark). South Asian condoms may prove small for the British traveller. Condoms should be stored away from heat and light.
- Alcohol and drugs affect your judgement and may precipitate an unwise sexual contact.
- Oral and visual reassurance that the other person is healthy is no reassurance at all; he or she may be infectious although looking and feeling well.
- Having sex with a prostitute (female or male) greatly increases the risk of contracting a sexually transmitted disease.
- The safest sex is with a faithful, life-time partner. Failing this, abstain.
- Sex with fellow travellers is not a safe option.
- Do not experiment/use injectable non-prescribed (illegal) drugs. If you do, never share equipment but take with you a supply of sterile needles and syringes.
- Never share razor shavers or toothbrushes.
- Avoid having a tattoo, acupuncture, or your ear or other parts of your body pierced. If you were to proceed to such action, be absolutely certain of the sterility of the equipment used—if not sure, do not have it.

- Avoid unnecessary medical or dental treatment abroad. Have a check up and complete any dental treatment well before you travel.
- If you need regular blood treatment (e.g. for haemophilia), bring your own supply of blood products and infusion, if it is possible and practical.
- Make sure that any medical equipment used for your treatment abroad, should this become necessary, is freshly sterilized or taken from a sealed pack and that any gloves worn are sterile and not used when treating others (a common problem in casualty departments in some countries).

Blood transfusion

Blood donated in Britain and most industrialized countries is tested for HIV. But the test only picks up antibodies to the AIDS virus, indicating its presence, usually 3 months after infection. The risk of acquiring HIV by such a mishap is estimated at one in a million. The more people carrying the virus in a geographical area, the greater the risk. High-risk areas are sub-Saharan Africa, New York, Los Angeles and Thailand. An additional problem is the quality of laboratories. Dr Guillermo Herrera, of the Federal Centre for Disease Control and Prevention in the USA, in the early 1990s, published research in the journal *East African* which showed that, when retested in sophisticated pathology laboratories in the USA, blood used in five Kenyan Government hospitals was in 25% of cases HIV-positive, while it was classified as safe and transfused to patients.

Systematic screening of blood donations is not yet feasible in all developing countries. On occasions travellers have requested blood or blood product from their home country available to them in case of urgent need. Apart from logistic, technical and ethical issues that such a request raises, the ultimate safety of the blood for them will depend on the quality of blood transfusion services in the host country.

The Blood Care Foundation, a registered British charity, can provide, by a specialist courier service, screened blood, sterile transfusion fluids and equipment needed for transfusion, for emergencies worldwide by simply calling one of its 24 h

alarm centres in Europe, North America or the Far East. The blood originates from internationally renowned sources in Western Europe. The Foundation's satellite blood banks receive screened blood every month, or more frequently if required. Unused supplies are donated to local hospitals. It does not provide blood for elective surgery abroad, while attempted suicide, self-inflicted injury, chronic blood disorder, war or nuclear risks are not included. An individual can join the Blood Care Programme by paying a fee either directly or via MASTA. Further details from the Blood Care Foundation, PO Box 7, Sevenoaks, Kent TN13 2SZ. Tel.: 01732 742 427, Fax: 01732 451 199. For information on membership: Tel.: 01293 425 485; Fax: 01293 425 488.

If you need a blood transfusion abroad, consider the following.

- Consider it only if there is no alternative.
- Try to ensure the donor blood has been screened. Talk to the attending physician.
- If blood cannot be adequately screened and your condition allows, request to be flown home or to another reliable country (ensure you are covered for emergency repatriation).
- Know your blood group and if travelling with your family or friends, find out who has a compatible blood group.
- Contact the British Embassy or if in a Commonwealth country the British High Commission for advice on where to obtain a safe supply of blood.
- Ask if any alternative to blood transfusion can be used instead, e.g. a plasma expander. This may also allow urgent evacuation home.
- Above all, try to avoid needing blood transfusion by minimizing the risk of injury (wear seatbelts whether front or back passenger, do not drive at night, etc.).
- If you are unwilling to accept the risk of treatment by local medical services in the event of a serious accident or other medical emergency, choose an alternative 'safer' destination for your holiday.
- Carry with you (one for each member of the family) a medical kit (see p. 288) that contains sterile needles and syringes for use in an emergency; keep all such equipment in its original case and carry it with you at all times, including your excursions at destination.

Contact with animals on land and sea

Avoid any contact especially with stray or wild animals—for action in case of suspected rabies see p. 208.

- Avoid snake bites by heeding the following:

  (a) do not walk in long grass areas, especially at night—carry a light;

  (b) never place hands into places you cannot first visualize;

  (c) wear boots and long trousers on hikes into the bush, especially at night—snakes tend to be active at night and in warm weather;

  (d) never handle snakes or pose with them for photographs;

  (e) if you encounter a snake, stay still until it is safe to move (snakes strike at moving objects); do not disturb or attack a snake;

  (f) if you have to sleep out or in a tent, raise your bed;

  (g) sleep under mosquito nets and shake clothing and shoes before putting them on, particularly in the morning; snakes and scorpions tend to rest in shoes and clothing;

  (h) remember sea snakes (the *Hydrophiidae*) can also be dangerous; avoid swimming in overgrown rivers or lakes, do not pick snakes off fishing nets.

If a person is bitten by a snake, wipe any visible venom from the skin and immobilize the limb with a splint if necessary, in order to avoid muscle contractions that will facilitate the systemic spread of the venom. Ensure the casualty is taken to a medical establishment as soon as possible and take the snake too if killed. For pain relief give paracetamol, avoid aspirin as it will increase the bleeding diathesis or may cause stomach bleeding.

The only specific remedy for snake bite is antivenom; signs that indicate systemic absorption of venom and need for antivenom are: bleeding from the gums or nose, haematemesis, generalized stiffness and myalgia, paralysis, ptosis (drooping of eyelids), drop in blood pressure and loss of consciousness.

The application of a tight tourniquet is only necessary if there is a definite bite by a dangerous neurotoxic species such as a cobra, mamba, coral snake, krait, sea-snake and Australian venomous snake. Do not leave the tourniquet on for more than 2 h—check that the pulse is present. An alternative is the use of a pressure pad over the wound or the firm application of a crêpe-bandage. The use of compression may increase the local effect of necrotic venoms (some cobras, *Viperidae*—vipers, adders and rattlesnakes).

Deaths from snake bites are relatively rare. Particularly dangerous are the coral and rattlesnakes in the Americas, the Australian brown snake, the carpet vipers in the Middle East, and the Russell's viper and cobras in Southern Asia.

An effective British antidote (Protherics) to rattlesnake venom received FDA approval in 2000. *CroFab* is the first new treatment for rattlesnake bite in more than 50 years. There are about 25 species and 44 sub-species of rattlesnake in the Americas and about 300 worldwide. The most poisonous tend to be those in Australia and South America.

- If stung by a jellyfish remove the stinging capsules from the skin of the victim with vinegar or alcohol—use seawater if necessary but avoid fresh water as it may activate them; seek medical advice.

The most dangerous bite is the one from the box jellyfish (*Chironex fleckeri*), which is found in the Indo-Pacific region; symptoms include diarrhoea and vomiting, rigors, hypotension, fits, paralysis of breathing muscles and loss of consciousness; apply a tight tourniquet and transfer to hospital immediately. If necessary, perform cardiopulmonary resuscitation. An Australian antivenom for box jellyfish is available.

- Fish stings can be very painful. Immerse the affected limb in hot water (just under 45 °C to avoid scalding) or inject the affected skin with a local anaesthetic such as lidocaine. Remove the stinging spine and membranes to avoid infection. Antivenom is available for *Scorpaenidae*, which include the stonefish and *Tachinidae* (Mediterranean basin and North Sea).

- Venomous spiders such as tarantula (*Latrodectus tredecemguttatus*) in the Mediterranean countries, the black widow spider (*Latrodectus mactans*) and the brown recluse spider (*Loxosceles reclusa*) of North America, the Australian red-back spider (*Latrodectus hasselti*), the Sydney funnel web spider

(*Atrax robustus*) of Australia and the banana spider (*Phoneutria keiserlingi*) found in South America, inject local anaesthetic; if neurotoxic symptoms occur apply a tight tourniquet or crépe-bandage and transfer to hospital for antivenom.

- Venomous scorpions are found predominantly in North and South Africa, Asia and the whole of America as well as the Caribbean. Similar precautions for snakes apply to scorpions. Treatment ranges from local anaesthetic to narcotic analgesics. An antivenom is available. Use atropine for severe bradydysrhythmias.

- Bees and wasps can deliver fatal stings, mainly as a result of the allergic reactions they induce, including anaphylaxis. Remove the sting by scraping it with a fingernail, razor or knife blade (do not grasp it with fingers). Advise travellers who are highly sensitive to bee or wasp stings to carry a Medic-Alert tag obtainable from the Medic-Alert Foundation International, 1 Bridge Wharf, 156 Caledonian Road, London N1 9UU. Tel.: 020 7833 3034.

Antimalaria prophylaxis

Lack of any antimalaria prophylaxis increases the traveller's chance of dying from malaria 20-fold. For specific advice see Malaria p. 375.

Combating stress

Travellers may be subject to various forms of stress such as overcrowding, long hours of waiting, changes in climate and time zones, disruption of eating habits, fear of flying. They need to plan ahead and allow sufficient time for journeys. They also need to plan when they are going to take their prescribed medications, such as insulin or diuretics. Stress and problems with medication contribute to the fact that cardiovascular disease is the most frequent cause of death occurring abroad in travellers aged 50–70 years. They should take adequate supplies of their prescribed medication and should not put all supplies in the baggage hold as baggage can be delayed or lost.

Medical kit

It is sensible to take a medical kit, especially if travelling to a remote destination. Sterile medical packs, which contain syringes, needles, dental needles, injection swabs, drip needles for blood transfusion, needle set for stitching, skin closure strips, dressings and gloves, are available commercially from travel clinics, some pharmacies and from organizations such as Homeway Ltd, MASTA and others (for addresses and telephone numbers see Sources of Travel Information, Chapter 64).

The contents of the medical kit will depend on the number of co-travellers, their health and potential health risks, the destination and availability there of quality medical supplies, the length of stay, the available space in the traveller's luggage and so on. Here is a list of items that can be included in a medical kit but it is by no means exhaustive.

- Material to treat cuts and bruises: disinfectant, alcohol swabs, cotton wool, dressings, plasters, scissors, bandages, antibiotic cream, safety pins, hot/cold packs, eye patch, disposable gloves, suture kit (sterile prepacked kit).

- Thermometer, tweezers, 2×5 mL syringes, 5 needles (preferably two sizes), 1 dental needle, 1 intravenous cannula, 1 skin suture with needle, 1 packet skin closure strips, 5 alcohol swabs for skin cleansing, 5×5 cm and 10×10 cm nonstick dressings, 1 roll surgical tape, condoms, blanket, candle, flash light, IV fluid kit, sterile drip set.

- Medication: regular medication, analgesics/antipyretics, anti-inflammatory agents, antihistamines, calamine, contraceptives, insect sting emergency allergy kit that includes adrenaline (EpiPen), antimalaria drugs for prophylaxis and standby, antibiotic, antacids, altitude sickness drugs (e.g. Diamox), motion sickness drugs, antidiarrhoeals, laxatives, rehydration powders, ear/eye drops, medication for period cramps and vaginal thrush if recurrent.

- Mosquito netting, appropriate insect repellent, container and water purification tablets/equipment, sunscreens and sanitary supplies.

Table 50.1 The countries of the European Economic Area—15 member states plus Iceland, Liechtenstein and Norway.

Austria	Belgium	Denmark	Finland	France	Germany
Greece	Iceland	Ireland	Italy	Liechtenstein	Luxembourg
Netherlands	Norway	Portugal	Spain	Sweden	UK

Medical insurance and cover

This is essential for any traveller no matter where the destination. With free healthcare in the UK we tend to forget the same will not apply abroad. The UK has a reciprocal healthcare agreements with some countries (see Chapter 63) but this agreement may not cover all the medical expenses the traveller may incur. Some will not cover treatment necessary after road traffic accidents or repatriation. On other occasions, in an emergency a patient may be sent across a border to another country for treatment that does not have such an agreement with the UK.

If the traveller is ordinarily resident in the UK and is a UK national or a national of any other European Economic Area (EEA) State, or stateless person or refugee, they are entitled to apply for form E111 (an application form can be found in 'Health Advice for Travellers'—see below) at the Post Office where it is stamped and signed. It entitles the bearer to free or reduced-cost emergency treatment in the EEA member states (see Table 50.1) and in addition in Iceland, Liechtenstein and Norway. It remains valid as long as the names on the form remain ordinarily resident in the UK. Some expenses and also repatriation in the event of illness or death are not covered. On many occasions travellers have been asked to pay part of hospital bills, which may or may not be refundable by the DoH here. Twenty per cent of a hospital bill for a family after a car crash in France may amount to many thousand of pounds.

Patients on renal dialysis should make advance arrangements before leaving the UK. In the case of Spain, obtain form P10 from the renal unit well before departure. For oxygen supplies in an EEA country contact the International Branch of the DoH on 020 7210 5318.

If a patient is going to another EEA country specifically for medical care, or if they require ongoing treatment of a pre-existing condition, form E112 should be obtained but it requires authorization from the DoH. Without it the traveller is likely to pay for treatment.

For medical treatment abroad in the EEA or an operation where the traveller is eligible to Form E111, the first application is to the Local Health Authority, which then forwards it to the DoH International Branch, for approval. The consultant will need to support the application and the Health Authority will need to agree to pay for the treatment.

If the traveller is travelling to an EEA country and needs medical care and/or treatment (blood tests, medication, injections), or antenatal care while there, they should apply directly by letter enclosing supporting evidence from their GP to: DoH International Branch, Room 512, Richmond House, 79 Whitehall, London SW1A 2NS, Tel.: 020 7210 5318, or for Northern Ireland: DoH and Social Services, Room 436, Dundonald House, Upper Newtownards Road, Belfast BT4 3SF, Tel.: 01232 520 000.

A comprehensive medical insurance is essential. The traveller should read the small print and especially the exclusions—some hazardous activities, road traffic accidents, bungee jumping or conditions such as pregnancy or chronic diseases may be excluded.

Ensure the insurance cover is adequate to meet the medical expenses in the country of destination, as well as repatriation if the need arises. If a credit card or employer provides medical insurance, check that it does not need 'topping up'. For frequent travellers an annual health policy is a good idea. Ensure the traveller understands that no health insurance guarantees a high enough standard of care, therefore prevention, where it is possible, is the best insurance. The most common causes of repatriation are cardiovascular and orthopaedic, followed by respiratory, neurological, psychiatric, gastrointestinal, dermatological and renal problems. Airlines will not carry travellers back unless they are fit to travel, otherwise the traveller may have to return to the UK by air ambulance. The cost can be considerable: approximately £15 000 from Spain, £22 000 from Turkey, £50 000 from the Caribbean or USA.

Fewer than 60 countries worldwide have any sort of agreement with the UK. More countries actually do not and include Switzerland, Turkey, Cyprus, Canada, USA, Mexico, most of the Caribbean islands, all South American countries, all countries in the Middle East, Africa and Asia, including India, Thailand, Japan, Hong Kong, the whole Pacific region (except for Australia and New Zealand), certain republics of the former Soviet Union.

Health Advice for Travellers

This very useful DoH publication, can be obtained free from the DoH (Freephone 0800 555 777). It contains travel advice and an application for form E111.

Some further travellers' tips

● Consult the doctor, or the specialist practice nurse, at least 2 months before departure. Keep immunizations up-to-date.

● If you have problems, have a medical and/or dental check-up well before departure date. Allow time for any necessary treatment.

● Take enough money, preferably in travellers' cheques, check the credit card expiry date and take with you the telephone number to ring if your card is lost or stolen. Place the money in a secure safe at your hotel/accommodation.

● Buy a return ticket.

● Check with the travel agent or embassy of the destination country (for telephone numbers see Chapter 65) well in advance to see whether a visa is necessary (remember to include the countries in transit). Have a passport photograph with you in case a hurried visa application is necessary.

● Ensure the passport is valid at least until the return date. Many countries require a valid passport for 6 months at least. Leave a photocopy of your passport behind with a friend who will be able to fax it to the British Embassy/High Commission if the need arises. Keep the names and addresses of relatives or friends with your passport too, in case they need to be contacted.

● Read in advance material about the country/ies of destination.

● While abroad:
  (a) keep money, tickets and passport in a safe;
  (b) carry only as much money as you may need when out;
  (c) do not wear 'provocative' jewellery/watches;
  (d) go out with others, avoid deserted streets;
  (e) obey the local laws;
  (f) avoid any direct or indirect involvement with illegal drugs.

● Do not forget your electrical adaptor and own shaving equipment.

● Take out a comprehensive medical insurance and take with you a copy of the policy and the 24 h emergency telephone number. Take with you form E111 if appropriate to your destination.

● If you are driving, do not leave home without your driver's licence, car insurance and breakdown recovery insurance.

● If you are flying and you are over 50 years of age or at risk of thrombosis, wear thigh-length, elasticated stockings, soft grip class I. Antiembolism stockings can be purchased from pharmacies. If you are at high risk of thrombosis, your doctor may wish to give you further advice and possibly arrange for injection of low-weight molecular heparin before departure and on arrival.

Chapter 51

Legal aspects of advice for travellers

The standard of care expected by a doctor or a nurse giving travel advice in a travel clinic setting is that of a reasonable practitioner exercising their particular skill of travel health care. The standard expected will be higher than that of just providing travel immunizations in a routine surgery. Patients at risk or with pre-existing medical problems need to be advised accordingly. Vaccinations are only a small part of the work that is undertaken in a travel clinic.

Published recommendations should be followed carefully. A decision not to follow such advice should be documented in the notes with reasons and warnings given.

The Medical Defence Union's advice to GPs states: 'There must be a very real possibility of a claim for negligence being made against a doctor who deliberately overrides a country's recommendations and the patient contracts one of the specified diseases. It is likely to prove extremely difficult to mount an adequate defence against this claim.'

After due consideration, if a doctor genuinely feels vaccination is contraindicated, he or she should provide the patient with a certificate giving full details of the reasons for nonvaccination or at least stating the traveller is exempted from immunization (see specimen on p. 392) In such cases an airline may permit travel but it is the Health Authority at the port of arrival which is the final arbiter on those arriving without valid certificates where they are required. Such travellers may be liable to inconvenience, delay and even quarantine at their final destination. Some risk having to receive vaccination at the border, sometimes with needles of questionable sterility.

For product liability purposes, the batch number of all vaccines/immunoglobulins should be recorded in the patient's notes. Vaccines and immunoglobulins should be stored under the conditions recommended by the manufacturers, usually at refrigerator temperatures of between 2 and 8 °C. Unused reconstituted vaccines or multi-dose vials should be discarded after a vaccination session.

For further information, see 'Medicolegal Aspects of Immunization and the Nurse' on p. 261.

Air travel—the problems, the doctor and the law

Another area with medicolegal implications regards the doctor who offers help to a patient on a flight. Under US law, a doctor who attends a patient during an in-flight emergency, could be sued where the aircraft is registered or where it is owned, where the incident took place, where the plaintiff lives, where the defendant lives or even, on some occasions, in more than one place at once.

The UK's General Medical Council's (GMC) advice to any doctor faced with an emergency situation is clear: doctors must offer anyone at risk the treatment they are reasonably expected to provide. This may mean that a psychiatrist might feel unable to carry out a procedure of which he or she has not had experience for many years. What is not very clear is what happens when it comes to medical emergencies on aircraft. A doctor will be required to respond to such an emergency on ethical grounds. Some airlines, such as British Airways, have indemnity cover built into their own insurance schemes. Medical defence organizations will usually cover doctors. Could a doctor be sued for not helping? The answer is not in English law, as there would be no duty of care. What the British doctor might face is a complaint to the GMC.

Litigation in such circumstances is thought to

be rare, with only two cases known of in the USA and none in the UK. About 40 USA states have Good Samaritan laws, which prevent cases being brought.

In general terms, airlines are keen to preserve an image of safety, so in-flight medical incidents can be underplayed. Rates on schedule carriers vary from one medical incident per 10 000 passengers (British Airways) to one per 100 000 (US carriers). A US Federal Aviation Administration report suggested four medical emergencies per million in 1993, with one in every 13 leading to diversion to another airport. Most emergencies are not flight related but everyday illnesses.

Indications for diversion and unscheduled landing include the following:
- acute breathing difficulties;
- severe unrelieved pain;
- uncontrolled bleeding;
- major injury with shock;
- continued unconsciousness;
- impending birth;
- disturbed behaviour with risk to passengers and crew.

Between April 1998 and March 1999, British Airways requested a doctor on board 872 times, on average more than twice every day. It had 3386 in-flight medical incidents reported out of a total of 36 million passengers worldwide and 43 flights were forced to divert for medical reasons. Asthma is the most frequently occurring chronic respiratory disease in air passengers (about 6% of in-flight medical incidents). Vomiting, diarrhoea and fainting account for one-third of total incidents. Head injuries and sunburns were other problems encountered. BA's medical kits were opened a total of 1395 times. Interestingly, doctors provided assistance in only 33% of these cases, which compares poorly with Air France, on whose flights the rate is reported to be 90%. This may be accounted for by the fact that it is illegal in France not to offer assistance.

Statistics from other airlines show the in-flight problems to be related to central nervous system (including stress and anxiety) in 16%, cardiovascular 15%, gastric 12%, respiratory 12%, while the remaining cases are other problems, including falls. Before deciding what treatment to recommend on board of an aircraft, ask the crew what is available. Aircraft medical facilities consist of emergency medical oxygen, variable medical and first aid kits, and variable flight-attendant training. Do not forget that passengers may carry a drug/s you may decide to recommend and/or, because of their training, may be able to assist.

The captain has the ultimate responsibility for the safety of the aircraft and well-being of all passengers and will make the final decision if a medical diversion is required. Of course, the doctor and the captain will usually discuss the seriousness of a medical issue should diversion be a possible option.

British Airways and Virgin Atlantic are among the many subscribers to MedLink, which connects flight crews and on-board volunteer doctors to specialist doctors on the ground operating from the emergency room at the private Good Samaritan Hospital in Phoenix. In 1998, MedLink received 2758 calls. A doctor was on board in 39% of cases. The most common problems were vasovagal 19%, cardiac 14%, neurological 13%, respiratory 12%, gastrointestinal 11% and others 31%.

GPs are sometimes asked to provide certificates of fitness to travel. A decision to issue such a certificate must be based on the patient's notes, history and examination. If a patient whom a doctor has declared fit does fall ill on holidays, the doctor might be liable to compensate the patient, the insurance company or a third party such as an airline—or all three—if the cause of illness was not predicted. In my practice, when issuing such certificates I write '... and I find no reason why this patient should not be travelling abroad today'.

In summary, a travelling UK doctor is under no obligation to respond with assistance. But, having volunteered, the doctor must offer the best standard of care possible.

Chapter 52

Air travel

Modern commercial aircraft cruise between 10 500 and 13 000 m (35 000–43 000 ft), maintaining cabin pressure at levels equivalent to those occurring at altitudes of 1500–2500 m (5000–8000 ft), which is not a problem for most people. The alveolar pressure of oxygen at sea level is 103 mmHg, but at 6000 ft it is reduced to 75 mmHg. Inside the aircraft, alveolar oxygen pressure drops from 13.7 kPa to 10.3 kPa, with arterial oxygen saturation falling by 3–10% (usually from 97% to about 89%), and gas in body cavities expanding by over 30%. The cabin humidity is low at 10–20% (comfortable level at home or the office is 55–65%).

Under these conditions patients with pre-existing disease, especially cardiovascular and respiratory may be compromised. In addition, cramped seating on aircraft, gastric distension following frequent in-flight drinks and meals, as well as the drowsiness frequently experienced by many passengers, may restrict the body's compensatory mechanism. Inactivity in particular, predisposes to venous thromboembolism.

The concept of cabin pressurization was developed towards the end of World War I and, by 1928, Junkers in Germany had developed a two-man removable altitude cabin for fighter aircraft. The first successful flight of an aircraft with an integral pressurized cabin (the American X-C35, a modified Lockheed Electra) took place in 1937. Pressurized Boeing 307 Stratoliners were in operation by 1939 and, from 1945 onwards, pressurized cabins were in routine use for passenger aircraft.

The International Air Transport Association (IATA) has introduced procedures for 'medical clearance' to travel by air (IATA—Resolution 700. Acceptance and carriage of incapacitated passengers. In: *Passenger Services Conference Resolutions Manual*, 14th edn. 1994). Passengers are required to notify the airline at the time of booking and obtain clearance by its medical officer if fitness is in doubt because of recent, current or chronic illness, injury or surgery. Also, if special services are required, i.e. oxygen, stretcher, authority to carry accompanying medical equipment. Some of the questions that need to be answered are the following.

● Will the patient be able to cope with the stress and anxiety at the airport (delays, long walks), the flight (enforced inactivity, confined space) and the jet lag afterwards?

● Will the patient present any risk to other passengers and crew (disturbed behaviour, infection)?

● What will the effect be on the patient of the 20% reduction in ambient pressure, and 10% reduction in arterial oxygen saturation?

● Is there a need for special provisions such as oxygen or an escort?

● Are there any contraindications that bar the patient from flying?

● Does the patient require advice on their medication (carriage abroad of opiates, taking anticonvulsants, insulin, diuretics, relief medicine such as glyceryl trinitrate, bronchodilators, etc.)?

A simple test that can be performed in general practice in order to assess the patient's cardiorespiratory fitness is to ask the patient to walk 50 m on the flat or climb one flight of stairs (10–12 stairs). If the patient becomes breathless or experiences angina, they need further assessment before they can travel by air.

Oxygen on board should be prebooked and the cost agreed in advance. It is delivered from portable cylinders at a fixed rate of 2–4 L/min (28%) via a Hudson mask (some airlines may also provide a nasal cannula and/or paediatric mask). The patient may be required to pay for the seat the oxygen cylinder will be secured on to as well as for the scheduled oxygen. Explain to the passenger that the emergency drop-down oxygen masks are exclusively reserved for aircraft emergencies when decompression is possible and it cannot be made available to individuals. Also, the first-aid small oxygen cylinder carried by most airlines is only for emergencies on board. Passenger's own oxygen is not allowed on board because of safety regulations. Pre-booked oxygen is provided only in-flight and there is no provision to supply oxygen in the airport while awaiting connections. Arterial gas measurement is not usually required for medical clearance but may have been performed by the patient's physician. Oxygen will be needed for those with respiratory disease in whom blood gases suggest arterial oxygen tension will fall to 7 kPa or less at cruising altitude. For further information see p. 317.

The key to minimizing hypoxia on long-haul flights is adequate hydration. Hypoxia causes leakage of water into the tissues resulting in ankle oedema and, in serious cases, confusion and disorientation. As fluid moves out of blood vessels, the blood becomes more sticky and prone to clotting. Swelling of limbs cannot be solely attributed to passenger immobility. In a survey carried out in New Zealand among flight attendants flying international routes [Criglington A. (1998) Do professionals get jet lag? *Aviation, Space and Environmental Medicine* 69, no. 8] it was found that 32% of flight attendants experienced swelling of limbs, but also dehydration (73%). This indicates that other factors such as changes in air pressure and dehydration contribute to limb swelling. Some passengers exposed to hypoxia can exhibit symptoms of increased aggressiveness, confusion, depressive mood, impaired memory/muscle coordination/vision, headaches, dizziness, euphoria, and reaction time delay.

A number of airlines have introduced automatic external defibrillators (with appropriate crew training) into aircraft. Pioneers were British Caledonian, Virgin Atlantic and Quantas, with American Airlines, Cathay Pacific, Ansett Australia, Air Zimbabwe, Air France, Air 2000, British Airways, Emirates, Delta, United and Singapore Airlines responding soon after.

Some countries require insecticidal measures for passenger aircraft to prevent the importation of insects such as mosquitoes. This may involve the spraying of the aircraft passenger compartment with insecticide while the passengers are on board. Although the WHO considers these procedures safe, they may aggravate certain health conditions such as allergies. Advise passengers who need to know what insecticidal procedures may be performed on a particular flight to contact their travel agent or the airline.

The quality of air on the aircraft

Air quality is subject to regulation. Fresh air is drawn in through the engines. Outside air enters the aircraft engine compressor section where it is heated to 200 °C and compressed to 28 kg/m². This air then enters the aircraft, passing to environmental control sections, which cool and condition the air before entry to all sections of the cabin from overhead distribution outlets above the windows or the middle of the ceiling. Airflow is laminar (side-to-side) with air flowing downward in a circular pattern to outflow grills in the sidewalls at floor level. In the modern aircraft air enters and leaves the cabin at about the same row with minimal side direction.

Because air at altitude is much thinner than at ground level, it has to be pressurized and cooled in special air packs, as described above. This uses fuel so airlines mix the treated, fresh air with filtered cabin air and recirculate. All newer commercial jets recirculate air, with between 10 and 50% of cabin air being filtered, mixed with fresh air taken in from the engines, and returned to the passenger cabin. The rate of recirculation is approximately 20 air changes per hour in flight, and seven changes during descent and while on the ground. The filters used in recirculation circuits are 'high efficiency particulate air' (HEPA), which can filter material as small as 0.3 μ. The US Federal Aviation Authority (FAA) regulation applying to all aircraft built after 1996, sets a statutory level of cabin ventilation. It requires a minimum of 10 cubic feet per minute (cfpm) of fresh air for every passenger. The aircraft manufacturers Boeing are trying to bring about change in the regulations in order to reduce this further to 5 cfpm. Some airlines try to economize in other ways. An example is turning off one of the three available air packs (which treat fresh air) on a Boeing 747 until a passenger complains.

Up to half the air passengers breath is recirculated. Concerns have been expressed about the possibility of transmission of tuberculosis from an infected person to other passengers and crew because of the high prevalence of the disease in some regions of the world. Such cases have been officially reported in the past. The WHO issued guidelines in 1998 intended to apply to all domestic and international airlines. They recommend tracing and informing passengers and crew members who were on a commercial flight with an infectious person, if the flight, including ground delays (during which passengers remain on board the aircraft with little or no ventilation), lasts more than 8 h. This is to be carried out if less than 3 months have elapsed between the flight and notification of the case to the health authorities. Anyone with infectious TB should postpone travel until they become noninfectious. Boarding can and should be denied to persons known to have infectious disease. For further information go to http://www.who.int/gtb/publications/aircraft/index.html

During an Australian senate inquiry in 2000, it was revealed by scientists that cabin air can be contaminated with oil fumes drawn in from engines with faulty seals—up to 300 flights worldwide face this problem every year. The passengers experience the smell of fuel.

Thromboembolism and air travel

For some passengers air (train and car) travel carries the risk of deep vein and other site thrombosis and/or pulmonary embolism. The incidence of this complication is estimated at less than 10% of all acute incidents and it mainly, but not exclusively, concerns passengers in 'economy' seats. In about 5–10% of all cases, deep vein thrombosis (DVT) may be linked to air travel—about 2500 per year.

The specific thromboembolic risk factors in air travel are: immobility for a prolonged period in a cramped position, compression of the popliteal vein by the metal bar at the front edge of the seat, leading to endothelial damage, shifts of body fluids with compensatory haemoconcentration, heightened blood viscosity, and stasis in the lower limbs, dehydration (beware of excessive consumption of alcohol and cases of diarrhoea), increasing age (especially over 40 years of age), previous history of thrombosis especially pulmonary embolism and inherited haematological abnormalities, thrombophilia, polycythaemia, being an unusually tall or short individual, malignancy, pregnancy, cardiac failure, recent surgery (especially on the lower limbs) oestrogen therapy, antipsychotic drugs, obesity (restricted mobility—a relative risk). Smoking is not a risk factor for venous thromboembolism, although it is for arterial thrombosis.

Some travellers with a history of venous thrombosis may require screening for haematological defects, which might predispose to thrombosis. Examples are individuals with a family history of thrombophilia or thromboembolism, recurrent venous thrombosis, thrombosis at an unusual site and early thrombosis (venous thrombosis under the age of 45 and arterial under 30 years).

Thrombosis may involve not just the lower limbs; cerebral venous thrombosis and arterial thrombosis have been associated with long-haul flights. Venous thrombosis in the lower limbs can involve the superficial as well as the deep veins, but also high up the common femoral as well as the iliac veins. The risk of pulmonary embolism is much greater when proximal veins are involved. Cerebral venous thrombosis often presents with headache and behavioural disturbances; it can progress to seizures as signs of increased intracranial pressure become more evident (rehydrate patient and administer steroids).

Most travel-related thromboembolic diseases are not recognised because the patient presents many days or weeks after the journey during which the thrombosis originally developed. Clinicians should always consider thromboembolism in cases where there is history of recent travel.

Over the past decade the seat pitch (the distance between the rows) in economy class has decreased, on average, from 86.5 cm (34 inches) to 79 cm (31 inches). As a result, the airlines have increased the number of seats by 13%. Problems that arise from long-term constrained sitting in a cramped position we now call 'Economy Class Syndrome', or, more appropriately, 'Travellers' Thrombosis' as it is not strictly confined to economy class.

The risk of thromboembolism increases with the length of the flight. It is small in flights under 5 h but rises considerably when the flight is of over 12-h duration, especially in individuals over the age of 40–50 years. Symptoms can manifest themselves during the flight or immediately after landing but more often these appear during the first 3 days after arrival. The next danger period for thrombosis, including pulmonary embolism, is the period of the first 2 weeks after a long-haul flight.

Prophylaxis against thromboembolic disease should be considered by at least those at risk (see above).

• Wear elasticated thigh length (closed toe), soft grip, class I support stockings. In order to stay up these support stockings require the use of a suspender belt—they have attachments for this purpose. Individuals can purchase the anti-embolism 'Rested' range of stockings with graduated support privately from pharmacists. These are not available on NHS prescription. Their support lies between the soft grip NHS stockings and the T.E.D. (thigh-length antiembolism stockings) purchased privately. Stockings prevent oedema in the legs and feet too. They should be put on just before, during and for at least 3 days after the flight including the return journey.

• Aspirin (adult) one tablet for every 12 h of flight. Aspirin reduces the risk of pulmonary embolism and deep-vein thrombosis by at least one-third throughout a period of increased risk [PEP Trial Collaborative Group (2000) Prevention of pulmonary embolism and deep-vein thrombosis with low dose aspirin: Pulmonary Embolism Prevention—PEP Trial. *Lancet* 355, 1295–302]. A meta-analysis of 55 clinical studies involving some 8500 surgical patients showed that asprin is of some prophylactic value and reduced the risk of thromboembolism by around 25% [Antiplatelet Trialists' Collaboration (1994) Collaborative overview of randomized trials of antiplatelet therapy III. Reduction in venous thrombosis and pulmonary embolism by antiplatelet prophylaxis against sur-

gical and medical patients. *Br. Med. J.* 308, 235–246]. To my knowledge, no trials of aspirin in air travellers have taken place. We can assume that these findings published in the *Lancet* and the *British Medical Journal* that concern orthopaedic patients and surgical patients could also apply to patients travelling. Asprin is a potent antiplatelet agent; however, platelets only play a minor role in the development of venous throbosis. None the less, the degree of risk reduction is significant but it is considerably less than acheived by compression stockings.

• Low-molecular weight heparin (LMWH) is reserved for individuals with a definite thrombotic risk. Give a single injection immediately before, and after the flight. The dose will depend on the product used.

• Adequate hydration during the flight. Avoid excess alcohol and coffee as they stimulate diuresis. Perform simple exercises during the flight (see opposite). Deep breaths can help the venous return and pulmonary circulation. Aisle seats and those by the emergency exits are better than window seats.

• Patients on warfarin should continue their medication. Compliance is very important. Its effect may be partially lost if the patient has diarrhoea. If the intention is to stay abroad for more than 2 weeks the warfarin control (INR—International Normalized Ratio) should be checked.

• Female passengers on hormone replacement therapy (HRT), overall should continue taking their medication but prophylactic measures should be considered.

The treatment of venous thromboembolism involves heparin followed by a coumarin such as warfarin (this agent shoulf not be used alone because of the high risk of extension, or recurrence of the thrombosis). The standard approach of the Oxford Churchill Hospital for the treatment of established venous thromboembolism is to initiate treatment with dalteparin (Fragmin®, a LMWH) either as a single dose of 200 IU/kg or 100 IU/kg twice daily (with a maximum daily dose of 18 000 IU). Warfarin treatment is started at the same time. Treatment with dalteparin is continued in parallel with oral anticoagulation for 5 days or until the INR is more than 2.0, whichever is longer.

Fitness to travel

Contraindications to flying

Disorder	Limits on flight
Cardiovascular	
● Uncomplicated myocardial infarction	Within 10 days
If any complications during recovery	4–6 weeks and stable on treatment
● Non-stabilized or severe heart failure	Until stabilized
● Unstable angina	Cannot travel
● Open heart surgery, e.g. CABG, valve surgery	Within 10 days if uncomplicated
● Angioplasty—no stenting	3 days
—with stenting	14 days
● Decompensated major valvular disease, congenital heart disease and cardiomyopathy	Cannot travel—careful assessment required
● Uncontrolled severe hypertension	Cannot travel
● Acute deep vein thrombosis	Until stabilized on anticoagulant therapy
● Peripheral vascular surgery	Cannot travel within two weeks
Central nervous system	
● Cerebrovascular accident (stroke)	Uncomplicated within 10 days
● Brain surgery	Within 10 days
● Epileptic fit (grand mal) within 24 h of flying	Cannot travel
● Subarachnoid haemorrhage	Within 10 days
Haematological	
● Severe anaemia—haemoglobin less than 7.5 g/dL but give special consideration to level < 8.5 g/dL	Cannot travel
● Sickling crisis within 10 days of travel	Cannot travel
● Sickle-cell disease (not trait)	Consider oxygen on board
Respiratory	
● Major chest surgery	Within 2–3 weeks
● Pneumothorax, pneumomediastinum	Cannot travel until lungs fully inflated
● Pleural effusion, pulmonary oedema	Cannot travel
● Pneumonia	Cannot travel
● Contagious chest infection e.g. Tuberculosis,	Cannot travel
Severe asthma, recent hospitalisation	Cannot travel until well
Severe chronic obstructive pulmonary disease and other pulmonary disease with hypoxia	Careful assessment required
● Dyspnoea at rest or after walking 50 m	Needs detailed assessment
● Requiring continuous oxygen therapy on the ground at more than 3 L/min	Cannot travel
● Requiring oxygen at less than 3 L/min	Give oxygen in flight at 2–4 L/min
Gastrointestinal and renal disorders	
● Abdominal operation including keyhole surgery	Within 10 days
● Laparoscopy, colonoscopy	Within 24 h and until bloating is absent
● Gastrointestinal bleed and haemoglobin ⩾ 10 g/dL	Within 3 weeks
● Rapidly progressing renal or liver failure	Cannot travel
Ear, Nose and Throat	
● Acute sinusitis, otitis media, middle ear effusion	Cannot travel until resolved
● Tonsillectomy	Within 1 week
● Middle ear surgery	Within 10 days
● Stapedectomy	Within 2 weeks
● Wired jaw	Unless escort present, trained and in possession of wire cutters, willing to use them in an emergency, e.g. vomiting

continued p. 298

Cont.

Disorder	Limits on flight
Ophthalmological	
• Intraocular surgery or penetrating eye injury	Within 1 week
• Eye surgery involving intraocular injection of gas	Until an ophthalmologist confirms complete resolution of the gas
• Acute retinal detachment	Cannot travel
Psychiatric	
• Psychosis and behavioural disorders	Unless escorted, and with medication
• With unpredictable behaviour, aggressive, disruptive or unsafe	Cannot travel
Infections	
• Infectious disease	While in the infective stage (see p. 24)
Terminal illness	
• Terminal illness	If there is a high risk of the patient dying on the aircraft
Decompression	
• Within 24 h of scuba diving	Cannot travel
• Within 12 hours of a single dive	Cannot travel
• Symptomatic cases (bends, staggers, etc.)	Within 10 days
Orthopaedics	
• Fractures in plaster (flight up to 2 h)	Within 24 h
• Fractures in plaster (flight over 2 h)	Within 48 h
• Plaster bivalved (split)	Can fly
Obstetrics	
• Pregnancy	Cannot travel after end of 36th week
• Neonates	Within 48 h (ideally 7 days) from birth

Main source: British Airways

Warfarin treatment is continued for 3 months (keep INR at 2.5 ± 0.5) in the case of an isolated venous thrombosis in the leg, and 6 months if there was evidence of pulmonary embolism. Treatment with warfarin can be stopped abruptly, there is no need to tail it off [Giangrande, P. (2000) Thrombosis and air travel. *J. Travel Med.* 7, 149–154].

Special notes

• *Fractures.* Air can be trapped in plaster casts, leading to limb compression as the air expands. No need to wait if the plaster is bivalved (split). Patients with full-length, above-knee plasters generally are required to purchase an extra seat in order to obtain the necessary leg room. The alternative is to travel by business or first class.

• *Pregnant women* cannot fly after the end of the 36th week—this refers to the return journey. The flight does not cause problems to the pregnancy itself. Flight attendants cannot and should not

have to attend obstetric emergencies on board. Advise a pregnant woman not to fly in the third trimester if: multiple pregnancy, history of premature delivery, cervical incompetence, bleeding, increased uterine activity that may result in premature delivery. Between the 28th and 36th weeks, a pregnant woman is required to carry a certificate stating that there are no complications and showing the estimated date of delivery. Intestinal gas expansion, especially during ascent, can cause additional discomfort to a pregnant woman; she should avoid gas-producing foods in the week before a flight.

• *Babies* should not fly until at least 2 days old (preferably 7 days) because their alveoli may not be fully expanded and significant hypoxaemia could occur at altitude (1988) Fitness to travel by air. In: Harding R.M. & Mills F.J. (eds) *Aviation Medicine*, 2nd edition. *Br. Med. J.* London.

• *Infants (especially up to 6 months) and travel.* There have been a number of cases of sudden infant death syndrome (SIDS) following long air flights, during which arterial oxygen saturation is known to fall in adults by 3% to 10% (usually from 97% to about 89%, see p. 293). In an interventional study in 34 infants exposed to 15% oxygen for a mean of 6.3 h, arterial oxygen saturation fell from 97.6% to 92.8% and episodes of apnoea increased in frequency 3.5-fold (p < 0.001). These data do not fully explain the occurrence of SIDS following prolonged flights [Parkins, K.J., O'Brien, L.M. *et al.* (1998) Effect of exposure to 15% oxygen on breathing patterns and oxygen saturation in infants: interventional study. *Br Med J* 316, 887–94]. Nonetheless, it is prudent to advise that infants with respiratory infections should not fly, and that the breathing status of babies should be observed frequently for 48 h after the flight to monitor apnoea.

● *Children with cystic fibrosis* are liable to marked oxygen desaturation. A specialist paediatrician should be consulted well in advance of flying. Consider pulse oximetry to monitor PaO_2.

● A patient who has suffered a *stroke* needs to be assessed with regard to mobility. If the traveller is unable to walk in the cabin and take care of all their own needs including lifting and toileting, then an escort is required who is capable and willing to assist with all aspects of in-flight requirements.

● Patients with well-controlled *epilepsy* can fly provided they have not suffered a grand mal epileptic fit within 24 h of travel. They should keep to the same dose of medication as at home and keep to 'home time' during the flight (as well as wearing an identity tag or bracelet). If recent epilepsy control has not been optimal, consider increasing the anticonvulsant dose temporarily during travel. Patients with epilepsy should be cautious about both sleep disruption and alcohol consumption before and during the flight.

● If an anxiolytic is required for *anxiety* during flight, it should be tried at home well before the flight, in order to ensure it is well tolerated.

● The same dose is continued by diabetic patients on insulin on journeys up to 8 h—for longer see The Diabetic Traveller' on pp. 318.

● *Respiratory disease*. If a prospective traveller develops dyspnoea on walking 50 m or climbing 10–12 stairs, he or she needs attention and further assessment. Current exacerbation of chronic obstructive pulmonary disease, excessive bronchospasm, severe breathlessness, very severe lung damage, large emphysematous bullae and lung cysts are contraindications to flying until the patient is stabilized and improved sufficiently. Two weeks after successful drainage of pneumothorax the patient can travel. Undetected pneumothorax may progress to a tension pneumothorax.

● Patients with *severe or unstable asthma* should consider oral steroids (adults: prednisolone 30–40 mg daily; children: up to 1 mg/kg bodyweight) starting 3 days before the flight and continuing until they reach their destination and are feeling well—usually about a week in total.

● *Coronary events* are three times more likely to occur while travelling. Postmyocardial infarction patients should wait for 10 days before flying. They should be able to walk 100 m on the flat, or climb 10–12 stairs without symptoms.

● Patients after *angioplasty* with stenting can travel earlier than 14 days if accompanied by an Assistance Company professional escort.

● During *CABG* surgery air is introduced. This takes about 9 days to be re-absorbed so travel can be contemplated from day 10 as long as there are no complications after the operation (serious dysrhythmia, residual angina, worsening heart failure).

● Adults with cyanotic *congenital heart disease* seem to tolerate the fall in arterial oxygen tension better. Their fitness to travel depends on whether they have other complications such as heart failure.

● *Cardiac pacemaker* patients are of low risk if medically stable. The risk of interaction with airport security devices is low but theoretically possible with the less common unipolar pacemakers. Patients should request a manual security check.

● *Drug- and alcohol-dependent* individuals need to undergo full detoxification before flying, to avoid withdrawal risk while on the aircraft.

● Patients with a *history of thromboembolism* should be considered for full anticoagulation or low weight molecular heparin (see thromboembolism and travel above) especially for flights over 11 h. Seats with space in the front for stretching the legs are ideal. Walk around. Thigh-length elasticated stockings, soft grip, class I or antiembolism stockings must be worn during the flight and for at least 3 days afterwards. Avoid large doses of diuretics, if possible, to reduce risk of haemoconcentration and drink plenty of still water.

- The risk of thromboembolism is particularly high after *orthopaedic operations*, especially on the lower limbs. Patients are advised not to travel by air for 3 months after hip or knee replacement operations.

- *Gas expansion* (in about 30%) can cause pain and perforation of the eardrum if the Eustachian tubes are blocked. On ascent, expanding air vents easily from the sinuses through their ostia. On descent, however, the sinuses' ostia are readily occluded, especially if the traveller has any degree of mucosal oedema, as occurs with the common cold. The symptoms of otic barotraumas develop during descent because air cannot pass back up the tubes so readily. Pain, which begins as a feeling of increased pressure on the tympanic membrane, quickly becomes increasingly severe unless the Eustachian tube is able to open and so equalize pressure between the middle ear cavity and the pharynx (i.e. the atmosphere). The traveller should attempt to open the Eustachian tube by:

    swallowing;

    yawning;

    moving the lower jaw from side-to-side;

    compressing air in the nasopharynx by the action of the muscles of the mouth and the tongue, with the mouth, nostrils and epiglottis closed—the Frenzel manoeuvre;

    raising pharyngeal pressure by swallowing while the mouth is closed and the nostrils occluded—the Toynbee manoeuvre.

- Gaseous expansion in the small bowel is aggravated by food and drinks that produce gas such as beans, curries, brassicas, carbonated beverages and alcohol. On occasions, expansion of gas within the small intestine can cause pain and can even lead to vasovagal syncope. The expansion of gas introduced during recent medical procedures (e.g. colonoscopy) or surgery can cause pain and may stretch suture lines, risking perforation and bleeding.

- Patients after *operations on the gastrointestinal tract* risk perforation and bleeding from suture sites as intraluminal gas expands and gastric or intestinal mucosa stretch at altitude. They should allow at least 10 days before they travel.

- Patients with *colostomies and ileostomies* should use a large colostomy bag, or carry extra bags on board and consider frequent changing in order to combat gas expansion and possible increase in faecal output.

- *Otitis media* should have been treated with antibiotics for at least 36 h and the patency of the Eustachian tubes assessed by a doctor before the patient can fly.

- Risk of *otic barotraumas* from flying with sinusitis, congested nose and upper respiratory tract infection.

- *Intraocular injection of gas*, if used during an operation (as in the case of retinal detachment), should resolve completely before flying. This may take approximately 2 weeks if sulpha hexafluoride is used and 6 weeks if perfluoropropane is used.

- *Burns*. Carriers require detailed information on each patient for assessment before acceptance.

- A *critically ill patient*, such as a terminally ill patient, who may die on board during the flight may not be accepted. Death of a patient during the flight is very distressing and results in complex administrative problems. Very short prognosis is not always a contraindication to travel. First class seating may be recommended by the airline's medical officer if the patient is very frail and needs to recline for long periods, if the flight is long, or if the patient needs extra space to accommodate equipment, which is approved by the airline's medical officer. Many aircraft can accommodate patients on stretchers, although this is expensive as one stretcher occupies nine economy class seats. All medication must be carried in the patient's hand luggage, in its original packaging and clearly labelled with the name of patient, the name of the drug and its dose, form and strength—this can be very helpful when going through security and customs. An escort sitting in the seat next to the patient may be insisted upon by the airline. A medically trained escort will be required if the patient:

    (a) has a syringe driver or surgical drains *in situ;*

    (b) needs significant analgesia or injections;

    (c) might need emergency treatment of symptoms;

    (d) has a long journey, involving transfers between airports or aircraft.

● Patients *travelling with controlled drugs*: in the UK, the maximum quantity of morphine sulphate that can be exported is 1.2 g. If there is a need for the patient to carry more than this amount, they must apply for a licence to the Home Office. A letter from the prescribing doctor is required, which gives details of the patient, the travel dates and specifies the exact name, form, strength and total quantity of each controlled drug to be exported. Such a licence may take 7 days to issue. The appropriate embassy should be contacted (for telephone numbers see Chapter 65) for information on arrangements for importing, as well as the availability of particular controlled drugs in the destination country.

● Patients with *chemotherapy lines* can travel if their general condition allows.

● Patients requiring *basic nursing on board* should travel with a trained escort as airline staff are not allowed to handle any human excreta (including colostomy and catheter bags) or help with the toilet because they also handle food.

● Patients with *continence problems* need assessment and advice before travel. Special continence pads may have to be used with the help of a trained escort. The patient may be catheterized, at least for the duration of the flight.

● If *jaundiced*, a traveller needs to carry a written confirmation that he or she is not infectious.

● In today's operations, including Concorde, there does not seem to be any radiation danger to passengers, including pregnant women.

● Never prescribe or advise *OTC medication for in-flight use* unless the would-be traveller has used it before or is prepared to try it well before flying.

For advice contact 'Passenger Clearance', British Airways Health Services Waterside, PO Box 365 (HMAG), Harmondsworth UB7 0GB. Tel.: 020 8738 5444; Fax: 020 8738 9644.

Advice for patients planning long-haul flights

● If you suffer from a chronic illness or have recently had injury, surgery or an infectious disease, notify the airline and obtain clearance.

● Take with you on board (in hand luggage) all your medication including relief medication.

● If you have a history of circulatory problems put on elasticated support stockings before getting on the aircraft and keep them on until you reach your destination and for at least 3 days afterwards.

● If you are elderly and/or at risk of thrombo-embolism, especially on flights over 4 h, consider elasticated support stockings as above and/or aspirin every 12 h during flight—unless contra-indicated, e.g. severe sensitivity or history of peptic ulceration. Keep stockings on for at least 3 hours after arrival at destination.

● During the flight drink plenty of nonalcoholic, noncarbonated fluids and eat just enough.

● Throughout the flight carry out exercises, particularly of the lower limbs, get up and walk about. Some airlines' magazines, such as the British Airways' in-flight magazine, include exercises to improve circulation.

(a) Gently lean head to one side. Rest for 3 s, breathe out. Repeat to the other side. Repeat three times.

(b) Lift hands, breathe in deeply and hold for 3 s. Place arms behind head. Breathe out. Repeat three times.

(c) Bend foot upwards, spread toes and hold for 3 s. Point foot downwards, clench toes and hold for 3 s. Repeat three times.

Air rage

Some passengers can respond to the tension of flying by becoming short-tempered, even aggressive. They disregard the constraints of normal behaviour in acts of irrational rage and violence. Factors that contribute to this are: low humidity and the air in the cabin, excess alcohol, nicotine withdrawal in heavy smokers who are unable to smoke on a flight (they could use nicotine gum or patch), taking illegal drugs, obsessional and/or schizoid personality, psychiatric illness such as mania, hypomania, schizophrenia. Two-thirds of air rage incidents are committed by drunken passengers.

British Airways recorded 266 incidents of disruptive behaviour on board its aircraft between April 1997 and March 1998. This represented a 400% increase over the previous year. American Airlines reported a 200% increase in passenger interference with flight attendants' duties between 1994 and 1995.

Fear of flying

About 28% of the population are thought to have a degree of fear of flying. Stress can worsen such fears. Factors that contribute to stress are the traveller's personal emotions (including work and home), the airport environment, the aircraft cabin environment both physical and social, pre-existing fear of flying, and past experiences. Counselling, cognitive therapy and relaxation sessions can usually help passengers who are unable to get on an aircraft. Diazepam (avoid alcohol) or a β-blocker can be of benefit.

Aviatours Ltd (see p. 399 for address) run two-monthly one-day (Saturday) courses in London and Manchester, designed to overcome fear of flying.

Jet lag

Jet lag is a syndrome related to travelling across time zones faster than the body can readjust. It affects 75–80% of travellers at any degree and results from rapid transition across time zones (usually more than three such zones) (for the world time zones in relation to Greenwich Mean Time see Fig. 57.2 on p. 321). This causes a conflict between the body's internal biological clock and the external time cues that guide it. This internal body clock, if isolated from external time cues such as daylight/darkness, is slower and about 25h in length. It is synchronized to the solar 24 h rhythm by these external cues as well as other cues such as social and work.

The internal clock is otherwise referred to as *circadian*, meaning occurring or recurring about once a day (from the Latin *circa* about and *dies* day). Adjustment of the body clock is taking place daily so that it runs in phase with solar time. Cues that help it to adjust come from the environment and our lifestyle and are known as *zeitgebers* (German for 'time givers'). In humans, the most important *zeitgeber* is the light/dark cycle.

Symptoms of jet lag include insomnia, reduced quality of sleep, daytime fatigue—especially dur-

ing the first 5 days after arrival, disorientation, decreased concentration, motivation, appetite and physical performance, irritability and some gastro-intestinal disturbances such as constipation. The traveller can become prone to accidents.

Recovery from jet lag is slow with advancing age, particularly in the over 50 year olds. Adaptation for east to west travel takes place at a rate of one and a half time zones per day, while for west to east travel this is slower, one time zone per day. Strengthening the cues in the new time zone and taking some precautions before and during the flight can enhance this adjustment. In general, sleep quality, alertness and performance efficiency take about 5 days to return to 'normal'.

Advice to travellers to combat jet lag

- For a few nights before you fly, go to bed earlier than usual if flying east, stay up later if flying west.
- Change your watch to destination time upon boarding the aircraft.
- If possible, plan arrival time to coincide with normal bedtime or break up your trip with a 24 h rest for every six time zones crossed.
- After arrival, allow time to readjust before important meetings, usually 1 day for each time zone crossed.
- If you arrive in the morning, expose yourself to daylight rather than go to bed. If you arrive in the evening, stay up at least until 22.00 h.
- During travel but also for 4–5 h before bedtime after arrival, avoid alcohol, caffeine and nicotine.
- Meals should not be heavy and should be regular and adjusted to local timetable.
- Avoid excess alcohol/hangover.
- Adopt local hours for sleep and wakefulness.
- Avoid catnapping during daytime.
- Take exercise during daytime.
- Telephone home daily.

Management of jet lag

Bright light therapy

This attempts to alter the relationship between the body clock and timing of sleep by exposing the traveller to bright light. Evening exposure to bright light delays the circadian clock. Exposure in the morning achieves a phase advance. Jet lag is lessened when the traveller is exposed to bright light at the time when exposure to natural daylight is beneficial.

When the traveller is exposed to sunlight at the 'wrong time', the endogenous circadian pacemaker will shift in the direction opposite to that desired. When travelling across more than six time zones:

Eastwards:
- shift bedtime 1 h earlier each night for 3 nights before departure morning;
- morning sunlight should be avoided for the first few days at destination;

Westwards:
- shift bedtime 1 h later each night for 3 nights before departure;
- late afternoon light should be avoided and morning sunlight increased at destination.

A computerized anti-jet-lag visor with integral light bulbs is commercially available (Circadian Travel Technologies, 7315 Wisconsin Avenue, Suite 1300 W, Bethesda, MD, USA 20814–3202, Tel.: 00 1301 9618559, Fax: 00 1301 9616407). The visor is programmed with the traveller's normal sleep pattern, time of day, season, point of departure, destination and time of arrival. The visor is then worn during the trip to deliver calculated doses of light. It is alternated with dark glasses to stimulate night.

For online ordering of Jet Lag Combat kit and Jet Lag trip calculator contact: http://www.outsidein. co.uk.

Melatonin

Physiological melatonin has a role in the regulation of the sleep–wake cycle and circadian rhythm in body temperature. Information is transferred to the pineal gland from the retina, via the suprachiasmatic nucleus of the hypothalamus, where the body's molecular clock seems to reside. This clock approximates to a day length, and strict 24 h timing is usually kept by light, a strong signal in resetting the 'clock'. Melatonin is produced by the pineal gland, at a rate of about 30 µg in 24 h, with almost all of it secreted during the hours of dark-

ness (it peaks at around 04.00 h). It is a weak signal in resetting the 'clock' and its action is exactly the opposite of that of bright light.

Melatonin synthesis and secretion is inhibited by bright light. Administration of melatonin in the morning causes phase delays and in the afternoon causes phase advances. Carefully timed doses of melatonin can improve, in a number of travellers, both the subjective and objective symptoms of jet lag. β-blockers given at an appropriate time can suppress endogenous melatonin secretion.

Melatonin can lower body temperature and causes some side-effects. Some people (8.3%) suffer some sedation at daytime, headaches (1.7%), nausea (0.8%), light-headedness (0.8%), giddiness (0.6%), and there may be some impact on driving performance.

In the USA melatonin is available from supermarkets and health food stores. It is a popular product largely because of claims that it can delay ageing, prolong sexual vitality and cure insomnia. The purity and origin is not always stated (it is synthetically produced as 1 million bovine pineal glands are needed to produce 10 mg of melatonin). In the UK, in October 1995, the Medicines Control Agency (MCA) ordered all suppliers to stop selling the product as it is medicinal by function. Melatonin does not occur normally in food and therefore one's diet cannot be deficient in it. It is not a licensed product (neither in Europe nor in Australia) therefore it is available on NHS prescription for an individual (named) patient or on a private prescription. In the UK melatonin is considered as an endogenous substance, which cannot be patented, although the process by which it is manufactured can. Information on how melatonin acts on the 'clock' and the identification of melatonin receptors 1 (phase shifting) and 2 (sedation) is leading to new drug development such as melatonin agonists.

On the limited evidence available, oral melatonin reduces the severity and duration of jet lag in some air passengers. We have very little data on the product's toxicity and long-term safety. How it should be taken has not been established. Despite this, oral administration of this hormone is believed to be the best pharmacological management for jet lag readily available today.

Dose of melatonin in the management of jet lag: 5 mg once daily (if 3 mg tablet take two).

Eastward travel

- 2 days preflight in early evening (it corresponds to about 02.00 h at destination).
- 4 days postflight at local bedtime (23.00 h or later).

Westward travel

- No preflight dose.
- 4 days postflight at local bedtime (23.00 h or later).

Short-acting hypnotics (half-life well under 5 h)

These are sometimes used to counteract jet lag and they may have a place in some passengers (zopiclone, zolpidem). Better effect is achieved in eastward than westward travel and in short journeys. They do not help readjustment in the new time zone. The combination of these hypnotics with melatonin is not recommended because of poor tolerability and increased side-effects, especially nausea, confusion and morning sleepiness.

Chapter 53

Tunnel travel

Millions of people now use the Channel Tunnel and the many other tunnels around the world. It is normal for all people to experience some slight discomfort when entering a tunnel in a train. There are rapid changes in ambient pressure when the train enters a tunnel at a rapid speed, or when two trains pass each other in a tunnel. This results in deflection of the intact tympanic membrane medially.

For most travellers this poses no problem or they equalize the relative pressures on each side of the tympanic membrane by swallowing, thus allowing air to pass through the Eustachian tube. Other measures that will achieve the same effect are blowing against pinched nostrils, yawning or rapidly moving the tongue against the soft palate.

The problem arises when the Eustachian tube is blocked by nasal congestion, as in the case of chronic nasal infection, rhinosinusitis and coryza.

The sudden increase in external pressure and the inability of the Eustachian tube to compensate result in a pain and increased risk of rupture of the tympanic membrane, often antero-inferiorly, and at the site of previous scars—usually it heals quickly. A worse complication is when the round window membrane ruptures or if there is a history of stapedectomy where the otosclerotic stapes was replaced by a prosthesis. In these cases there is an increased risk of ear damage. The patients who will not feel pain are those with fluid in the middle ear cavity or with perforations or aerating tubes (grommets).

Contraindications to tunnel travel

- Ear surgery within 2 months.
- Especially stapedectomy within 2 months.

Chapter 54

Motion sickness

Motion sickness is a debilitating but usually short-lived illness. Only deaf mutes with nonfunctioning labyrinths are known to be immune to this problem. It is considered to be a physiological vertigo. Motion sickness appears to arise from stimulation of the labyrinthine sense organs in an intense manner to which the body is not accustomed. Of the normal population, 5% will suffer severely, 5% will hardly be affected, and the rest (90%) will suffer moderately.

It is a common problem in children (especially among those aged 3–12 years) and adults. Women are more commonly affected than men. The ancient Greeks called it *nausia* (*naus* meaning 'ship'). It can affect sea, land, air and space travel. The characteristic symptoms are feelings of warmth, light-headedness, drowsiness, yawning, cold sweats, belching, nausea, vomiting, tachycardia and the patient may look pale. What can bring it on are movements up and down and their frequency, sight or smell of food or petrol (for example on a boat). With continuous exposure, the severity of symptoms is usually progressively reduced.

Advice to individuals that experience motion sickness may include the following.
- Avoid reading or doing puzzles during travel.
- Avoid looking out of the side-windows. Sit in the front. Do so also in a bus, by a window.
- If it is practically possible, be the car driver.
- Look straight ahead, at the direction of travel, at the horizon.
- Open the car window for fresh, cool air.
- Lie down—horizontal position. It can help if you shut your eyes too.
- Avoid the smell of fuel or similar substances (as on a boat).
- Have frequent breaks, especially if travelling with children.

- Drink an adequate amount of fluids.
- Avoid alcohol.
- Take only light meals when travelling.
- Carry a vomit bag.
- On a plane, the seats over the wings or wheels are the most suitable because the aircraft moves least. Tilt the seat back, close your eyes and keep your head still against the headrest. Avoid alcoholic drinks and a large meal before take-off.
- On a boat, try to get a midship cabin close to the waterline.
- Consider taking a drug to prevent or treat motion sickness.

The most effective preventive drug is hyoscine hydrobromide. It should not be given to anyone with glaucoma and cannot be used when alcohol is consumed. It may affect driving for up to 24 h after the last dose was taken. Exercise caution with elderly patients with a history of cardiovascular disease, urine retention, bowel obstruction, hepatic or renal impairment. Possible side-effects are drowsiness, dizziness, dry mouth, difficulty with micturition and blurred vision. Pregnant women should not use hyoscine unless the expected benefits to the mother outweigh the potential risks to the fetus. It should not be used in lactation as it is not known whether it passes into breast milk.

A 1.5-mg hyoscine patch (Scopoderm TTS) releases an average of 1 mg, over 72 h when in contact with skin and can be applied to a hairless area of skin behind the ear 5–6 h before the journey or in the evening before travel (not recommended for children under the age of 10 years). It is available on prescription only. When kept in contact with skin its action lasts 72 h. If longer protection is required, a fresh patch should be applied behind the other ear. If required for shorter time, it can be removed after the journey is completed. Advise the traveller to wash their hands after handling hyoscine so that it is not transferred accidentally to eyes. Limited accidental contact with water should not affect the patch efficacy. It can be used in the elderly, although they are more prone to side-effects.

The over-the-counter (OTC) available preparations are Joy-Rides chewable tablets (0.15 mg) for children aged 3 years and over, Junior Kwells (0.15 mg) from age 4, and Kwells tablets (0.3 mg) from age 10 and for adults—doses are clearly given on their boxes.

Antihistamines are generally better tolerated than hyoscine but slightly less effective.

- Cinnarizine (Stugeron) 15-mg tablet: adults 2 tablets 2 h before travel, then 1 tablet every 8 h during the journey if necessary. Children age 5–12 years half the adult dose. Available on prescription and OTC. Side-effects are drowsiness, dry mouth, blurred vision and tiredness.
- Meclozine hydrochloride (Sea-Legs) 12.5 mg is available OTC and has similar side-effects to cinnarizine.

- Promethazine hydrochloride (Phenergan) 10-mg and 25-mg tablets as well as 5 mg/5 mL syrup, is available on prescription and OTC. It is a sedative antihistamine. For best results take the recommended dose (2–5 years: 5 mL; 5–10 years: 10 mL; over 10 years: 25 mL/25 mg) the night before and repeat 6–8 hourly as necessary. For parenteral administration it is available in 25-mg ampoules—available on prescription only.
- Acupressure with the aid of two elasticated bands (Sea-Band, Acuband)—one on each forearm, three fingers width anteriorly and above the wrist, over the acupuncture point 'Pericardium Six' (the Nei-Kuan point) can be tried, especially if drugs need to be avoided.
- The best herbal remedy is ginger—in capsules, sweets, drinks or biscuits. Take it regularly throughout the trip. Homeopathic remedies are 'Petroleum 6' or 'Cocculus'.

Chapter 55

Sea cruises

Sea cruises are now increasingly becoming popular, especially among the retired population. Cruise ships offer a protected environment with few physical demands on the passengers but an emergency can occur well away from hospital facilities. It is important that cruise passengers carry enough drugs with them, in their hand luggage and if possible some information about their past medical history. They accept a degree of risk, as hospital facilities may not be readily available. The close environment encourages the spread of such diseases as influenza, gastroenteritis, tuberculosis, etc. Consider influenza immunization for travellers on cruises, as well as all other immunizations required for the countries they intend calling at. They may wish to take land tours.

The majority of cruise ships have a doctor on board. Medical conditions should be notified to the shipping line. The majority of passengers needing attention during a cruise are over 65 years of age and female (2 : 1 female to male ratio). A comprehensive medical insurance is very important as the passenger may need the services of a hospital at a port visited or may require airlifting to a hospital on land.

The USA Centres for Disease Control and Prevention (CDC) established in 1975 the 'Vessel Sanitation Program' (VSP) as a cooperative activity with the cruise ship industry. Every vessel with a foreign itinerary that carries 13 or more passengers is subject to twice-yearly inspections, and when necessary re-inspection. It covers the following:

- water supply, storage, distribution, backflow protection and disinfection;
- food handling during storage, preparation and service, and product temperature control;
- potential contamination of food, water and ice;
- employee practices and personal hygiene;
- general cleanliness, facility repair and vector control;
- the ship's training programmes in general environmental and public health practices.

A score of 86 or higher at the time of the inspection indicates that the ship is providing an acceptable standard of sanitation. The score of each ship is published biweekly in the *Summary of Sanitation Inspections of International Cruise Ships*, commonly known as the 'green sheet'. This is available via the internet at http://www.cdc.gov/nceh/programs/vsp or by the CDC fax information service by dialling 00–1-888-232-6789 and requesting Document 510051.

Chapter 56

High altitude sickness

Altitude sickness (acute mountain sickness) is associated with rapid ascent to altitudes over 2500 m above sea level. This may already be happening at altitudes of between 1500 and 2500 m. The patient experiences light-headedness, headaches, nausea, vomiting, loss of appetite, lethargy and sleep disturbances. This may then progress to cough, altered behaviour, unsteadiness on the feet, peripheral oedema, disorientation, confusion, breathlessness, pulmonary oedema, cerebral oedema and coma. Retinal haemorrhages occur in a third of trekkers at 5000 m, especially first timers.

If a person is experiencing symptoms, they should stop further ascent and wait until all symptoms have disappeared. If there is no improvement, they should descend until feeling well again (a few hundred metres may be all that is needed). Descent should be immediate if there are any signs of pulmonary and/or cerebral oedema. Acetazolamide (Diamox 250 mg) one tablet every 8 h may be useful (contraindicated in individuals who are allergic to sulphonamides). It should never be used as an alternative to a gradual ascent. Paracetamol or aspirin can be used for headaches. Anti-emetics can be of use in the case of nausea. Avoid hypnotics.

To prevent symptoms occurring, acetazolamide may be considered at a dose of 250 mg twice a day, starting a day or two before ascent or the latest before ascending above 2500 m. It can make the climber pass more urine and can cause 'pins and needles' especially in fingers and toes. Carbonated drinks may taste 'flat'. In no way should this be used as a substitute for proper acclimatization.

At above 4000 m and with an ascent rate of 500 m per day, prophylactic acetonolamide 750 mg or dexamethasone 8–16 mg daily should be considered.

If a person is intolerant of acetazolamide and drug prophylaxis is necessary, dexamethasone can be used at a dose of 4 mg every 6–8 h starting at least 24 h before ascent above 2500 m. It is relatively safe to use, although steroid psychosis can sometimes occur.

The incidence of headaches at high altitude increases when arterial oxygen saturation and associated oxygen partial pressure decline with increasing altitude. The use of aspirin (if not contraindicated) is advocated as a preventive measure—it raises the headache threshold. Because acute hypoxia augments prostaglandin concentrations, aspirin probably prevents headaches by diminishing the sympathetic activity mediated by prostaglandins.

In an emergency, parenteral dexamethasone can be used. This is of great value in the case of acute cerebral oedema when dexamethasone, 8 mg initially followed by 4 mg every 6 h, should be given parenterally, or orally if this is impractical. Alternatively, prednisolone 40 mg daily. Oxygen and hyperbaric treatment may need to be given while arranging evacuation.

Climbers who have previously experienced pulmonary oedema at high altitude could consider nifedipine 20 mg slow release every 8 h. In case of acute pulmonary oedema, break a capsule of nifedipine and give 10 mg sublingually, followed by 20 mg slow release capsule by mouth every 6 h. Hypotension can sometimes be a problem. Oxygen often produces immediate and dramatic improvement. A portable hyperbaric chamber (Gamov bag) may relieve symptoms and facilitate descent. Dexamethasone is given if there are signs of accompanying cerebral oedema.

Climbers experiencing insomnia at high altitudes could consider acetazolamide 250 mg, taken a few hours before bedtime.

Thrombosis at high altitudes can be encouraged by factors such as dehydration, cold, hypoxia and decreased physical activity. As a result of hypoxia at altitude polycythaemia can occur. Raised haematocrit and increased blood viscosity may then contribute to thrombosis. The problem can be made worse by smoking, previous personal history or family history of thrombosis and, in the case of female climbers, oestrogen- and some progesterone-containing contraceptives (especially at 4500 m and above). There do not appear to be any changes in the coagulation cascade nor in platelet count nor function as a result of hypoxia, although disseminated intravascular coagulation in patients with altitude sickness has been observed. Reported incidences of thrombosis include peripheral and cerebral venous thrombosis and pulmonary embolism, especially at altitudes above 6000 m.

Advice to travellers intending to climb to high altitude

- Discuss with your doctor prophylaxis if climbing to altitudes over 2500 m.
- Ascend slowly, e.g. up to 400 m per day to 4300 m; above this level 150–300 m per day with every third day a rest day.

- Do not overexert yourself and ensure you take adequate fluids.
- Avoid alcohol and sedatives.
- Take food low in salt and high in carbohydrates.
- Sleep at no more than 400 m further above sea level than the previous night's stop.
- If female and intending to climb to 4500 m and above, ensure you are not on the combined oral contraceptive pill (COCP). See own GP 3–6 months before travel so that an alternative method can be used (oral progesterone-only pill and depot injection may be used but better to use the cap, condoms or fit a coil).
- Consider UVA + UVB sunscreens, hat, long-sleeved clothing and goggles to protect against ultraviolet radiation and its consequences (sunburn, snow blindness).
- Appropriate clothing must be worn to combat hypothermia, frostbite, etc.
- Adequate hydration and measures to protect from heat are important. The temperature in the sun can be 30 °C, while in the shade of a mountain it can be below freezing.
- Diabetic patients should consider short-acting insulin and regular glucose monitoring, with sugar and glucagon at hand (ensure companions are trained in glucagon administration).

Table 56.1 The height of some elevations worldwide.

Europe	Asia
Elbrus (Russia) 5633 m	Mount Everest (Nepal/Tibet) 8848 m
Mont Blanc (France/Italy) 4807 m	K2 (Pakistan) 8611 m
Monte Rosa (Switzerland/Italy) 4633 m	Everest Base Camp (Nepal) 5300 m
Matterhorne (Switzerland/Italy) 4478 m	Mount Fuji (Japan) 3776 m
Ben Nevis (Scotland) 1343 m	Kathmandu (Nepal) 1220 m
Africa	*North America*
Kilimanjaro (Tanzania) 5895 m	Mount McKinley/Denali (USA) 6194 m
Mount Kenya (Kenya) 5199 m	Mount Logan (Canada) 5950 m
Johannesburg (South Africa) 1760 m	Mount Rainier (USA) 4392 m
Nairobi (Kenya) 1660 m	Mexico City (Mexico) 2350 m
South America	*Oceania/Pacific/Antarctica*
Aconcagua (Argentina) 6959 m	Carstensz Pyramid (Indonesia) 5030 m
Huascarán (Peru) 6768 m	Mauna Kea (Hawaii) 4205 m
Quito (Ecuador) 2850 m	Mount Cook/Aoraki (New Zealand) 3750 m
Bogota (Colombia) 2640 m	South Pole 3000 m

Chapter 57

Travellers at risk

The woman traveller

There are some issues in travel that are specific to women travellers.

Oral contraceptive pill

Crossing time zones or forgetting pills may result in the combined oral contraceptive pill (COCP) being taken more than 12 h from the usual time. If this happens, the following measures should be taken:

- the last of the forgotten pills should be taken immediately (if more than one pill has been forgotten, the last one only should be taken) and the traveller should revert to normal pill-taking time;
- abstain or use condoms for a week;
- in addition, if forgetting the pill for 12 h has occurred during the last week of pill-taking, there should be no break between the present and next packet;
- this action should also be taken if the traveller is taking an antibiotic that will extend into the pill-free week;
- if the traveller misses the first two or more pills in the first week of a new packet and she has unprotected intercourse, there is a need to take 'emergency contraception' too.

If a traveller on the progesterone only pill (POP) misses a tablet for more than 3 h, she should:

- take the missed pill as soon as she remembers, and the next pill at the usual time;
- abstain or use condoms for a week;
- in addition, if the traveller has had unprotected intercourse up to 72 h after the 3 h pill delay, there is a need to take 'emergency contraception' as well. (It takes two pills to restore the cervical mucous contraceptive effect of the POP.)

Motion sickness, diarrhoea and vomiting may interfere with the absorption of the contraceptive pill. If a woman on the pill suffers from diarrhoea and/or vomiting, she should continue taking the pill and should also use condoms or abstain until a week after the symptoms have ceased. Ensure an adequate supply of pills and condoms in the luggage. If taking mefloquine, the pill or other contraceptive method should be continued and conception avoided for 3 months after the last tablet of mefloquine was taken.

As the safe time to 'forget' the POP is up to 3 h (as opposed to 12 h for COCP), a careful planning of time when crossing a time-zone is required so that the POP is taken within the 3 h allowance. It is better to reduce the time between pills than elongate the period. If in doubt, the traveller should use condoms for a week before and after the start of the holiday while continuing the POP. Another method is to keep an additional watch on 'home-time' for pill-taking purposes.

Postponement of menstruation on a short holiday

Women on the oral contraceptive: if on COCP, take the next packet without a break. If on a biphasic or triphasic pill, repeat the last 'phase' in the packet.

For a woman who is not on the pill, nor-ethisterone can be considered, 5 mg three times daily, starting 3 days before the anticipated period and continuing until home return; menstruation usually occurs 2–3 days after discontinuing it.

Women on hormone replacement therapy (HRT) and menstruating, if expecting to have a period during a short holiday, could consider taking the oestrogen-only containing tablets for longer (some extra tablets) before the combined oestrogen/progesterone tablets, so that their period will occur on their return home.

Unprotected sex

Whether on the pill or not, if there is any possibility that the traveller may indulge in a sexual relationship while abroad, advise that she should carry with her good quality condoms and use them on every occasion. Quality control of condoms manufactured in some countries may not be up to standard, equally the standard sizes may differ. Condoms available in developing countries may be older than those available in developed countries, and evidence suggests that older condoms are less reliable. In addition, latex deteriorates more rapidly in tropical climates.

Emergency contraception

The 'morning after' pill may not be available at the country of destination. If it is available, it should be sought within 72 h of unprotected sexual intercourse. A barrier method should be continued until the next period, which may be late, on time or early. Some travellers may need to take with them a hormonal preparation to take in an emergency—it should not be relied upon as a contraceptive method.

One method is the Yuzpe regimen and it involves taking 'PC4' (ethinyloestradiol 50 µg plus levonorgestrel 0.25 mg) two tablets taken as soon as possible after sexual intercourse and up to a maximum of 72 h, followed by another two tablets 12 h after the first dose. If taken before ovulation, it tends to delay ovulation rather than prevent it, so the traveller must use a barrier method until her next period. If given after ovulation, it works mainly by preventing implantation. The main side-effects are nausea (50%) and vomiting (20%)—take the tablets with food. If vomiting occurs within 2 h of a dose, another should be taken, if possible with an anti-emetic. Main contraindications are pregnancy, past thromboembolism and current focal migraine. Caution if previous ectopic pregnancy. Certain factors may increase the risk of thrombosis, e.g. smoking, obesity, varicose veins, cardiovascular disease, diabetes and migraine. WHO clinical trials have shown that, overall, PC4 prevents 57% of expected pregnancies although the manufacturer quotes

75%. Follow-up should be undertaken 3–4 weeks later. Patients who, having taken PC4, still become pregnant should be monitored for ectopic pregnancy.

The other method is the 'progestogen-only emergency contraception' (POEC). The preparation available in the UK is Levonelle-2 (levonorgestrel 750 µg). One tablet is taken as soon as possible after sexual intercourse and up to a maximum of 72 h afterwards, and another one tablet 12 h after the first dose. Nausea (20%) and vomiting (5%) can also be a problem but less than with the combined preparation above. Repeat the dose if vomiting occurs within 2 hours of any one dose. Monitor for ectopic pregnancy if period does not occur. Clinical trials under the WHO have shown it to prevent 86% of expected pregnancies, or 95% if used within 24 h. It does not interfere with lactation.

An intrauterine contraceptive device (the coil) can be inserted up to 120 h (5 days) after unprotected intercourse—if there are no contraindications to its insertion. If more than 5 days have elapsed, the device can still be inserted up to 5 days after the earliest likely calculated ovulation (expected 2 weeks before the earliest time the period is anticipated). So, for example, in a regular 28-day cycle it can be fitted until day 19. This is the most effective postcoital method. It is suitable in cases of multiple 'exposure', where there is repeated vomiting after hormonal postcoital method or when it is too late to repeat the dose. It is contraindicated if there is current pelvic inflammatory disease (PID). Relative contraindications are past PID (if it is to be fitted, take swabs and give antibiotic cover) and history of ectopic pregnancy—in both cases, remove the coil after the next period.

Travellers can obtain information on the internet about emergency contraception by connecting to the Emergency Contraception Website run by the Office of Population Research at Princeton University: http://www.not-2-late.com

Women travellers should be reminded to take with them adequate supplies of their pill in their hand luggage, and personal hygiene materials—it may prove unwise to rely on local supplies. Also condoms in case they get diarrhoea and/or vomiting while taking the contraceptive pill. A common problem encountered by a woman traveller is the theft of her handbag where she may be keeping all her supplies and pills.

Deodorants, perfumes, scents and hair sprays appear to attract mosquitoes in warm countries. Some women suffer from recurrent monilial vaginitis (candida—thrush)—exclude diabetes. Taking an antibiotic, such as doxycycline for malaria prophylaxis, can 'provoke' an attack. Such travellers should consider taking with them an oral antifungal such as fluconazole (Diflucan, Pfizer) or itraconazole (Sporanox, Janssen-Cilag)—not to be used if pregnant or lactating. If the problem is consistent, consider lowering the pH of the vaginal mucosa with daily applications of acetic acid 0.94% (Aci-Jel Janssen-Giloag)—it can interact with barrier contraceptives.

A healthy woman about to go climbing or trekking at high altitudes should not be taking the COCP if she intends to spend more than a week above 4500 m. If she is spending a shorter time above 4500 m, or not going over 4500 m, she should be made aware that she is at increased risk of thrombosis if on the COCP and advised about alternative methods of contraception. The POP or the injectable contraceptive may be a good choice but barrier methods or the coil are preferable. She should consult her family planning advisor 3–6 months before travel so that she is well controlled using the method chosen. The reason for the increased risk of thrombosis is the increased blood viscosity resulting from the raised haematocrit. Polycythaemia occurs as a response to hypoxia (thinner air) at altitude. Dehydration can worsen the situation. Check that the female traveller on the COCP does not have any other risk factors for thrombosis, such as smoking, personal or family history of thrombosis, in which case she should not be taking the COCP.

Advise the traveller using the diaphragm (the cap) of the need to ensure the device is washed with clean, safe water that normally the traveller will use for drinking.

The child traveller

Children are usually more adventurous travellers. They tend not to adopt health and safety precautions, relying mainly on the parents for this task. They may stroke an animal, eat and drink liberally, play in the sun for long periods and have fun with the waves. Continuous observation of children on holiday is very important. Always think on behalf of the child. Check the height and safety of the balcony rail, inspect the cot, beware of the lifts. Apply adequate sunscreen lotion, give them a hat, and be with them all the time.

If a child develops pyrexia or feels unwell, parents should seek medical advice. They should treat diarrhoea promptly with rehydration powder/fluids as children have a greater tendency to dehydration. The European Society of Paediatric Gastroenterology and Nutrition recommends early feeding when managing acute gastroenteritis. A consensus view is emerging that optimal management of mild to moderately dehydrated children consists of:
- oral rehydration with oral rehydration solution over 3 to 4 h (replacing deficit);
- reintroduction of normal diet after 4 h (breast-feeding to be continued throughout);
- continuing supplementation with oral rehydration solution to compensate for fluid and electrolytes lost in the stool while diarrhoea lasts, to prevent dehydration.

Sound advice is not to travel to malaria-endemic areas with young children unless it is unavoidable. The WHO advises against taking babies and young children to these areas, in particular where there is transmission of chloroquine-resistant *Plasmodium falciparum*. Children are at special risk as they can rapidly become seriously ill with malaria. If they must travel, they should take malaria prophylaxis (see Malaria p. 381 according to their weight rather than age. Take every measure to avoid mosquito bites. In the under-5-year-olds use DEET mainly on clothing rather than directly on the skin. Mosi-guard Natural containing derivatives of eucalyptus oil appears to be safe for children. Autan Family is an insect-repellent that can be used by children over 2 years of age. Use mosquito cot nets for babies and bed nets for all other ages.

Before travelling, parents should obtain some information about the local health system and take some important medication such as paracetamol, rehydration powders, sunscreen lotions of at least SPF 15, calamine lotion for itchy skin. Children can dehydrate very quickly in hot tropical climates so give plenty of fluids. They also burn very easily in the sun. Take some toys and games for the plane and the airport lounges and some food and drink in the hand luggage. For sedation or to combat motion sickness (see p. 306), if necessary use promethazine hydrochloride (Phenergan, Rhône-Poulenc Rorer)—for dosage, see p. 307. Warn the mother that the effect of antihistamines can be unpredictable. Younger children may be encouraged to sleep if they take with them their favourite blanket or pillow.

On the airline, if an alternative can be found, avoid the harness system that straps the baby onto the same seat belt as the parent. An accident report into a plane crash in Leicestershire in 1989 questioned the safety of these belts—they have been shown to cause harm to both child and adult as a plane slowed down quickly. For children over 6 months and up to the age of 3 years request in advance a carrier (British Airways and Virgin can provide them) and use it on an empty seat or purchase a seat for this purpose (children over 2 years pay for a ticket). The rigid shell of the carrier provides more protection than a lap belt. Back-facing carriers for infants offer more safety benefits but are only used for infants up to 9 kg.

Cot port may be available in the front seats at each cabin section.

Failing all this and in case of severe turbulence or an impending crash landing, attach the baby's strap onto your belt, place the child on the front edge of the seat between your legs, and bend over as far as possible, bending the child over in the process. Children over 3 years of age should have a seat and use normal lap belts. A child should not be placed inside a standard seatbelt with an adult, as the child may be crushed in an emergency.

If during take off or landing a child happens to be crying, it may help to equalize the air pressure in the middle ear cavity and relieve pain. Give infants the breast, if breast fed, a bottle, or a pacifier. Some children, especially with ear disease, may benefit from a small dose of decongestant before departure and landing.

Full appropriate immunization should be considered for every child traveller. Table 57.1 shows the minimum age for the first dose of vaccine. For the traveller with HIV, see p. 234. The doctor or nurse should not forget to check that all scheduled childhood vaccinations have been given.

High altitudes pose problems for children. A conservative approach in remote areas is to climb no higher than 2000 m if children are under 2 years and no more than 3000 m if older.

Breast-feeding a baby during travel is very

Vaccine	Minimum age for first dose (months)
DTP	2
Polio	2
Hib	2
MMR	13
Hepatitis B	Birth
Hepatitis A (Havrix)	12
Typhoid parenteral (Typhim Vi)	18
Meningococcal A + C (AC Vax)	2
Meningococcal C conjugate	2
Tuberculosis (BCG)	Birth
Pneumococcal (polysaccharide)	24
Rabies	12
Tick-borne encephalitis (under 12 months if imminent risk of infection)	12
Japanese B encephalitis	12
Yellow fever	9

Table 57.1 The child traveller—minimum age for first dose of vaccine in the UK.

important and the mother will need to maintain a high fluid intake. Avoid fluid supplements as long as the mother herself drinks plenty. Children on formula milk are at risk of taking contaminated feeds if the water is not safe. Crossing time zones may cause disruption in feeding habits.

Children may be visiting a farm, zoo or park while abroad (or at home). Some simple precautions should be taken in order to avoid infection such as:

• wash and dry their hands thoroughly after touching animals, and after they leave the farm;

• do not let them touch animal droppings but if they do, they should wash and dry their hands immediately;

• tell children not to put their fingers in their mouth after they touch an animal;

• they should not to put their faces against an animal;

• children should not eat or drink while going around the farm, zoo or park;

• they should clean shoes after they leave the farm.

Travellers with pre-existing conditions or health problems

The elderly

As people retire earlier and live longer, it is inevitable that numbers of elderly travellers will increase. Indeed, the elderly now make up one-quarter of airline passenger lists. It is important that the conditions of travel are suited to their physical condition. Elderly travellers may need to book a wheelchair at the airport, request help for getting on and off the aeroplane, oxygen during travel, a special diet, help with the toilet facilities on the plane. They should carry their regular prescribed drugs in their hand luggage. Hypoxia (see 'Air Travel' p. 284) can be a problem for the elderly when flying. Ensuring they drink plenty of still water, walk about, and also wear elasticated, thigh-length stockings (and for 3 days after arrival at their destination) soft grip, class I, can to a large extent prevent hypoxia and tendency to thromboembolism. Once they arrive at their destination they may

need help with getting to the hotel. Difficulties with communication can frustrate an elderly traveller. Some may present with a degree of confusion on arrival at their destination.

For advice on how to cope with the flight, see 'Air Travel, advice for patients planning long-haul flights' on p. 310. At the other end, warn the elderly not always to expect the medical facilities and quality of medical care they are accustomed to at home, if travelling to developing countries. It is most important for the elderly to have adequate and comprehensive medical insurance cover with no exclusions applying to them. They should pay attention particularly to the rules on repatriation. Even then, there is no guarantee that they will receive skilled medical attention when they need it or that air evacuation will be practical and available. On some occasions a medical certificate of fitness to travel may be required—the patient's doctor should be able to give such opinion. Any medical problem should be notified to the airline in advance, as it may be necessary to have a preflight clearance by the airline's medical officer. Special facilities, such as a wheelchair at the airport, or oxygen on board, should be requested in advance and the price of oxygen agreed.

With heart disease

Air travel, although the fastest mode of transport, poses particular problems for the heart patient. Long waiting times at airports, long walks to the flight gate, climbing stairs to the aircraft, anxiety, cabin pressurization, arterial oxygen desaturation, forced immobility, dehydration and other factors, can induce a dysrhythmia, chest pain, pulmonary embolism, pulmonary oedema and general deterioration. Hypoxia may be prevented by supplementary oxygen. Avoiding alcohol, taking adequate fluids, wearing elasticated, thigh-length stockings and undertaking leg exercises regularly during the flight is important advice.

Patients on angiotensin-converting enzyme (ACE) inhibitors and diuretics (but also on other groups of drugs such as lithium) may become hypotensive and dehydrated if adequate fluids are not taken. If an elderly person omits the diuretic on the day of travel in order to avoid frequent visits to the toilet, they may drift into worse heart failure or suffer worse ankle/foot oedema. The problem mainly arises with the loop diuretics (frusemide, bumetanide). Their action is most evident in the first 4–6 h. If the elderly traveller is taking a morning flight, advise him or her to take the diuretic on the plane soon after take off. Similar advice could also be given if most of the morning is taken by travelling in a car or coach to the airport. The diuretic can be taken at the airport or on the aircraft. Otherwise, loop diuretics should be taken at their usual time.

When should heart patients not travel? If they have angina at rest or on minimal exertion, they should best avoid travel by air. To be fit for air travel they should be able to walk 110 m on the flat at a normal pace without severe breathlessness. Patients with unstable angina, nonstabilized or severe heart failure, or within 10 days of an uncomplicated myocardial infarction or open-heart surgery, cannot travel by air.

At the holiday destination they may be exposed to hypoxia at high altitudes, a different diet (beware of sodium imbalance), excessive heat, sweating, dehydration, gastrointestinal upset. Any fluid-losing complications, such as diarrhoea and/or vomiting, could lead to hypotension, particularly if patients are receiving ACE inhibitors and diuretics, with all other consequences such as oliguria, failure to fully excrete the ACE inhibitor and renal failure. A rule of thumb is to consider omitting the diuretic and ACE inhibitor if they lose 3 kg in weight. At the same time they should be seeking medical advice.

Marked increases in sodium intake may precipitate pulmonary oedema and/or peripheral oedema in patients with heart failure. Changes in diet can alter anticoagulant control as a result of changes in gut flora because of different food. Patients on warfarin staying abroad for more than 2 or 3 weeks should consider having a blood test at destination for international normalized ratio (INR).

Patients with paroxysmal atrial fibrillation and anxiety may benefit, in the absence of contra-indications, from a small dose of a β-blocker (i.e. 25–50 mg atenolol, 5–10 mg bisoprolol) about an hour or two before take-off to help prevent attacks.

An alternative in patients with respiratory disease is verapamil 80 mg. The patient should take a dose some days before departure in order to ascertain tolerance. Both these drugs can be self-administered by the patient, which will terminate some attacks and control ventricular rate. They should never be used in combination. Most patients return to sinus rhythm within 24 h. As long as regular pulse is not restored, the patient is at increased risk of thromboembolism and local medical opinion should be sought urgently. Ensure the patient knows of various manoeuvres that may terminate an attack. These are the Valsalva manoeuvre, quickly taking a large ice-cold drink of water or plunging the face into cold water.

Patients with angina and anxiety not on a β-blocker could benefit from this class of anti-anginal medication provided they are not contra-indicated.

Patients having undergone cardiac surgery are at increased risk of thromboembolism. They should avoid long journeys, especially air travel, during the first 6 weeks and particularly during the first 2 weeks after surgery.

Counsel patients about excessive alcohol intake. Unless heart disease has been induced by alcohol, patients should be allowed a modest daily intake with a maximum of two units for a female and three units for a male.

Photosensitivity can be a problem in patients on agents such as thiazides and amiodarone. Doxycycline (used in some areas for malaria prophylaxis) can also cause photosensitivity. Cardiac patients should be advised to wear a sunhat and keep arms and legs covered when going out in strong sunlight. They should also consider sunscreens.

Thigh-length elasticated stockings and walking/exercising the limbs on board the plane should be advised. Patients on warfarin are at a lesser thromboembolic risk. Adequate hydration to combat hypoxia is very important. If oxygen is necessary, it should be arranged with the airline in advance.

Sea travel is not advisable during the first 3 months after myocardial infarction or stroke. Lifestyle and diet on board a ship may have an impact on the patient's cardiovascular status.

Adequate medical insurance is essential. Contact the British Heart Foundation, 14 Fitzhardinge Street, London W1H 4DH, Tel.: 020 7935 0185, Fax: 020 7486 1273, for information on 'sympathetic' insurance companies.

With respiratory disease

Patients with respiratory disease may suffer worse in an aircraft because of lower arterial oxygen desaturation, lower humidity (10 20%), cigarette smoking (when allowed usually it is at the back) and sometimes because medication has been left behind. Patients with chronic obstructive pulmonary disease (COPD) are likely to have problems during the flight and they should inform the airline before they fly. Furthermore, higher altitudes, cold climates, dry climates, airborne dust particles during overland travel, traffic fumes, smoky establishments such as bars, increased physical exertion may all trigger an increase in asthma symptoms in many patients. In addition, atmospheric pollutants can prove a problem for a patient with asthma. They are better advised to take holidays by the sea.

The airline is interested to know whether the traveller can walk 50 m on the flat without becoming short of breath. Another way to assess the traveller is to ask them to climb 15 stairs.

Adequate supplies of 'preventers' and 'relievers' should be carried, with reserve supplies to allow for loss or nonfunctioning of inhaler devices. Not all supplies should be in one piece of luggage.

Ideally, the traveller with asthma should carry a large plastic volume spacer device (nebuhaler, volumatic), a supply of oral steroids and a peak flow meter. They should continue the prophylactic medication ('preventer') as prescribed (usually 12 hourly) and should check their peak flow. If the peak flow readings drop to below 75% of the patient's normal reading, the prophylactic medication should be doubled and 'reliever' used more frequently. If it drops to below 50% of normal, they should take a course of oral steroids (30–40 mg of prednisolone daily for 7–10 days—children could take 1 mg/kg bodyweight). The 'reliever' is best taken via the plastic volume spacer in such a situation: eight puffs of salbutamol or terbutaline first

and another eight if no distinct improvement occurs 15 min later. This may be considered as a substitute for a nebulizer dose if one is not available. Seek local medical advice if not improving.

Commercial aircraft fly at altitudes of between 10 500 and 13 000 m (35 000–43 000 ft). Cabin pressure is set at a level equivalent to an outside altitude of 1500–2500 m (5000–8000 ft). This gives an inspired partial pressure of oxygen (PaO_2) of 15–18 kPa compared with the normal 21. In healthy subjects PaO_2 would fall to about 8.7 kPa. Patients with respiratory disease who are hypoxic at ground level would inevitably become much more hypoxic in flight.

Short-term hypoxia can worsen undiagnosed cardiac or cerebrovascular disease, or COPD. Asthma is consistently the fourth or fifth most common in-flight illness. About 6–10% of in-flight deaths or requests for medical aid relate to respiratory disease.

If oxygen will be necessary on board, it should be prebooked (see 'Air Travel' for more details). It can be purchased at a variable cost, often with an extra seat to house the oxygen cylinder. The patient's own oxygen is not permitted on board. Patients request continuous oxygen from the airline's medical department using the INCAD form obtainable from the travel agent. The doctor completes the MEDIF form, which includes information on diagnosis, prognosis, treatment, clinical state and oxygen requirements. Airlines cannot supply oxygen before boarding the aircraft, after landing or at stopovers, so arrangements will need to be made if such therapy is necessary. Direct flights are best. Only battery-operated nebulizers can be used on board. British Airways has about 1000 requests per year to supply oxygen. Charter airlines may not be able to provide this service.

The asplenic patient

Patients with anatomical or functional asplenia (patients after bone marrow transplantation, with sickle-cell disease and some other haemoglobinopathies) are particularly at risk of malaria. They should be advised of this risk. They should take malaria prophylaxis and strict precautions against mosquito bites. Children up to the age of 16 years should receive prophylactic penicillin V twice daily. Asplenic patients should be immunized with the pneumococcal, *Haemophilus influenzae* b, influenza and meningococcal A + C vaccines. For further details see 'Asplenia' on p. 204.

The diabetic traveller

Before setting off

Vaccinations

Diabetic patients should ensure they have all the required vaccinations for the countries they are going to visit. Diabetes itself is not a contra-indication to vaccination, and diabetics are no more or less likely to contract illnesses abroad. On the other hand, if they become ill, the consequences could be more serious than in non-diabetics.

A day or two of feeling somewhat unwell as a result of local or systemic reaction may follow immunization. There can be a temporary rise in blood sugar. These problems are rarely of any concern.

If travelling to an area where malaria is endemic, the patient should remember to start appropriate antimalarial tablets 1 week before departure and continue to take them until at least 4 weeks after leaving that area.

Insurance

The diabetic patient may require hospital or other medical care while abroad, be it as a result of accident, the diabetes or some other illness, and treatment may be expensive. In addition, the diabetic patient may have to cancel their holiday for a reason beyond their control or as a result of illness. Comprehensive travel insurance that does not exclude diabetes must be obtained. For UK residents, Form E111 will enable the diabetic patient to receive emergency medical care within the European Economic Area (EEA) for short stays of less than 1 year. Some non-EEA countries also have reciprocal healthcare agreements with the UK (see Chapter 63 and also Medical Insurance, p. 289). The Diabetes UK (British Diabetic Association)

can give excellent advice about insurance for travellers.

Medical supplies

Adequate supplies of medication should be packed so that the patient does not run short and is able to replace lost items. Double or triple the estimated requirements of supplies should normally be taken to cover such emergencies. This applies not only to insulin or oral hypoglycaemics but also to blood glucose testing strips, extra battery for the glucose testing apparatus, urine glucose and ketones testing strips, finger-pricking devices and lancets, cotton wool, insulin syringes, glucagon, glucose tablets, Hypostop Gel and needle-disposal container (in an emergency a soft drink can will do). During the flight needles should be disposed of safely and never in seat pockets or toilets.

For longer stays, the diabetic patient could make arrangements for continuous supplies of insulin abroad if necessary. Some larger pharmacies can send insulin abroad by prior arrangement if there is no suitable insulin in the country of destination. In Europe some countries still have insulin 40 rather than 100 units/mL strength. If the patient runs out of U-100 and gets U-40 insulin, they should be instructed to ask for U-40 syringes so that the lines on the syringe will correspond to the units of insulin. Countries that may use U-40 insulin include France, Germany, Italy, Spain, the Czech and Slovak Republics, Morocco, Russia, Tunisia, Algeria, Kenya, Nigeria, Egypt, Syria, China, Japan and Korea. The British Diabetic Association can provide a conversion chart.

Transporting and storing insulin

Insulin will remain stable, even if partly used, for up to 2 years or more (depending on the expiry date) if stored in a refrigerator that normally has a temperature of 2 to 8 °C. Insulin should not be stored in or close to the freezer compartment, as freezing will damage it, with loss of effectiveness. Exposing the vials to sunlight or high temperature will do similar damage.

If kept below room temperature (20–25 °C), insulin (including cartridges for pen devices) will remain stable for up to 1 month—it should not be used after that (some reports have suggested insulin can be kept at 25 °C for up to 10 months losing 5% effectiveness and at 40 °C for several weeks). If travelling for longer, or to particularly hot or cold parts of the world, patients should carry their insulin in a polystyrene container or a wide-necked vacuum flask which can be rinsed out with cold water or ice in the morning. Alternatively, if freezer facilities are available, an insulated storage bag with a frozen plastic insert can be used, but the vials of insulin should not come into contact with the frozen plastic container as the insulin may freeze.

It should be noted that insulin generally can last for up to 6 months in hot countries without a refrigerator, with only partial loss of its effectiveness. Insulin that has a brownish colour as a result of exposure to bright sunlight, or is cloudy, grainy and sticky on the side of the glass vial because of damage by heat should not be used. A frequent visual check of the insulin should be made. If soluble insulin looks cloudy or 'clumpy' in appearance it should be discarded. Isophane, Lente and premixed insulins normally have a cloudy appearance. When such insulin is damaged, the cloudiness is uneven, with solidified pieces appearing as clumps when the vial is gently rotated.

Other considerations before setting off

Storage of glucagon should pose no problem as it comes as a powder with a vial of water for dilution. The patient should bear in mind that some blood-glucose testing strips over-read in very hot climates and under-read in very cold (check with manufacturers). Check the expiry date. Glucometers operate best at temperatures of 15–30 °C. Advise taking some blood-glucose testing strips in case of failure of the meter to work.

The USA and some European countries use milligrams per 100 millilitres (mg%) instead of millimoles per litre (mmol/L) to measure serum glucose. Table 57.2 provides information on conversion.

The patient should carry identification in the form of a bracelet, pendant, disc or identification card, or a letter from their physician stating the tablet or insulin dosage and the patient's details.

Table 57.2 Blood glucose units conversion table.

mmol/L	mg%	mmol/L	mg%
1	18	11	198
2	36	12	261
2.5	45	13	234
3	54	14	252
3.5	63	15	270
4	72	16	288
4.5	81	17	306
5	90	18	324
5.5	99	19	342
6	108	20	360
7	126	21	378
8	144	22	396
9	162	23	414
10	180	24	432

Moreover, the address and telephone number of the diabetic association in the country of destination and the nearest hospital to the resort should be noted.

Some Muslim countries may not allow use of porcine insulin. The patient on such insulin should check with the appropriate embassy, preferably in writing, and if it is necessary and possible, the patient should change to human insulin well before departure. Some countries do not use 'pen' insulins.

The inclusion of a medical kit, sunscreens, sunhat and mosquito nets in the luggage, as appropriate, is advisable. Travel guides from diabetic associations will provide details about food and other important information for many tourist destinations.

During the journey

A journey can be unexpectedly delayed. The diabetic patient should carry emergency snacks for such eventualities. If prone to travel sickness, medication to prevent it could be taken. When passing through customs the patient may be required to account for needles and syringes he or she is carrying. Airport X-ray machines will not damage insulin. Alcoholic drinks during travel will affect the blood glucose level and are best avoided.

Luggage

Insulin and testing equipment should not be

packed in suitcases. Aeroplanes fly at altitudes that can cause freezing in the baggage hold. In addition, baggage can be delayed or lost. Insulin and testing equipment should therefore be packed in hand-held luggage.

Immobility

Long journeys on buses, trains or aeroplanes can cause feet to swell and predispose to leg thrombosis because of the enforced immobility. The diabetic patient should therefore be advised to walk up and down the aisle whenever possible and to take some comfortable shoes or slippers to wear on the journey.

Adjustments to insulin dose and monitoring

Diabetic patients on insulin and travelling for up to 8 h, could consider keeping to 'home time' with their meals and injections and accept a degree of hyperglycaemia during the flight rather than risk hypoglycaemia.

If travelling for over 8 h, the dose of insulin and timing of injections need to be varied (see Fig. 57.1). Four methods of such readjustments are described below of which the first and fourth are the simplest and most popular. The amount of insulin to be changed (reduced or decreased) is equivalent to 2–4% of the daily dose per hour of time shift (see Fig. 57.2).

● *Method 1.* Leave out the medium or long-acting injection entirely and rely on short-acting injection before meals until the patient is safely back on a 24-h clock at destination.

Take 20% of the total daily insulin dose as a short-acting insulin, with each of the three meals.

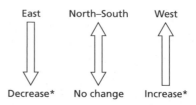

Fig. 57.1 Insulin dose change when travelling. *By 2–4% of daily dose of insulin per hour of time shift.

Monitor blood glucose frequently and make minor adjustments if necessary, allowing for blood glucose levels to be moderately raised. As soon as daily routines return to normal at destination, return to usual insulin regimen.

● *Method 2.* Travelling across several time zones changes a patient's schedule for insulin injections (Fig. 57.1). As a general rule the international traveller needs to increase their dose of insulin when travelling west and decrease it when travelling east. Frequent monitoring by blood testing, at least every 6 h, is advisable. There is no need to adjust insulin for north–south travel. Generally, it is necessary to increase or decrease by 2–4% the daily dose of insulin for each hour of time shift for each westward or eastward flight (Table 57.3).

For westward travel the shift in time zone should be covered by one or two extra injections of short-acting insulin on the plane. The total additional dose is 2–4% of the total daily dose per time-shift hour.

For eastward travel, a late evening meal on the plane is covered with an extra dose of short-acting insulin (2–6 units). The subsequent breakfast dose of intermediate-acting insulin should be reduced by 20–40% (3–5% per time-shift hour), but the usual dose of short-acting insulin can be injected.

Table 57.3 Insulin dose changes—method 2.

Going west (longer day)
Extra short-acting insulin on the plane
2–4% per time-shift hour (one or two doses)

Going east (shorter day)
Short-acting insulin (2–6 units) for late evening meal on flight
Breakfast dose on arrival:
● on short-acting insulin, no change
● on intermediate-acting insulin, reduce dose by 3–5% per time-shift hour
● if also on lunchtime dose, omit it

Adapted from Sane *et al.* (1990) *Br. Med. J.* 301, 421–2.

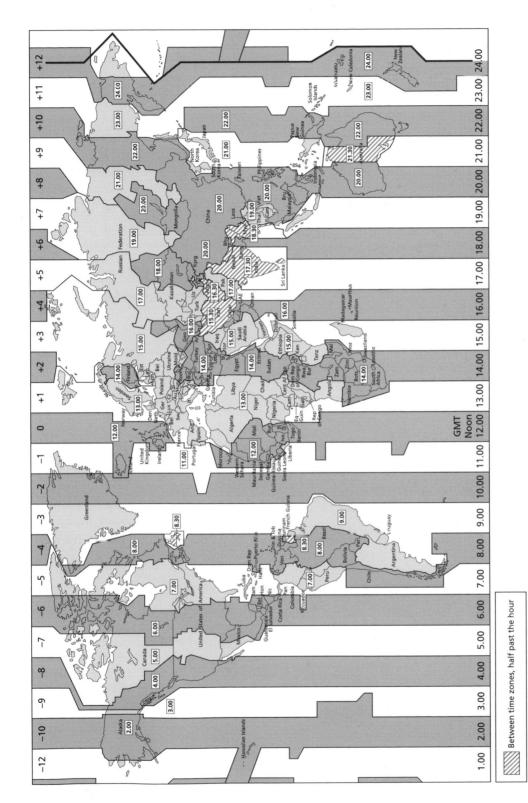

Fig. 57.2 The world time zones in relation to Greenwich Mean Time.

321

	Table 57.4 Dose of insulin if crossing six or more time zones.

Going west
Check glucose 18 h after morning dose—if elevated, give extra insulin

Going east
Reduce regular insulin dose by one-third
Check glucose 10 h later—if elevated, give extra insulin

Adapted from Benson *et al.* (1984–85) *Bull. Mason Clin.* 38, 145–51.

Table 57.5 Common infections in diabetic patients.

Foot ulcers and osteomyelitis
Pneumonia (incidence not increased but infection may be more severe)
Various staphylococcal and group B streptococcal infections
Mucocutaneous conditions
In females: urinary tract infections (reduced fluid intake during travel, increased sexual activity). Candida infection secondary to doxycycline (used in some circumstances for malaria prophylaxis) or other antibiotics, and cutaneous infection of the perineal region can both extend candida infection from the vulvovaginal tract to the urinary tract

The late timing (in local time) of the morning injection means that an injection before lunch is not necessary in patients who normally have one.

• *Method 3.* Another formula for insulin dose readjustment is for westbound travellers who cross six or more time zones to adjust their insulin dose for the longer day (Table 57.4). If the blood glucose is elevated 18 h after the morning injection, an extra dose of insulin is given. For eastbound travel, adjustment should be made for the shortened day. The regular insulin dose should be reduced to two-thirds on the first morning of arrival (at local time); testing and readjusting the dose should be carried out 10 h later if the blood glucose is elevated.

• *Method 4.* For westbound travel increase the time between injections by 2–3 h twice. The total daily insulin dose may need to be increased by 2–4% for each hour of time shift.

For eastbound travel shorten the time between injections. As this will lead to lowering of the blood sugar, the daily dose of insulin will need to be decreased by 2–4% for each hour of time shift.

See Fig. 57.2 for time zones according to Greenwich Mean Time.

Travellers injecting insulin on an aircraft are advised not to inject until their food tray has been delivered to them. Sudden turbulence or other factors may delay meal times on the aircraft.

Patients on oral hypoglycaemics could consider staying on home time for medication and meals until they can adjust on arrival.

Alcohol should be avoided while travelling as it can lead to dehydration.

At destination

Physical activity

Undertaking unaccustomed physical activity increases the likelihood of hypoglycaemia, so diabetic patients may need to increase carbohydrate intake. Inactivity while lying on the beach all day and overeating may increase blood glucose level and this can be compensated for by extra insulin. On the other hand, the absorption of insulin in hot climates is faster and can precipitate hypoglycaemia. In such situations frequent blood test monitoring should be carried out.

Trauma and infection

Walking barefoot on hot sand and other trauma (cuts, abrasions) to the feet should be avoided. Neuropathy involving the foot could contribute to the diabetic patient not being able to appreciate the temperature of the ground. They are also at increased risk of infection and slow healing. Table 57.5 shows common infections in diabetic patients.

Fluids and food

In some countries it may not be safe to drink the

local tap water, so sterilizing tablets or bottled water are recommended. Adequate fluid should be ensured. Alcohol can be dangerous in hot, humid climates and can lead to dehydration. Fruit and vegetables should be washed in sterilized or bottled water if the local water is suspect. Avoid adding ice to drinks in such circumstances unless it is prepared with safe water.

Gastrointestinal illness

Most problems arise from ingestion of contaminated food or water. In the case of vomiting and/or diarrhoea the diabetic traveller should be advised not to stop taking his or her insulin or tablets but to monitor blood glucose levels frequently and adjust the insulin dose accordingly. In case of diarrhoea, solid food and milk should be substituted with carbohydrate-containing proprietary salt and sugar solution. In an emergency, a solution can be made by mixing 1 level teaspoonful of salt and 8 level teaspoonfuls of sugar in 1 L of safe water. If vomiting/or diarrhoea persists, medical advice should be sought locally.

By following relatively simple rules and careful planning there is no reason why a diabetic patient cannot have just as enjoyable a holiday abroad as anyone else. The spouse or friend travelling with the diabetic patient needs to be trained in recognition and management of diabetic emergencies.

Diabetes UK (10 Queen Anne Street, London W1M 0BD) is a very useful source of support and information including special insurance. It can provide insulin users with an identification card that allows the carrier to verify his/her need to carry syringes and medical equipment (it has a photograph of the carrier on it). Its Careline telephone number is 020 7636 6112, while the Association can be contacted on 020 7323 1531. For identification bracelets or necklace, diabetic patients should contact the Medic Alert Foundation on 020 7833 3034.

A comprehensive website for diabetic patients is provided by the Diabetes Centre at the Western General Hospital, Edinburgh: http://www.qmuc.ac.uk/travel/htm/page01.htm

The disabled traveller

Increasing numbers of people with disabilities are making journeys, travelling either independently or with tour operators. Those who have done it before are usually confident but the newly disabled person may lack such confidence to travel for fear of embarrassment or the unknown.

Travellers using a wheelchair may not get any assistance in some airports. Airlines should be given prior notification if they are required to dismantle or reassemble a wheelchair, especially battery-operated electric wheelchairs.

In order to arrange appropriate seating, the airline should be notified well in advance. Ensure arrangements refer to the return journey too. Aisle wheelchairs can be used to take a disabled passenger to the toilet but further help inside the toilet may not be available as airline staff are food handlers.

Immobility can greatly increase the risk of thrombosis. Disabled travellers should exercise their limbs on board, massage the legs and elevate them where possible to minimize ankle oedema.

A disabled person that travels frequently and who has stable disabilities, could consider completing a Frequent Traveller's Medical Card, obtainable from some airlines such as British Airways.

Disabled travellers will find these sources of information helpful:
- another disabled person who has travelled before;
- publications such as *Holiday, Disabled Traveller* by Alison Walsh (written for the BBC Holiday programme and available from Disabled Traveller, PO Box 7, London W12 8UD) and *Nothing Ventured: Disabled People Travel the World*, Penguin Books (1991);
- organizations such as the Royal Association for Disability and Rehabilitation (RADAR) (020 7250 3222);
- TRIPSCOPE (020 8580 7021), helpline: 08457 585 641;
- Air Transport Users Committee, Care in the Air gives advice for handicapped travellers (020 7242 3882);
- Heathrow Travelcare (020 8745 7495);

- Wheelchair Travel (01483 233 640), http://www.wheelchair-travel.co.uk/;
- The British Airport Authority booklet *Travellers information, Special Needs Edition* (1995), as well as other brochures and audiotapes (01233 211 207);
- The Disabled Living Foundation (020 7289 6111) http://www.dlf.org.uk (for information on all aspects of travel for the disabled)
- The Automobile Association (020 8954 7373) can provide a free *Traveller's Guide for the Disabled*;
- The British Red Cross (020 7235 5454) for loan of equipment such as wheelchairs;
- The Holiday Care Service (01293 774 535)—travel advice and information for elderly, disabled and carers;
- John Groom Association for the Disabled (020 7452 2000).

The traveller with epilepsy

The object of treatment of epilepsy is to prevent occurrence of seizures by maintaining an effective plasma concentration of the anti-epileptic drugs. Every effort should be made for this to be maintained during travel. Patients not under control with their condition should ensure they achieve good control before they travel. An epileptic fit on the aircraft is not an infrequent reason for aircraft diversion.

Crossing time zones poses a problem with timing of medication. Ideally, the patient with epilepsy should remain on 'home time' until arrival at destination—do not change the time, or wear an additional watch on home time on the other wrist. They could then readjust to local time. When travelling *westwards* (longer day) on arrival they could bring the next dose forward rather than prolong the interval between doses. When travelling *eastwards* (shorter day) they could shorten the interval between doses.

All medication, including supplies for the length of the holiday, should be taken in the hand luggage with them rather than placed in a suitcase in the hull; it is not unusual for the suitcase not to follow the traveller. Emergency medication (usually in the form of rectal diazepam) could be carried if it is thought it may be necessary and the parent or companion should know how and when

to administer it. For malaria prophylaxis and epilepsy see p. 376.

'Trigger factors' should be avoided. Many situations during travel can trigger an epileptic attack in susceptible individuals, such as television screens, flashing lights in discos, excess alcohol, forgetting to take medication after a night out, etc.

For identification bracelet or necklace, patients with epilepsy should contact the Medic Alert Foundation on 020 7833 3034. It is important that they do wear an identification disc. The British Epilepsy Association's helpline can be accessed by ringing 0808 800 5050.

The HIV-positive and AIDS traveller

An HIV-positive/AIDS traveller needs to be managed with great sensitivity and thought. Such travellers are at a higher risk than immunocompetent travellers, their immune system is compromised to varying degrees and appropriate immunization needs to be undertaken on time so that titres can be checked. Some studies have shown that immunization of HIV-positive individuals can cause a transient rise in HIV viral load. However, these increases are small and short-lived and are probably not clinically significant [Glesby M. *et al.* (1996) The effect of influenza vaccination on human immunodeficiency virus type 1 load: a randomised, double-blind, placebo-controlled study. *J. Infect. Dis.* 174, 1332–6].

They should be counselled on all preventative measures with regard to food, water, beverages, insect precautions, sex, etc. There are no data to suggest that those with HIV are at increased risk of malaria, so standard malaria advice should be given. They should take appropriate malaria prophylaxis, including mefloquine. Consider starting mefloquine 3–4 weeks before travel so that problems can be identified very early. Beware of simultaneously prescribing proguanil (a folate antagonist) in individuals taking co-trimoxazole because of the additive effect on folate.

Some infections are only endemic in certain geographical locations and may be encountered for the first time by an HIV-positive traveller. Such infections, for example *Penicillium marneffei* (a fungus endemic in parts of South-East Asia), may be acquired when abroad and subsequently present as a clinical problem some time later at home.

HIV-infected persons should plan for the possibility of having to use healthcare facilities at the country of destination. Embassies (see Chapter 65 for contact numbers) are usually able to give such information but they are not always able to indicate how welcome an AIDS patient will be at their hospitals.

According to Article 81 of the International Health Regulations, the only health document that port authorities may permissibly require of travellers as a condition of entry is an International Certificate of Vaccination for Yellow Fever. A footnote to this article provides that countries may request a health certificate if the visit is for a 'protracted' period, but no definition of 'protracted' period is given. Based on this note, 20% of the world's countries currently have HIV test requirements.

Travellers are advised to inquire about HIV test requirements at the appropriate embassy/ies, as well as ascertain whether a test conducted in their home country, prior to travel (and how long before travel), will be accepted. Some countries demand serological screening of incoming travellers, especially those with extended visits (work, studies). Some deny entry to persons with AIDS and those with test results indicating infection with HIV. An unofficial list of country requirements has been compiled by the USA State Department and can be found on the Internet (http://www.travel.state.gov/HIVtestingreqs.html). If a test is required to be performed upon arrival in a developing country, advise the traveller to purchase sterile blood-taking equipment before departure in case it is needed.

The HIV-infected traveller should not receive the following vaccines.
● BCG—danger of dissemination; tuberculin test to assess risk;
● Yellow fever—uncertain safety and efficacy in HIV-infected persons. Consider supplying the traveller with a letter of exemption. Travellers with asymptomatic HIV infection who cannot avoid potential exposure to yellow fever could be offered the choice of immunization. The WHO recommends yellow fever vaccination in asymptomatic

HIV infection, and they state that there is insufficient evidence to permit a definitive statement on whether administration of this vaccine poses a risk for symptomatic HIV-infected persons [*International Travel and Health*. WHO (1999) p. 66]. Most physicians caring for people with HIV would be reluctant to give yellow fever vaccine to patients with CD4 lymphocyte counts below $500/mm^3$ and would offer waiver letters for travel purposes.
● Oral typhoid.
● Varicella—its effect is unknown in this situation.
● Oral polio (should also not be given to their household members or close contacts).
● Oral cholera vaccine—currently not available in the UK.

The following vaccines can be given to HIV-infected travellers:
● tetanus;
● hepatitis A;
● hepatitis B;
● MMR (unless severely immunocompromised—see below);
● DTP/DT/Td;
● influenza;
● pneumococcal;
● meningococcal;
● injectable polio;
● injectable typhoid;
● rabies;
● tick-borne encephalitis;
● Japanese B encephalitis;
● immunoglobulin;
● Hib for children. For adults—weigh the risk of the disease against the effectiveness of the vaccine at a given stage of HIV infection.

Vaccine efficiency in HIV-positive patients may be reduced. Check titres and take appropriate action before travel. Consider immunoglobulin (HNIG) after exposure to measles, varicella/herpes zoster. Symptomatic HIV-infected patients exposed to measles should receive HNIG regardless of vaccination status, unless they have received immunoglobin within 3 weeks of exposure. Severely immunocompromised patients with HIV infection should not receive the MMR vaccine—low CD4+ T-lymphocyte count or low percentage of total lymphocytes.

Prophylactic antimicrobial agents against *traveller's diarrhoea* are not recommended routinely for HIV-infected persons travelling to developing countries. These agents, apart from their adverse effects, can promote the emergence of drug-resistant organisms. There may be some special circumstances (e.g. very high risk of infection) when a physician may advise an antimicrobial agent for prophylaxis, i.e. ciprofloxacin 500 mg once a day. On the other hand, HIV-infected travellers to developing countries should carry with them a supply of an appropriate antibiotic (e.g. ciprofloxacin 500 mg twice daily for 3–7 days) to be taken should diarrhoea develop. If they carry antiperistaltic agents such as loperamide or diphenoxylate, they should not be used in the presence of high fever or if there is blood in the stools. They should also be discontinued if symptoms persist beyond 48 h. Preventive measures against *malaria* are very important and appropriate chemoprophylaxis (including mefloquine) should be taken.

Advice to the HIV-infected traveller should include the following:
- discuss risks of travel plans 6–8 weeks prior to travel exposure;
- check there are no contraindications to travel;
- check CD4 count, viral load, maximize antiviral regimen before travel;
- consider water filtration—commercial filters should have pore size of 1 μ or less. Water obtained from deep wells or a spring is less likely to be contaminated with *Cryptosporidia* than water obtained from rivers and lakes;
- discuss daily quinolone for prevention of diarrhoea during high risk travel and discuss self-administration in the case of diarrhoea occurring;
- consider the well-being of others; do not spread the disease. The only safe sex is no sex.

For information on HIV and AIDS see p. 350. For addresses/telephone numbers of various agencies see Sources of Travel Information, Chapter 64.

Transplant recipients

Transplant recipients take immunosuppressive medication to prevent graft rejection. Drugs such as cyclosporin, have profound effects on T-lymphocytes. Azathioprin also affects T-cells and impairs neutrophil function. Steroids increase the risk of infection, primarily through their effect on neutrophils.

Patients with transplants are less likely to respond to immunization than healthy individuals, and the responses can be weaker and less durable [Versluis D. *et al.* (1986) Impairment of the immune response to influenza vaccination in renal transplant recipients by cyclosporin, but not azathioprin. *Transplantation* 42, 376–9]. There is no evidence to suggest that immunization leads to a greater risk of graft rejection.

Live vaccines should be avoided. Because of the T-cell impairment in these patients, the administration of a live vaccine such as polio or yellow fever, may put the patient at risk of disease from the vaccine strain. Patients who have undergone bone marrow transplantation have a more severe immunosuppression than solid organ recipients. They should be considered functionally as asplenic (see p. 204).

All transplant recipients probably carry an increased risk of bacteraemia if they contract traveller's diarrhoea, especially salmonella or campylobacter. Consider supplying these patients with a quinolone antibiotic to take if necessary or as prophylaxis. Renal transplant patients should avoid dehydration in hot climates or if they get traveller's diarrhoea.

Advise transplant recipients to use sunscreens, hats and generally avoid excess sunlight. They have an increased risk of skin cancer, that is further augmented by exposure to sunlight.

Patients receiving chemotherapy

Chemotherapy patients respond less well than healthy individuals. Patients with myeloma or chronic lymphatic leukaemia are functionally antibody-deficient and do not overall respond adequately to vaccines. Use immunoglobulin in case of exposure to a virus such as measles or varicella. Consider supplying them with antibiotics to use as necessary or for prophylaxis.

Live vaccines should be avoided until 6 months after chemotherapy or generalized radiotherapy has been completed.

Patients on immunosuppressive drugs

A number of patients have to take long-term oral steroids and other immunosuppressive drugs, such as methotrexate and cyclophosphamide. These patients exhibit weaker responses to vaccinations, to a large extent because of their underlying disease. Administration of live vaccines should be postponed for at least 3 months after immunosuppressive treatment was stopped, or 3 months after levels have been reached that are not associated with immunosuppression.

The pregnant traveller

It is important that women of child-bearing age who travel have completed immunization courses against measles, mumps, rubella, tetanus, diphtheria, poliomyelitis and hepatitis B before they consider pregnancy, ideally during their childhood. In antenatal clinics pregnant women should be screened for rubella antibody and antibody to hepatitis B surface antigen. This is particularly important for rubella because of the consequences of infection for the development of the fetus in a mother susceptible to infection. A pregnant mother may be a carrier of the hepatitis B virus unknown to her, as she could have had a subclinical infection in the past, thus risking perinatal infection of her newborn infant.

The question of vaccination of a pregnant woman usually arises in relation to travel. Ideally, all vaccine courses should have been completed well before the onset of pregnancy. They should generally be avoided during pregnancy but if considered necessary, when possible, postpone until the second or third trimester.

The risks associated with vaccination are largely theoretical, so the advantages of vaccination may outweigh the potential risk to the fetus. More recent information continues to confirm the safety of vaccines given inadvertently in pregnancy.

The clinician should take into consideration the degree of possible exposure to infection and its consequences to the mother and the fetus. If the mother cannot postpone her travel and the benefits of preventing infectious disease during pregnancy clearly outweigh concerns about the safety of a vaccine, immunization should be considered.

Live viral vaccines

Live viral vaccines should be avoided during pregnancy unless specifically indicated (pregnant mothers at particularly high risk).

• *Yellow fever.* Vaccine is not recommended in pregnancy unless travel to areas of very high risk is unavoidable. In such cases vaccination should be considered, as the risk to the mother of yellow fever infection may far outweigh the small theoretical risk of fetal infection from the vaccine. The WHO advises that vaccination against yellow fever is permitted after the sixth month of pregnancy when justified epidemiologically [*International Travel and Health*, WHO (1999) p. 88]. As yellow fever immunization is a requirement for entry into certain countries, the clinician should provide the patient with an explanatory letter where a decision has been taken not to immunize a pregnant woman.

• *Measles/mumps/rubella (MMR), or rubella monovalent.* Should not be given during pregnancy and 3 (minimum 1) months before. May be given in the postpartum period.

• *Oral poliomyelitis.* Should be avoided in pregnancy especially during the first 16 weeks, unless there is a high risk of infection to the mother (DoH). The injectable inactivated polio vaccine can be considered instead—see below. The WHO advises that oral immunization against poliomyelitis is not contraindicated in pregnancy [*International Travel and Health*, WHO (1999) 88].

• *Varicella.* Not given during pregnancy and for 3 months before. Susceptible pregnant women exposed to varicella virus may be given varicella-zoster immunoglobulin, which may prevent or modify serious maternal illness.

Live bacterial vaccines

• *Tuberculosis (BCG).* Should be avoided, particularly in the early stages and if possible be delayed until after delivery. However, where there is a significant risk of infection, the importance of vaccination may outweigh the possible risk to the fetus.

- *Typhoid (oral)*. The oral typhoid vaccine should not be given in pregnancy. If the mother is travelling to a very high-risk area, the parenteral vaccine should be considered.

Inactivated viral vaccines

- *Influenza*. Should not normally be given in pregnancy unless there is a specific risk or an underlying high-risk condition, although there is no evidence that inactivated influenza vaccine causes damage to the fetus.
- *Poliomyelitis (injectable)*. If a pregnant woman needs to be vaccinated against polio because of high risk exposure during unavoidable travel, the inactivated injectable polio vaccine (IPV) should be preferred. If less than 10 years have elapsed since the pregnant woman completed a primary series of polio vaccinations (oral or injectable) or had a booster, there is no need for the vaccine to be given. If more than 10 years have elapsed, a single dose of the IPV will boost immunity to all three poliovirus agents. If a pregnant woman has not previously been immunized and risks exposure to poliovirus infection, at least two doses of the IPV should be given, 1 month apart. Otherwise, it is prudent to avoid IPV vaccination during pregnancy (in common with all other vaccines).
- *Hepatitis A*. Not recommended in pregnancy unless there is a very definite risk of hepatitis A infection, in which case vaccination should not be withheld.
- *Rabies*. Pre-exposure vaccine should be given in pregnancy if the risk of exposure to rabies is high. Postexposure prophylaxis should be given.
- *Tick-borne encephalitis*. May be given in pregnancy if indicated.
- *Japanese B encephalitis*. The manufacturer does not recommend the vaccine in pregnancy unless there is a definite high risk of infection.

Inactivated bacterial vaccines

- *Cholera*. Should be avoided in pregnancy unless there is a definite risk of infection. No cholera vaccine is currently available in the UK.
- *Pertussis*. Avoid, unless a young, nonimmunized mother is at high risk.

Toxoids

- *Tetanus*. May be used in pregnancy if necessary.
- *Diphtheria*. Avoid in pregnancy (no data available) unless the mother is at increased risk, in which case the low-dose diphtheria vaccine (preferably with tetanus if indicated) should be used. Where possible, waiting until the second trimester of pregnancy is a reasonable precaution for minimizing any theoretical concerns. It is not necessary to boost the immunity if the primary course or a booster was given 10 or less years previously.

Bioengineered

- *Hepatitis B*. Not routinely recommended for pregnant travellers unless there is a very definite risk of hepatitis B infection, in which case vaccination should not be withheld if the mother is screened and found to be seronegative for antibody to hepatitis B surface antigen.

Polysaccharide extracts

- *Haemophilus influenzae* b. Avoid (no data available).
- *Meningococcal A + C*. Avoid unless the mother is at high risk.
- *Pneumococcal*. Avoid (no data). If a pregnant woman is at high risk, if possible wait until after first trimester of pregnancy (the safety of the vaccine during the first trimester of pregnancy has not been evaluated).
- *Typhoid (Vi antigen)*. Avoid, unless the mother is at high risk—not enough data available.

Malaria

A pregnant woman should not travel to a malarious area unless her trip is unavoidable, in which case she should take every precaution to avoid mosquito bites (use insect repellents containing DEET on the skin sparingly). A pregnant woman is more likely to develop life-threatening malaria and may lose the pregnancy or go into premature labour.

During pregnancy, blood flow to the skin increases, which helps heat dissipation, particularly in the hands and feet. In addition, a pregnant woman is likely to leave the protection of her bed-net at night to urinate twice as frequently as a non-pregnant woman. It has been shown that pregnant women attract twice the number of *Anopheles* [Linday, S. *et al.* (2000) Effect of pregnancy on exposure to malaria mosquitoes. *The Lancet*, 355, 1972].

It is safer for a pregnant woman to take anti-malarial medication than to risk catching malaria. Choroquine and proguanil are regarded as safe. Proguanil is an antifolate agent so folic acid, 5 mg daily on alternate days, should be taken, especially during the first trimester. They are both regarded as safe in breast-feeding. Mefloquine should be avoided in pregnancy—if indicated, may be safe in the second and third trimesters. Avoid doxycycline.

Breast-feeding and immunization

If a mother is breast-feeding and may become exposed to infectious disease through travel or otherwise, immunization should be considered. Breast-feeding offers considerable protection to the neonate.

Avoid mefloquine and doxycycline in breast-feeding mothers.

Chapter 58

The returned traveller

The care of the returned traveller starts before the travel begins. Advise on the risk and disease avoidance, appropriate immunization and advise to report to their doctor if, on return from their holiday, they feel unwell, particularly with fever—even after a year if they had travelled to a malarious area. With increasing numbers of business and pleasure travellers worldwide, general practitioners and nurses are often faced with the returned traveller who has a raised temperature. Although viral upper respiratory tract infections are the most common cause of fever, malaria should always be excluded. Symptoms are often nonspecific and the problem is made worse by our unfamiliarity with many tropical diseases. Having a high index of suspicion can save lives.

A good clinical history is very important. What are the presenting symptoms and how long have they been present? Any other symptoms preceding them? Details of pretravel immunization and any chemoprophylaxis taken—which one; how long before and after travel taken; compliance? What medication was taken while abroad? Any invasive procedures (injections, transfusions, dental or surgical procedures, tattoos, ear piercing, etc.)? The patient's travel itinerary will allow the doctor or nurse to focus on some diseases and exclude others—remember to inquire about brief stopovers.

The duration of the trip will point to the degree of exposure risk and give a clearer picture when considering the incubation periods of imported diseases. The conditions during travel are important: travel through rural areas, type of accommodation, meals (and where taken), milk and milk products (whether unpasteurized), seafood, water and its source (drinking and bathing), exposure to parasitic disease (walked barefoot, close contact with domestic/wild animals, bites from mosqui-

toes, sandfly, tsetse fly, tick), use of local travel and additional areas visited, the geographical conditions of the visit (savannah, rain forest, rice fields, mountains, desert, major city, rural area or combinations), hotel (and what class), camping, mission compound, with locals. Sexual behaviour during travel should be discussed.

The physical examination will differ according to the indications given by the clinical history and may range from a screening to an in-depth examination. Care should be taken to assess the skin, rashes or insect bites, and the abdomen for discomfort and hepatosplenomegaly. If the patient reports fever but is apyrexial at the time of the examination, suspicion of malaria should still remain high.

Noninfective conditions sometimes produce fever and they need to be borne in mind: inflammatory bowel disease, connective tissue disease, pulmonary embolus and infarction, neoplasms, reactions to drugs.

Among the 'non exotic' conditions that may present with fever in the returned traveller are: upper respiratory tract infections, pneumonia, urinary tract infections, prostatitis, cholecystitis, infective endocarditis. If the diagnosis does not seem to be apparent, instead of observation in general practice it may be preferable to seek advice from a specialist or a specialist centre.

Laboratory testing and the level of investigations will be determined by the history and examination including the most likely diagnosis. These may include: a full blood count with platelets and a white cell differential count; thick and thin blood films; faecal examination for ova, cysts and parasites; urine multistix analysis and culture; blood cultures; chest X-ray; serum electrolytes and liver function tests. Specific serological tests according to suspicion for arboviral infections, brucellosis,

Table 58.1 Diseases presenting with fever and their incubation periods.

Fever within 3 weeks of infection	Fever more than 3 weeks after infection
Malaria	Malaria
Hepatitis A	Hepatitis A, B, C and E
Typhoid	Typhoid
Rickettsial infection (spotted/typhus fevers, Q fever)	Amoebic liver abscess
Dengue fever and other arboviral infections	Tuberculosis
Brucellosis	Brucellosis
Legionnaire's disease	Filariasis
Trypanosomiasis	Visceral leishmaniasis
Leptospirosis	Schistosomiasis (Bilharziasis)
Lyme disease	HIV and AIDS
Plague	
Haemorrhagic fevers (Lassa, Ebola, Marburg)	
Sometimes *Shigella*, *Salmonella* and *Campylobacter*	

schistosomiasis, filariasis, HIV, etc. At least two further blood films should be examined 24 and 28 h later if the initial film is negative and malaria is suspected.

The incubation period can be particularly helpful when considering the cause of illness in the returned traveller with fever. It is convenient to divide pyrexial diseases into those with an incubation period of less than 3 weeks and those with longer than this (see Table 58.1).

Skin rashes

Skin rashes are not uncommon in the returned traveller. They may be a result of medication (including prophylactic) the traveller has taken, infected skin injuries, fungal infections on moist skin surfaces, sunburn, mosquito bites. Streptococcal and staphylococcal infections are the cause of about 25–30% of skin problems in travellers.

A maculopapular rash may be seen in several infectious diseases, including rickettsial infections, dengue fever, brucellosis, leptospirosis, hepatitis B and HIV. Rose spots present in typhoid fever, mainly on the trunk (rarely seen on dark skins), pale in colour, slightly raised, fade on pressure. Petechial rashes can be associated with dengue haemorrhagic fever, meningococcal and rickettsial infections. The erythema chronicum migrans of early Lyme disease is an annular rash with pale centre and spreading erythema. Cutaneous leishmaniasis is the most important ulcerating condition in the world (nodules and ulcers on the exposed regions).

Jaundice may indicate hepatitis, malaria, yellow fever, leptospirosis.

Cutaneous larva migrans is caused by the dog hookworm *Ancylostoma braziliensis*, which penetrates the skin and causes characteristic intensely itchy tracks, usually on the feet. The larva penetrates the epidermis but is not able to develop further and just wanders aimlessly through the skin until it dies a few weeks later. It leaves behind a very itchy, red track, which the patient has frequently scratched. Usually there is a single track on one foot. It may be seen on the buttocks and even trunk depending on whether the patient had just walked or lain down on the sand.

It is seen in travellers returning from tropical areas, especially the Caribbean, less commonly from Africa or Asia, where the larva is often present in the sand and soil contaminated with dog faeces. Treat by local freezing of the proximal end of the eruption with ethyl chloride spray, or systemically with albendazole 400 mg twice daily for 5 days (available from IDIS on a named-patient basis) or thiabendazole 500 mg chewable 3 tablets twice daily with meals (under 60 kg, 25 mg/kg body weight) for 3 days. The larva can be destroyed by freezing it with liquid nitrogen. Prevention is by wearing shoes along beaches where dogs play.

Loiasis is confined to west Africa. The worm may present as it migrates across the eye beneath the bulbar conjunctivae, leading to pain, irritation and periorbital swelling.

Larva cerrens is caused by the soil helminth *Strongyloides stercolis*. Larvae can migrate through the skin, resulting in a recurrent, pruritic, serpinginous weal on the trunk, which lasts several hours.

Myasis is the development of fly larvae in living tissue. There are several flies, most notably the bot fly (*Dermatobia hominis*) in Central and South America, and the tumbu fly (*Cordylobia anthropophaga*) in Africa, whose larvae develop in the flesh of living animals. Myasis can affect the ear, nose, eyes, anus, vagina or wounds. Eggs hatch and the maggots of these insects need to penetrate tissues to develop further. Cover the lesions with vaseline. As they come up to the surface to breath they can be removed, usually by gently squeezing them out.

Scabies is not uncommon in travellers. It is caused by the mite (acarus) *Sarcoptes scabiei* var. *hominis*. The mites are transferred from person to person by close bodily contact, including sexual contact. The chance of getting the mite from clothing and bedding is small, as mites found in the environment die quickly. Any mites on clothing not worn for a week will die. A fertilized female mite burrows through the stratum corneum and deposits about three eggs each day in its tunnel. Within about 2–3 weeks these will turn into sexually mature mites. For the first 4–6 weeks after infestation there may be no pruritus present. Once the host skin is sensitized to the mites and their products, the characteristic eruption and pruritus appear on the limbs, trunk but also vulvae and nipples. Apply malathion (aqueous solution if traveller is pregnant) to the whole body below the neck once. A hot bath before treatment should be avoided; it increases absorption of the scabicide into the bloodstream. The itching of scabies may last for several days or weeks. This is not an indication for further application of the scabicide as long as it was correctly applied the first time. Calamine lotion can help with combating pruritus.

Pubic (crab) lice (*Phthirus pubis*) is usually transmitted by sexual contact and, rarely, from clothing and bedding. The presenting symptom is severe irritation in the pubic area. It can affect hair elsewhere, particularly in the axillae. The diagnosis is established by demonstrating the presence of the lice or the nits, which adhere to the hair. Malathion treatment should be repeated after a week in order to kill lice that are hatching from eggs. Sexual partners (if known) need treatment too.

Malaria

Malaria should be considered as a medical emergency and the patient admitted to hospital. In 1996, 1659 cases of malaria were reported in England and Wales. In 1997 the number of reports dropped to 1476, and in 1998 down to 1110. Every year in the UK an average of seven to nine people die of malaria they contracted abroad. Nine out of 10 travellers from the tropics who have acquired malaria will not develop symptoms until they are back in the UK. At the other end of the spectrum are the 10% of cases of *Plasmodium vivax* that do not present until a year after exposure. For details on malaria see Chapter 59.

The hepatites

For details on hepatitis A and hepatitis B see pp. 141 and 153, respectively.

Hepatitis C virus (HCV)

This was discovered in 1989. It is a spherical, enveloped, single-strand, linear RNA genome. HCV has the ability to change its genomic composition over time. This takes place also within the infected person, so the HCV creates a family of closely related viruses with minor differences, called 'quasi-species'. Antibodies formed for one 'quasi-species' do not necessarily afford protection against another and they respond differently to interferon-α. This is one of the challenges facing scientists attempting to develop a vaccine. Of the six HCV genotypes known today, numbers 1–3 are found worldwide, 4 and 5 mainly in Africa, and number 6 mainly in Asia.

Its world prevalence is estimated by the WHO to be 3%; 0.2–0.5% in northern Europe, 1.2–1.5% in southern Europe, 0.5–1% in the UK, around 2% in the USA, 6.5% in parts of Africa. In Egypt, the prevalence of antibody to HCV in the general population is 15–20%; this is probably because of the widespread use of parenteral antischistosomal therapy (and inadequate sterilization procedures employed), a practice that was discontinued in the 1980s. Figure 58.1 shows the prevalence of HCV antibodies among blood donors around the world

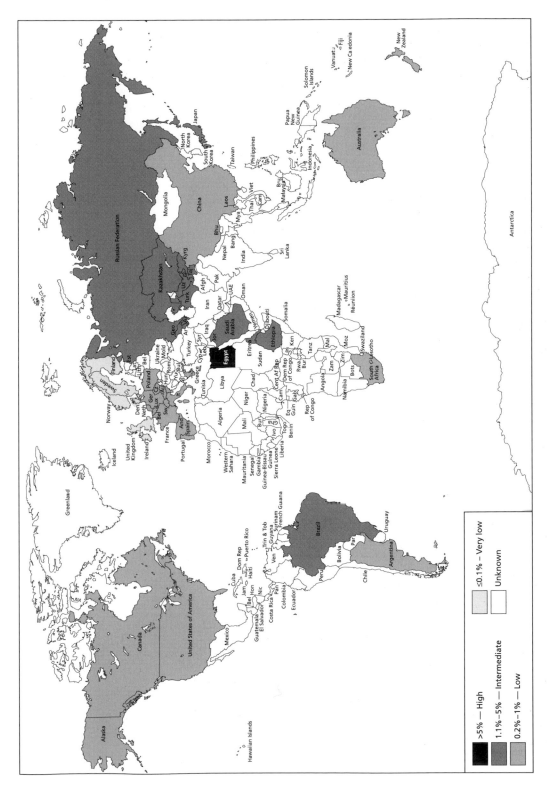

Fig. 58.1 Prevalence of antibody to hepatitis C virus among blood donors. (Source: CDC.)

333

Table 58.2 Numbers of people worldwide infected by the hepatitis C virus in 2000.

China	50.8 million
Egypt	10.5 million
France	667 000
Italy	278 000
Japan	2.8 million
Pakistan	20% of blood donors
Spain	288 000
UK	250 000
USA	4.5 million
Vietnam	4.5 million

according to the CDC. Another source, the Roche website, gives information on the number of people infected with HCV (Table 58.2).

HCV is more infectious than HIV, and four times more common than HIV in the USA.

The mean incubation time of hepatitis C is 6–7 weeks but it ranges from 2 to 26 weeks. The acute course of infection is mild, and the peak serum alanine aminotransferase (ALT) elevations are less than those encountered with hepatitis A or B. Only 25–30% of patients develop jaundice. In about 0.1% of cases it follows a fulminant course. About 15–20% will recover and the infection will clear. Another 20% develop inactive liver disease, and 60% develop active liver disease that includes cirrhosis of the liver (10–20% of patients) over 10–

30 years, and primary hepatocellular carcinoma (6.7% of patients). It is estimated that there are about 300 million cases of hepatitis C worldwide with 170–200 million being chronic carriers.

Transmission of HCV is mainly by intravenous drug abuse. Injecting drug-users should be tested for this condition, as well as patients with elevated liver enzymes, such as ALT, of unknown aetiology. Laboratory-based surveillance of hepatitis C virus infection in England and Wales between 1992 and 1996 has identified injecting drugs as the main route of transmission in up to 80% of cases, while receipt of blood or blood products was the cause in 10%. Transfusion services in the UK introduced routine screening for HCV in September 1991. Recipients of blood transfusions and blood products (e.g. patients with haemophilia, thalassaemia) before this date could have been at risk of HCV infection. Table 58.3 shows the number of laboratory-confirmed cases and notifications of hepatitis C infection in England and Wales.

Other parenteral routes capable of HCV transmission include tattooing, ear-piercing, acupuncture. Unlike hepatitis B, sexual activity seems to be a less important route of infection—infection rate of less than 5% in sexual partners. Vertical transmission (mother to baby) occurs in less than 7% of infected mothers, the risk being related to

Table 58.3 Laboratory-confirmed cases and notifications of hepatitis C infection: 1996–98 England and Wales.

	History of travel			Number	
	Yes	No	No information	Notified	Laboratory confirmed
1996	15	73	2456	194	2544
1997	9	41	3008	333	3058
1998	40	166	4298	616	4504

Source: ONS; PHLS Communicable Disease Surveillance Centre.

Injecting drugs
Blood transfusion, blood products, transplantation, from infected donor
Haemodialysis
Sharing needles/syringes
Accidental injury with needles or sharps
Fights, human bites, tattooing, body piercing, acupuncture
Sexual/household exposure to a chronically infected person (anti-HCV-positive)
Multiple sex partners
Birth to a HCV-infected mother

Table 58.4 Risk associated with transmission of hepatitis C virus.

the level of viraemia (viral load), and is 3.8 times higher if mother is co-infected with HIV [Gibb, D.M. *et al.* (2000) Mother-to-child transmission of hepatitis C virus: evidence for preventable peripartum transmission. *The Lancet* 356, 904–907]. The type of delivery affects the risk (higher in vaginal and emergency caesarian than elective caesarian section). Breast-feeding has not been associated with spreading the infection. In about 40% of cases the origin of the infection is unclear. It is important to enquire about human bites or fights which the patient may not remember. Within the family, patients should not share toothbrushes or razors—there is no transmission risk from household activities such as cooking, eating, etc. Table 58.4 shows the risk associated with transmission of HCV.

Occupational exposure in the healthcare setting accounts for about 2% of cases, while the prevalence of anti-HCV among healthcare workers in the UK is 0.28% [Zuckerman J. *et al.* (1994) Prevalence of hepatitis C antibodies in health care workers. *Lancet* 343, 1618–20]. HCV-infected surgeons in the UK associated with proven transmission are recommended not to perform exposure-prone procedures (two cases of transmission from surgeon to patient have been reported in the UK in 1995 and 1997).

'Travellers' risk of contracting HCV infection depends on their potential risks for exposure to blood, such as injecting drugs, needing medical care that may involve blood transfusion. Also, engaging in high-risk sexual practices especially with commercial sex workers, body piercing, tattooing.

HCV infection is primarily detected with antibody tests. An enzyme-linked immunosorbent assay (ELISA), which detects HCV antibodies in the blood, can detect about 95% of chronically infected patients. However, the long interval between infection and the appearance of antibodies in the blood (6 months and over), reduces the detection rate of acute infection to 50–70% when this test is used. A more sensitive test is the recombinant immunoblot assay (RIBA) or 'Western blot'. As the antibody test may be negative for several months following HCV infection, specialist units use the polymerase chain reaction (PCR) test to detect minute quantities of HCV RNA in order to confirm the diagnosis—this last test is also used in infants.

Available treatment is α-interferon alone or in combination with ribavirin. The aim is to reduce liver inflammation and thus possibly reduce the risk of development of cirrhosis. Short courses (6 months) of interferon can lead to a loss of detectable hepatitis C virus RNA in about 40% of patients, but most relapse when treatment is stopped. In about half of these patients a sustained response can be achieved by using combination therapy [report in *Lancet* (1999) 354, 655]. Previously untreated patients receiving combination therapy for 6 or 12 months achieve sustained response in 31 and 38%, respectively [McHutchison J. *et al.* (1998) Interferon alpha-2b alone or in combination with ribavirin as initial treatment for chronic hepatitis C. *N. Engl. J. Med.* 339, 1485–92].

In the USA, postexposure use of immunoglobulin is not recommended in prophylaxis against HCV infection. Furthermore, immunoglobulin is currently manufactured from plasma documented to be negative for anti-HCV antibodies.

Prevention

No vaccine is available to protect against hepatitis C, and it is unlikely one will be available in the near future. The virus has not been cultivated *in vitro* so it is not yet possible to develop inactivated or attenuated vaccines. It is safe to immunize patients with HCV infection against hepatitis B but do check sero-conversion. Prevention is by:

● requesting that infected persons avoid donating, and screening of donors of blood, organs or tissues;
● high-risk behavioural modification;

Anti-HCV-positive individuals should be counselled on the need that:

● they do not donate blood, organs, tissue, or semen, share household articles such as toothbrushes, razors;
● they should consider themselves potentially infectious:

  (a) keep cuts and skin lesions well covered;
  (b) be aware of the potential for sexual as well as perinatal transmission (no evidence at the moment to advise against pregnancy and breastfeeding).

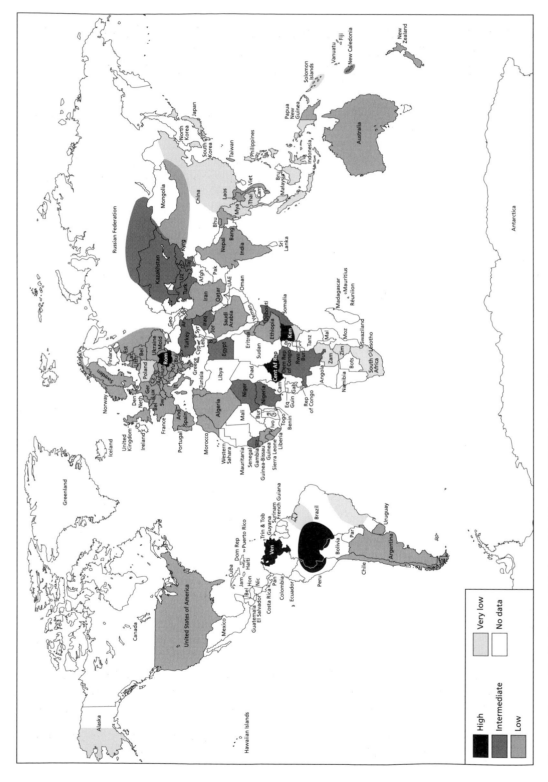

Fig. 58.2 Geographic distribution of the hepatitis delta virus (HDV) infection. (Source: CDC.)

Table 58.5 Laboratory-confirmed cases and notifications of hepatitis E infection: 1996–98 England and Wales.

	History of travel			Number
	Yes	No	No information	laboratory confirmed
1996	47	0	4	51
1997	11	0	8	19
1998	23	0	33	56

Source: ONS; PHLS Communicable Disease Surveillance Centre.

For up-to-date information on hepatitis C visit the website http://www.roche-hepc.com

Hepatitis delta virus

Hepatitis delta virus (HDV) is a defective virus, too small to replicate itself. It behaves like a parasite on the hepatitis B virus, using the surface antigen of HBV to multiply. It can only therefore infect patients infected with HBV. Five per cent of HBsAg carriers worldwide (around 18 million people) are estimated to be infected with HDV. Intravenous drug users are at increased risk of contracting HDV infection.

Main modes of HDV transmission are:
● percutaneous exposure—blood, blood products, body piercing, injecting drugs;
● permucosal exposure—unprotected sex.
Delta hepatitis is common in the Mediterranean, parts of Eastern Europe, the Middle East, Africa and South America (see Fig. 58.2). HDV is rare but when it infects HBV carriers, it can lead to fulminant hepatitis or severe chronic liver disease. Hepatitis B immunization can prevent co-infection with HDV.

Hepatitis E virus

Hepatitis E virus (HEV) was first described in the early 1980s in India and is now recognized to be the primary agent responsible for enterically transmitted non-A, -B, -C hepatitis. It is endemic in many areas of the world, especially in India, Bangladesh, Myanmar, Mexico, Somalia, Ivory Coast, Sudan, Algeria and China (see Fig. 58.3). Premonsoon and monsoon seasons are high-risk periods for epidemics.

The incubation period is 15–60 days (average 40 days). The symptoms include jaundice, fatigue, anorexia, nausea, vomiting, abdominal pain, diarrhoea, headaches, fever, pruritus, arthralgia, hepatomegaly and splenomegaly. The bilirubin and aminotransferases are raised. 1–2% go on to develop fulminant hepatitis. The mean recovery time is just over 8 weeks with an overall case fatality rate of 0.5%, rising to 1–3% during epidemics. The main cause is fulminant hepatic failure. Its severity rises with age. Among pregnant women in the third trimester mortality is 15–25%. Hepatitis B carriers also have a high mortality rate. There is no carrier state for hepatitis E, although biochemical and histopathological evidence of mild chronic hepatitis may be recorded in 20% of the patients who recover from subacute hepatic failure. Subclinical infection appears to be common.

Anti-HEV IgM is present from about 10–12 days of acute illness until about day 50. Anti-HEV IgG appears about 10–12 days from the beginning of the illness and remains detectable for a longer period.

The main mode of transmission is the faecal-oral route, that is faecal contamination of drinking water and food, generally in areas of poor sanitation and hygiene. Person-to-person transmission is possible, where a person comes into direct contact with an infected person's faeces. Much rarer modes of transmission are vertical and through blood and blood products.

Sporadic outbreaks occur from time to time. Where it does circulate, seroprevalence in industrialized countries is 1–5% and in other countries about 20%. The prevalence of hepatitis E is greatest among young adults (15–40 years of age). In England and Wales in 1998, 56 cases of hepatitis E were notified (see Table 58.5). There is a possibility of an animal reservoir.

● The disease can be controlled through the provision of safe water and food.

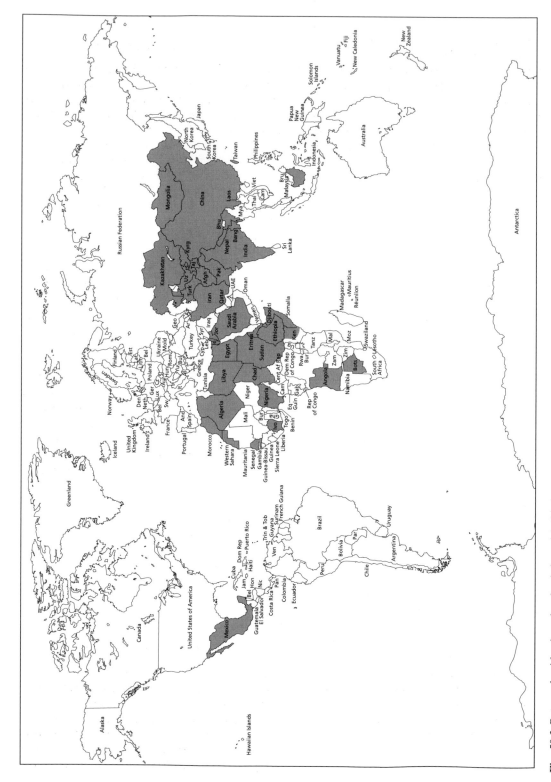

Fig. 58.3 Reported epidemic and endemic hepatitis E infection. (This map generalizes available data.)

- Travellers visiting endemic areas are at risk of contracting HEV infection.
- Pregnant women, particularly in the third trimester, should consider postponing nonessential visits to endemic areas.
- There is no vaccine available. A vaccine has been tested on volunteers and has been found to be safe and immunogenic (SmithKline Beecham)—it is undergoing tests.
- Strict food/water precautions are the only available means of prevention.

Hepatitis G virus

Hepatitis G virus (HGV) was identified in 1995. In fact, three viruses have been identified; GBV-A, GBV-B and GBV-C. Hepatitis G represents an independent isolate of GBV-C. It is distantly related to HCV and is spread parenterally. It is associated with acute and chronic hepatitis but its role in cirrhosis and hepatocellular carcinoma has not as yet been clarified. HGV exists in a chronic carrier state.

HGV and HCV infection can be simultaneously transmitted and may result in co-infection. Among blood donors its prevalence is 1–2% and among patients who have multiple blood transfusions is 16%. Seroprevalence of 15.2% has been reported in West African residents. Most at risk are patients who receive frequent blood transfusions or are on haemodialysis, as well as persons abusing drugs parenterally. There is now some evidence for perinatal transmission.

Typhoid

The number of cases of typhoid fever reported in England and Wales was 175 in 1996, 140 in 1997 and 122 in 1998. About 80% are reported by travellers returning from abroad, especially the Indian subcontinent. Some cases (20 in 1996, 16 in 1997 and 13 in 1998) are contracted in the UK from carriers who have been exposed to the disease in the past. It is important to remember typhoid can present with constipation before the diarrhoea. For further details please see Chapter 40.

Rickettsial infections

The *Rickettsia* have mammals (therefore humans too) as their reservoir and are transmitted by the bites, body fluids or faeces of arthropods such as mites, ticks, lice or fleas. They include *Rickettsia conori* (tick typhus), *R. tsutsugamushi* (scrub typhus), *R. prowazeki* (louse-borne epidemic typhus), *R. typhi* (murine endemic typhus) and *R. rickettsii* (Rocky Mountain spotted fever). Another rickettsial organism, *Coxiella burnetii*, causes Q fever and its most common animal reservoirs are cattle, sheep and goats. They have a worldwide distribution.

The symptoms they cause are common to other diseases: headaches, fever and myalgia. They need to be distinguished from conditions such as meningitis, hepatitis, leptospirosis, dengue fever or drug allergy. A widespread erythematous maculopapular or petechial rash (most prominent on the extremities) may be characteristic, accompanied by regional lymphadenopathy. Patients with tick and scrub typhus often have a painless eschar (scab) at the site of the insect bite. Diagnosis is by clinical exclusion, skin biopsy and specific serological testing. Treatment is with tetracyclines (doxycycline), chloramphenicol or quinolone (ciprofloxacin) antibiotics. Prevention is by personal measures to avoid insect bites, wearing protective clothing and sleeping on camp beds when out camping, as well as inspecting the skin regularly for ticks.

Q fever, a widespread zoonosis, spreads by inhalation of contaminated dust as well as drinking unpasteurized milk and, occasionally, from tick bites. Suspect Q fever in a patient with prolonged pyrexia of unknown origin (PUO) or atypical pneumonia. The diagnosis is made serologically.

Arboviral infections

There are over 400 such viruses transmitted by arthropod vectors (mosquitoes, sandflies or ticks). Of them, 127 are named. The reader will find information on yellow fever in Chapter 42, tick-borne encephalitis in Chapter 39 and Japanese B encephalitis in Chapter 35. Most of them cause nonspecific febrile illness with myalgia. Some

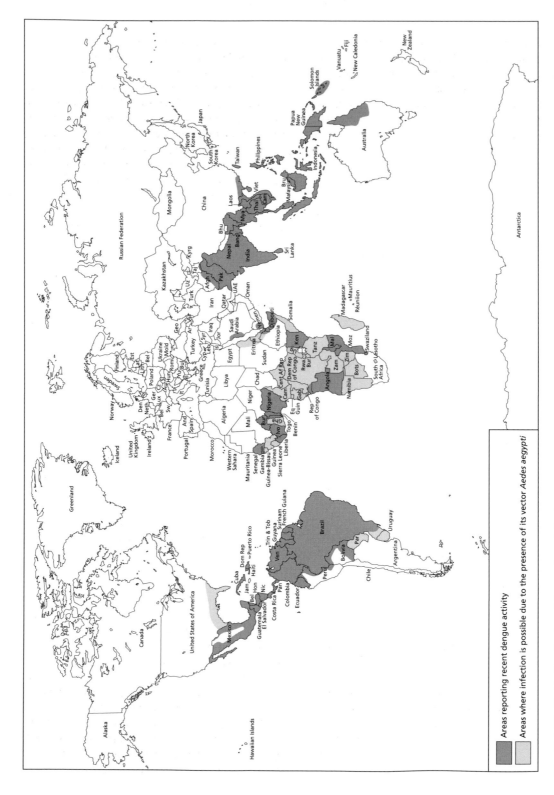

Fig. 58.4 Worldwide distribution of dengue fever infection.

Areas reporting recent dengue activity

Areas where infection is possible due to the presence of its vector *Aedes aegypti*

cause haemorrhagic and some encephalitic illness. In Australia the Ross River virus infection is now the most common arboviral infection of humans and symptoms include headaches, fever, myalgia, malaise, depression, rash and, most characteristically, arthritis of varying severity of hands, knees and feet.

Dengue fever

This is now the world's most important arboviral infection in humans. It is transmitted by the mosquito *Aedes aegypti*, which flourishes in conditions of poor housing, overcrowding and inadequate sanitation. The mosquito is domestically adapted and circulates in communities. Its larvae are mostly found where there is an accumulation of water, especially discarded cans, water jars, flower vases/pots, discarded tyres, barrels, buckets, blocked rain gutters, wells, water tanks, tree holes and coconut shells. A second mosquito, *A. albopictus*, can also transmit dengue and is found mainly in discarded tyres in West Africa and other areas. A third mosquito is *A. polynesiensis*. The female mosquito has a predilection for human blood and it bites mainly early in the morning and late afternoon (day-biting), especially indoors, in shady areas, or when it is overcast.

A new programme, sponsored by the Governments of the UK and Australia, has been successful in reducing the risk of dengue fever in parts of Vietnam, where 170 000 people are infected every year. It involves the use of a mesocyclops crustacean, a 1-mm long organism that devours the larvae of the mosquitoes that carry dengue fever, in their breeding grounds.

Dengue fever has been on the increase worldwide during the last few years (Fig. 58.4). This is facilitated by climatic changes to a warmer environment, the growing urban populations, expanding mosquito breeding sites, transportation and international travel. About 2.5 billion people live in areas at risk of infection, in about 100 tropical and subtropical countries in South-East Asia, the Pacific, east and west Africa, the Caribbean and subtropical regions of the Americas. The incidence of severe disease, dengue haemorrhagic fever (DHF), has increased dramatically in South-East

Asia in the past 20 years, with major epidemics occurring in most countries every 3–4 years. DHF is an emerging disease in the Americas.

An estimated 100 million cases occur each year, causing a huge strain on local medical services. About 500 000 are haemorrhagic, with 25 000–30 000 fatalities—case fatality of its haemorrhagic form is 2–5%. It is not long since dengue fever was present in the Mediterranean Sea area—10 000 cases of DHF were reported in Greece in 1927/8.

The Dengue flavivirus has four serotypes: dengue 1, 2, 3 and 4. Infection confers lifelong immunity to a particular serotype but there is no cross-immunity. A second infection with a different serotype is usually associated with an increased risk of DHF, although DHF may occasionally occur after one primary infection. Increasing age is another risk factor for DHF. The disease has been noted in adults revisiting endemic areas but the risk seems to be extremely low.

The disease is usually benign and self-limiting, although convalescence may be prolonged. The vast majority of infections, particularly those in children, are overall asymptomatic. The severity tends to increase with the patient's age and repeated infections.

The incubation period is 3–8 days and fever lasts 4–5 days. The onset is abrupt, with rigors, frontal headaches, pain behind the eyes, which worsens with movement, nausea, vomiting, arthralgia, severe myalgia and often a transient macular rash with a secondary maculopapular rash appearing between days 3 and 6. Dengue is often referred to as 'breakbone fever' because of the severe joint and muscle pains.

Lymphadenopathy and leukopenia with relative lymphocytosis may be present. In the haemorrhagic form there may be gastrointestinal bleeding as well as bleeding from the nose, gums and mouth as a result of haemorrhagic diathesis, hypotension, hepatomegaly, generalized lymphadenopathy, excessive thirst, difficulty in breathing and shock. On testing, hypoalbuminaemia, thrombocytopenia and clotting abnormalities are found.

The diagnosis is based on clinical manifestations, negative malarial films and arboviral serological tests that rely on detecting the virus and antibodies in the blood. This is carried out by viral culture, PCR and detection and follow-up of the levels of antibodies in the blood. The virus itself remains detectable only for a short period of about 5 days during which time the patient is pyrexial.

Treatment is by management of the fever (avoid aspirin so as not to increase the bleeding diathesis—use paracetamol), replacement of fluid, serum proteins and electrolytes. Most patients recover fully following rest and symptomatic treatment. Severe bleeding requires a combination of medical and surgical treatment. Prevention is primarily by avoiding daytime-biting mosquitoes, and vector control by eliminating domestic breeding places.

Efforts to develop a vaccine include combining all four serotypes of the dengue virus. Such live-attenuated tetravalent vaccines have been developed but not yet licensed. Research now is attempting to develop a second generation of recombinant vaccines that will potentially be safer and more immunogenic.

In 1995, we witnessed the worst dengue epidemic in Latin America and the Caribbean for 15 years. It spread to 14 countries, causing more than 250 000 cases of dengue fever and about 6000 cases of DHF. The first outbreak in the American continent was in Cuba in 1981.

In the UK, between 1994 and 1996, 15 cases of dengue were confirmed, mainly ethnic travellers visiting India. The risk to travellers is about 1 per 1000 travellers and depends on degree of exposure (lower risk during short visits, in air-conditioned hotels with well-kept grounds). The self-limiting nature of the disease may mean that much dengue fever in travellers goes unreported. Travellers to dengue-endemic areas can reduce the probability of mosquito bites by wearing clothes that reduce the amount of exposed skin and using mosquito repellent and, if necessary, aerosol insecticides in rooms.

Dengue should be considered in returning travellers from endemic areas, presenting with 'flu-like' illness, especially when accompanied by a rash and fever. Patients with dengue typically have a low or normal white cell count, mild thrombocytopenia, and negative blood cultures and blood films for malaria. Renal impairment and elevated liver enzymes are seen in more severe disease. The diagnosis is aided by virus isolation in tissue culture,

detection of viral RNA using PCR or, more often, by demonstrating rising serological titres between acute and convalescent blood samples. It is unlikely that a traveller will have dengue if symptoms start more than 2 weeks after leaving the dengue-endemic area, or if the fever lasts more than 2 weeks.

Travellers to dengue fever areas should be advised to cover up in the daytime too (not just at night), use mosquito repellents and stay away from areas where there are containers in which water can collect. They should clear their living areas of any containers, such as buckets, flower pots, etc.

Brucellosis

Human brucellosis is a bacterial disease caught from farm animals such as cattle, goats, sheep, pigs and dogs. Transmission occurs when contaminated meat, milk or cheese are ingested, infected material from animals is inhaled or inoculated onto broken skin or mucous membranes. Very rarely, sexual, vertical or via blood transfusion transmission is reported. The four different animal species are: *Brucella abortus* (cattle present worldwide), *B. melitensis* (goats—mainly in the Middle East, Mediterranean, Latin America and Asia), *B. suis* (pigs) and *B. canis* (dogs).

It is now rare in most European countries, North America and Australasia. It is rapidly increasing in the eastern Mediterranean and the Middle East. Brucellosis is reported in at least 86 countries and accounts for 500 000 cases worldwide every year—about 20–30 cases are reported in the UK. It has an important impact on the animal industry.

The incubation period is from 1 to 3 weeks (acute) to several months (chronic form). Symptoms of acute infection include headaches, fever, myalgia, backache, vomiting, hepatomegaly and lymphadenopathy. The diagnosis is established by the history of contact (e.g. consumption of untreated milk or unpasteurized cheeses), leukopenia, raised erythrocyte sedimentation rate (ESR), blood cultures and serological tests. Treatment is by combining rifampicin and doxycycline for 6 weeks.

Legionnaire's disease

Legionella pneumophila was first recognized as the cause of an outbreak of severe pneumonia in 1976 in the USA, and was subsequently identified as the cause of several earlier outbreaks. In the UK, 279 cases were reported in 1988 and 200 in 1996. Transmission is by inhalation of contaminated, airborne water droplets generated from air-conditioning cooling water towers for offices and industry, hot-water taps and showers, humidifiers, domestic and recreational whirlpool spas. The ideal environmental temperature for the organism is 10–50 °C.

A flu-like illness follows a short incubation period of 1–2 days. The patient complains of headaches, rigors, fever and myalgia. There may be abdominal pain, diarrhoea and confusion. Chest symptoms follow in the form of a dry cough, breathlessness and haemoptysis. Crepitations are present on auscultation and chest X-ray shows signs of consolidation. There is raised ESR, leukocytosis, raised liver transaminases, hyponatraemia and a rise in antibody titres. Treatment consists of a 2-week course of erythromycin to which ciprofloxacin or rifampicin is added. The mortality rate ranges between 10 and 25% of cases. Prevention is by adequate chlorination of water supplies stored in cold water storage systems, and heating hot water to above 60 °C. Just under half of cases reported in the UK result from travel, the most common destinations being Spain and the Spanish islands, Turkey, Greece, Italy, the Caribbean, France, Portugal, USA, and other European countries.

African trypanosomiasis (sleeping sickness)

The parasite *Trypanosoma brucei* causes African trypanosomiasis and is restricted to localized areas in Africa. There are two distinct forms: the western and central African *gambiense* which currently seriously affects Angola, Cameroon, Central African Republic, Chad, Congo, Sudan, Uganda and the Democratic Republic of Congo (former Zaire) where 2% of the population carry the disease, with prevalence in some countries reaching 70%. The *rhodesiense* is found in east Africa in countries such as Tanzania, Malawi, Mozambique, Uganda, Ethiopia and Zambia. It is confined to tropical Africa between 15 degrees north and 20 degrees south latitude.

It is transmitted to humans by the bite of an infected tsetse fly, a grey-brown insect about the size of a honeybee. It is found only in parts of Africa and inhabits rural areas only, living in the woodland and thickets of the savannah and the dense vegetation along streams. Travellers to urban areas only are not at risk. The tsetse fly feeds on the blood of animals and humans. It is attracted to moving vehicles and dark, contrasting colours. It is not affected by insect repellent and can bite through lightweight clothes. About 60 million of the 400 million people inhabiting 36 sub-Saharan African countries are at risk. In 1997, 45 000 cases were reported among the 5–10% of the population under surveillance. This indicates that more than 450 000 carry the disease today.

The incubation period is up to 28 days, shorter in the east African disease. The early symptoms are headaches, fever, myalgia, itching and weakness. There may be a transient macular rash. There follows lymphadenopathy, hepatosplenomegaly, anaemia, cardiovascular and renal complications. In the later stage the parasite invades the central nervous system where it causes meningoencephalitis. This causes intractable headaches, ability to concentrate diminishes, the mood changes unpredictably, the patient becomes ataxic, drowsy, confused and drifts into coma. Death can follow. The *gambiense* form develops slowly with death occurring several years after infection, while the rhodesiense form is more acute with symptoms developing within a few days and death following within a few weeks to a year.

Serology will indicate part contact with the disease. The essential test is examination of the cerebro-spinal fluid (CSF). Effective drugs are suramin (before the central nervous system is affected), melarsoprol (80% effective) and pentamidine (93% effective). Prevention is by vector control and avoiding tsetse fly bites. Travellers should wear clothes of colours similar to the background environment, of medium-weight fabric, covering ankles and wrist. No vaccine is available.

American trypanosomiasis (Chagas' disease)

American trypanosomiasis appears in an acute and also a chronic form where principally the heart is affected. The parasite, *T. cruzi*, is found both in domesticated and wild animals that infect a blood-sucking triatomiid (usually cone-nosed) bug that is usually found in areas where living conditions are poor. Infection takes place via contaminated bug faeces (bug defecates while taking blood) when they come into contact with mucous membranes (e.g. the conjunctivae) or damaged skin. The disease can also be transmitted via contaminated blood or blood products (in some areas blood may not be screened for *T. cruzi*), vertically (mother to baby *in utero*, during breast-feeding), from organ transplantation and nosocomially.

It is present only in the Americas. Cases are mainly reported in Mexico, Argentina, Peru, Brazil, Venezuela and Chile. Other Central and South American countries also report cases, as well as the Caribbean islands and the United States. About 100 million people are at risk of contracting the disease, already 18 million are infected, with 2 million people having complications. The death toll of the disease is around 45 000 people annually.

Symptoms of the acute form include fever, malaise, anorexia, headaches and myalgia. There may be oedema of the face and the lower limbs, lymphadenopathy and hepatosplenomegaly. Early complications include myocarditis and meningo-encephalitis. A third of those infected progress to develop chronic Chagas' disease, and 30% become incapacitated as a result of cardiac complications, which can lead to death—it is the leading cause of cardiac death among young adults in parts of South America. The digestive and peripheral nervous system can also be involved.

Laboratory diagnosis is by serology, feeding laboratory-reared triatomine bugs with the patient's blood to see whether they subsequently have the parasite, mouse inoculation or blood culture. For treatment in the acute phase, nifurtimox or benznidazole is used. Prevention is by vector control, living conditions improvement and screening of donated blood.

Travellers should avoid overnight stays in dwellings that may be infested by the vector, such as those constructed of mud, adobe brick or palm thatch, particularly those with cracks or crevices in the walls and roof. No vaccine is available.

Leptospirosis

Leptospirosis is a zoonotic disease (infects animals—rats, mice, dogs, pigs, cattle) caused by a variety of *Leptospira* spp. with worldwide distribution except the polar regions. It is particularly common in the tropical and subtropical areas. Weil first described it in 1886. Animals are the natural reservoir and in the UK the principal reservoirs are in the rat (*L. icterohaemorrhagiae*) and cattle (*L. hardjo*). Approximately 60 cases are reported each year in the UK.

The infected animal sheds the organism in its urine. Transmission occurs when damaged skin or mucous membranes and conjunctivae come into contact with infected animal urine directly or indirectly (fresh water contaminated with animal urine). The occurrence of flooding after heavy rainfall facilitates the spread of the organism as *Leptospira* present in the soil pass directly into surface waters. Exposure is usually occupational (farmers, vets, sewage workers, river fishermen) or recreational (swimming, canoeing, rafting, windsurfing, fishing).

The incubation period is 7–21 days. In 90–95% of cases it runs a mild course but in 5–10% this is severe. During the first phase of the illness the patient experiences a sudden severe headache that comes on suddenly and is the predominant feature, also rigors, fever and myalgia (sometimes the patient is unable to walk). Occasionally there may be abdominal pain, nausea, vomiting, chest pains, cough, haemoptysis, maculopapular rash and confusion. Many patients recover.

If the patient goes into the second phase, the fever returns after 2 or 3 days, the conjunctivae become red because of engorged blood vessels (almost pathognomonic), there is uveitis, neck stiffness, there may be jaundice, renal impairment with proteinuria, and aseptic meningitis. The patient may present with gastroenteritis or respiratory disease. Most deaths occur within 2 weeks and mortality is 5–10% in severe disease (higher with increasing age—30% in 70-year-olds). Mild and subclinical infections are common. Leptospirosis in pregnancy can cause abortion and intrauterine death.

The diagnosis is supported by serology and cultures of blood and cerebrospinal fluid during the first 10 days of illness (if negative repeat), and urine after the first week of illness. Warn the laboratory you suspect leptospirosis as they need to set up special cultures. The platelet count is reduced while the ESR, white cell count (neutrophils) and prothrombin time are raised. The bilirubin may be raised while the transaminases are relatively low. Creatinine kinase is raised because of myalgia.

Benzylpenicillin is the drug of choice with amoxycillin, ceftriaxone, doxycycline and erythromycin as alternatives. It is resistant to chloramphenicol. Intravenous fluids, transfusion and vitamin K are administered. Complications such as renal failure are treated appropriately.

Prevention is by wearing protective clothing and footwear during occupational exposure. Any damage to the skin should be covered with a waterproof dressing before exposure to suspect water. Treat water with iodine—some water filters may not be adequate. Avoid submersion in water, keep head above water. Diving can introduce water to the nasal mucosa, eyes and mouth. Doxycycline may be used for prevention of leptospirosis: 200 mg once each week throughout the stay in the area and 200 mg on completion of the trip—not recommended for children under 12 years of age, and not for pregnant or lactating mothers.

Vaccines are available for animals. Human vaccines are associated with a high incidence of adverse reactions and give only limited protection. Rodent control and periodic immunization of domestic pets and cattle are important measures. Chemoprophylaxis is with doxycycline 200 mg once weekly starting 1 week before entering the endemic area and 1 week after departing. In malarious areas where doxycycline is indicated, 100 mg twice daily may cover both malaria and leptospirosis.

Leptospirosis is a notifiable disease.

Lyme disease (Lyme borreliosis)

Lyme disease was first described in 1975 when there was a close clustering of cases in Lyme, Connecticut, USA. It is caused by a spirochaete, *Borrelia burgdorferi*, with different strains in the USA (more likely to produce carditis) and Europe (more neurological involvement). Animal reservoirs are small rodents, deer, dogs, cats, chipmunks, racoons, voles and humans. In the USA, robins have been found to act as a reservoir for Lyme disease spirochaetes. American robins become infectious for vector ticks as do reservoir mice, but infectivity in robins wanes more rapidly.

It is transmitted to humans by the bite of an infected hard tick of the genus *Ixodes ricinus* complex. This disease has been reported in the USA, Canada, Africa, Asia, Australia and Europe—including Britain where transmission has been recorded in the New Forest and deer parks in London and the south-east and in Scotland. Up to 20% of the ticks in Switzerland, France and Southern Germany are carriers of *Borrelia*.

About 3–30 days after a tick bite, in about 80% of cases, a characteristic rash appears at the site of the bite (erythema chronicum migrans). It reaches a size of 5 cm or more and as it expands the centre clears to produce a ring-shaped eruption ('bull's eye'), although other forms can also appear. This rash grows over a period of days (2–4 weeks) during which time patients often complain of fever, headaches, fatigue, myalgia, arthralgia and neck pain (meningism).

A few weeks or even months after the rash (and sometimes without a rash preceding) the patient may develop neurological complications (cranial nerve palsy, meningoencephalitis, neuropathies, meningitis, encephalopathy, neuropsychiatric disorders), cardiovascular symptoms (conduction defects, myocarditis, pericarditis), musculoskeletal (most commonly arthritis involving the knee) and ophthalmological symptoms.

The clinical diagnosis can be supported by serological tests. Treatment is with a 3-week course of doxycycline, or amoxicillin plus probenecid. The macrolite, azithromycin, can be used with good response. Late Lyme disease, and especially where neurological complications are present, requires intravenous ceftriaxone.

Prevention for travellers includes wearing protecting clothing (permethrin may be used on clothing) and skin applications of repellents containing DEET or Mosi-guard Natural preparations. Travellers should inspect their skin daily for ticks and if found they should be removed. A blunt-tip, fine-point tweezers is generally the best tool for tick extraction. Get as close to the tick's mouthparts as possible and pull the tick straight back.

A safe and effective (78% protection rate, 90% in those under 65 years of age) recombinant OspA vaccine (LYMErix—SmithKline Beecham) is available in the USA for use in the endemic areas, in people aged 15–70 years (3 doses over a 1-year period—0, 1 and 12 months). This vaccine is not likely to be efficacious outside North America because of the strain diversity that causes Lyme disease in Europe and Asia. Information on recommendations for vaccine use in travellers to high-risk areas of the USA is available on the Internet at: http://www.cdc.gov/ncidod/dvbid/lymeinfo.htm

Surveillance for Lyme disease—USA: http://www.cdc.gov/epo/mmwr/preview/mmwrhtml/ss4903al.htm.

Plague

For details on this disease see Chapter 36.

Viral haemorrhagic fevers

Lassa fever

The natural reservoir of the Lassa virus is the multi-mammate rat *Mastomys natalensis*, which is found in the rural areas of West Africa where the disease is endemic (Sierra Leone, Liberia, Nigeria). Transmission of the virus from asymptomatically infected rodents to humans causes severe disease, often in the form of fatal haemorrhagic fever. There are about 300 000 cases and 5000 deaths annually. No vaccine is available.

Marburg disease

This disease is caused by a filovirus and has been transmitted to laboratory workers by monkeys. The main route of transmission is via blood and body fluids.

Ebola virus

This virus emerged with simultaneous outbreaks in Sudan and the Democratic Republic of Congo (former Zaire) in 1976. It re-emerged with an outbreak in southern Sudan in 1979, and again in southern Congo in 1995, when the mortality rate reached 77%.

Consider these viral haemorrhagic fevers if a traveller to Africa presents within 3 weeks of travel with fever, headaches, myalgia, haemorrhagic features, thrombocytopenia and clotting abnormalities. If such a suspicion should arise, the local consultant in communicable disease control should be notified immediately, as the patient will need to be placed in a special isolation unit.

Hantavirus infection

Hantaviruses of the family *Bunyaviridae* are widely distributed throughout the Americas, Asia and Europe. The vector is the rodent population. Infection occurs by inhaling aerosols of rodent excreta, while person-to-person transmission is rare. These viruses cause two major human diseases: hantavirus pulmonary syndrome (HPS) exclusively in the Americas, and haemorrhagic fever with renal syndrome (HFRS) mainly in the Old World.

The symptoms are fever, myalgia, nausea, vomiting and diarrhoea. Thrombocytopenia, the presence of immunoblasts, and haemoconcentration point to the diagnosis. Death results from shock and cardiac complications. HFRS starts abruptly with backache, headaches, fever, rigors, and sometimes haemorrhage. In severe HFRS there is albuminuria. There is no specific treatment although ribavirin is promising.

Under development are vaccines against Sin Nombre, the predominant hantavirus strain in

North America, and the Hantaan in China where the virus causes 100 000 cases of severe HFRS each year. In Europe, HFRS is associated with Puumala (PUU) and Dobrava (DOB) hanta-viruses. PUU causes a mild disease mostly in northern Europe and in Russia, while DOB has been connected to a more severe form in Slovenia, Albania, Greece and Bosnia Herzegovina.

West Nile fever

West Nile fever is a mosquito-borne, febrile illness, endemic in Africa, the Middle East and South-Eastern Asia. The flavivirus has also been isolated in Australia and sporadically in Europe including Israel and, recently, the USA. Clinical features are acute fever with myalgia, arthralgia, headaches, conjunctivitis, a roseolar rash and lymphadenopathy. Occasionally (up to 15% of cases), it is complicated by meningitis or encephalitis.

Laboratory findings are slightly raised ESR, mild leukocytosis. It can be cultured (peak viraemia 4–8 days after infection). Recovery is complete, often accompanied by long-term myalgia and weakness. Most fatal cases occur in people over 50 years of age.

West Nile virus is a member of the Japanese encephalitis antigenic complex of the genus *Flavivirus*, family Flaviviridae. The virus was first isolated from the blood of a febrile woman in the West Nile district of Uganda in 1937 and was subsequently isolated from patients, birds and mosquitoes in Egypt in the early 1950s. It was soon to be found to be a widespread infection in Africa but also Europe and Asia. The virus has been isolated from 43 mosquito species, predominantly of the genus *Culex*. It affects mainly birds and, rarely, mammals such as camels, cattle, horses and dogs.

Amoebic liver abscess

Entamoeba histolytica infection of the bowel can be complicated by formation of an amoebic abscess, usually in the right liver lobe. The presenting symptoms may be fever and malaise. Bowel symptoms can be absent in over half of patients. The alkaline phosphatase is raised. The diagnosis is made by ultrasound, aspiration of the abscess and serology.

Cholera

Details can be found in Chapter 29.

Tuberculosis

Details can be found in Chapter 27.

Leprosy

Leprosy is an ancient disease that is often feared by travellers. It is a chronic granulomatous disease caused by the bacterium *Mycobacterium leprae*. It is spread by nasal secretions from lepromatous patients. Well over 90% of people are not susceptible to leprosy and after typical exposure will not develop it. Those who do, after an incubation of several years (5–10), may have a single lesion which often self-heals. When this does not happen or the single lesion is not treated, the disease may progress to the formation of further skin lesions. The diagnosis is usually established by the clinical picture and biopsy of the skin lesions. Six effective antileprosy drugs are available today but only rifampicin, dapsone and clofazimine are widely used. The others are minocycline, ofloxacin and clarithromycin. The BCG vaccine gives some protection against the disease.

Registered cases have fallen from 5.4 million worldwide in 1985 to below 1 million in 1998. The incidence, however, has changed very little; 685 000 new cases were registered in 1997. Most cases (92%) are detected in just 16 countries, led by India and Brazil. The disease is widespread in Asia, and also in Africa and South America. It occurs sporadically in other areas. About 10 cases have been notified each year in the past 10 years in England and Wales.

Leprosy is a notifiable disease.

Filariases

There are three main clinical forms of human filariasis.

Lymphatic filariasis

Lymphatic filariasis is caused by the nematode worms *Wuchereria bancrofti* and *Brugia malayi*. An infected mosquito bite injects larvae, which then migrate to the lymphatic system of humans. Six to 12 months later the new mature and pregnant female worms release a large number of microfilariae, which reach the peripheral blood to be ingested by a blood-sucking mosquito to complete their life cycle. Each adult worm lives for 4–6 years in the lymphatic system.

The patient may remain asymptomatic. If symptoms appear, it will usually be 9–12 months after infection. The patient may be asymptomatic or may suffer from episodic fevers lasting a few hours, rigors and sweating. Recurrent lymphangitis leads to chronic lymphatic obstruction and lymphoedema manifested as thickened, oedematous, hard skin, involving the breast, scrotum (testicular hydrocoele) and legs (elephantiasis). Demonstrating microfilariae in blood specimens taken at night, and serology supports the diagnosis. Treatment is with diethylcarbamazepine. Prevention is by vector control, and avoiding mosquito bites.

The disease is endemic in sub-Saharan Africa, Egypt, Arabian peninsula, southern and East Asia, the Indian subcontinent, Iran and Iraq, the northern coast and central areas of South America and the Caribbean. Generally, lymphatic filariasis affects an estimated 120 million people in 80 countries, and 1 billion people are at risk of infection in tropical regions. In recent years there has been an increase in Bancroftian filariasis in the Nile delta, around breeding sites of the *Culex pipiens* mosquitoes.

Long-term travellers to endemic areas are at greater risk of contracting the disease. No vaccine is available. Avoidance of mosquito bites is very important.

Onchocerciasis

Onchocerciasis is caused by the prelarval (microfilaria) and adult forms of *Onchocerca volvulus* and it is transmitted to humans by the bite of an infected female blackfly (Simulium fly) that breeds near fast-flowing water and bites at daytime. The larvae mature within a few months and produce microfilariae, which migrate to the skin (dermatitis, disfiguring skin changes) and eyes (conjunctivitis, keratitis, anterior uveitis), weight loss, growth arrest, epilepsy. There is lymphadenopathy and vision is affected (river blindness). Treatment is by a single yearly dose of ivermectin. Prevention is by vector control and avoiding blackfly bites (nets, insect repellents such as Mosi-guard Natural, wearing long-sleeved clothing, etc.).

The disease is endemic in 34 countries in a broad band across the central part of Africa, small areas in the Arabian peninsula (Yemen), and Latin America (Brazil, Colombia, Ecuador, Guatemala, Venezuela, southern Mexico). An estimated 17.7 million persons are infected with the parasite, the vast majority in Africa. The WHO has undertaken a programme of community-based annual administration of ivermectin and selective aerial spraying of insecticide in Africa. It aims to treat 50 million people and eliminate the disease in the 16 participating countries by the year 2002.

Long-term travellers to endemic areas are at greater risk of contracting the disease. No vaccine is available. Avoidance of blackfly bites is very important.

Loaisis

Loaisis is caused by the worm *Loa loa*. Infected horsefly or deerfly of the genus *Chrysops* inject the larvae into humans. Once mature they release microfilariae which concentrate in subcutaneous tissues, especially the periorbital skin and distal extremities. Involvement of the conjunctivae, sclerae, urticaria and fever are not uncommon. Treatment and prevention are as for lymphatic filariasis. It is mainly seen in central African rainforests.

Leishmaniasis

This is a term given to diseases caused by protozoa of the genus *Leishmania*, mainly transmitted by sandflies. The disease appears in the form of two syndromes; the visceral (kalaazar) and the cutaneous. A tenth of the world's population is at risk of infection with *Leishmania*. The WHO estimates that globally about 1.8 million new cases occur every year. There are no vaccines currently available and prevention is mainly by avoiding contact with sandflies—they are most active between dusk and dawn, although infection may be acquired during the daytime if resting sandflies are disturbed. Use protective clothing and insect repellents, as well as bed nets impregnated in permethrin, insecticide sprays and appropriate window screens.

Visceral leishmaniasis (kala-azar)

This leishmaniasis is caused by *Leishmania donovani* (seen in India and east Africa), *L. infantum* (Mediterranean) and *L. chagasi* (central and southern America). The reservoirs are humans in India (accounts for half of the world's cases), rodents in east Africa, and dogs in the Mediterranean, Central and South America, China and Asia. The incubation period is 2–4 months, after which a constant fever appears for a few weeks and then becomes intermittent. Weight loss, diarrhoea and malaise follow. Over several weeks the skin becomes darker as a result of increased pigmentation that gives the disease the name 'kala-azar' meaning 'the black sickness'. There is hepatomegaly and considerable splenomegaly, as well as pancytopenia and a raised ESR. The diagnosis can be confirmed by examining splenic aspirations and serology. Kala-azar behaves like an opportunistic infection in immunosuppressed patients such as those with advanced HIV disease. The treatment of choice is stibogluconate or amphotericin B.

Cutaneous leishmaniasis

This is common in tropical countries, the Middle East, the Mediterranean, China and the Indian subcontinent. After an incubation period of 2–6 weeks (sometimes a few months) a circular ulcer appears, usually on the face or extremities, with indurated edges and satellite lesions, associated with lymphadenitis. Most heal with a scar within a year. In the mucocutaneous form, months or years after the healing of the primary ulcer, mucosal lesions reappear, affecting the mouth, nose and pharynx.

Control of leishmaniasis is by vector control and avoiding bites of sandflies. Mosi-guard Natural can be effective as a repellent of sandflies.

Leishmania Genome Network provides up-to-date information on the current state of the physical mapping of the *Leishmania major* genome: http://www.ebi.ac.uk/parasites/leish.html

Schistosomiasis (bilharziasis)

Schistosomiasis is caused by parasitic flatworms, *Schistosoma*, that cause damage by their egg deposition in blood vessels. Three species commonly affect humans.

- *S. mansoni* causes intestinal schistosomiasis in Africa, the Middle East, the Caribbean and parts of South America (especially Brazil).
- *S. haematobium* causes urinary schistosomiasis in Africa (particularly along the Nile valley) and the Middle East (particularly along the Euphrates and Tigris rivers).
- *S. japonicum* causes intestinal schistosomiasis in the Far East and South-East Asia (particularly China and the Philippines).

The main host of the first two is humans while *S. japonicum* is hosted by various other mammals such as water buffalo, cattle, pigs, dogs and rodents. The intermediate host is the snail. In the case of *S. mansoni* and *S. haematobium* the freshwater snails found in pools, small lakes, irrigation canals or slowly flowing streams or rivers. Dam construction in three African river deltas—the Nile, the Senegal and the Volta, has led to a 75% increase in schistosomiasis infection in local villagers as well as upstream of the dams as far as 500 km away. For *S. japonicum* the intermediate host is an amphibious snail found in rice paddy fields and damp fallow land.

Once the eggs come into contact with fresh water they hatch to release larvae. They, in turn, infect the snail where they replicate asexually forming cercariae after about 1 month. The snail remains alive for a further 1–2 months producing cercariae and releasing them as free-swimming larvae in the water, at a rate of 1000 per day. The cercariae then penetrate the skin of the human host and become schistosomula. These migrate via the bloodstream, initially to the lungs and eventually to the hepatic portal system where they mature into adult worms, and migrate further into small venules of the inferior mesenteric vein—bowel (*S. mansoni*, *S. japonicum*) or vesical plexus—urine bladder (*S. haematobium*).

Six to 12 weeks after infection, the female worms are laying hundreds of eggs in the blood vessels every day for an average of 5 years. The eggs are transported by blood to the liver, lungs, spinal cord and central nervous system, where they cause fibrosis and inflammation leading to portal hypertension, lung fibrosis, cor pulmonale, transverse myelitis and epilepsy. In the urine bladder wall, fibrosis can lead to a form of cancer, which is the primary cause of death among men under 44 years in Egypt. Eggs are also released in the lumen of the bowel or bladder and pass out in the excreta (faeces or urine), thus completing the cycle.

Transmission is greatest during the rainy season and the peak prevalence of infection is in children aged 5–15 years. About 200 million people have acquired this infection from bathing or wading in infested rivers, lakes and irrigation systems. Every year 20 000 people die from this disease. About 40% of the world's school-age children (400 million) are infested with intestinal worms. Eighty-eight million children under 15 years of age are infected with schistosomiasis. For global distribution of schistosomiasis see Fig. 58.5.

When cercariae invade the skin, the swimmer may experience an itch a day or two later and even a rash. During the visceral invasion the patient may complain of a cough and abdominal discomfort. There is eosinophilia in the blood and the spleen may be palpable. Once there is significant infiltration the patient develops an acute illness (Katayama fever) characterized by fever, generalized aches, headaches, urticaria, abdominal pain, diarrhoea, lymphadenopathy and hepatosplenomegaly. There is marked eosinophilia. The patient's stools can be blood-stained or there is haematuria (depending on the species).

The clinical diagnosis is supported by the demonstration of eggs in stools, urine, or biopsy (liver, rectal, bladder). Serology fails to distinguish between present or past infection. None the less it is helpful when dealing with travellers.

The drug of choice for all three species is a single oral dose of praziquantel. Prevention is by targeted, selective chemotherapy especially of school-age children, improvement in sanitation and water supplies. Travellers should be advised not to swim in fresh water (the deep middle of the lake is safer than the shores), if visiting endemic areas (oceans and seas are safe, adequately chlorinated pools are virtually always safe). High-risk regions include the Nile and Lakes Victoria, Malawi, Tanganyika and Kariba in Africa. Also, along the Euphrates and Tigris rivers in the Middle East, and parts of the Amazon in Brazil.

Available tests for antibody detection are highly sensitive and specific. Tests for *Schistosoma* antigen in serum or urine are also available and offer the added advantage of close correlation with intensity of infection and disease activity.

There is no vaccine available. Bathing water should be heated to 50 °C for 5 min, or be treated with iodine or chlorine in a similar manner to precautions recommended for preparing drinking water (see p. 280), or allow the bath water to stand for 3 days (cercariae rarely survive longer than 48 h).

HIV infection and AIDS

The human immunodeficiency virus (HIV) is a retrovirus with two distinct serological types—HIV-1 and HIV-2. HIV-1 is responsible for most cases worldwide. HIV-2 was originally predominant in west Africa but has gradually spread beyond. Acquired immunodeficiency syndrome (AIDS) is a clinical syndrome characterized by progressive damage to the body's immune system, the development of opportunistic infection and tumours, in the presence of evidence of HIV infection. Indeed, the hallmark of HIV disease is a profound immunodeficiency. Each day more than a billion CD4+ cells (T4—subset of thymus-derived T-lymphocytes) are produced, infected and destroyed by the virus, eventually exhausting the patient's immune system, thus allowing opportunistic infection and encouraging certain forms of cancer (Kaposi's sarcoma, lymphoma, cervical and anal neoplasia).

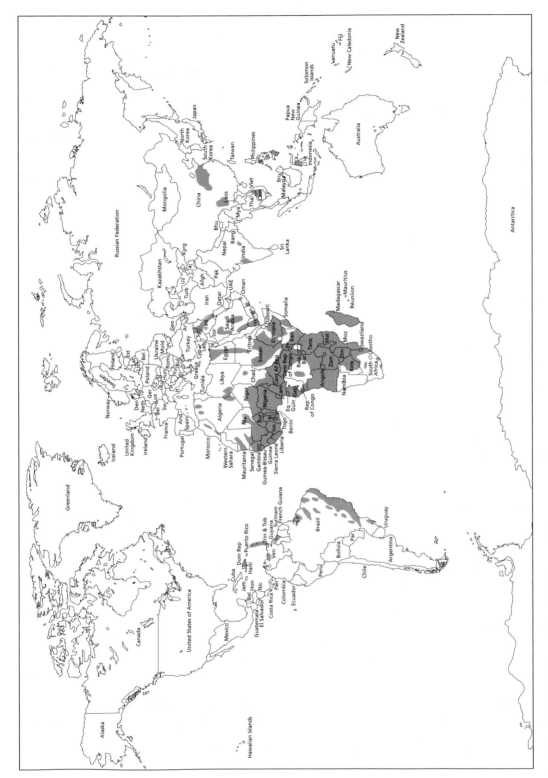

Fig. 58.5 The global distribution of schistosomiasis.

351

Transmission of the HIV virus is through the following.

- Sexual intercourse—vaginal, oral or anal. There is an increased risk of transmission during receptive anal intercourse and in the presence of a genital ulceration such as that of herpes virus infection.
- Vertical transmission—from mother to fetus *in utero*, at the time of delivery and, less commonly but still possible, during breast-feeding. In the absence of specific antiretroviral therapy, about 20% of nonbreast-feeding HIV-infected mothers in the UK, and up to 40% in Africa, transmit HIV to their children. Most babies become infected in the third trimester or during delivery. Current evidence indicates that caesarean section reduces the risk of transmission by half.
- Transfusion of blood or blood products—since 1985 all blood and blood products in the UK have been screened for HIV antibodies. This has had a dramatic positive effect on this mode of transmission (only 7 cases out of 34 000 in 1998). The risk of contracting HIV infection from blood and blood products is now very small. Nevertheless, the possibility exists of collecting blood from an infected donor before HIV antibodies have developed (the 'window period'). HIV antibody in the serum can take up to 3 months to develop after infection. Two such cases have been reported since 1985, one in Scotland in 1986 and one in England in 1997. This risk is reduced by advising individuals who are at increased risk of HIV infection not to donate blood. There have been no reports of HIV transmissions in the UK since the introduction of heat treatment of blood products.
- Travellers receiving blood transfusions should be aware that there is a higher risk that donors may be seroconverting if they have negative antibody test on screening in areas of high HIV prevalence. For supplies of safe blood prospective travellers may contact the Blood Care Foundation (see p. 286, and Sources of Travel Information on p. 400).
- The WHO estimates that medical treatment with blood-infected needles results in 80 000–160 000 cases of HIV infection a year worldwide.
- Sharing contaminated needles, syringes or other equipment.
- Occupational—increased risk among hospital

and laboratory staff. This may occur after a splash of infected material on mucous membranes or damaged skin. The risk of HIV transmission following a single skin puncture from a contaminated needle is approximately 1 in 300 (0.33%), and following a single mucocutaneous exposure it is 1 in 3000 (0.03%) [(2000) Preventing HIV infection. *Prescriber's Journal*, 40 (No. 1), 4–9].

Diagnosis

The detection of HIV infection requires testing for HIV antibody with standard ELISA or Western blot assays. The development of DNA and RNA PCR techniques has enabled researchers to document the presence of HIV in virtually all patients with AIDS and at all stages. The limitation is that PCR measures viral replication in the blood but does not indicate the degree of HIV replication in other parts of the body, such as the brain, eyes and testis. As a result, a patient could appear to be free of the virus following treatment, while still developing AIDS. Patients have to wait for a month for their results and it costs around £1000. A new test, announced in December 1999 by researchers from the London Hammersmith Hospital, uses waste products of HIV replication to determine whether HIV is still present and replicating in patients taking antiretroviral drugs. It targets peripheral white blood cells containing viral circles of HIV DNA, indicating they had 'visited' hidden sites on infection. The results of this test are available within 24 h at one-tenth of the cost of the PCR test.

Infection

Infection with HIV can be asymptomatic or associated with a variety of clinical symptoms.

- *Prodromal seroconversion illness*—within 4–12 weeks of infection the patient develops pyrexia, with the clinical picture resembling glandular fever. There can be mild lymphadenopathy present and often there are atypical mononuclear cells in the blood. These symptoms coincide with the development of HIV antibodies. A minority of patients will present with pyrexia and a painless rash that is not itchy, a few with lymphocytic meningitis. Occasionally there may be opportunistic infections such as candidal oesophagitis or *Pneumocystis carinii*, pneumonia.

• *Latent HIV infection*—the patient may remain asymptomatic from 18 months to 15 years (60% for up to 10 years). Towards the end of this period many patients develop generalized lymphadenopathy. The CD4 (T4) count starts to fall below 400 $\times 10^9$/L.

• *Symptomatic HIV infection*—symptoms are overall related to skin and mucous membranes: varicella zoster infection, oral candidiasis, oral hairy leukoplakia, seborrhoeic dermatitis, persistent generalized lymphadenopathy, cervical dysplasia, pelvic inflammatory disease, vaginal candidiasis, recurrent minor infections, fatigue, fever, headaches, myalgia, arthralgia, retro-orbital pain, weight loss, diarrhoea and night sweats.

• *Progression to AIDS*—eventually the patient's immune system is exhausted and he or she develops a specified opportunistic infection or a secondary cancer. Among these are: oropharyngo-oesophageal candidal infection, *P. carinii* pneumonia, tuberculosis (a lethal partnership), cerebral toxoplasmosis, *Cryptococcus neoformans* meningitis, chronic diarrhoea as a result of *Cryptosporidium*, lymphomas, *Salmonella* recurrent infection or septicaemia, cervical carcinoma, Kaposi's sarcoma, wasting syndrome. The patient goes on to develop forgetfulness, loss of concentration, loss of balance, dementia and confusion. AIDS has a very long and variable incubation period, ranging from a few months to many years. Some persons infected with HIV have remained asymptomatic for more than a decade. Once the diagnosis of AIDS is made, the mean time to death in the UK is 20 months (6 months in 1985).

Medication

There are drugs licensed for HIV and AIDS in the UK—GPs are not required to prescribe them and only specialist pharmacies stock them. The treatment overall is supervised by hospital specialists.

Prevention of HIV infection is most important. Travellers are at much higher risk than when they remain at home, not only because of often different behaviour in travellers but also because of the fact that there may be poor medical and hygiene conditions in the destination country. At risk are the long- as well as short-term travellers, people visiting relatives and people working abroad. Current data indicate that 75% of heterosexually contracted HIV is attributable to having sex while abroad.

The scale of the HIV/AIDS problem

Although AIDS does not kill as many millions as other diseases, such as tuberculosis or malaria, it does kill young people in their most productive years. Many developing countries are deprived of skilled and managerial workers they cannot afford to lose. The cost of preventing AIDS and caring for people with the disease can be beyond what some developing countries could possibly afford.

Around 90% of new infections arise in poorly resourced countries, which together account for only 10% of global gross national products. Commonwealth countries are disproportionately affected and contain 60% of prevalent HIV infections worldwide. The WHO estimates that about nine out of 10 people living with HIV are unaware of their infection.

At the end of 1999, it was estimated there were about 33.6 million people in the world alive and living with HIV/AIDS infection (see Fig. 58.6). Of them, 23.5 million live in Africa, 6 million in South and South-East Asia and 2.2 million in the Americas. About 14 million people have died already from HIV/AIDS.

Figure 58.7 shows the estimated number of new HIV infections in 1999 by region (estimated total 5.6 million). The steepest increase in reports of HIV infection has been in the newly independent states of the former Soviet Union where the number of people living with HIV infection is estimated to have doubled in the 2 years to December 1999. The main group of new cases are intravenous drug users. In 1998/9, Ukraine accounted for around 90% of all AIDS cases reported in the WHO's Eastern European Region. Cases in Russia are rising alarmingly too.

The region most affected by HIV infection remains sub-Saharan Africa, which accounts for

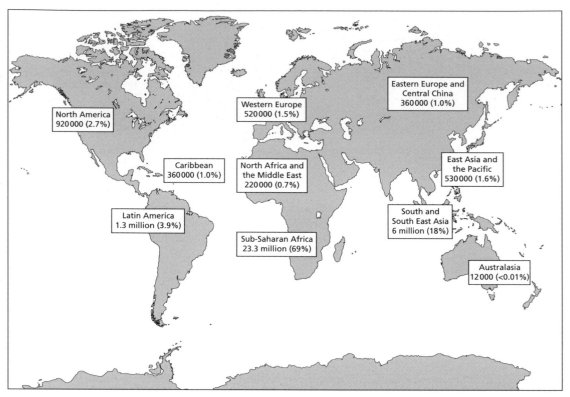

Fig. 58.6 UNAIDS/WHO estimated number and distribution of people living with HIV/AIDS at the end of 1999. (Reproduced with permission of the PHLS Communicable Disease Surveillance Centre © PHLS.)

69% of all prevalent infections, and 68% of transmission (Fig. 58.7), even though it accommodates only about 10% of the world's population. Southern Africa fares badly. One in seven new infections in sub-Saharan Africa is thought to occur in South Africa. In Botswana, Namibia, Swaziland and Zimbabwe up to 30% of all adults aged 15–49 years are infected with HIV (*Communicable Disease Report*, Vol. 9 no. 52, 25 Dec. 1999). The WHO estimates that in Kenya, over 1.5 million people are HIV-positive, and over half a million people have died from AIDS. In Thailand, the WHO estimates that 7.8 million people are HIV-positive, and nearly a quarter of a million have died from AIDS (WHO's website—http://www.who.int).

The number of cases of AIDS in 1997 estimated by the WHO was 12 940 000, with sub-Saharan Africa being the biggest contributor (10 457 000) followed by South and East Asia (850 000), North America (690 000) and Latin America (510 000).

The number of adults living in England, Wales and Northern Ireland with diagnosed HIV infection had risen by 29% between the end of 1995 (14 200) and the end of 1998 (18 300). Most of this increase occurred in 1997 and 1998, when annual increases of 12 and 13% were observed. Numbers of HIV infection diagnosed in the UK in 1999 are the highest recorded in the last 10 years (3300 new cases), with the number of heterosexually acquired infection overtaking those of infection acquired through sex between men.

By the end of 1999, it was estimated that over 60 000 individuals had tested HIV-positive, with around 18 000 cases of AIDS. There have been 12 800 AIDS/HIV-related deaths, and over 10 000 people are alive with undiagnosed HIV infection. One of the reasons the number of patients with HIV/AIDS is rising is the available antiretroviral therapy, which is delaying the onset of AIDS and deaths in many of those treated.

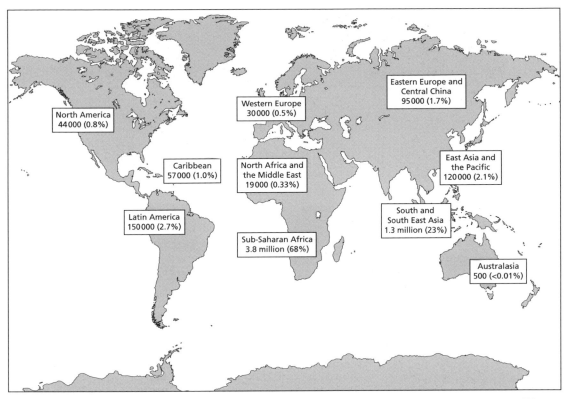

North America
44 000 (0.8%)

Western Europe
30 000 (0.5%)

Eastern Europe and
Central China
95 000 (1.7%)

Caribbean
57 000 (1.0%)

North Africa and
the Middle East
19 000 (0.33%)

East Asia and
the Pacific
120 000 (2.1%)

Latin America
150 000 (2.7%)

South and
South East Asia
1.3 million (23%)

Sub-Saharan Africa
3.8 million (68%)

Australasia
500 (<0.01%)

Fig. 58.7 UNAIDS/WHO estimated number of new HIV infections in 1999 by region (estimated total 5.6 million). (Reproduced with permission of the PHLS Communicable Disease Surveillance Centre © PHLS.)

By 31 December 2000, all Health Authorities in England should be offering and recommending an HIV test as an integral part of their antenatal care. The aim is to reduce the transmission of HIV infection to neonates. The administration of zidovudine to HIV-infected women during pregnancy and in labour, and to the neonate for the first 6 weeks of life, greatly reduces mother to child transmission of HIV. This, as well as a large increase in the proportion of elective caesarean section deliveries, has contributed a fall in HIV vertical transmission from 19% in 1995 to 2% in 1998 among mothers whose diagnosis had been known during pregnancy. Further guidance on mother-to-baby transmission of HIV as well as HIV and infant feeding can be found on the DoH's website: http://www.doh.gov.uk/coinh/htm. Africa bears approximately 70% of the worldwide burden of AIDS.

Treatment

Up-to-date *Guidelines on the Use of Antiretroviral Agents in HIV-Infected adults and Adolescents*, by the USA Panel on Clinical Practices for the Treatment of HIV Infection (a joint effort of the Department of Health and Human Services and the Henry J. Kaiser Family Foundation) is available to clinicians on http://www.hivatis.org. Single copies may be ordered by calling (301) 519 0459, or by E-mail: atis@hivatis.org

Postexposure prophylaxis

Healthcare staff exposed to blood that is potentially HIV-positive as a result of an accident, e.g. needle stick or splash injury, are recommended in the USA and most European countries to have 4 weeks' treatment of triple antiretroviral therapy: zidovudine 200 mg three times daily, plus lamivudine 150 mg twice daily, plus indinavir 800 mg three times daily.

The UK guidelines on HIV postexposure prophylaxis 2000

The Expert Advisory Group on AIDS (EAGA) published its guidelines on the use of post-exposure prophylaxis for HIV in July 2000 [UK Health Departments (2000) *HIV postexposure prophylaxis; guidance from the UK Chief Medical Officers' EAGA.* DoH, London. http://www.doh.gov.uk/eaga]. They replace those published in 1997 [UK Health Departments. (1997) *Guidelines on postexposure prophylaxis for health care workers occupationally exposed to HIV. Recommendations of the Expert Advisory Group on AIDS.* DoH, London].

Serious side-effects have been noted with the previously recommended drug combination of zidovudine, lamivudine and indinavir (especially with the latter). The new guidance suggests nelfinavir or soft gel saquinavir as alternative protease inhibitors to indinavir. When the results of anti-retroviral resistance testing in the source patient are available, it is recommended that these should be taken into account when selecting postexposure prophylaxis drugs—seek specialist advice in such circumstances.

The guidance includes new sections on health care workers from the UK seconded overseas, and exposures outside the health care setting. Recommended drug regimens, drug resistance, interactions and the special considerations for health care workers who are, or may be, pregnant are included in new annexes.

HIV vaccine

The development of an HIV vaccine poses one of the biggest challenges to scientists. Among the problems they face is the fact that stimulating neutralizing antibody formation is not sufficient to prevent HIV-1 infection (high titres in HIV patients do not alter the disease progression) and does not prevent the latent phase. Furthermore, the HIV undergoes frequent antigenic variations, making it difficult to achieve the right strain composition.

There is a need to identify unique vaccine immune-response markers so that immunity from the vaccine can be distinguished from natural infection. Testing the vaccine is also a problem as it takes on average 10 years from infection to development of AIDS. To solve these problems, scientists are employing DNA technology. Indeed, US scientists have reported [(1997) *Nature Medicine* 3, 526–32] successful blockage of transmission of HIV-1 in chimpanzees (the closest relative to humans in terms of immunological response) with a new vaccine based on DNA technology. The vaccine was developed from the genes of a weakened virus, rather than the proteins produced by those genes. This DNA vaccine was shown to be capable of interrupting the establishment of persistent infection in the chimpanzees.

The US FDA has approved the first phase III trial of the VaxGen's AIDSVAX. This vaccine consists of recombinant gp120 envelope antigens from two HIV-1 strains. In earlier trials, AIDSVAX induced strong circulating antibody responses. Phase III trials will now find out to what extent these antibodies protect against HIV-1.

The vaccines now under development and/or under trials are:

- live attenuated virus;
- subunit peptide vaccine, e.g. gp120;
- synthetic peptide vaccine of gene sequences, e.g. gag;
- bacterial or viral vectors with HIV DNA inserts, e.g. canarypox;
- plasmids with HIV DNA inserts.

The first human trials of a new HIV vaccine are to begin simultaneously in South Africa and USA in February 2001. The vaccine, Alphavax, is a hybrid of HIV and Venezuelan equine encephalitis, a disease contracted by horses, which is designed to trigger a huge human immune response against HIV. This vaccine will tackle type C HIV, the strain that affects more than 90% of South Africans that have the virus. If successful, the vaccine could be made available by 2005.

Further information can be found on the Internet: International AIDS Vaccine Initiative—http://www.iavi.org and the WHO's UNAIDS website: http://www.unaids.org

Health advice for travellers with HIV/AIDS

For advice to the HIV-positive and AIDS traveller see p. 324.

For advice on Safer Sex for Travellers see p. 385.

For special leaflets published by the DoH, Tel.: 0800 555 777. Also contact the Terence Higgins Trust Helpline, the National AIDS Helpline and MASTA—for addresses and telephone numbers see Sources of Travel Information in Chapter 64.

The revised *Guidance to Reduce Risks to Patients from Healthcare Workers Exposed to HIV Infection* was published in December 1998 and is available from the DoH. It can also be accessed via the Internet on http://www.open.gov.uk/doh/aids.htm

Advice for health professionals

The Journal of the American Medical Association (*J. Am. Med. Assoc.*) maintains a website with information on HIV, prevention and treatment, as well as articles published, daily updates on HIV from CDC, coverage of conferences, etc. http://www.ama-assn.org

Travellers' diarrhoea

Travellers' diarrhoea is by far the most common illness to afflict travellers, especially those travelling to tropical or semitropical regions from industrialized countries. The incidence varies according to destination (up to 55% in some countries) (see Fig. 58.8). Between 30 and 40% of travellers develop traveller's diarrhoea [McKee M. (1996) *Br. Med. J.* 312, 925–6].

According to the WHO, diarrhoeal disease caused more than 3.3 million deaths worldwide in 1995, of which 80% were children under the age of 2 years. In the same year, the WHO estimated that there were over 1 billion episodes of diarrhoea in children. Food is responsible for up to 70% of diarrhoea episodes and water as well as person-to-person spread accounting for the rest. It is important that breastfeeding is promoted, as it is an effective way of the infants in developing countries avoiding the disease. Food hygiene and the provision of clean water are very important. In addition, vitamin A supplementation reduces diarrhoea mortality by 30% in young children.

Definition

A traveller is said to have travellers' diarrhoea if, while abroad or within 10 days after returning home, they experience a syndrome that is characterized by diarrhoea (twofold or greater increase in the frequency of unformed stools per day, usually three or more) and at least one of the following accompanying signs or symptoms: abdominal pain/cramps, nausea, vomiting, faecal urgency, tenesmus (straining) and sometimes fever and frank dysentery (passage of bloody stools). Milder forms are characterized by one or two unformed stools per day with or without additional symptoms.

Symptoms usually start on the third day (most cases within the first week) after arrival at destination, and 20% will have a second episode in the second week. It usually begins suddenly and, if untreated, lasts on average 5 days, with the severity varying widely. In approximately 10% it lasts longer than a week, in 2% of cases the diarrhoea and other signs and symptoms will last longer than 1 month, even a year. In these cases consider intestinal protozoa such as *Giardia lamblia*, *Cryptosporidium* or *Cyclospora*.

Bacterial enteropathogens, including enterotoxigenic *Escherichia coli* (ETEC), may cause illness that lasts over 2 weeks and therefore the traveller may return symptomatic. If symptoms persist in a well patient, with no weight loss and with negative stool culture and microscopy, the patient may be suffering from a postinfective irritable bowel syndrome (IBS) that may take as long as 1 year to subside. Individuals with a past history of IBS may suffer a recurrence of their symptoms.

Travellers at higher risk are those who have not travelled to the tropics in the previous 6 months, those with high socioeconomic status, young children and the elderly, those staying and/or sharing food with locals, with achlorhydria (postgastrectomy, on acid-suppressant medication), with chronic inflammatory bowel disease, and the

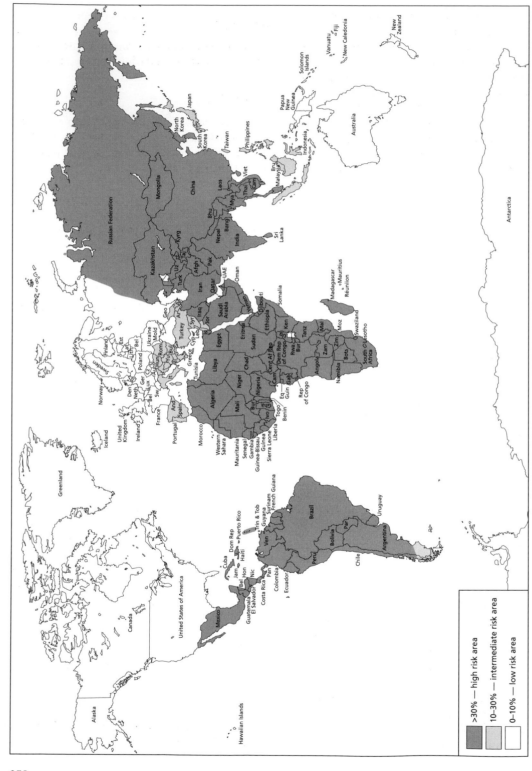

Fig. 58.8 Estimated rate and comparable risk of travellers' diarrhoea infection according to the area visited. (This map generalizes available data.)

>30% — high risk area

10–30% — intermediate risk area

0–10% — low risk area

immunodeficient travellers (because of treatment or disease—AIDS patients are particularly at risk of infection with intestinal protozoa such as *Giardia* and *Cryptosporidia*).

Transmission of the pathogens causing travellers' diarrhoea is mainly by the faecal–oral route through contaminated food, water and also by direct person-to-person spread. Poor personal health, immunity and hygiene, inadequate sanitation and lack of clean water are important factors.

Aetiology

Bacteria

Bacteria are responsible for over 80% of cases.

Enterotoxigenic Escherichia coli

Enterotoxigenic *Escherichia coli* (ETEC) is a major cause of diarrhoea. In high risk areas it accounts for over half of the cases and is spread mainly in contaminated food and water. Other *E. coli* infections are rarer but it is worth mentioning *E. coli 0157:H7*. Its reservoir is the gastrointestinal tract of cattle and possibly other domesticated animals. Meat can become contaminated during slaughter and organisms can be thoroughly mixed into beef when it is ground. Drinking unpasteurized milk and swimming in or drinking sewage-contaminated water can also cause infection. Children under 5 years of age and the elderly are particularly at risk of complications such as haemolytic uraemic syndrome. Countries such as the USA or UK do not escape from this infection.

Campylobacter jejuni

This organism was identified as early as 1913 in fetal tissues of aborted sheep. It is now the leading cause (2.1–2.4 million cases every year) of bacterial gastroenteritis in the USA, where its resistance to quinolones has risen from 1.3% in 1992 to 10.2% in 1998. Its reservoir is the gastrointestinal tract of birds (particularly poultry) and animals such as cattle and domestic pets (raw, undercooked meat, unpasteurized milk or even bird-pecked milk on the doorstep, contact with infected pets).

Shigella spp.

These are transmitted via the faecal–oral route from cases with diarrhoea as well as by food and water.

Salmonella spp.

These are transmitted from contaminated, insufficiently cooked meat, eggs, milk, dairy products, also person-to-person during the acute phase. For typhoid see Chapter 40.

Aeromonas spp., Plesiomonas spp.

Transmitted by water and contaminated food. Vomiting and diarrhoea.

Vibrio parahaemolyticus and other noncholera vibrios

Contaminated food, shellfish. Diarrhoea and fever.

Clostridia

Contaminated cooked meat and poultry dishes.

Yersinia spp.

Contaminated food. Diarrhoea, fever, arthritis.

Listeria monocytogenes

Unpasteurized milk, cheese, pâté, contaminated vegetables and meat products. Known to grow at refrigeration temperatures—keep high-risk foods such as soft cheese and pâté at temperatures below 4 °C. Neonates can acquire the disease from an infected maternal birth canal, when it carries a mortality rate of up to 30%.

Viruses

Viruses are responsible for about 8% of cases.

Rotavirus A, B and C

Person-to-person by faecal–oral route. Especially common in children.

Small round viruses (e.g. Norwalk and other agents)

Person-to-person by faecal–oral route, contaminated food and water. Mild, short-lived diarrhoeal illness, often associated with vomiting.

Enteric adenoviruses and astrovirus

Diarrhoea in children.

Protozoa

Protozoa are responsible for 10–15% of cases.

Giardia lamblia

Faecally contaminated water, food, person-to-person via the faecal–oral route. Boiling the water will kill the infective cysts. The incubation period is 5–25 days. Acute and persistent abdominal pain, diarrhoea, bloating, fatigue, flatulence ('eggy burps'), metallic taste in the mouth, anorexia, nausea, weight loss. Symptoms last for over 5 days. Fever and vomiting are uncommon.

Up to 6% of persons having traveller's diarrhoea have *Giardia lamblia*. About 200 million people have giardiasis, 500 000 new cases a year, the vast majority of them in children. In some developing countries 20–30% of the population can be infected. Widespread in Latin America, Africa, Asia and Russia but outbreaks can occur anywhere and in developed countries (Sweden, Australia). There is no effective chemoprophylaxis. Metronidazole or tinidazole (2 g once daily for 2 days) can be used for treatment. Asymptomatic carriers need to be treated if they come into contact with pregnant women, cystic fibrosis or immunocompromised patients.

Entamoeba histolytica

Faecally contaminated food, water, person-to-person, mainly among male homosexuals. Diarrhoea develops over 1–3 weeks and contains blood and mucus. Symptoms persist over several weeks. Among the complications is amoebic liver abscess. It occurs throughout tropical and subtropical Africa, Asia, the Middle East, Central and South America. Up to 6% of persons with travellers' diarrhoea have *Entamoeba histolytica*. It is estimated that 480 million people are infected, of whom 90% are asymptomatic.

Cryptosporidium spp.

Recognized in humans since 1976. A six-continent infection, it affects all ages—more common in those over 2 years of age. Exclusive breast-feeding protects. Faecally contaminated water or food, direct contact with an infected person (particularly through sexual oro–anal contact) or animal, swallowing water while swimming in contaminated waters. From asymptomatic to severe life-threatening disease. Diarrhoea and slight fever usually for 3–7 days in immunocompetent individuals. In immunocompromised patients it can be fatal—particularly a problem in patients with AIDS. The organism is highly infectious and can survive routine water chlorination. Rehydration is important. Azithromycin may be beneficial for some people. Water should be boiled. No vaccine is available.

Microsporidia

These are an important cause of chronic diarrhoea in immunocompromised HIV patients.

Isospora belli infection

First described in 1915. This is an important cause of chronic diarrhoea among HIV-infected patients in sub-Saharan Africa and generally in immunosuppressed patients, in whom we see a relapse of the order of 5%. In immunocompetent people it is a self-limiting condition.

Cyclospora cayetanensis

First observed in the 1980s. Can be contracted by ingesting food or water contaminated with the parasite. It can be asymptomatic or can cause protracted diarrhoea for several weeks or months, with weight loss, dyspepsia, flatulence, nausea, vomiting, fatigue, myalgia, and low-grade fever. Direct person-to-person transmission is less likely with this organism. Immunocompromised patients fare worse.

Treatment—prevention

Best treatment is prevention. For advice on food and water hygiene for travellers see Chapter 50.

Treatment starts with pretravel advice, which has been shown to be effective in reducing the need for medical assistance while abroad. Only very clean water should be used for drinking and tooth brushing. Carbonated bottled water/drinks with intact seals are ideal when the drinking water source is in question. Undercooked meat, salads, raw shellfish and ice-cubes should be avoided. Warn travellers that intimate sexual contact can transmit enteropathogens (especially homosexual contact).

Advise the traveller with diarrhoea to rest and drink plenty of clear fluids but to avoid milk. If proprietary sugar and salt solutions are not available, travellers can make one up by adding 1 level teaspoon of salt and 8 level teaspoonfuls of sugar to 1 litre of clean, safe water. This solution may be flavoured to taste with squash concentrate. The minimum water intake should be one glass after every motion and another glass every hour. If vomiting occurs sip water frequently. For food, if it is necessary, they could try bananas, salted crisps, clear soups, and rice. Breast-fed babies should continue feeding from their mother.

Antidiarrhoeals

Loperamide (Imodium): Administer two capsules initially, followed after 1 h by one capsule with each diarrhoea motion, up to a maximum of eight per day. Children aged 4–8 years, 5 mL and 9–12 years, 10 mL or 1 capsule three or four times daily. Diphenoxylate (Lomotil): four tablets initially then two every 6 hours in adults. Children aged 4–8 years one tablet three times daily, 9–12 years, one four times a day and 13–16 years, two three times daily. They can be given if the adult or a child traveller over 4 years of age experiences diarrhoea, especially with painful spasms. Adequate hydration is of paramount importance. They can be taken for a short period, up to 3 days (young children) to 5 days, before a local physician should

be contacted. They should not be used where invasive disease is suspected, e.g. in the presence of blood or mucus in the stools and/or fever.

Antibiotics

These should be considered in the immunocompromised or those in whom, because of their age or medical condition (e.g. cardiac disease), even a small degree of dehydration may have health implications. Treatment can range from a single dose to a course of 3–5 days.

Ciprofloxacin (or any other quinolone) is the drug of choice as it covers ETEC, as well as *Salmonella* and *Campylobacter* (normally contraindicated in children and growing adolescents except where benefits exceed risks—also contraindicated in pregnancy). For mild to moderate disease, a single dose of 500 mg is given and perhaps repeated if diarrhoea is still present after 4–8 h. An alternative dose is 250–500 mg twice daily for 1–3 days. For severe disease (diarrhoea with systemic symptoms) it should be given twice daily for 5 days. Ideally, the traveller that is to take ciprofloxacin if needed should purchase the preparation in the UK, as the quality of the product including the dissolving ability of the capsule cannot be guaranteed in a developing country.

Erythromycin covers *Campylobacter* well. Metronidazole (2 g daily for 3 days—no alcohol) or tinidazole (2 g—4 tablets in a single dose) are indicated if giardiasis (abdominal distension) or amoebic dysentery is suspected. Other antibiotics that can be used are doxycycline 100 mg twice daily or trimethoprim 100 mg twice daily. Prolonged therapy is not usually recommended. The usual course is 2–5 days.

Antimicrobial chemoprophylaxis

A number of broad-spectrum antibiotics have been shown to reduce the incidence of travellers' diarrhoea by 70–90%. Their indiscriminate use could increase resistance to them. Routine antibiotic chemoprophylaxis is not needed or recommended for most travellers. It may be considered for the following cases.

• Travellers with an underlying illness such that

an attack of diarrhoea could compromise the patient's health (e.g. immunocompromised patients such as with AIDS, malignancy, insulin-dependent diabetes mellitus, postgastrectomy, on antacids such as proton pump inhibitors or H_2 blockers and generally hypochlorhydria, cardio-vascular disease, history of stroke/TIA, inflammatory bowel disease, elderly infirm, etc.). Assess each patient individually.

- History of severe repeated travellers' diarrhoea.
- VIPs or other travellers that cannot afford to lose any time because of very important commitments.
- A traveller who is making a very short trip (3–5 days) during which loss of any time would seriously impact on the success of their visit.

Antibiotics that can be used are quinolones (e.g. ciprofloxacin 250 mg daily—90% effective, ofloxacin once daily), doxycycline 200 mg on the first day, then 100 mg daily, trimethoprim 100 mg daily and, in some instances, such as travel to Mexico during rainy summertime, co-trimoxazole one tablet daily can be considered. They are given once daily, beginning on the day of travel and continuing until after return home. Such treatment is usually 70–90% effective.

The WHO does not recommend antibiotics in children, especially in the under-5-year-olds. Antibiotics are effective in children too and the usual contraindications should be observed. Hospitalization of a child in a developing country may put that child at risk. Appropriate rehydration in the young as well as the elderly is very important. Avoid antispasmodics in children.

Warn female patients on the oral contraceptive pill (combined or progesterone-only) of the need to continue taking their pill during an attack of diarrhoea and in addition to use condoms or abstain from sexual intercourse until 1 week after the diarrhoea has ceased (see the Woman Traveller, p. 311).

Bismuth subsalicylate

Bismuth subsalicylate (two tablets four times daily at meal times and before bedtime—in the UK the liquid (87.6 mg/5 mL) formulation is available—30 mL four times daily for adults) may be used as an alternative nonantibiotic chemoprophylactic agent; it has an overall efficacy of about 60%. There are concerns about bismuth toxicity following long-term ingestion. Side-effects include temporary blackening of tongue and stools, constipation, nausea, tinnitus. Avoid in aspirin sensitivity, renal failure, gout, and during warfarin or methotrexate use. It should not be used for over 3-week periods and it should not be given to children under 3 years of age.

Probiotics

The concept of colonizing the gastrointestinal tract with a protective and harmless microflora is an attractive approach to the prevention of travellers' diarrhoea. *Lactobacillus GG* has been shown to produce modest protection. *Lactobacillus acidophilus* and *L. fermentum* were no better than placebo when evaluated in British servicemen in Belize.

Vaccines

We do not currently have a multivalent vaccine. Measles immunization is very important. An oral, killed, whole-cell ETEC preparation, plus cholera toxin B subunit vaccine is now available (not in the UK) see Chapter 29.

Rotavirus

Rotavirus is the most common cause of severe dehydrating diarrhoea in infants worldwide. It is responsible for 600 000 to 800 000 of the 3 million deaths of children worldwide caused by diarrhoea every year. The tetravalent rhezus vaccine Rota-Shield (Wyeth-Ayerst) was introduced to the USA childhood immunization programme in August 1998. The trials in the USA and Finland had shown that the vaccine had an efficacy of 49–68% in preventing rotavirus diarrhoea overall and, importantly, 69–91% efficacy in preventing severe disease. The vaccination programme was suspended in the summer of 1999 after cases of bowel obstruction (intussusception) were reported in infants in the weeks after vaccination, representing an additional risk of 1 in 10 000 for this complication. Soon after the manufacturer withdrew the vaccine from the market.

A new oral rotavirus vaccine (Avant Immunotherapeutics—licensed to SmithKline Beecham) has shown 89% efficacy in a Phase II study and will be proceeding to Phase III trials. This compares with efficacy ranging from 49% in the largest US study of RotaShield to 68% in a Finnish trial.

Breast-feeding

Diarrhoea is less common in breast-fed babies and this should be encouraged. Parents of infants are best advised not to travel with their children to high risk areas. Breast-feeding should be continued during diarrhoea. Non-breast-fed babies should receive clear fluids in small amounts to start with, building up the dose as the child is tolerating the fluids.

Patients who return home from foreign travel with diarrhoea of over 5 days' duration should have a stool examination by microscopy and culture (ideally three separate samples). If antibiotics were taken before the onset of diarrhoea, the possibility of infection with *Clostridium difficile* (pseudomembranous colitis) should be borne in mind and appropriate cultures requested. If the stools contain blood, request culture for *Salmonella, Shigella, Campylobacter* and *Escherichia coli* (especially 0157). Febrile travellers returning from a region where malaria is endemic must have malaria excluded. Bloody diarrhoea persisting for more than 14 days should be investigated (sigmoidoscopy/colonoscopy) in order to investigate possible inflammatory bowel disease.

Helicobacter pylori infection

Helicobacter pylori infection is one of the world's most common bacterial infections. It was first shown to be associated with gastritis in Perth, Australia in 1982. The organism is present in virtually all patients with duodenal ulcer and more than 80% of those with gastric ulcers. Also in 92% of patients with mucosal-associated lymphoid tissue (MALT) lymphoma and may be associated with gastric carcinoma (about 550 000 new cases a year). The WHO has declared *H. pylori* as a Class 1 carcinogen. Although the aetiology of gastric carcinoma is multifactorial, it has now been established that *H. pylori* infection may eventually lead to the development of this cancer.

The geographical distribution of *H. pylori* is closely related to socioeconomic conditions. In developing countries, seroprevalence rises steeply after 1 year of age to reach around 50% among 10-year-olds and 80% by young adulthood in poor socioeconomic conditions. In industrialized countries it is relatively uncommon in earlier years, increasing to 40–70% among the elderly. Thus socioeconomic deprivation and increasing age are important risk factors for *H. pylori*. A crowded environment (e.g. sharing beds) has also been identified as a risk factor. Prevalence of infection is increased in the families of infected children.

Transmission of the organism is thought to be from person-to-person, via the faecal–oral and oro–oral route, as the bacterium is found in saliva, in dental plaque, vomitus and faeces. About 1% of *H. pylori* is caught from animals, such as cats and dogs. The frequency of transmission in adults is low, while it is higher among children.

Sixty per cent of *H. pylori* strains are cytotoxic, while 40% are not. The observation that some strains of the organism may have characteristics that make them inherently more pathogenic may explain why not all people with *H. pylori* infection develop peptic ulcers.

Treatment is by a combination of a proton pump inhibitor, e.g. omeprazole or lansoprazole, and one (clarithromycin or amoxycillin) or two (add metronidazole or tinidazole) antibiotics.

As yet, there is no effective vaccine against this infection.

Chapter 59

Malaria

The popular view before 1897 was that malaria was caused by contaminated air (hence malaria) or through infected water. During that year Ronald Ross worked out how the parasite spreads and how to prevent the disease by killing mosquitoes or preventing them from biting or breeding. Ross won the Nobel Prize in 1902, was knighted in 1911 and died in 1932. Malaria was common in England between the times of Elizabeth I and Victoria. It disappeared between 1860 and 1930. The English word for malaria was ague (Shakespeare mentioned ague in eight of his plays), a term that remained in common use until the nineteenth century. Oliver Cromwell died of ague in 1658. In 1975, the WHO declared Europe free from malaria. The last indigenous case in England had been in the 1950s and in Brueghel's Holland in 1961.

Malaria is one of the more common and serious of the tropical diseases. About 40% of the world's population live where there is a risk of malaria. Children under 5 years old and pregnant women in malaria-endemic areas are at greatest risk of dying from the disease. There are about 300–500 million new clinical cases of malaria and about 1.5–2.7 million deaths worldwide every year [American Academy of Paediatrics (2000) *Red Book*, p. 382], the majority (90%) of them in sub-Saharan Africa, where young children are the most affected—it is responsible for one in five deaths in children [WHO (1999) *The World Health Report 1999, 'Making a difference'*]. Indeed, in this area of Africa, 74% of the population live in highly endemic areas and a further 18% live in epidemic areas; about 550 million people are at risk, there are about 270 million new cases, with almost 1 million deaths every year according to the WHO.

Malaria has been re-emerging at an alarming and unprecedented rate in Africa. Factors that appear to be contributing to the resurgence of malaria are:

- rapid spread of resistance of malaria parasites to chloroquine and the other quinolones;
- frequent armed conflicts and civil unrest in many countries, forcing populations to settle under difficult conditions, sometimes in areas of high malaria transmission;
- migration for reasons of agriculture, commerce, and trade, from areas with no or low malaria levels to high transmission areas;
- changing rainfall patterns;
- water development projects such as dams and irrigation schemes at low altitudes, which create new mosquito breeding sites (other vector-borne diseases of concern include schistosomiasis, filariasis, onchocerciasis);
- changes in the behaviour of the vectors, particularly in biting habits, from indoor to outdoor biters;
- high birth rates leading to a rapid increase in the susceptible population under 5 years of age;
- adverse socioeconomic conditions leading to a much reduced budget and gross inadequacy of funds for drugs and prevention.

Despite the fact that malaria continues to be one of the biggest contributors to disease burdens in terms of death and suffering, research into the disease is suffering from lack of funds. In its 1996 report the Wellcome Trust's unit for Policy Research in Science and Medicine points out that total global expenditure on malaria research in 1993 was only about $84 million, compared with over $900 million for HIV/AIDS and $127–158 million for asthma. Over half the funding for malaria comes from the USA. The economic burden, especially for the countries in sub-Saharan Africa is enormous and estimated at around 1% of the gross domestic product (GDP) of these coun-

Table 59.1 Number of notifications and deaths from malaria in England and Wales during the decade 1990 to 1999.

	1990	1991	1992	1993	1994	1995	1996	1997	1998	1999*
No. of cases notified	1493	1553	1189	1198	1139	1300	1659	1476	1163	1039
No. of deaths	3	11	9	4	11	4	11	11	8	12

Source: PHLS Communicable Disease Surveillance Centre. * Figures for 1999 are provisional.

tries according to the WHO. The Multilateral Initiative on Malaria in Africa (WHO/World Bank/UN) launched in 1997, aims to increase the funding for research on malaria and bring together scientists, funding agencies, the pharmaceutical industry and governments to identify common research priorities.

The number of 'imported' malaria cases associated with travel worldwide is put at 20 000–50 000 per annum. The UK leads the world in numbers (5%), while Germany has the highest case : fatality ratio (7.4%).

About 2500 cases of malaria were 'imported' into the UK in 1996 (1659 in England and Wales). The *Plasmodium falciparum* malaria cases are steadily rising (1283 in the UK in 1996—the vast majority acquired in Africa, very few in the Indian subcontinent). Over one-third of cases concerned immigrants settled in the UK who had travelled back home to visit friends and relatives. We now expect 7–10 deaths from malaria every year involving travellers (Table 59.1). Almost all of these deaths are preventable.

Epidemiology

Malaria in humans is caused by one of four protozoan species of the genus *Plasmodium* (mean incubation period): *P. falciparum* (12 days), *P. vivax* (13 days), *P. ovale* (17 days) and *P. malariae* (28 days). Of these, *P. falciparum* is the most dangerous and often called 'malignant malaria', while the other three are referred to as 'benign malaria'. It is also the parasite most common in Africa.

Infection is usually acquired by the bite of an infected female *Anopheles* mosquito, usually between sunset/dusk and sunrise/dawn. Transmission peaks at around midnight in Latin America and Asia, and about 2 h earlier in Africa. The *Anopheles* mosquito will feed at daytime only if unusually hungry. Of the 800 *Anopheles* species, at

least 80 are able to transmit malaria, half of which are considered important vectors.

The wet seasons in tropical areas, the lakes, rice fields, etc., create breeding sites for the mosquitoes whose numbers rise rapidly with high humidity, high rainfall and high atmospheric temperature. They usually fly approximately a mile from the breeding sites, but strong seasonal winds can disperse them far away. Figure 59.1 shows the life cycle of the parasite.

Other less common modes of transmission include transfusion of blood and blood products, such as platelets and fresh frozen plasma, flushing intravenous lines (nosocomial infection) in wards with malaria patients, contaminated needles and congenitally from mother to fetus. Transmission of malaria from patients to healthcare workers is possible but unusual. When it happens it is usually associated with a needle stick injury and the preparation of blood smears. Clearly mark all requests for blood in suspected cases so that the phlebotomist and the laboratory staff are aware of the need to avoid any contact with the patient's blood.

Plasmodium vivax and *P. ovale* may persist in a dormant stage in the liver (hypnozoites) despite treatment with chloroquine, causing periodic relapses for as long as 5 years. Chloroquine has no effect on the dormant parasite in the liver. *P. falciparum* does not have the ability to remain dormant in the liver, therefore it rarely causes a first attack of malaria more than 3 months after infection. On the other hand, it can be carried without symptoms for over 3 years—in some countries history of malaria is a contraindication to blood donation.

It is important to recognize that malarial illness may be delayed until several weeks or months after exposure. Equally important to remember is the fact that the shortest mean incubation period of malaria is about 12 days so short-term holidaymakers are most likely to develop the disease after their return. In fact the vast majority of travellers

Fig. 59.1 The life cycle of *Plasmodium* spp.

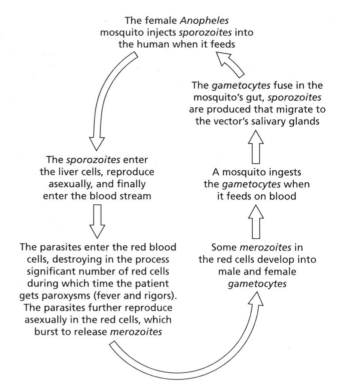

The female *Anopheles* mosquito injects *sporozoites* into the human when it feeds

The *gametocytes* fuse in the mosquito's gut, *sporozoites* are produced that migrate to the vector's salivary glands

The *sporozoites* enter the liver cells, reproduce asexually, and finally enter the blood stream

A mosquito ingests the *gametocytes* when it feeds on blood

The parasites enter the red blood cells, destroying in the process significant number of red cells during which time the patient gets paroxysms (fever and rigors). The parasites further reproduce asexually in the red cells, which burst to release *merozoites*

Some *merozoites* in the red cells develop into male and female *gametocytes*

who acquire malaria in the tropics develop symptoms after their return home. *Plasmodium malariae* also does not have the ability to persist in the liver but infections may occur 20 or more years after leaving an endemic area, as a result of extrahepatic parasitaemia.

Malaria transmission occurs in large areas of Africa, Central and South America, the Indian subcontinent, South-East Asia, the Middle East and other areas. Ninety per cent of cases of *P. falciparum* malaria originate from Africa and become symptomatic within 2 months of departure from the endemic area. Almost 90% of *P. vivax* malaria cases originate in Asia, particularly in India, and 50% become symptomatic within 2 months of departure.

Frequent travel to endemic areas does not convey useful immunity against malaria. Only those people who have survived childhood in a malaria-endemic area may be considered to be immune, as long as they do not leave that area for more than a few months. Immune immigrants resident for a year or more in the UK, who then visit their home country, can be susceptible to severe malaria.

The risk of contracting malaria is proportional to the length of stay in the malaria-endemic area. Heavy rains considerably increase malaria transmission. Exposure time is important; travellers to Africa tend to spend considerable time, including evening and night-time hours, in rural areas where malaria risk is higher. Travellers to Asia and South America tend to spend most of their time in urban resort areas where there is limited, if any, risk of exposure and travel to rural areas mainly during daytime hours, when the risk of infection is limited. Tourists staying in air-conditioned hotels may be at lower risk than backpackers or adventure travellers.

Plasmodium falciparum is developing resistance to antimalarial drugs and the mosquito host is becoming resistant to insecticides, enjoying an increase in breeding sites because of deforestation and irrigation projects. The disease is closely related to poverty therefore another problem in malaria control is shortage of resources.

Plasmodium vivax malaria was endemic in the UK in the nineteenth century. It disappeared between 1860 and 1930. During the past 30 years, two cases of malaria were reported in the UK in persons living 6 and 10 miles from an airport, as a result of the importation of infected mosquitoes on aircraft that arrived at Gatwick ('airport malaria'). Since 1997, 75 cases of airport malaria have been observed in Western Europe, 28 of which occurred in France.

Apart from the infected vector being accidentally flown to Europe in aircraft, other local vectors in Europe can have a role. A reported case in Italy [Baldari M. *et al.* (1998) Malaria in Maremma, Italy. *Lancet* 351, 1246–7] involved a 60-year-old woman who had never travelled abroad, received transfusions or shared contaminated syringes. She acquired malaria by mosquito transmission from an infected person in August 1997. A girl with unrecognized, self-limiting *P. vivax* malaria, who had come from India 4 months earlier, was living nearby. The vector was *Anopheles labranchiae*, a mosquito that used to contribute to the transmission of malaria in Italy before the disease was eradicated. Here in Britain, *Anopheles phimbeus*, a species present in many parts of the country, has been found to be able to carry malaria in laboratory experiments.

Clinical presentation

The classic symptoms are malaise, myalgia, headaches, high fever, rigors and sweats. Also nausea, vomiting, diarrhoea (experienced by one-third of patients), abdominal pain, back pain, joint pains, anaemia after several days, and jaundice caused by haemolysis and anaemia. A common presentation in children is cough, pyrexia, tachypnoea followed by febrile convulsions. Severe infection with *P. falciparum* can result in severe anaemia, pulmonary oedema, renal and hepatic failure, coagulopathy, convulsions, encephalopathy, coma and death.

After several days fever fluctuates so a patient may be afebrile when seen. Episodes of fever consist of cold, hot and sweating phases lasting 6–8 h. There is hepatosplenomegaly in about 35% of cases. Differential diagnosis includes influenza, hepatitis, gastro-enteritis, haemolytic anaemia, acute psychosis (in early cerebral malaria), menin-

gitis, meningococcaemia, pneumonia, influenza, typhoid fever. In children, acute respiratory infections because of the respiratory symptoms of malaria in children.

Pregnant women should be discouraged from travelling to endemic areas as *P. falciparum* infection in pregnancy poses serious problems, such as miscarriage, stillbirth and risk of maternal death. The organism adheres to chondroitin sulphate A on the surface of syncytiotrophoblasts, and sequesters in the placenta. Thus, pregnant women are at increased risk of infection. The same advice (do not travel) should be given to asplenic patients. The WHO advises against taking babies and young children, or pregnant women travelling to malaria-endemic areas, in particular where there is transmission of chloroquine-resistant *P. falciparum*.

Mortality in *P. vivax*, *P. ovale* and *P. malariae* infection is rare and is mainly associated with rupture of the spleen in vivax malaria. In complicated *P. falciparum* infection, mortality overall is 4%. Among the over 40 year olds the mortality rate is 6% and in those over 70 years of age is 30%.

Major complications of severe malaria in children are cerebral involvement, respiratory distress, anaemia, convulsions, metabolic acidosis, hypoglycaemia and shock. In addition, in those who survive cerebral malaria, 10% (4–21%) of children and 5% of adults are left with neurological sequelae. Many children with these complications seem to make a complete recovery within 6 months.

Major complications of severe malaria in adults include cerebral malaria, pulmonary oedema, acute renal failure, anaemia, jaundice, spontaneous bleeding, metabolic acidosis, hypoglycaemia, convulsions and collapse.

In travellers, most of the deaths follow delay in presenting to medical services and in arriving at the correct diagnosis, hence it is important to have a very high index of suspicion and always inquire about recent (within 1 year at least) travel abroad in the case of history of fever. The case fatality in European travellers who do not take malaria prophylaxis and become infected is 2%. In the UK the current mortality rate for cases of falciparum malaria is about 0.4% [Winstanley P. & Behrens R. (1999) Malaria prophylaxis with mefloquine: neurological and psychiatric adverse drug reactions. *Prescriber's Journal* 39 (No. 3), 161–5].

In 1997, a multinational team reported that the risk of severe childhood malaria was lowest in areas with the highest parasite transmission, and proposed that exposure early in life 'furnishes a child with an acquired resistance to the consequences of infection' [(1997) *Lancet* 349, 1650–4]. One explanation of this is that in areas of high transmission, infants are more likely to be exposed to infection when they are protected by maternal immunity than in areas of low transmission. These infants emerge from this period of clinical protection with more immunity than those exposed to fewer parasites.

A question often asked by travellers in the travel clinic is whether the *Anopeles*, having fed on a hepatitis B carrier, can transfer the hepatitis B virus to another person on a subsequent feed. I have never found any evidence that this has occurred.

Laboratory diagnosis

Diagnosis in the laboratory is by microscopic examination of stained fresh blood thick and thin films. Blood should arrive at the laboratory ideally within 2 h of venepuncture. Negative findings do not exclude malaria entirely and at least two further samples should be examined 24 and 48 h later in the presence of clinical suspicion. Serological tests for antibodies against individual *Plasmodium* species cannot differentiate current from past infection therefore these tests are not appropriate for the diagnosis of acute malaria. More recent tests, based on antigen detection, may prove to be useful adjuncts to standard microscopy. Thrombocytopenia is found in 50–80% of patients with malaria and is a useful clue where blood films are negative.

Rapid diagnostic tests for malaria

Rapid diagnostic tests are malaria tests that use finger-prick whole blood. Currently available strip tests detect only *P. falciparum*. In the UK, Ireland, USA, Australia and elsewhere the MalaPac test (MalaQuick in Europe) (Launch Diagnostics) is available. It is a rapid *in vitro* immunochromatographic test for the qualitative detection of circulating *P. falciparum* histidine-rich protein-2 antigen in whole blood. The manufacturers claim over 86% specificity (much lower in the presence of low parasitaemia).

An immunographic dipstick test for the detection of *P. falciparum* antigen to diagnose malaria in travellers who develop fever in at-risk areas is available in several European countries. It is the ICT Malaria Pf from ICT Diagnostics, Sydney, Australia. A survey was carried out in Mombasa, Kenya, where patients reporting with febrile illness were asked to use the stick test with no assistance apart from the manufacturer's leaflet instructions. Patients experienced problems in obtaining blood from a finger prick. Only 68% were able to carry out the test, and 10 out of 11 with malaria failed to diagnose themselves correctly. However, when health professionals did the test, all 11 cases showed the same results as microscopy. The conclusion is that the use of a dipstick test for malaria diagnosis by travellers should be recommended only after appropriate instruction and training [Jelinek T. *et al.* (1999) Self-use of rapid tests for malaria diagnosis by tourists. *Lancet* 354, 1609]. The ICT Malaria Pf was found to be 100% sensitive and 84.5% specific vs. microscopy for *P. falciparum* in a study in India.

A UK multicentre study organized by the London Hospital for Tropical Diseases found ParaSight F strip tests to be 92% sensitive and 98% specific for the initial diagnosis of *P. falciparum* when compared to microscopy. It does not remove the need for a blood film examination where possible because it is not 100% sensitive at low parasitaemias.

Malaria is a notifiable disease.

Treatment of malaria infection

The GP should admit to hospital without delay all cases where malaria is suspected or proven, especially *P. falciparum* malaria because of the risk of complications, including death. Advice on treatment can be obtained from the London Hospital for Tropical Diseases, Tel.: 020 7387 4411 (ask for the Duty Doctor).

The oral regimens below are given for information only and for those cases where there is no hospital nearby. Patients suspected of or with malaria in the UK should be admitted to hospital for treatment.

Treatment of falciparum 'malignant' malaria

- *Quinine* (300 mg tablet) 600 mg (400 mg if nausea, tinnitus or deafness occurs) three times daily for adults (10 mg/kg bodyweight three times daily for children) for 7 days. At the end of day 7 give a single dose (if the patient is not pregnant) of sulfadoxine/pyrimethamine (Fansidar, Roche)—three tablets for adults (children: up to 4 years, half a tablet; 5–6 years, one tablet; 7–9 years, one and a half tablets; 10–14 years, two tablets); avoid if patient is allergic to sulphonamides. If there has been previous sensitivity to Fansidar, use doxycycline (100 mg) 200 mg daily for at least 7 days (not for a child under 12 years, and not for a pregnant woman). Quinine on its own is the treatment of choice for pregnant women.
- *Mefloquine* (Lariam, Roche, 250 mg tablet): for all ages the dose is 20–25 mg/kg (maximum: 1500 mg) as a single dose or preferably divided into 2–3 doses, 6–8 h apart (not for pregnant women, especially in the first trimester, patients with psychiatric disease or epilepsy, or those on β-blockers, digoxin, calcium-channel blockers, quinine, quinidine or before halofantrine). Skin rashes and cardiac conduction defects are rare. Mild ataxia and nausea are common. If the patient vomits within 30 min after receiving the drug, repeat the dose. If vomiting occurs 30–60 min after a dose, give an additional half-dose. Dizziness and disturbed sense of balance are possible. Advise the patient to avoid tasks that require fine co-ordination, such as driving, for at least 3 weeks following therapy. It is not necessary to give Fansidar or doxycycline after mefloquine.
- *Halofantrine* (Halfan, SmithKline Beecham Pharmaceuticals, 250 mg tablet) 500 mg for adults, 8 mg/kg for children (not if under 23 kg) every 6 h for three doses, repeat after 1 week. It is rarely used nowadays. Do not use this drug if mefloquine was used for prophylaxis (danger of potentially fatal prolongation of the electrocardiographic Q–T interval). Do not use halofantrine for standby self-treatment of malaria.
- Atovaquone 250 mg plus proguanil hydrochloride 100 mg (Malarone, GlaxoWellcome) is currently licensed in the UK for the treatment of malaria (it is not as yet licensed in the UK although it is effective for prophylaxis). It is particularly effective against *P. falciparum* malaria. Adults and children over 40 kg: four tablets, once daily, for three consecutive days, with food; children under 11 kg—no suitable dose; children between 11 kg and 20 kg: one tablet daily on three consecutive days; children between 21 kg and 30 kg: two tablets as a single dose on three consecutive days; children between 31 kg and 40 kg: three tablets as a single dose on three consecutive days. Avoid in lactating mothers.

Treatment of 'benign' malaria

Chloroquine is the drug of choice. Initially 600 mg, then a single dose of 300 mg 6–8 h later, followed by 300 mg once daily for 2 days. Children should receive an initial dose of 10 mg/kg, then a single dose of 5 mg/kg 6–8 h later, followed by 5 mg/kg once daily for 2 days. This regimen is adequate for *P. malariae* infections.

For *P. vivax* and *P. ovale* further treatment to follow chloroquine is required with primaquine in order to destroy parasites in the liver (hypnozoites) and thus prevent relapses. Adults should receive 15 mg daily for 14–21 days. Children receive primaquine at a dose of 250 µg/kg BW daily for 14–21 days. This treatment should not be given to pregnant women who should, instead, continue to receive chloroquine at a dose of 600 mg each week during the pregnancy. Before primaquine is used, glucose-6-phosphate-dehydrogenase (G6PD) deficiency should be ruled out by appropriate laboratory testing.

Doxycycline 200 mg daily for at least 7 days can be considered for the treatment of chloroquine-resistant falciparum malaria. Due to the potential severity of the infection, a rapid-acting schizonticide such as quinine should always be considered in conjunction with doxycycline.

Medicine for Malaria Venture

With regard to the global picture of malaria treatment, a joint public–private sector initiative, the 'Medicines for Malaria Venture' (website: http://www.mim.nih.gov/partnerships/index.html), aims to develop antimalarial drugs and drug combinations and make them available in poor countries. Effective drugs, such as mefloquine, are expensive but appropriate for multiresistant falciparum malaria. Resistance against them is growing. Artemisinin (from the Chinese antipyretic plant *Artemisia annua L.*) and its derivatives have proved the most rapidly acting and potent of all agents. In large trials they have been shown to be safe and effective, both in severe and uncomplicated malaria. Using combinations of these drugs may reduce the ever-increasing resistance problem. Combining artemisinin derivatives with mefloquine has been shown to halt the increase in mefloquine resistance on the western border of Thailand (WHO—*The World Health Report 1999*).

Stand-by (emergency) treatment

Antimalarial measures and chemoprophylaxis do not always give total protection to everybody in all parts of the world, especially in areas of resistance to chloroquine or mefloquine. A number of travellers may therefore contract malaria. Some frequent travellers to endemic areas (e.g. business people, airline flying crews) do not always take their chemoprophylaxis. 'Breakthrough' malaria is also a problem in those taking prophylaxis. In some areas prompt medical attention (within 24 h of becoming ill) or suitable drugs may not be available. Other travellers are advised not to take chemo-prophylaxis for certain areas but to take every precaution against mosquito bites. Such travellers should be advised to carry with them a stand-by emergency treatment for use in the case of fever. They must seek medical advice as soon as practically possible, which usually means returning to base or to a town. The use of rapid diagnostic tests for malaria (see above) can aid self-diagnosis provided they are used correctly.

Quinine is the only stand-by drug that is safe for pregnant women. Stand-by treatment is not necessary for those overseas for less than 1 week (it takes at least 9 days from bite to becoming ill with malaria at the earliest). Inform the traveller what symptoms to expect in case of malaria and urge them to carry a thermometer. Instructions on how and when to take stand-by treatment should be clear and written. Stress to the traveller that this treatment is only a first-aid measure, and that medical advice must be sought as soon as possible.

Quinine (300-mg tablet)

Two tablets three times daily for 7 days. Alternatively, two tablets three times daily for 3 days followed by three tablets once of Fansidar (this alternative option is not for pregnant women). The children's dose for quinine is 10 mg/kg bodyweight 8 hourly, and Fansidar single dose (see below for dosage). This regimen could cover *P. falciparum* well.

An alternative regimen (not for pregnant women or children under 12 years) is quinine, two tablets three times daily for 3 days, together with doxycycline 100 mg twice daily for 7 days—this regimen is appropriate for travellers taking mefloquine for prophylaxis.

Possible side-effects include tinnitus, nausea, headaches, rash, confusion and visual disturbances such as blurred vision and temporary blindness. Use with caution in patients with cardiac problems or G6PD deficiency. Few people complete a 7-day course because of increasing side-effects.

Sulfadoxine 500 mg and pyrimethamine 25 mg (Fansidar, Roche)

Three tablets once only. The corresponding dose for children is: 2–11 months, quarter of a tablet; 1–3 years, half a tablet; 4–6 years, one tablet; 7–9 years, one and a half tablets; 10–14 years, two tablets; > 14 years, three tablets. Possible side-effects include rashes, insomnia, depression of haematopoiesis, Stevens–Johnson syndrome and toxic epidermal necrolysis. Contraindicated in pregnancy and lactation.

Table 59.2 Which drug for standby treatment?

Chemoprophylaxis taken	Area of chloroquine resistance	Standby treatment
None	Yes	Quinine plus doxycycline
None	No	Chloroquine
Proguanil	No	Chloroquine
Chloroquine	No/Yes	Fansidar or mefloquine
Mefloquine	No/Yes	Quinine plus doxycycline or quinine plus Fansidar (Africa, south of the Sahara only)
Area with chloroquine resistance		Fansidar or mefloquine or quinine plus another drug
Pregnant women		Quinine for 7 days. Avoid situations in which stand-by treatment may be needed

Chloroquine 150-mg base (Nivaquine, Rhône-Poulenc Rorer)

In chloroquine-sensitive areas, four tablets on the first and second day, and two tablets on the third day or 10 mg/base kg BW for 2 days, then 5 mg base/kg BW on the third day. It is useful in individuals who are semi-immune. Details on adverse effects can be found on p. 376.

Mefloquine 250 mg (Lariam, Roche)

The dose of mefloquine depends on bodyweight and the extent of mefloquine resistance in the area concerned. The total therapeutic dose for non-immune patients is 20–25 mg/kg, not exceeding six tablets, in split dose, 6 h apart. A total single dose of 15 mg/kg, not exceeding four tablets, may be sufficient for partially immune individuals. The 1997 British malaria guidelines recommend 15 mg/kg, not exceeding four tablets in split dose, 6 h apart. Mefloquine is not very useful as a stand-by therapy when it is being used for prophylaxis. Details on adverse effects can be found on p. 379.

Antimalarial chemoprophylaxis should be resumed 7 days after the first dose of a stand-by treatment (Table 59.2).

Malaria prophylaxis

Immunization

The development of the ideal malaria vaccine is beset by the complexities of the different stages in the life cycle of the malaria parasite and the differ-ing needs and responses to a vaccine in different populations. Two kinds of vaccine are necessary to prevent malaria: transmission blocking vaccine and a vaccine to protect the individual.

During its life cycle within the human host, the malaria parasite undergoes several distinct stages of development. Studies in humans and animals indicate that immunization with one stage of the parasite generates an immune response to that stage alone. In other words, malarial immunity is stage-specific. An effective malaria vaccine will probably need to contain epitopes from multiple stages of the parasite's lifecycle and to elicit both T- and B-cell responses.

The best known vaccine to date has been developed by Manuel Patarroyo of the Bogota, Colombian group. In randomized blind trials, his vaccine SPf66 protected a group of children against malaria. These trials have indicated that clinical attacks of falciparum malaria could be reduced by 34% (1993) in South American (Colombian) vaccinees aged 1–45 years, by 31% (1994) in Tanzanian children aged 1–5 years, and 8% (1995) in infants aged 6–11 months in the Gambia. No efficacy (1996) was shown in Thailand in children aged 2–15 years. Nonetheless, the Patarroyo vaccine has so far proved to be safe, immunogenic, and able to reduce clinical attacks, although at varying levels in different countries.

Researchers from the US Centers for Disease Control and Prevention (CDC), Bethesda, have constructed a vaccine containing 12 B-cell, six T-cell, and three cytotoxic T-cell epitopes from nine stage-specific *P. falciparum* antigens. Their pre-liminary results are encouraging.

DNA technology is also entering the field of malaria. The first clinical trials of *P. falciparum* DNA vaccines, designed to induce protective CD8+ T-cell responses against infected hepatocytes started in 1997. Almost all vaccine trials have had to focus on only two of the estimated 6000 *P. falciparum* proteins. Already, a DNA vaccine made by 'Powderject' of Oxford Science Park is being evaluated in Europe in healthy volunteers and in Africa.

Quite a number of other malaria vaccines are in development. The 'Quilimmune-M' by Aquila in Massachusetts has completed safety trials in humans and is undergoing Phase II trials. San Diego-based Epimmune Inc. is testing a malaria vaccine in preclinical trials, although this could be 1 or 2 years away from being tried in humans. The Johns Hopkins School of Public Health in Baltimore, and the US CDC is also working on a vaccine together with scientists from India.

A high-resolution linkage map of all the *P. falciparum* genome has been constructed. The map should help in the localization of genes for such traits as drug resistance [*Science* (1999) 286, 1351–3]. This discovery may lead to new, clinically useful directions in vaccine development as well as in diagnosis, treatment and overall control of malaria.

Advice to travellers on protection against mosquito bites

Emphasize to the traveller that strict adherence to effective measures for preventing contact with mosquitoes and bites is most important as no malaria chemoprophylaxis is totally effective.

● Wear long-sleeved clothing, long trousers or skirts and socks when going out between dusk and dawn (sunset and sunrise) when malaria mosquitoes commonly bite (to avoid dengue fever as well, do so day and night).

● Avoid dark colours as they attract mosquitoes—wear light colours.

● Avoid perfume, aftershaves, hair sprays, etc., as they attract mosquitoes.

● Choose air-conditioned accommodation.

● Use a knockdown insecticide spray before evening to kill any mosquitoes that may have entered the room during the day.

● Remain in well-screened areas: mosquito screens on windows, doors closed especially from late afternoon onwards.

● If mosquitoes can enter during the night, use an electrically heated mat that heats a tablet impregnated with synthetic pyrethroids (remember to take the appropriate adaptor to suit voltage and sockets) or burn mosquito coils (they burn slowly and contain a mixture of repellent and insecticide). Electronic buzzers are of no value.

● If accommodation allows entry of mosquitoes or sleeping in a tent or outside, use a mosquito net while sleeping at night, especially one that is impregnated every 6 months with synthetic pyrethroids. Tuck the edges of the net under the mattress during the day so as to ensure that no mosquitoes are trapped inside. Repair holes promptly. If the net is not long enough to fall to the floor all around the bed, tuck it under the mattress.

● Remember to re-impregnate the mosquito bed net with permethrin every 6 months as per manufacturer's instructions. As permethrin-treated bed nets kill the mosquito, they reduce the mosquito population in a room, thus they indirectly protect other occupants too. Such bed nets have achieved striking reductions of childhood mortality in the natives. The WHO-sponsored campaign 'Roll Back Malaria' aims to provide every child in Africa with a net, as these can cut malaria deaths by a quarter and cost less than $4 each. For the traveller, they offer the additional advantage of also killing most biting insects such as mosquitoes, fleas, bedbugs, ticks and sandflies.

● Apply to exposed skin only (face, hands and ankles) a mosquito repellent containing diethyl toluamide (DEET) which is available as a spray, cream, gel, stick or liquid. To be effective these repellents require repeated application. The DEET concentration determines the length of action: 3 h (25%), 8 h (55%), 10 h (100%). A 60 mL spray used twice in 24 h will last one person approximately 1 week. Follow the manufacturer's recommendations as they can be toxic when used in excess, especially in children who, very rarely, may suffer from encephalopathic reactions. Wash off when indoors. Keep DEET away from eyes, mouth and any mucous membranes.

• DEET may damage synthetic fabrics and plastics, e.g. watch straps. It can be applied to appropriate clothing. For application on all types of fabrics (not harmful to plastics) use a preparation that is made from the pyrethrum plant only such as 'Repel Clothing Treatment' available in pump spray and wrist bands.

• Consider using wrist and ankle bands impregnated with DEET. Most have a material backing so the DEET is expelled outwards. They usually last for 100–120 h. Wear them when necessary and place them in their container at all other times.

• Concern about toxicity of DEET, particularly in children, has led to the production of a non-DEET-based insect repellent that offers effective protection similar to DEET. It comes under the name of Mosi-guard Natural and has a pleasant lemon, eucalyptus aroma. It does not damage plastic, or synthetic fabrics (as DEET does), lasts for up to 6 h, and can be used by the whole family, including babies and children. It is available in spray, cream and stick. It is approved and recommended by the London School of Hygiene and Tropical Medicine.

• Autan is a non-DEET-based effective mosquito repellent that contains Bayrepel. It gives up to 8 h protection against insect/mosquito bites from a single application. It is available in aerosol spray, pump spray or stick form. The Autan Family lotion with aloe vera moisturiser can be used from the age of 2 years.

• Avoid evening visits to or spending nights near ponds or rivers—areas where mosquitoes breed.

Antimosquito equipment can be obtained from, among others, British Airways Travel Clinics, Homeway Ltd, other companies and many pharmacists. (For addresses and contact telephone numbers see Sources of Travel Information in Chapter 64.)

General advice to travellers on chemoprophylaxis against malaria

• Take chemoprophylaxis against malaria, starting at least 1 week before arrival and continuing without interruption until at least 4 weeks after leaving the malaria-endemic area.

• Proguanil and doxycycline can be started the day before travel, mefloquine can be started up to 3 weeks prior to travel (better chance for side-effects, if any, to occur before travel). Explain the need to continue chemoprophylaxis for 4 weeks after leaving the malaria-endemic area—the parasites do not enter the bloodstream until the completion of a phase of multiplication in the liver (it lasts a minimum of 10 days) and available chemoprophylaxis has no effect on parasites prior to their entering the bloodstream.

• Prophylactic antimalarial drugs should be taken after food and swallowed with plenty of water. Doxycycline should not be taken before lying down (may cause oesophagitis/heartburn). If for any reason the traveller vomits the drug for prophylaxis within 30 min of swallowing it, a second full dose should be given, and if between 30 and 60 min, an additional half dose should be given. Vomiting and diarrhoea together may render the drug ineffective.

• Take tablets on the same day each week or, in the case of tablets to be taken daily, at the same time each day.

• Comply fully with chemoprophylaxis; nearly three-quarters of travellers who develop malaria do so because they do not comply or do not take chemoprophylaxis. This applies also to regular travellers to endemic areas—they often think they have developed immunity. British primary care surveys have shown that a large number of travellers (up to two-thirds) do not comply fully.

• Natural immunity is rapidly lost. If a traveller was born and brought up in a malaria-endemic area but has lived away from home for more than 6 months, he or she should comply fully with malaria chemoprophylaxis.

• No chemoprophylactic regimen gives total protection to everybody at all times—warn patients that they may still contract malaria despite correct antimalarial prophylaxis.

• Young children, infants, pregnant women and patients with anatomical or functional asplenia should not travel to malaria-endemic areas unless their trip is unavoidable. If they do, they must use chemoprophylaxis and fully comply.

• Any febrile, flu-like illness occurring after the first week of stay, or in the weeks or months (even

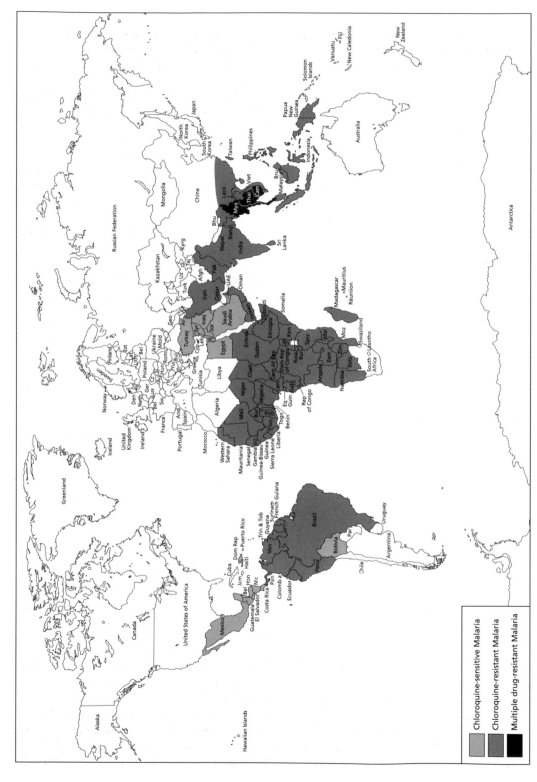

Fig. 59.2 Malaria endemic areas and drug resistance.

Chloroquine-sensitive Malaria

Chloroquine-resistant Malaria

Multiple drug-resistant Malaria

a year) after travelling to a malaria-endemic area (Fig. 59.2), should arouse suspicion. They should report to their doctor and malaria should be excluded.

● While in a malaria-endemic area seek medical advice for fever, especially if associated with rigors. Malaria can kill if the treatment is delayed.

● Inform the traveller that some of the essential antimalarial drugs can, very rarely, cause serious adverse reactions. In such a case the traveller should stop the drug and seek medical advice locally on an alternative drug.

● Women of child-bearing age should avoid falling pregnant while taking, and for 3 months after the last dose of mefloquine, and 1 week after doxycycline prophylaxis is stopped.

● Consider taking drugs for stand-by treatment if prompt medical help is not available (within 24 h) in the area of travel.

● Antimalarial prophylaxis should be resumed 7 days after the first dose of a stand-by (emergency) treatment.

● Malaria chemoprophylaxis is necessary in situations where a traveller is advised that it is not necessary to take it because he or she is staying in a large town only but, while there, he or she decides to go on safari even for a few hours. Indeed, the main risk to business travellers is a short unexpected trip to visit a game park or to eat or stay in the country. Risk exists in most African cities, with the exemption of central Nairobi and cities at high altitude such as Addis Ababa and cities in southern Africa.

● Report any unexplained pyrexial illness to the GP, within 3 months of returning from a *P. falciparum* area, and at least a year from all areas.

Chemoprophylaxis against malaria

In considering a particular drug, consider the risk of malaria and the levels of drug resistance in the area(s) to be visited and the medical condition/s of the individual receiving it. The risk for malaria is proportionate to the length of stay in the malaria-endemic area. Point out to the traveller the risk of malaria—especially the possibility of death—which needs to be balanced against the concerns over drug toxicity.

For medicolegal purposes, doctors and nurses should ensure they record in the traveller's notes their recommendations and the patient's final choice.

Chemoprophylaxis should generally be started at least 1 week (the day before travel in the case of doxycycline and proguanil) before arrival and continued without interruption until at least 4 weeks after leaving the malaria-endemic area.

Travellers who develop any serious side-effects while taking antimalarial chemoprophylaxis should consider stopping it and seeking local medical attention.

● For *infants and children* the dose is calculated according to the child's weight. Breast-fed babies are not protected by their mother's prophylaxis, and require their own. The WHO advises against taking babies and young children to malaria-endemic areas, in particular where there is transmission of chloroquine-resistant *P. falciparum*. If they must travel, every precaution should be taken to avoid mosquito bites in addition to chemoprophylaxis. Chloroquine and proguanil can be given safely to babies and young children (may be crushed and given with food, fruit or jam—chloroquine is available in syrup 50 mg/5 mL). Fansidar can be given from the age of 2 months, or Maloprim under 5 years of age. Doxycycline is contraindicated under the age of 12 years (under 8 years in some other countries; Mefloquine for babies over 5 kg in weight). Parents should take care of antimalaria drugs, which should be in child-proof containers.

● Malaria in a *pregnant woman* increases the risk of maternal death, miscarriage, stillbirth and low birth weight with associated risk of neonatal death. She should not travel to a malaria-endemic area. If a pregnant woman must travel to a malaria-endemic area, she could take proguanil (with folic acid 5 mg daily) and chloroquine. She should not take pyrimethamine (Fansidar, Maloprim), mefloquine (Lariam), except on explicit medical advice. Mefloquine or Maloprim may be taken in the second and third trimesters if it is absolutely necessary. Additional folic acid 5 mg daily with Maloprim. Inadvertent use of mefloquine in early pregnancy is not viewed as an indication for termination of pregnancy. Avoid doxycycline throughout the pregnancy. Medical advice should be sought immediately if pyrexial and/or feeling unwell. Stand-by treatment should be considered if appropriate.

- *Women of child-bearing age* should take adequate contraceptive precautions while taking mefloquine and for 3 months after the last dose. Avoid doxycycline in the week before falling pregnant.
- *Breast-feeding mothers* should not take mefloquine and doxycycline (see p. 378).
- In *epilepsy* avoid mefloquine and chloroquine. Use doxycycline in areas with, and proguanil (200 mg daily) in areas without chloroquine resistance. Alternatives are weekly Maloprim (add folic acid 5 mg daily if the patient is on phenobarbital or phenytoin) and azithromycin (not licensed for this purpose) for children.
- *Renal failure* patients can take mefloquine or doxycycline in areas of chloroquine resistance. Chloroquine can be given as it is mostly metabolized in the liver, although some is excreted in urine. Proguanil is excreted by the kidney therefore use a full dose if serum creatinine is up to 150 µmol/L, half the dose if between 150 and 300 and seek specialist advice if above 300 µmol/L.
- *Liver failure* patients can take proguanil, and possibly chloroquine in mild failure. Mefloquine and doxycycline are metabolized in the liver. Seek specialist advice.
- *Splenectomy* patients, whether anatomical or functional, should not travel to malaria-endemic areas. If they must, they must take meticulous precautions against mosquito bites and appropriate chemoprophylaxis.

None of the drugs available for use for malaria chemoprophylaxis in the UK are prescribed on the NHS. The NHS Executive issued FHSL(95)7 on 14 February 1995, in which it informed GPs of an addition to the 'Terms of Service' paragraph 38 which gives GPs power to charge patients for the prescribing or providing of drugs for malaria prophylaxis for travel. A necessary consequent amendment to paragraph 40 to cross-reference the charge has been made. This means that private prescriptions should be used to prescribe such drugs. These regulations apply to dispensing doctors too.

Chloroquine (Avloclor, AstraZeneca; Nivaquine, Rhône-Poulenc Rorer)

Chloroquine should be started 1 week before entering the malaria-endemic area. In patients with psoriasis it may precipitate a severe attack. Caution should be exercised in patients with hepatic and renal disease (see above). It should not be used in patients with epilepsy. Chloroquine frequently causes itching in black-skinned people. In some people it may cause blurring of vision (reversible), headaches, convulsions, loss of hair, depigmentation, gastrointestinal disturbances, pruritus, bone marrow suppression, dizziness and occasionally a rash. It may aggravate severe gastrointestinal disorders, G6PD deficiency, and myasthenia gravis. Chloroquine is safe in pregnancy and lactation. Individuals who need to take chloroquine for long periods should consider changing the drug once they reach a total dose of 100 g—because of the danger of corneal and retinal changes. For dosage, see Tables 59.4 and 59.5.

Proguanil (Paludrine, AstraZeneca)

Proguanil should be started not later than 24 h before entering a malaria-endemic area. It may cause gastric symptoms and diarrhoea, aphthous-like mouth ulcers, stomatitis, skin reactions and hair loss. If on warfarin, re-stabilize control before travel. It is safe in pregnancy (add folic acid 5 mg daily). If the renal function is impaired (serum creatinine > 50 µmol/L) seek specialist advice. For dosage, see Tables 59.4 and 59.5.

Proguanil and chloroquine combined

Proguanil (200 mg daily) and chloroquine (300 mg weekly) combined achieve efficacy of protection of the order of 70%. The rate of serious adverse effects (fatal, life-threatening, hospitalization or severe/permanent disability) is similar to that seen with mefloquine and is of the order of 1 in 10 000. Mild to moderate adverse events are also similar in number to mefloquine but they are more related to the gastrointestinal tract. This combination can be given to pregnant women (with folic acid), and infants.

Age (years)	Paludrine tablets (once daily)	Avloclor tablets (once weekly)
1–4	0.5	0.5
5–8	1.0	1.0
9–14	1.5	1.5
> 14 and adults	2.0	2.0

Table 59.3 Doses of combined proguanil/chloroquine (Paludrine/Avloclor, AstraZeneca).

A proprietary combined preparation is available. Paludrine/Avloclor (AstraZeneca). It contains (98) proguanil (Paludrine) 100-mg tablets, and (14) chloroquine (Avloclor) 250-mg tablets, which is equivalent to 155 mg chloroquine base. One pack is enough for 7 weeks prophylaxis for one adult. It is not licensed for children under 1 year of age. The tablets should be taken at the same time of the day, with water after food (for young children crush the tablet and mix it with milk, honey or jam), at the dosage given in Table 59.3.

Doxycycline

Doxycycline is now licensed in the UK for malaria prophylaxis (and for the treatment of malaria). If used for prophylaxis, it should be prescribed on a private prescription, and started no later than 48 h before entering and continued for 4 weeks after leaving the malaria-endemic area.

In two small studies, doxycycline was found to have similar efficacy to mefloquine—over 90% [Anderson S. *et al.* (1998) Successful double-blinded, randomised, placebo-controlled field trial of azithromycin and doxycycline as prophylaxis for malaria in Western Kenya. *Clin. Infect. Dis.* 26(1), 146–50].

Doxycycline may cause skin photosensitivity (manifested as an exaggerated sunburn reaction) in 3–10% of travellers taking it. The risk of such reaction can be minimized by avoiding prolonged direct exposure to the sun and by using sunscreens that absorb long-wave ultraviolet (UVA) radiation. Diarrhoea is possible, while nausea and vomiting may be improved if the drug is taken with a meal. It

should not be given to children under the age of 12 years (in some other countries under 8 years of age), or pregnant, or lactating mothers. It may provoke vaginal candidiasis in susceptible females (consider supplying the patient with fluconazole 150 mg capsule on a private prescription to be taken if it becomes necessary).

Doxycycline must be taken after meals (preferably after breakfast) with copious quantities of fluid and the traveller should not lie down immediately after taking the drug as there is a risk of oesophagitis. Avoid using it for more than 3 months. It is active against *P. falciparum* malaria, and partly against *P. vivax*. In areas of mefloquine-resistant malaria, in South-East Asia (areas of Thailand bordering with Myanmar (Burma) and Cambodia) it is the drug of choice. Compliance with the daily dose regimen of doxycycline needs to be strictly observed. When used, it is also effective against leptospirosis and rickettsia.

Pyrimethamine with dapsone (Maloprim, Glaxo Wellcome)

Pyrimethamine with dapsone is contraindicated if the patient is allergic to sulphonamides and caution should be exercised in patients with G6PD deficiency. It is contraindicated in pregnancy, especially in the first trimester—folate supplements should be prescribed later in pregnancy if it has to be used. There is a risk of blood dyscrasias, including agranulocytosis. Do not exceed one tablet weekly in adults. Other side-effects are: jaundice, psychosis, pneumonia with eosinophilic pulmonary infiltration, and in long-term therapy hypoalbuminaemia.

Pyrimethamine with sulfadoxine (Fansidar, Roche)

Fansidar is no longer recommended for malaria prophylaxis because of severe side-effects in long-term use. It has a place in stand-by treatment but not for pregnant women.

Azithromycin

Azithromycin suspension can be used for children if necessary (but it is not licensed in the UK for this purpose). Issue a private prescription if it is to be used. This agent is an alternative to doxycycline when that cannot be taken. Azithromycin has to be taken daily. Its efficacy is probably about 70–80%.

Mefloquine (Lariam, Roche)

Mefloquine is the preferred antimalarial prophylaxis for those travelling to areas of multiple drug-resistant *P. falciparum*, such as east and sub-Saharan Africa. Its protective efficacy is approximately 90% in Africa and the Pacific, but in Thailand is 50% and on the Thai border of Myanmar (Burma) and Cambodia resistance is widespread. Struc-turally, mefloquine is related to quinine. Like quinine, its exact mechanism of action is not known. It probably works by interfering with the asexual blood forms of the human malaria parasite.

Dosage

Adults and children weighing more than 45 kg: one tablet once weekly. When body weight is less than 45 kg, the dose is as follows:
- 5–19 kg (3 months to 5 years) quarter tablet;
- 20–30 kg (6–8 years) half tablet;
- 31–45 kg (9–14 years) three-quarter tablet.

The tablet should be swallowed whole, after a meal with plenty of liquid. Taking it after the evening meal may overall be associated with less immediate side-effects at the point of highest serum level— 6 h post dose.

Length of prophylaxis

Adverse effects usually occur early—41% after the first dose, 69% within the first 2 weeks and 78% within the first 3 weeks of use as prophylaxis [van Riemsdijk M. *et al.* (1997) Neuro-psychiatric effects of antimalarials. *Eur. J. Clin. Pharmacol.* 52, 1–6]. Mefloquine taken for the first time should be started 2.5 to 3 weeks prior to travel. Otherwise, it should be started 1 week prior to travel. It should be continued until 4 weeks after departing from the malaria-endemic area. The maximum licensed duration for prophylaxis in the UK is 12 months. The earlier commencement of mefloquine prophylaxis allows for the pretravel detection of side-effects in most cases (another drug for malaria prophylaxis can then be started).

Contraindications

Contraindications to mefloquine are:
- history of convulsions (ever);
- epilepsy—it can increase the risk of convulsions (see below);
- history of epilepsy in a first-degree relative (parents, siblings);
- history of psychiatric disease (including depression);
- severe impairment of liver function;
- pregnancy especially in the first trimester—its use in the second and third trimester should be considered only if there are compelling medical reasons;
- avoid pregnancy within 3 months after taking the last mefloquine tablet—women of child-bearing age should take reliable contraceptive precautions for the entire duration of therapy and for 3 months after;
- breast-feeding; the data sheet does not indicate whether a breast-feeding mother whose infant is over 5 kg in weight could take mefloquine. About 3–4% of the drug is excreted in the breast milk;
- severe hypersensitivity to mefloquine or related compounds, e.g. quinine;
- infants less than 3 months old or weighing less than 5 kg (because of limited experience);
- administration of halofantrine at the same time or after mefloquine (danger of potentially fatal

prolongation of the electrocardiographic Q–T interval); no data available for when mefloquine was given after halofantrine;

• within 12 h (DoH) or 3 days (data sheet) of administering the oral live typhoid vaccine (or any other live oral bacterial vaccine such as the oral live cholera vaccine which is not as yet available in the UK).

Caution should be exercised in the following cases.

• If the patient suffers from cardiac conduction disorders (transient cardiac alterations have been observed with mefloquine). If given, monitor the patient (including ECGs) during the 3 weeks of therapy, before departure.

• Concomitant administration of mefloquine and other related compounds, e.g. quinine, quinidine, chloroquine—may produce ECG abnormalities and increase the risk of convulsions. The use of halofantrine after mefloquine may cause significant prolongation of the Q–T interval.

• Coadministered with other drugs known to alter cardiac conduction such antiarrhythmic or β-blockers, digoxin, calcium-channel blockers, antihistamines, tricyclic antidepressants, phenothiazines, as they may also contribute to a prolongation of the Q–T interval.

• If used in people who have to drive or carry out tasks demanding fine coordination and precision such as piloting aircraft or operating machines, as dizziness, a disturbed sense of balance or neuropsychiatric reactions have been reported during and for up to 3 weeks after use of mefloquine.

• Impaired renal function (although dose adjustment is not necessary, caution in the use of mefloquine is recommended).

• May lower the plasma levels of anticonvulsants (e.g. phenytoin, phenobarbital, carbamazepine, valproic acid)—dosage adjustments of antiseizure medication may be necessary. Do not use mefloquine for chemoprophylaxis in patients with epilepsy.

• Before departure, check control of patients on oral hypoglycaemic agents, anticoagulants.

• Coadministration of metoclopramide causes faster absorption of mefloquine and raised levels. Monitor patients closely for side-effects.

• An interaction with alcohol is not suspected (it

has been suggested) although they share some common side-effects. Alcohol, if taken, should be in moderation.

Adverse reactions

Mefloquine has a long half-life (average 21 days in white people). Its elimination from the body is very slow therefore adverse reactions may occur or persist up to several weeks after the last dose. There is no specific antidote to mefloquine and the drug is non-dialysable. Between 17 and 25% of users develop some side-effects, most of which are mild and self-limiting. An independent review [(1998) Mefloquine and malaria prophylaxis. *Drug. Ther. Bull.* 36(3), 20–2] concluded there was no evidence of increased incidence of serious central nervous system (CNS) side-effects compared to other regimens.

Common adverse reactions are nausea, vomiting, loose stools, diarrhoea, abdominal pain, dizziness, vertigo, headaches, drowsiness, insomnia, nightmares and fatigue.

Uncommon adverse reactions:
• *general:* anorexia, fatigue, fever and chills;
• *psychiatric:* depression, suicidal ideation, anxiety, panic, restlessness, forgetfulness, confusion, hallucinations, paranoid delusions and agitation;
• *neurological:* convulsions, tinnitus and vestibular disorders, abnormal coordination, ataxia, visual disturbances, motor neuropathies, paraesthesia;
• *cardiovascular:* hypo- and hypertension, flushing, syncope, tachycardia, palpitations, extrasystoles, dysrhythmias;
• *musculoskeletal:* myalgia, muscle cramps, muscle weakness and arthralgia;
• *dermatological:* rash, exanthema, urticaria, pruritus, hair loss, erythema multiforme, Stevens–Johnson syndrome;
• *laboratory abnormalities:* leucopenia or leucocytosis, thrombocytopenia, transient elevation of transaminases.

Very rare adverse reactions are encephalopathy, AV-block.

The discontinuation rate of mefloquine prophylactic therapy is about 2% (similar to the rate observed with proguanil plus chloroquine). Warn travellers to discontinue mefloquine if they experience fits, unusual changes in mood or behaviour, such as feelings of worry or anxiety, restlessness, agitation or confusion. They should seek local medical advice, including an alternative antimalarial drug.

Warn the traveller that about one-quarter of people who take antimalarial prophylaxis report some side-effects, irrespective of what they take. At the same time stress the importance of taking prophylaxis and complying fully.

Severe neuropsychiatric reactions, such as coma, convulsions and psychotic disturbances have been reported in 0.01% (1 in 10 000) taking prophylactic doses, and more commonly in women than in men.

The overall frequency of adverse reactions, regardless of type of severity, with prophylactic use of mefloquine has been reported to be 17–22%. This is not so dissimilar to the frequency for chloroquine and proguanil (they tend to cause mainly gastrointestinal symptoms such as nausea, diarrhoea, anorexia). Mefloquine may cause restlessness, dizziness and disturbed sleep.

In a study by Professor Robert Steffen *et al.* [Mefloquine compared with other malaria chemoprophylactic regimens in tourists visiting east Africa. *Lancet* (1993) 341, 1299–303] the rate of side-effects was 18.8% for mefloquine users, 17.1% for chloro-quine 300 mg base, 18.6% for 600 mg base per week, 30.1% for chloroquine plus proguanil, and 11.7% for sulfadoxine and pyrimethamine. They concluded the mefloquine was more effective than chloroquine plus proguanil for malaria prophylaxis in short-term tourists visiting east Africa and that it has a tolerance similar to that of chloroquine used alone.

In a British study [Barrett P., Emmins P., Clarke P. & Bradley D. (1996) Comparison of adverse events associated with the use of mefloquine and combination of chloroquine and proguanil as antimalarial prophylaxis: postal and telephone survey of travellers. *Br. Med. J.* 313, 525–8] disabling neuropsychiatric adverse effects occurred in 0.7% (70 in 10 000) of all travellers taking mefloquine and 0.09% (9 in 10 000) in those taking chloroquine plus proguanil. They found that both regimens had similar rates of any side-effects occurring (40%), although most side-effects were trivial.

The 1997 *Guidelines for the prevention of malaria in travellers from the UK* (see below) mention that between 0.1 and 1% of people taking mefloquine suffer 'unpleasant and temporarily disabling neuropsychiatric adverse events'. They go on to suggest that 'travellers spending two weeks or less in well screened accommodation may be better advised to take proguanil plus chloroquine rather than mefloquine, but the consequences of reducing the number of neuropsychiatric reactions (probably difficult to document) will be a rise in the number of cases of malaria.' They advise prompt reporting of febrile illness on return.

The persistence of neuropsychiatric adverse events after ceasing to take mefloquine varies. A substantial proportion (45%) disappear within 20 days, but persist for 2 months in about 25% of cases. Very few travellers have described symptoms after 6 months from mefloquine discontinuation.

If a decision is taken to stop mefloquine because of adverse reaction, it should be replaced with an alternative drug (chloroquine plus proguanil, doxycycline) if the patient remains at risk of malaria transmission. If the patient is no longer at risk of transmission, but is taking postexposure prophylaxis after returning to the UK, an alternative regimen may not always be necessary; seek expert advice if in doubt.

UK media interest in adverse effects of mefloquine has contributed to a drop in use of this drug. This may prove disastrous for British visitors to east Africa, as mefloquine has, independently of other factors, contributed to a threefold reduction in imported malaria from Kenya between 1993, when the British Malaria Guidelines recommended for the first time the use of mefloquine as an alternative to chloroquine plus proguanil, and 1996 [Behrens R. *et al.* (1996) *Lancet* 348, 344–5]. Mefloquine continues to be most effective in preventing malaria in British tourists to Kenya but already there are reports of developing resistance in areas such as western Kenya and Tanzania.

Mefloquine is not contraindicated in HIV patients.

Malarone (Glaxo-Wellcome)

Malarone's licence for use in malaria prophylaxis is

expected in the spring of 2001. It contains atovaquone 250 mg and proguanil 100 mg. The prophylactic dose is likely to be one tablet daily, continuing for 7 days after leaving the malarious area.

Antimalarial chemoprophylaxis— recommendations

Recommendations on appropriate antimalarial chemoprophylaxis are published weekly in the UK medical press. Furthermore, expert centres all over the UK (see below) and other organizations worldwide are able to give up-to-date advice. Prevention against mosquito bites applies to all areas.

Drugs used for prophylaxis against malaria should be started 1 week before travel—2.5 to 3 weeks before if taking mefloquine for the first time, the day before travel if taking proguanil or doxy-cycline.

They should be taken with unfailing regularity while in the malaria-endemic area and should be continued for 4 weeks after leaving the area. All antimalarials should be taken with or after food, with plenty of water. Doxycycline should not be taken lying down or immediately before lying down. Tables 59.4 and 59.6 give the drug regimens recommended for malaria chemoprophylaxis. The new British Malaria Guidelines expected in 2001 (Advisory Committee on Malaria Prophylaxis) and will be advocating child doses of antimalarial prophylactics according to the child's age and weight—see Table 59.5.

Table 59.4 Children's prophylactic doses for antimalarials.

Age	Weight (kg)	Chloroquine (C) plus proguanil (P)	Mefloquine	Dapsone plus pyrimethamine (Maloprim)
0–5 weeks	< 5	⅛ adult dose	Not recommended	Not recommended
6 weeks–1 year	5–10	⅛–¼ adult dose	¼ tablet	No paediatric formulation available
1–5 years	10–19	½ adult dose	¼ tablet	No paediatric formulation available
6–11 years	20–39	¾ adult dose	½ tablet (20–30 kg) ¾ tablet (31–39 kg)	½ adult dose
12 years to adult	> 40	Adult dose: C: 2 tablets once weekly P: 2 tablets daily	Adult dose ¾ tablet (40–45 kg), then 1 tablet once weekly (over 45 kg)	Adult dose 1 tablet once weekly

Table 59.5 Proportion of adult dose required for adequate child dose of antimalarial prophylactics according to the child's weight (from The new British Malaria Guidelines, expected to be published in 2001)

Weight in kg	Chloroquine 150 mg base weekly	Proguanil 100 mg weekly	Mefloquine 250 mg weekly	Doxycycline 100 mg weekly	Maloprim [one size] weekly	Age approximate
Under 6.0	0.125 dose ¼ tablet	0.125 dose ¼ tablet	NR	NR	NR	Term to 12 weeks
6.0 to 9.9	0.25 dose ½ tablet	0.25 dose ½ tablet	0.25 dose ¼ tablet	NR	0.25 dose ¼ tablet	3 months to 11 months
10.0 to 15.9	0.375 dose ¾ tablet	0.375 dose ¾ tablet	0.25 dose* ¼ tablet	NR	0.25 dose* ¼ tablet	1 year to 3 yrs 11 months
16.0 to 24.9	0.5 dose 1 tablet	0.5 dose 1 tablet	0.5 dose ½ tablet	NR	0.5 dose ½ tablet	4 years to 7 yrs 11 months
25.0 to 44.9	0.75 dose 1½ tablets	0.75 dose 1½ tablets	0.75 dose ¾ tablet	adult dose from age 12yrs 1 tablet†	0.75 dose ¾ tablet	8 years to 12 yrs 11 months
45 kg & over	Adult dose 2 tablets	Adult dose 2 tablets	Adult dose 1 tablet	Adult dose 1 tablet	Adult dose 1 tablet	13 years and over

Caution: In other countries tablet size may vary. NR: Not Recommended

* For these two medicines at this age/weight, 0.375 dose would be preferable, but cannot be safely provided by breaking the adult tablet.

† The adult dose is necessary as doxycycline is only available in capsule form and a 0.75 dose is not feasible.

Table 59.6 Oral prophylaxis against malaria.

Drug	Trade name	Tablet/capsule (mg)	Prophylactic dose	
			Adult	Paediatric
Chloroquine	Avloclor*	250 (155 base)	Two tablets once	5 mg base/kgBW once weekly
	Nivaquine†	200 (150 base)	weekly	
Proguanil	Paludrine*	100	Two tablets	< 1 year: 0.25 tablet
			once daily,	1–4 years: 0.5 tablet
				5–8 years: 1 tablet
				9–14 years: 1.5 tablet
Mefloquine	Lariam	250 (228 in USA)	One tablet once	< 5 kg: not recommended
			weekly	5–19 kg: 0.25 tablet
				20–30 kg: 0.5 tablet
				31–45 kg: 0.75 tablet
Doxycycline	Nordox	100	One tablet daily	Not recommended
	Vibramycin	100		under 12 years
Dapsone plus	Maloprim	100 + 12.5	One tablet	< 5 years: not recommended
pyrimethamine			once weekly	5–10 years: 0.5 tablet
				> 10 years, 1 tablet once weekly

*A combined proprietary preparation 'Paludrine/Avloclor' is available (see Table 59.3).
†Nivaquine is available as a syrup-chloroquine sulphate 68 mg/5 mL (= chloroquine base 50 mg/5 mL) in 100-mL bottles. Note: in France a once daily combined preparation is available ('Savarine'–AstraZeneca) that gives a higher weekly dose of chloroquine as the tablet taken daily contains proguanil 200 mg plus chloroquine 100 mg (base).

Advice on malaria

Expert up-to-date advice should be obtained before travelling. Health professionals should seek advice when necessary. Among sources for information are the following.

The Malaria Reference Laboratory. For the public, Tel.: 0891 600 350—24-h Helpline (payline). For advice to doctors and nurses, Tel.: 020 7927 2437.

London Hospital for Tropical Diseases, Mortimer Market, Capper Street, off Tottenham Court Road, London WClE 6AU. Main switchboard for University College Hospital, Tel.: 020 7387 9300. Fax: 020 7388 7645. Clinical services, Tel.: 020 7387 4411 (ask for the duty doctor). Travel Clinic—pretravel advice on prophylaxis, Tel.: 020 7388 9600; Fax: 020 7383 4817. Department of Clinical Parasitology, Tel.: 020 7387 9300 ext. 5418. Healthline provides recorded verbal advice, Tel.: 0839 337733 (payline as above).

London School of Hygiene and Tropical Medicine, Keppel Street, London WClE 7HT, Tel.: 020 7636 8636. Advice for medics, Tel.: 020 7530 3500. Medics for advice on malaria prophylaxis, Tel.: 020

7927 2437 (09.00–16.30 h). Continuous pre-recorded tape with malaria advice for travellers, Tel.: 0891 600350 (payline).

Malaria, a website mainly concerned with southern Africa, but the advice may be considered good, and there is also a link to British Airways Travel Clinics, which is worth looking at for information: http://www.africasafari.co.za/malaria1.htm

Medical Advisory Service for Travellers Abroad (MASTA), Room 28, Denton House, 40–44 Wicklow Street, London WC1 9HL, Tel.: 020 7837 5540; Travel Health Line, Tel.: 0906 822 4100 (24 h advice, payline, 60p per minute); visa and passport information line, Tel.: 0906 5501 100 (calls charged at £1.00 per minute). MASTA Marketing and sales: Moorfield Road, Yeadon, Leeds LS19 7BN, Tel.: 0113 2387 500; Fax: 0113 2387 501. Website: http://www.masta.org/index.html

Health professionals only can obtain advice from the following centres:
Glasgow: 0141 9467 120
Liverpool: 0151 7089 393
Birmingham: 0121 7666 611
Oxford: 01865 225 570 (Ward). 01865 225 217

London: (Outpatients 14.00–17.00 h)
020 7927 2437 (09.00–16.30 h on weekdays). PHLS Communicable Disease Surveillance Centre, Tel.: 020 8200 6868 ext. 3412 (09.00–12.30 h on weekdays).

Travel Health, a website for advice to nurses: http://www.TravelHealth.co.uk

Visiting Africa, Asia, South America? Think Malaria—information leaflet for travellers from the DoH. For copies, write to: DoH, PO Box 410, Wetherby LS23 7LN.

Malaria Foundation: http://www.malaria.org

Medicines for Malaria Venture (MMV): http://www.malariamedicines.org

American University of Beirut: information on malaria prophylaxis, countries listed alphabetically: http://www.aub.edu.lb/uhs/chm/travel

Centres for Disease Control and Prevention: details recommendations for the prevention of malaria are available from US CDC 24 h a day from the voice information service (001 888 2323228), the Fax information service (001 888 2323299) or the Internet: http://www.cdc.gov/travel/index.htm

SCIEH *Fit for Travel* is a colourful and informative website from SCIEH free for the public. It gives country-specific information on immunizations and other preventive strategies, including information on malaria: http://www.fitfortravel.scot.nhs.uk

The Yellow Book: Health Information for Overseas Travel. A new edition was expected in spring 2001. Edited by G. Lea and J. Leese. HMSO.

The Yellow Book: International Travel and Health—vaccination requirements and health advice 2000, WHO. http://www.who.int/ith/english/index.html.

Malaria Guidelines—UK, the 1997 British Malaria Prophylaxis Guidelines (see below): http://www.phls.co.uk/advice/cdrr1097.pdf

The British malaria prophylaxis guidelines

The need to balance the risk of malaria and the risk of adverse reactions to antimalarials, as well as the need to provide up-to-date, easy to understand information was achieved with the publication of the new *British Malaria Guidelines* in September 1997 [Bradley D.J. & Warhurst D.C. on behalf of an expert group of doctors, nurses and pharmacists. (1997) Guidelines for the prevention of malaria in travellers from the United Kingdom *Commun. Dis. Rep. CDR Rev.* 7, R137–52, and on the web: http://www.phls.co.uk/advice/cdrr1097.pdf]. The material in Tables 59.7–59.12 refers to these guidelines (Fig. 59.3 contains information on malaria from the WHO).

The preferred chemoprophylaxis recommendations for each country are followed by an alternative regimen for those people who cannot tolerate or are unwilling to follow the recommended regimen. These guidelines give general guidance. For specific guidance on particular areas or up-to-date advice, the reader should consider contacting the Malaria Reference Laboratories and other specialist organizations (see above).

North Africa and the Middle East

Travellers in north Africa and the Middle East who are advised no chemoprophylaxis but avoidance of mosquito bites should remember the possibility of malaria if they get fever even after a year of returning to the UK—this advice applies to all of north Africa (except for the El Faiyum area of Egypt south-west of Cairo) and to most tourist areas in Turkey, as far as east of Antalya (see Table 59.7). Vivax malaria predominates eastwards along the Turkish coast from Antalya to the Syrian border and further inland in east Turkey (about 100 000 cases of malaria reported every year), and in parts of Syria and Iraq. Falciparum malaria with varying degrees of resistance to chloroquine occurs in Iran, Afghanistan, Oman, Yemen and some Emirates.

Africa south of the Sahara

The risk of falciparum malaria (much of it

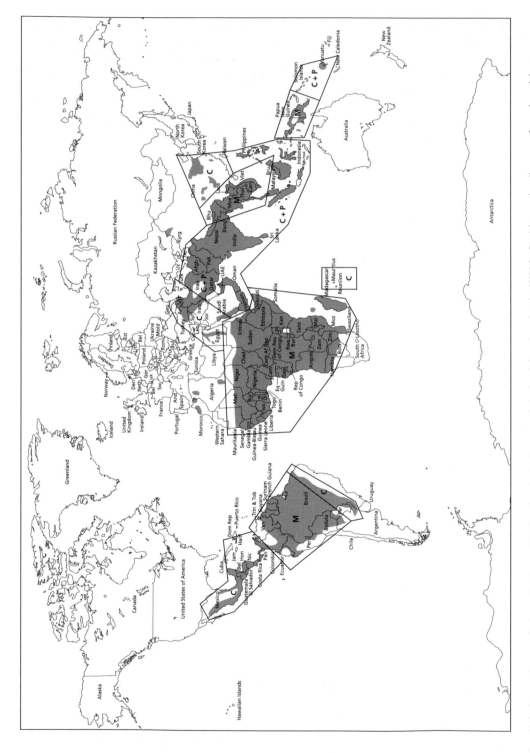

Fig. 59.3 Areas where malaria can be transmitted and malaria drug prophylaxis advice given by the WHO. C, chloroquine (in case of very low risk no prophylaxis); C + P, chloroquine plus proguanil (in case of very low risk no prophylaxis); M, mefloquine—first choice; chloroquine and proguanil—second choice; border areas near Cambodia/Myanmar/Thailand—doxycycline (in case of very low risk no prophylaxis). (Adapted from *International travel and health vaccination requirements and health advice.* Geneva: WHO, 1999.)

Table 59.7 Malaria in North Africa and the Middle East (reproduced with permission of the PHLS Communicable Disease Surveillance Centre © PHLS).

Risk	Country	Preferable approach/drug(s)	Alternative drug(s)
Very low	Abu Dhabi, Algeria, Egypt (tourist areas) Libya, Morocco, Tunisia Turkey (most tourist areas)	Avoid mosquito bites	
Low	Azerbaijan (southern border areas), Egypt (El Faiyum only, June-Oct.), Iraq (rural north, May-Nov.), Syria (north border, May-Oct.), Turkey (plain around Adona, Side, south-east Anatolia; Mar.–Nov.) Tajikistan (south border areas)	Chloroquine	Proguanil
Present chloroquine resistance	Afghanistan (below 2000 m, May-Nov.), Iran (Mar.-Nov.), Oman Saudi Arabia (except northern, eastern and central provinces, Asir plateau, and western border cities, where there is very little risk), United Arab Emirates (northern rural areas only), Yemen	Chloroquine plus proguanil	

Table 59.8 Malaria in sub-Saharan Africa (reproduced with permission of the PHLS Communicable Disease Surveillance Centre (© PHLS).

Risk	Country	Preferable approach/drug(s)	Alternative drug(s)
Risk very high, or locally very high. Chloroquine resistance very widespread	Angola, Benin, Burkina Faso, Burundi, Cameroon, Central African Republic, Chad, Comoros, Congo, Djibouti, Eritrea, Equatorial Guinea, Ethiopia, Gabon, Ghana, Guinea, Guinea-Bissau, Ivory Coast, Kenya, Liberia, Madagascar, Malawi, Mali, Mozambique, Niger, Nigeria, Principe, Rwanda, São Tomé, Senegal, Sierra Leone, Somalia, Sudan, Swaziland, Tanzania, The Gambia, Togo, Uganda, Zaire, Zambia	Mefloquine 2001*	Proguanil plus chloroquine (doxycycline used with efficacy for some exposed to high risk)
Risk in parts of country. Some chloroquine resistance	Botswana (only in the northern half of the country, Nov.–June), Mauritania (year round in the south; in north, July–Oct.) Namibia (northern third only, Nov.–June) South Africa (north-east, low altitude areas of north-eastern Transvaal, and eastern Natal down to 100 km north of Durban) Zimbabwe (areas below 1200 m, Nov.–June; all year in Zambezi valley where mefloquine is preferable)	Chloroquine plus proguanil	Maloprim or mefloquine
Low risk	Cape Verde (remember low risk exists if fever develops) Mauritius (except rural areas where chloroquine prophylaxis is appropriate)	Avoid mosquito bites	

* New guidelines suggest mefloquine is recommended, and doxycycline or malarone are good alternatives. For short trips malarone may be preferred (continued for only 7 days after exposure).

resistant to chloroquine) in sub-Saharan Africa is very high, except in the extreme south of Africa (see Table 59.8). Mefloquine gives the best protection. Breakthrough malaria may occur on all regimens. The Seychelles and some highland areas of Ethiopia (Addis Ababa) and Kenya (includes central Nairobi but not its surroundings) are malaria-free. Tourists to South Africa who stay only in major cities only do not need to take chemoprophylaxis but they should report fever promptly, especially in the first 3 months of their return.

East Africa

Visitors to tourist resorts on the coast of Kenya and Tanzania (but not rural Tanzania) for periods of 2 weeks or less, the Gambia in January to May, and local areas known to be low risk, can take proguanil plus chloroquine, although protection will be incomplete (they must remember to report unexplained fever for at least 3 months after their return). They should not leave the tourist resorts for rural areas or safari. Mefloquine is recommended for longer visits, higher risk activities (backpacking, safaris, staying/visiting rural areas). Stress to these travellers that even a short trip away from the coastal resort could expose them to malaria. If they are unwilling to take mefloquine or cannot take it because of contraindications, in the absence of contraindications they may consider doxycycline. When the traveller intends to stay for over 2 weeks in east Africa, the benefits of taking mefloquine far exceed the risks of adverse effects.

West Africa

The risk of falciparum malaria in the forest zone of west Africa is 4% per fortnight if the traveller is unprotected. In these forest areas high rates of transmission are observed throughout the year. Chloroquine resistance is patchy. Mefloquine is the drug of choice, especially during the transmission season (June to December—as in the Gambia), with proguanil plus chloroquine being an alternative regimen, especially between January and May, but it is generally a less effective combination.

South Asia (Table 59.9)

Plasmodium vivax predominates in this area but *P. falciparum* is often present and resistant to chloroquine. Immigrants to the UK returning to south Asia to visit friends and relatives are at particular risk.

South-East Asia (Table 59.10)

The risk in much of Thailand, Bangkok, Chiang Mai, and the main coastal holiday resorts of Pattaya, Phuket and Ko Samui is low and tourists may consider no chemoprophylaxis but they should

Table 59.9 Malaria in south Asia (reproduced with permission of the PHLS Communicable Disease Surveillance Centre © PHLS).

Risk	Country	Preferable drug(s)	Alternative drug(s)
Risk variable, chloroquine resistance usually moderate	Bangladesh (except Chittagong Hill Tracts; no risk in Dhaka city) Bhutan (southern districts only) India (no risk in mountain states of north) Nepal (below 1300 m; no risk in Kathmandu) Pakistan (below 2000 m) Sri Lanka (no risk in and just south of Colombo)	Chloroquine plus proguanil	Will vary locally
Risk high, chloroquine resistance high	Bangladesh (only in Chittagong Hill Tracts)	Mefloquine	Chloroquine plus proguanil

Table 59.10 Malaria in South-East Asia (reproduced with permission of the PHLS Communicable Disease Surveillance Centre © PHLS).

Risk	Country	Preferable approach/drug(s)
Risk very low, remember malaria possible if fever	Bali, Brunei, China (main tourist areas), Hong Kong, Malaysia (except Sabah and deep forest where chloroquine plus proguanil), Sarawak, Thailand, Bangkok, and main tourist centres	Avoid mosquito bites
Risk variable, some chloroquine resistance	Indonesia (other than Bali and cities where there is low risk and Irian Jaya, where mefloquine is recommended) Sabah Philippines (rural below 600 m; no risk in Cebu, Leyte, Bohol, Catanduanes) Deep forests of peninsular Malaysia and Sarawak	Chloroquine plus proguanil
Risk substantial and drug resistance common	Cambodia China (only in Yunnan and Hainan; chloroquine in other remote areas of China) Irian Jaya, Laos, Myanmar (formerly Burma), Vietnam (except no risk in cities, Red River delta area, coastal plain north of Nha Trang)	Mefloquine
Risk great, mefloquine resistance prevalent	Cambodia, western provinces Thailand, borders with Cambodia and Myanmar	Doxycycline

Table 59.11 Malaria in Oceania (reproduced with permission of the PHLS Communicable Disease Surveillance Centre © PHLS).

Risk	Country	Preferable drug(s)	Alternative drug(s)
Risk high, chloroquine resistance high	Papua New Guinea, below 1800 m Solomon Islands Vanuatu	Doxycycline	Mefloquine or Maloprim plus chloroquine

take every precaution against mosquito bites and report fever promptly. Travellers to Ko Chang should take chemoprophylaxis. Singapore is malaria free. Travellers to China may not take chemoprophylaxis other than for travel to South Yunnan and Hainan Province, where mefloquine (or doxycycline) is appropriate. Kunming, Dali and Lijiang are malaria-free. On the borders of Thailand with Cambodia and Myanmar (Burma) as well as in the western provinces of Cambodia, the malaria parasite exhibits multidrug resistance, including mefloquine, so doxycycline is recommended for these areas.

Kalimantan (Borneo) is part of Indonesia (Sabah and Sarawak north of Kalimantan are part of Malaysia). The recommended regimen is chloroquine plus proguanil.

Oceania

See Table 59.11.

Latin America and Caribbean

The basin of the river Amazon is a high risk, highly chloroquine-resistant malaria area and mefloquine is the drug of choice. Central America is free of chloroquine resistance, predominated by vivax malaria. Falciparum malaria is a risk on the island that includes Haiti and the Dominican Republic but it is sensitive to chloroquine, which should be taken (see Table 59.12).

Since the publication of the *British Malaria Guidelines*, the prevailing by consensus advice for visits to sub-Saharan Africa is that mefloquine should

Table 59.12 Malaria in Latin America and the Caribbean (reproduced with permission of the PHLS Communicable Disease Surveillance Centre © PHLS).

Risk	Country	Preferable drug(s)	Alternative drug(s)
Risk high, marked chloroquine resistance	Brazil ('legal Amazon' area, Amazon basin, Mato Grosso, and Maranhão only; very low risk and no chemoprophylaxis elsewhere) Colombia (most areas below 800 m) French Guiana, Guyana (all interior regions), Surinam (except Paramaribo and coast), Amazon basin area of Bolivia and Venezuela	Mefloquine 2001*	Chloroquine plus proguanil
Risk variable or high, chloroquine resistance present	Bolivia (rural areas below 2500 m) Ecuador (areas below 1500 m) Panama, east of canal Peru (rural areas below 1500 m) Venezuela (rural areas other than coast, Caracas free of malaria)	Chloroquine plus proguanil	Mefloquine or Maloprim 2001*
Risk variable to low, no chloroquine resistance	Argentina (small area in north-west only), Belize (rural except Belize district), Costa Rice (rural below 500 m), Dominican Republic, El Salvador, Guatemala (below 1500 m), Haiti, Honduras, Mexico (in some rural areas not regularly visited by tourists), Nicaragua, Panama (west of canal), Paraguay (rural October–May)	Chloroquine	Proguanil

* New guidelines suggest doxycycline or malarone are recommended as alternatives. For short trips malarone may be preferred (continue for 7 days after exposure).

be reserved for visits of over 2 weeks, and chloroquine plus proguanil for visits of up to 2 weeks in tourist areas. These travellers should be reminded of the need to report any pyrexial illness, especially in the first 3 months after their visit to Africa.

Part 6

Immunization and Travel Information Resources

Chapter 60

International Society of Travel Medicine

European Charter for Travel Health

Minimum standards for travel health advice to be provided by the travel trade (agent) at the time of booking prior to travel.

General
- Verbal/written advice to traveller to seek medical advice at least 4 weeks (if possible) prior to travel
- Supplementary information leaflets provided

Malaria
- Highlight whether malaria precautions are necessary
- Advise on measures against mosquito bites
- No reference to specific drugs
- Advise medical consultation if fever is present on return

Vaccination
- Required: yellow fever
- Recommended: Update of basic vaccination, i.e. tetanus; diphtheria; polio
- Travel related, i.e. hepatitis A, typhoid

Other
- Food/beverages
- Hygiene
- Animal bites
- Sunburn
- Accidents

Chapter 61

Specimen immunization exemption certificate

The Ringmead Medical Practice
Birch Hill Medical Centre
Bracknell, Berkshire RG12 7WW
United Kingdom
Tel.: + 44 1344 456 535

Date:

Immunization Exemption Certificate

Name:

Address:

Date of Birth:

Destination:

The traveller named above is my patient and under my medical care. Having considered his/her medical details, I am exempting this traveller from the requirement of being immunized against

. . . .

Faithfully,

Dr George Kassianos
General Medical Practitioner

Chapter 62

Notifiable diseases

The notification system in England and Wales is the oldest national system for the collection of morbidity statistics on communicable diseases (see Table 62.1 for list). It came about with the introduction of the Infectious Disease (Notification) Act 1889, which aimed to identify and prevent the spread of infectious disease. The responsibility for processing data on notifications of infectious disease now rests with the Public Health Laboratory Service (PHLS) Communicable Disease Surveillance Centre (CDSC).

● A fee is payable to doctors in the UK who notify any of the above diseases. The average GP notifies fewer than 12 infectious diseases each year.

● Acquired immune deficiency syndrome (AIDS) is not a notifiable disease in the UK. None the less, doctors are advised to report new cases to the Director, PHLS Communicable Disease Surveillance Centre, London.

● Doctors looking after patients who have, or are suspected of having a notifiable disease, are legally required by the Public Health Acts to notify such cases to their Local Authority proper officer (consultant in communicable diseases, the Local Authority environmental health officer). Such notification is not dependent upon laboratory confirmation.

● In Scotland and Northern Ireland the appropriate officer is the chief administrative medical officer (CAMO) or the director of public health.

Table 62.1 Notifiable diseases within the UK.

England and Wales	Year when made notifiable in England and Wales	Northern Ireland	Scotland
Anthrax	1960	Acute encephalitis	Anthrax
Cholera	1889	Acute meningitis	Chickenpox
Diphtheria	1889	Anthrax	Cholera
		Cholera	Diphtheria
Dysentery (amoebic or	1919	Diphtheria	Bacillary dysentery
bacillary)		Dysentery	Food poisoning
Encephalitis (acute)	1918	Food poisoning	Legionellosis
Food poisoning (all sources)	1949	(all sources)	Leptospirosis
		Gastroenteritis	Malaria
Leprosy	1951	(children under 2 years)	Measles
Leptospirosis	1968	Infective hepatitis	Membranous croup
		Lassa fever	Meningococcal infection
Malaria	1919	Marburg disease	Mumps
Measles	1940	Paratyphoid fever	Paratyphoid fever
Meningitis	1968	Plague	Puerperal fever
Meningococcal septicaemia	1988	Poliomyelitis: paralytic	Rabies
(without meningitis)		and nonparalytic	Relapsing fever
Mumps	1988	Relapsing fever	Scarlet fever
Ophthalmia neonatorum	1914	Scarlet fever	Smallpox
		Smallpox	Tetanus

continued p. 394

Table 62.1 *cont.*

England and Wales	Year when made notifiable in England and Wales	Northern Ireland	Scotland
Paratyphoid fever	1889	Tuberculosis: pulmonary	Tuberculosis
Plague	1900	Rabies	Rubella
Poliomyelitis (acute)	1912	and nonpulmonary	Typhoid fever
Rabies	1976	Typhoid fever	Typhus fever
Relapsing fever	1889	Typhus	Viral haemorrhagic fever
Rubella	1988	Viral haemorrhagic fever	Viral hepatitis
		Whooping cough	Whooping cough
Scarlet fever	1889	Yellow fever	
Smallpox	1889		
Tetanus	1968		
Tuberculosis	1912		
Typhoid fever	1889		
Typhus	1889		
Viral haemorrhagic fever	1976		
Viral hepatitis	1968		
Whooping cough	1940		
Yellow fever	1968		

Chapter 63

Reciprocal healthcare agreements between the UK and other non-EEA countries

People who normally live in the UK can obtain a certain level of treatment while visiting countries outside the European Economic Area (EEA) with which the UK has a reciprocal agreement—it may not apply if the person is going to live or work in that country. This agreement provides for urgently needed medical treatment at reduced cost or, in some cases, free in over 40 countries around the world. Points to remember are the following.

- Only urgently needed treatment is provided.
- The UK traveller is treated on the same terms as residents of that country.
- The range of services may be more restricted than under the NHS.
- If charges are involved, these cannot be refunded by the British Government.
- Extra travel insurance is strongly advisable.

- To obtain treatment the traveller will need to produce his/her passport or some proof of UK residence, such as a driving licence or medical card.
- Requirements vary from country to country and are shown in Table 63.1.
- Renal dialysis is not provided as 'urgently needed treatment' under the reciprocal agreement, except in Australia. The full cost of dialysis has to be paid.

In Table 63.1 you will find the full country-by-country checklist, as it was published in March 2000 in the DoH booklet *Health Advice for Travellers*, which can be obtained by phoning the Health Literature Line on 0800 555 777 any time, free of charge. I am grateful to the DoH for allowing me to reproduce this checklist.

Table 63.1 Reciprocal healthcare agreements: country-by-country checklist of countries outside the European Economic Area.

Country	Documents needed to get medical treatment	What is normally free	What you pay charges for	Other information
Anguilla	Proof of UK residence (e.g. NHS medical card or UK driving licence)	Minor emergency treatment	Hospital in-patient and outpatient treatment. Hospital accommodation. Dental treatment. Prescribed medicines. Ambulance travel	Family doctor-type treatment is available at outpatient clinics. A charge is made
Australia	Proof of UK residence (e.g. UK passport or NHS medical card) and temporary entry permit	Hospital treatment (including renal dialysis but arrangements must be made before departure—further details from NHS renal units)	Treatment at most doctors' surgeries. Prescribed medicines. Ambulance travel. Dental treatment	You will need to enrol at a local Medicare office but this can be done after you get treatment. Some doctor's charges may be partially refunded by the Medicare scheme. Claim at the local office before you leave

continued p. 396

Table 63.1 *cont.*

Country	Documents needed to get medical treatment	What is normally free	What you pay charges for	Other information
Barbados	UK passport (or NHS medical card if not a UK national)	Hospital treatment. Treatment at polyclinics. Ambulance travel. Prescribed medicines for children and the elderly	Dental treatment. Prescribed medicines	
British Virgin Islands	Proof of UK residence (e.g. NHS medical card or UK driving licence)	Hospital and other medical treatment for persons aged 70 or over and school-age children	Other visitors are charged for all services at rates applicable to residents	
Bulgaria	UK passport and NHS medical card	Hospital treatment. Other medical and dental treatment	Medicines supplied by public pharmacy	
Channel Islands—if staying less than 3 months	Proof of UK residence (e.g. driving licence or NHS medical card)	*On Guernsey/Alderney:* Hospital treatment.	Some prescribed medicines. Accident and emergency hospital treatment. Emergency dental treatment. GP and other medical care. Ambulance treatment.	No outpatient department at Guernsey General Hospital
		On Jersey: Hospital in-patient and outpatient treatment. Ambulance travel *On Sark:* Medical treatment	Treatment at a doctor's surgery. Dental care. Prescribed medicines	Free treatment at a family doctor-type clinic is available most weekday mornings at the General Hospital. Hospital treatment provided in Guernsey
Czech Republic	UK passport	Hospital treatment. Dental treatment	Other medical care	
Falkland Islands	Proof of UK residence (e.g. medical card or UK driving licence)	Hospital treatment. Dental treatment. Other medical treatment. Prescribed medicines. Ambulance travel		
Hungary	UK passport	Treatment in hospital, polyclinic or at a doctors' surgery	Dental and ophthalmic treatment. Prescribed medicines (flat rate charge)	
Isle of Man	No documents needed	Treatment as for UK National Health Service	Dental treatment. Prescribed medicines	
Malta —up to 30 days stay	UK passport	Immediately necessary medical treatment in a government hospital, area health centre (polyclinic) or district dispensary	Non-government hospital dispensary or polyclinic treatment. Treatment at a private doctor's surgery. Prescribed medicines	

continued

Table 63.1 *cont.*

Country	Documents needed to get medical treatment	What is normally free	What you pay charges for	Other information
Montserrat	Proof of UK residence (e.g. NHS medical card or UK driving licence)	Treatment at government institutions for persons aged over 65 and under 16. Dental treatment for school-age children	Hospital in-patient and outpatient treatment. Hospital accommodation. Most prescribed medicines. Dental treatment. Ambulance travel	Family doctor-type treatment is available at government clinics and the hospital casualty department. A charge is made
New Zealand	UK passport	Dental treatment (persons under 16). Public hospital in-patient treatment	Treatment at hospitals (outpatient). Treatment at a doctor's surgery. Prescribed medicines. Dental treatment	Ask hospital or doctor if a refund is due. If not, claim at the local health office. Cash benefits from New Zealand Department of Health reduce charges
Poland	NHS medical card	Hospital treatment. Some dental treatment. Other medical treatment	Doctor's visit (e.g. to your hotel). 30% of cost of prescribed medicines from a public pharmacy	
Romania	UK passport	Hospital treatment. Some dental treatment. Other medical treatment	Medicines supplied by public pharmacy	
Russia	UK passport	Treatment in state hospitals	Prescribed medicines	
Slovak Republic	UK passport	Hospital treatment. Other medical care	Prescribed medicines	
St Helena	Proof of UK residence (e.g. NHS medical card or UK passport)	Hospital treatment in outpatient clinics during normal clinic times	Hospital in-patient treatment. Dental treatment. Prescribed medicines. Ambulance travel	Family doctor-type treatment is available at the hospital outpatient clinic
Turks and Caicos Islands	Proof of UK residence (e.g. NHS medical card or UK driving licence)	All treatment to those under 16 and over 65 *On Grand Turk Island*: Dental treatment (at dental clinic). Prescribed medicines. Ambulance travel *On Outer Islands*: Medical treatment at government clinics. Prescribed medicines	*On Grand Turk Island*: Hospital in-patient treatment. Other medical treatment and the Town clinic	*On Outer Islands*: No hospital services available on the outer islands

continued p. 398

Table 63.1 *cont.*

Country	Documents needed to get medical treatment	What is normally free	What you pay charges for	Other information
This agreement applies to the following republics of the former USSR: Armenia, Azerbaijan, Belarus, Georgia, Kazakhstan, Kirgizstan, Moldova, Russia, Tajikistan, Turkmenistan, Uzbekistan, Ukraine	UK passport	Hospital treatment. Some dental treatment. Other medical treatment	Prescribed medicines	This agreement does not apply to Latvia, Lithuania, Estonia
Yugoslavia, i.e. Serbia and Montenegro and successor states Croatia, Bosnia, Slovenia, Macedonia	UK passport if you are a UK national. If you are a UK resident but not a UK national you will need a certificate of insurance, obtainable from Inland Revenue National Office, International Services, Longbenton, Newcastle-Upon-Tyne, NE98 1ZZ	Hospital treatment. Some dental treatment. Other medical treatment	Prescribed medicines	If you are a Yugoslav national resident in the UK you will need to show your Yugoslav passport and a certificate of UK social security insurance, obtainable from Inland Revenue National Office, International Services, Longbenton, Newcastle-Upon-Tyne, NE98 1ZZ or Social Security Agency, Overseas Benefits Unit, Block 2, Castle Buildings, Stormont, Belfast BT4 3SP, Tel.: 02890 520520. If you are not an UK/Yugoslav national but are the dependant of someone who is, you should also apply for a certificate. The agreement applies to all the successor republics

Chapter 64

Sources of travel information: useful addresses/telephone numbers/websites

- **African Medical Research Foundation.** Tel.: 020 7201 6070. Website: http://www.amref.org.
- **Age Concern.** Tel.: 020 8679 8000. Provides advice on travel insurance for the elderly and all aspects of travel.
- **Airports. Heathrow Travelcare.** Tel.: 020 8745 7495. **Gatwick:** Airport services for the disabled—North Terminal Tel.: 01293 507 147 and South Terminal Tel.: 01293 502 337.
- **Air Transport Users Committee.** (Advice for disabled travellers) Care-in-the-Air, 1229 Kingsway, London WC2B 6NN. Tel.: 020 7240 6061.
- **Alertness Solutions.** Advice on jetlag in association with British Airways: http://www.alertness-solution.com
- **Alliance Group** (includes Bill and Melinda Gates): http://www.vaccines.org
- **Alpine Club,** 55/56 Charlotte Road, London EC2 3QT. Tel.: 020 7613 0755. Website: http://www.alpine-club.org.uk
- **American Academy of Paediatrics.** 141 North-west Point Blvd, Elk Grove Village, IL 60007-1098. Tel.: 001 847 228 5005. Fax: 228 5097. http://www.aap.org. For the current USA shedule of routine childhood immunizations, go to http://www.aap.org/family, then click on *Immunization Information*, followed by *Immunization Schedule* that is preceded by the year in numeric.
- **American Association of Immunologists,** 9650 Rockville Pike, Bethesda, MD 20814; Tel.: 001 240 264 8600; Fax: 001 301 571 1816; Website: http://www.aai.org
- **American Digestive Health Foundation**'s website reviews the hepatites very well: http://www.mars.gastro.org/adhf/viral-hep.html
- **American Home Products.** http://www.ahp.com
- **American Society of Microbiology,** 1752 N Street, NW Washington, DC 20036-2804; Tel.: 001 202 942 9356; Fax: 942 9340; Website: http://www.asmusa.org
- **American Society of Tropical Medicine and Hygiene.** http://www.astmh.org. Go to questions and answers. Connections to other websites.
- **American University of Beirut.** Information on malaria prophylaxis, countries listed alphabetically. Also, information on yellow fever: http://www.aub.edu.lb/uhs/chm/travel
- **Asia Source.** Developed by the US-based Asia Society to meet the need for timely, reliable, unbiased information for travellers about Asia: http://www.asiasource.org
- **AstraZeneca,** King's Court, Water Lane, Wilmslow, Cheshire SK9 5AZ. Tel.: 01625 712 712. Fax: 01625 712 581.
- **Automobile Association (AA).** Produces a free Travel Guide for the Disabled. Tel.: 020 8954 7373.
- **Aventis Pasteur MSD Ltd,** Mallards Reach, Bridge Avenue, Maidenhead, Berkshire SL6 1QP. Tel.: 07000 822 2463. Fax: 01628 671 722. Vaccine Information Service: Tel.: 07000 766 73 847. Orders: 0321 2 8222 463. Freefax order number: 0321 329 8222 463. Website: http://www.aventis-pasteur-msd.com
- **Aviation Health Institute.** Oxford. Tel.: 01865 739 681. Website: http://www.aviation-health.org.
- **Aviatours Ltd,** Pinewood, Eglinton Road, Tiford, Surrey GU10 2DH. Tel.: 01252 793 250. Manchester Office Tel.: 01618 327 972. Two-monthly one-day (Saturday) courses in London and Manchester, designed to overcome fear of flying.
- **Bayer—Diagnostics Division,** Bayer House,

Strawberry Hill, Newbury, Berkshire RG14 1JA.
Tel.: 01635 563 000.
- **Baxter Healthcare Ltd**. See Hyland Immuno,
Baxter Healthcare Ltd.
- **BBC2 Ceefax** p. 470
- **BBC Travel Pages**. http://www.takeoff.beeb.com
- **BCB Ltd**, Moorland Road, Cardiff CF24 2YL.
Tel.: 029 20 464 464. Fax: 029 20 481 100. Website:
http://www.bcb.ltd.uk For the 'Wilderness First
Aid Kit', disposable personal urination pouches
and other products.
- **BHAN (Black HIV/AIDS Network)**, St Ste-
phen's House, 41 Uxbridge Road, London W12
7LH. Tel.: 020 8749 2828.
- **Birmingham Heartlands Hospital—
Department of Infection and Tropical Medi-
cine**, Bordesley Green East, Birmingham B9 5ST.
Tel.: 0121 766 6611 ext. 4382/4403.
- **Bio Products Laboratory**, Dagger Lane,
Elstree, Herts WR6 3BX. Tel.: 020 8905 1818. Fax:
020 8207 4824.
- **Blood Care Foundation**, PO Box 7, Seve-
noaks, Kent TN13 2SZ. Tel.: 01732 742 427. Fax:
01732 451 199. Information and Membership
details Tel.: 01293 425 485. Fax: 01293 425 488. E-
mail: JulianBruce@compuserve.com
- **Blood Transfusion Services**, Scotland
  Aberdeen: Forester Hill Road, Aberdeen AB9
  2ZW, Scotland. Tel.: 01224 681 818.
  Dundee: Ninewells Hospital, Dundee DD1 9SY,
  Scotland. Tel.: 01382 645 166.
  Edinburgh: Department of Transfusion Medi-
  cine, Royal Infirmary, Laurison Place, Edin-
  burgh EH3 9HB, Scotland. Tel.: 0131 536 5360.
  Glasgow: Law Hospital, Carluke NL8 5ES,
  Scotland. Tel.: 01698 373 315/8.
  Inverness: Raigmore Hospital, Inverness IV2
  3UJ, Scotland. Tel.: 01463 704 21213.
  Scottish National Blood Transfusion Service, 21
  Ellens Glen Road, Edinburgh EH17 7QT. Tel.:
  0131 664 2317S.
- **British Airways Health Services** Waterside
PO Box 365, Harmondsworth UB7 0GB. Tel.: 020
8738 5444. Fax: 020 8738 944. The 'Passenger
Clearance Department' will answer questions
about concerns with travellers. Patients may ring
directly for advice too.
- **British Airways Travel Clinics**. For details of

nearest clinic Tel.: 01276 685 040. Website: http://
www.british-airways.com or for common ques-
tions and answers on travel health http://
www.british-airways.com/travelqa/fyi/health/
health.shtml
- **British Diabetic Association. Now Diabetes
UK**
- **British Epilepsy Association**, 40 Hanover
Square, Leeds LS3 1BE. Helpline: 0800 800 5050.
- **British Heart Foundation**, 14 Fitzhardinge
Street, London W1H 4DH. Tel.: 020 77935 0185.
- **British Liver Trust**. Tel.: 0808 800 1000 (10 am
to 2 pm Monday to Friday).
- **British Malaria Advisory Panel**, the 1997
British Malaria Prophylaxis Guidelines: http://
www.phls.co.uk/publications/CDReview/
cdrr1097.pdf
- **British Medical Association**, Tavistock
Square, London WC1P 9PJ. Website: http://
www.bma.org.uk Tel.: England—020 7387 4499;
Scotland—0131 662 4820; Wales—01222 766 277;
Northern Ireland—01232 663 272.
- **British Mountaineering Council**, Informa-
tion Service, 177–179 Burton Road, Manchester
M20 2BB. Tel.: 0161 445 4747. Fax: 0161 445 4500.
Website: http://www.thebmc.co.uk
- **British National Formulary** online: http://
bnf.org/
- **British Red Cross Society**, 9 Grosvenor
Crescent, London SW1 7EJ. Tel.: 020 7235 5454.
For loan of equipment such as wheelchairs.
- **British Travel Health Association (BTHA)**,
c/o Scottish Centre for Infection and Environ-
mental Health, Clifton House, Clifton Place,
Glasgow G3 7LN. Tel.: 0141 300 1174. Fax: 0141 300
1170. E-mail: btha@scieh.csa.scot.nhs.uk Website:
http://www.btha.org
- **CABI Publishing**, Cab International, Wall-
ingford, Oxon OX10 8DE (for CD-ROMS on
Topics in International Health). Tel.: 01491 832 111.
Fax: 01491 829 292. E-mail: publishing@cabi.org
Website: http://www.cabi.org
- **Canada—Division of Immunization**:
http://www.hc-sc.gc.ca/hpb/lcdc/bid/di
- **Canadian Pediatric Society (CPS)**, 2204
Walkley Road, Ste 100, Ottawa, Ontario K1G 4G8.
Tel.: 001 613 526 9397. Fax: 526 3332. Website:
http://www.cps.ca/.

- **Centers for Disease Control and Prevention (CDC), USA Department of Health and Human Services**. National Centre for Infectious Diseases, 1600, Clifton Road, Atlanta, Georgia 30333, USA. Tel.: 001 404 332 4555.

  Website: http://www.cdc.gov

  For travel information and advice, including current yellow fever requirements, website: http://www.cdc.gov/travel

  CDC's Advisory Committee on Immunization Practices (ACIP) publishes statements for each recommended childhood vaccine: http://www.cdc.gov/nip/publications/acip-list.htm

  Vaccine Information Statements developed by CDC: http://www.cdc.gov/nip/publications/VIS

  CDC Morbidity and Mortality Weekly Report (MMWR): http://www2.cdc.gov/mmwr/ and http://www.cdc.gov/mmwr

  Information on hepatites: http://www.cdc.gov/ncidod/diseases/hepatitis

  Notifiable Diseases/Deaths in Selected Cities Weekly: http://www.cdc.gov/epo/mmwr/preview/mmwrhtml/mm4916md.htm

  Geographical areas for which vaccination is recommended: http://www.cdc.gov/travel/ Information on all vaccines: http://www.cdc.gov/nip/publications/acip-list.htm

  Malaria: detailed recommendations for the prevention of malaria are available from US CDC 24 h a day from the voice information service (00 1888 232 3228), the fax information service (00 1888 232 3299) or the internet: http://www.cdc.gov/travel/index.htm

  CDC—National Immunization Programme: http://www.cdc.gov/nip.

  Information on influenza pandemic (FluAid): http://www.cdc.gov/od/nvpo/pandemics/

- **CIA (Central Intelligence Agency)**: http://www.odci. gov/cia/publications/pubs.html and select 'World Factbook'.

- **Cheap flights and holidays**: http://www.cheapflights.com/; http://www.teletext.co.uk/holidays; http://www.lastminute.com; http://www.bargainholidays.com; http://www.laterooms.com; http://www.holidaybank.co.uk for self-catering; http://www.lski.com

- **Chiron Vaccines, Chiron Behring GmbH & Co**, PO Box 1630, 35006 Marburg, Germany. Tel.: 00 49 6421 39-4132. Fax: 00 49 6421 39-5497.

- **Committee on the Safety of Medicines**, 1 Nine Elms Lane, London SW8 5NQ. Tel.: 020 7273 3000.

- **Communicable Disease Surveillance Centres (CDSC)**.

  London: 61 Collingdale Avenue, London NW9 5HT. Tel.: 020 8200 6868.

  Wales: Abton House, Wetal Road, Roath, Cardiff CF4 3QX, Wales. Tel.: 029 20 521 997.

  Scotland: Scottish Centre for Infection and Environmental Health, Ruchill Hospital, Bilsland Drive, Glasgow G20 9NB, Scotland. Tel.: 0141 946 7120 (ext: 1277 for TRAVAX service).

- **Contraception and Sexual Health**, advice for women travellers: http://www.mariestopes.org.uk

- **Contraception—emergency advice**: website: http://www.not-2-late.com Operated by the Office of Population Research at Princeton University. Good advice on emergency contraception included.

- **Corona travellers** (advice on living and working abroad), c/o Commonwealth Institute, Kensington High Street, London W8 6NQ. Tel.: 020 7610 4407.

- **Cotswold.** (Water purification equipment, bed nets and other travel clinic accessories) Main Office: Broadway Lane, South Cerney, Gloucestershire GL7 5UQ. Tel.: 01285 860612.

- **Council for Disabled Children**, 8 Wakley Street, London EC1V 7QE. Tel.: 020 7843 6000.

- **Dental travel kits** are available from: Dentanurse UK, Hereford. Tel.: 01981 500 135. Fax: 01981 500 115.

- **Department of Health, UK**, Skipton House, 80 London Road, London SE1 6LH. Tel.: 020 7972 2000. Office of Immunization and Communicable Disease: Tel.: 020 7972 1522. For advice on vaccine refrigerators: Tel.: 020 7972 1430. Vaccine supply team Tel.: 020 7972 1426. Website: http://www.doh.gov.uk Travel: http://www.open.gov.uk/doh/hat/index.htm Advice for travellers: http://www.doh.gov.uk/hat/

- **Department of Health and Human Services, USA**: A website with information for parents on childhood immunizations. It includes the current US schedule of childhood vaccinations: http://www.ecbt.org/parents.htm#guide

● **Diabetes UK**. 10 Queen Anne Street, London W1M 0BD. Tel.: 020 7323 1531. Fax: 020 7637 3644. Website: http://www.diabetes.org.uk Careline: Tel.: 020 7636 6112. E-mail for Careline: careline@diabetes.org.uk

● **Diabetes Centre**, Western General NHS Trust, Edinburgh. Excellent advice for diabetic travellers on their special website: http://www.qmuc.ac.uk/travel/html/page01.htm

● **Disabled Living Foundation**. Tel.: 020 7289 6111. Fax: 020 7266 2922. Provides information on aspects of travel for the disabled. Website: http://www.dlf.org.uk

● **Diving emergencies**. The Royal Navy operates a 24-h emergency advice service. Telephone from anywhere in the world 0831 151523 (cell phone) and if there is no answer Tel.: 023 9276 8026.

● **Durex**. Advice on safe sex and contraception: http://www.durex.com/

● **Electronic Medicines Compendium**. Up-to-date summaries of product characteristics and patient information leaflets: http://emc.vhn.net

● **Emerging Infectious Diseases**. A peer-reviewed journal published by the National Centre for Infectious Diseases, Department of Healthcare and Human Services USA. Website: http://www.cdc.gov/ncidod/EID

● **Eurosurveillance** Weekly: http://www.eurosurv.org/jhp/—Outbreak Information. website: http://www.euroserv.org/main.htm

● **Eurotunnel**. Tel.: 0990353535 (passenger services). Tel.: 01303 273 747 (special needs customers). Fax: 01303 288 784. E-mail: callcentre@eurotunnel.com

● **Expedition Advisory Centre, Royal Geographical Society**, 1 Kensington Gore, London SW7 2AR. Tel.: 020 7591 3030. Fax: 020 7591 3031. Website: http://www.rgs.org/eac

● **Farillon Ltd**, Ashton Road, Romford, Essex RM3 8UE. Tel.: 01708 379 000. Fax: 01708 376 554. Customer service Fax: 01708 378 771; information on deliveries and vaccine returns Tel.: 01708 330 200. Website: http://www.farillon.co.uk

● **Food and Drug Administration (FDA), USA**: http://http://www.fda.gov. Vaccine Adverse Event Reporting System: http://www.fda.org/cber/vaers/vaers.html

● **Foreign and Commonwealth Office**. Advice on safety for travel abroad. Tel.: 020 7270 4129. Public enquiry line Tel.: 020 7228 4503. Website: http://www.fco.gov.uk Also on BBC2 Ceefax page 470.

– British Foreign Office Safety Information for Travellers: http://www.fco.gov.uk/travel/default.asp

● **Frio Cooling Products**, PO Box 10, Haverford west SA62 5YG. Tel.: 01437 741 700. Fax: 01437 741 781. Website: http://www.friouk.com

● **Gatwick Airport**. Tel.: 01293 535 353.

● **Gatwick Airport, Port Health Unit**, London Gatwick, West Sussex RH6 0NP. Tel.: 01293 533 229/502 358. Fax: 01293 502 503.

● **Gatwick Express**. Tel.: 0990 301530 (information line). Tel.: 020 7922 6206 (to arrange assistance). Website: http://www.gatwickexpress.co.uk

● **General Medical Council**, Tel.: 020 7580 7642. Website: http://www.gmc-uk.org/

● **Glaxo Wellcome Ltd**, Stockley Park West, Uxbridge, Middlesex UB11 1BT. Tel.: 020 8990 9444.

● **Global Alliance for Vaccines and Immunization (GAVI)**: http://www.vaccinealliance.org and http://www.who.int/gpv-aboutus/gavi. GAVI's quarterly publication online can be found on: http://www.vaccinealliance.org/newsletter/may2000/contents.html

● **Global HIV/AIDS & STD Surveillance**: http://www.unaids.org/hivaidsinfo/documents.html E-mail: unaids@unaids.org

● **Greer Laboratories Inc**, PO Box 800, Lenoir, NC 28645-800, USA. Tel.: 001 704 754 5327.

● **Guillain–Barré Syndrome Support Group**: Patients: http://www.gbs.org.uk/support.html Professionals can go directly to: http://www.gbs.org.uk/Prof.html

● **Haelix/clinnix**, Portland House, Aldermaston Park, Aldermaston, Reading RG7 4H. Tel.: 0118 981 6666. Fax: 0118 981 9082. News desk Fax: 0118 981 9082. Updated via telephone line travel advice for individual countries. Computer and modem necessary. E-mail: healix@ibm.net Website: http://www.healix.co.uk

● **Haemophilia Society**. Tel.: 0800 018 6068 (9 am to 5 pm Monday to Friday).

- **Health Care Advice for Travellers** and other leaflets such as HIV and AIDS. Department of Health. Freephone: 0800 555 777.
- **Health and Safety Executive** (information on occupational health risks). Tel.: 01742 892 345.
- **Health Education Authority**. Information and fact sheets on the national childhood immunization programme on the website: http://www.immunisation.org.uk
- **HealthFax**. Up-to-date advice on travel issues for patients, GPs and nurses. It has links to other related sites: http://www.healthfax.org.au For 'Travel Health' that includes advice on some individual countries go straight to: http://www.healthfax.org.au/travind.htm
- **Heathrow Airport** Tel.: 01233 211207 (brochure line). Textphones for terminals: 020 8745 5184 (Terminal 1), 020 8745 4094 (Terminal 2), 020 8745 6646 (Terminal 3), 020 745 1024 (Terminal 4).
- **Heathrow Airport, Port Health Unit**, Terminal 3 Arrivals, Heathrow Airport, Hounslow, Middlesex TW6 1NB. Tel.: 020 8745 7419. Fax: 020 8745 6181.
- **Heathrow Express**. Tel.: 0845 600 1515. Website: http://www.heathrowexpress.co.uk
- **Help for the World Traveller**:
  Electricity. Among other information, there is a guide to electricity around the world, including the kind of plugs used: http://www.kropla.com
  Telephone sockets: http://www.teleadapt.com
  Currency converter: http://www.oanda.com
  Bank Holidays: http://www.national-holidays.com
  Cyber Cafes: Find the nearest e-cafe to the destination: http://www.cybercafes.com
  Travel-vault. Deposit information on passport, visa, credit cards, etc. in case they are lost or stolen. Remember the Ekno password: http://www.lonelyplanet.co.uk
  Weather at destination: http://www.weather.com
  Time and lighting up times at destination: http://www.hilink.com.au/times
  Health Advice: http://www.doh.gov.uk/hat/index.htm and http://www.fitfortravel.scot.nhs.uk
  Telecare: 24 h free phone access for advice by English speaking professionals, e.g. pharmacist, nurse, midwife (£19.95 per family for 21 days):

http://www.interglobe.co.uk
Passport Agency, for getting a new passport quickly: http://www.ukpa.gov.uk
BAA Airport's duty free service, car parking, to order currency: http://www.baa.co.uk
Airport parking: http://www.bcponline.co.uk
Foreign currency, collect at the airport: http://www.travelex.co.uk
Travel Insurance with Columbus Direct: http://www.columbusdirect.net
Locator of cash machines abroad: http://www.visa.com/pd/atm/main.html or http://www.mastercard.com/atm

- **Hepatitis B, Group B patient helpline** Tel.: 020 7244 6514.
- **Hepatitis B USA** Websites: http://www.cdc.gov/hepatitis/index.htm http://www.cdc.gov/ncidod/diseases/hepatitis, http://www.liverfoundation.org and http://www.immunize.org. Hepatitis B Foundation: www.hepb.org
- **Hepatitis Foundation** international website for patients: http://www.hepfi.org/infomenu.htm
- **Hepatitis Information Network, Canada**: website: http://www.hepnet.com
- **Herpes Zoster**. Patients: http://www.medinfo.co.uk/conditions/shingles.html
- **High Altitude Medicine Guide**. Website: http://www.gorge.net/hamg/
- **Himalayan Rescue Association Nepal**, PO Box 4944, Thamel, Kathmandu, Nepal. Tel.: (9771) 418755. Website: http://www.nepalonline.net/hra
- **Holiday Care Service (HCS)**, 2 Old Bank Chambers, Station Road, Horley, Surrey RH6 9HW Tel.: 01293 774 535. Fax: 01293 784 647. Offers travel advice and information to anyone who asks, including people who are elderly or disabled, lone parents, carers and those who have financial problems.
- **Home Office**, Immigration and Nationality Departments, India Building (3rd Floor), Water Street, Liverpool L2 0QN.
- **Homeway Ltd**, West Amesbury, Salisbury, Wiltshire, SP4 7BH. Tel.: 01980 626 360. Tel.: for orders: 01980 626 361. Fax: for orders: 01980 626 362. Website: http://www.travelwithcare.co.uk
- **Hospital for Tropical Diseases**, Mortimer Market, Capper Street, off Tottenham Court Road, London WC1E 6AU. Main switchboard for Uni-

versity College Hospital Tel.: 020 7387 9300. Fax: 020 7388 7645. Clinical services Tel.: 020 7387 4411 (ask for the duty doctor). Travel Clinic Tel.: 020 7388 9600. Fax: 020 7383 4817. Department of Clinical Parasitology Tel.: 020 7387 9300 ext. 5418. *Healthline* provides recorded verbal advice. Tel.: 0839 337 733 (payline as above).

● **Hoverspeed.** Tel.: 0990 240241. E-mail: info@hoverspeed.co.uk

● **Hyland Immuno, Baxter Healthcare Ltd,** Wallingford Road, Compton, Newbury, Berkshire RG20 7QW. Tel.: 01635 206 000. Customer service Tel.: 01635 206 265. Fax: 01635 206 126. Medical Information Tel.: 01635 206 373.

● **IDIS Ltd,** Millbank House, 171 Ewell Road, Surbiton, Surrey KT6 6AX. Tel.: 020 8410 0700. Fax: 020 8410 0800.

● **Immunization Action Coalition & the Hepatitis B Coalition,** 1573 Selby Avenue, Suite 234, St Paul, MN 55104, USA. Tel.: (651) 647 9009. Free registration for health professionals—you get occasional e-mail: messages containing up-to-date information on immunization and/or hepatitis B. Website: http://www.immunize.org/express

● **Immunization Information System,** The University of Manchester: http://www.immunise.man.ac.uk

● **Immunization Resource for Parents— Public Health, Seatle & King County:** http:// www.metrokc.gov/health/immunization/ childimmunity.htm

● **Immunization Resource for Adults—Public Health, Seatle & King County:** http:// www.immunizeseniors.org

● **Infectious Disease Society of America** *Vaccine Initiative*: http://www.idsociety.org

● **Infectious disease statistics and news** on: http://www.phls.co.uk and http://www.eurosurv.org Eurosurveillance is available at: http://www. ceses.org/eurosurv

● **Institute for Social and Preventive Medicine University of Zurich (ISPM),** Sumatrastr. 30, CH-8006 Zurich, Switzerland. WHO Collaborating Centre for Travellers' Health. Director: Professor Robert Steffen. Tel.: 00 41 1 634 46 08/21. Fax: 00 41 1 634 49 84. E-mail: travclin@ifspm.unizh.ch

● **Institute for Vaccine Safety:** http://www.vaccinesafety.edu

● **International Aids Vaccine Initiative:** http:// www.iavi.org

● **International Association for Medical Assistance for Travellers,** 417 Centre Street, Lewiston, NY 14092, USA. Tel.: 001 (716) 754 4883 Website: http://www.sentex.net/ ~ iamat OR 57 Voirets, 1212 Grand-Lancy-Geneva.

● **International Dialysis Organization,** 9, ruelle du Pont, 69390 Vernaison, France. Tel.: 00 33 4 72 30 12 30. Fax: 00 33 4 78 46 27 81.

● **International Network for the Availability of Scientific Publications (INASP).** Access to reliable information for health care workers in developing and transitional countries. Its website provides useful links to information resources, mainly in Africa and Latin America, including local library links: http://www.inasp.org.uk/

● **International Society for Mountain Medicine:** Arztpraxis, CH 3822 Lauterbrunnen, Switzerland. Fax: 00 41 33 856 2627. Website: http:// www.ismm.unige.ch and http://daedalus74.mc. duke.edu/ismm/

● **International Society of Travel Medicine (ISTM),** PO Box 871089, Stone Mountain, GA 30087–0028, USA. Tel.: 001 770 736 7060. Fax: 001 770 736 6732. E-mail: bcbistm@aol.com Website: http://www.istm.org *Travel Medicine News-Share.* Website: http://www.istm.org/newsshare.html

● **International Union of Alpine Associations,** Dr Charles Clarke, St Bartholomew's Hospital, 38 Little Britain, London EC1A 7BE.

● **International Vaccine Institute,** website: http://www.ivi.org

● **ISOsafe Ltd,** Units 3 & 4, Woodlands Business Village, Basingstoke, Hants RG21 4JX. Tel.: 01256 362 700. Fax: 01256 869 911. Verifiable temperature control technology equipment.

● **Janssen-Cilag Ltd,** PO Box 79, Saunderton, High Wycombe, Bucks HP14 4HJ. Tel.: 01494 567 567. Fax: 01494 567 568.

● **John Bell and Croyden** 50, Wigmore Street, London W1H 0AU. Tel.: 020 7935 5555.

● **John Groom Association for the Disabled.** Tel.: 020 7452 2000.

● **John Radcliffe Hospital,** Headley Way, Oxford OX3 9DU. Tel.: 01865 741 166.

● **John Hopkins University's** website gives information on the hepatites: http://www.hopkins-id.edu/diseases/hepatitis/index_hep.html

- **Laboratories, The**. Belfast City Hospital, Lisburn Road, Belfast BT9 7AB, Northern Ireland. Tel.: 028 90 329 241.
- **Launch Diagnostics Ltd**, Ash House, Ash Road, New Ash Green, Longfield, Kent DA3 8JD. Tel.: 01474 874 426. Fax: 01474 872 388.
- **Leishmania Genome Network** provides up to date information on the current state of the physical mapping of *Leishmania major* genome: http://www.ebi.ac.uk/parasites/leish.html/
- **Lifescan**, Enterprise House, Station Road, Loudwater, High Wycombe, Buckinghamshire HP10 9UF. Tel.: 01494 450423.
- **Lifesystems Ltd** (water purification equipment for travellers) 4 Mercury House, Calleva Park, Aldermaston, Berkshire RG7 4QW. Tel.: 0118 981 1435.
- **Links to Key Clinical Tropical Medicine Sites**: http://info.dom.uab.edu/gorgas/geomed/links.htm
- **Liverpool School of Tropical Medicine**, Pembroke Place, Liverpool L3 5QA. Tel.: 0151 708 9393. Website: http://www.lshtm.ac.uk/home.html
- **London School of Hygiene and Tropical Medicine** Keppel Street, London WC1E 7HT. Tel.: 020 7636 8636. Advice for medics Tel.: 020 7530 3500. Medics for advice on malaria prophylaxis Tel.: 020 7927 2437 (09.00–16.30 h). Continuous prerecorded tape with malaria advice for travellers Tel.: 0891 600350 (payline).
- **Lonely Planet**: http://www.lonelyplanet.com
- **Malaria**, a website mainly concerned with southern Africa, but the advice may be considered good, and there is also a link to British Airways Travel Clinics, which is worth looking at for information: http://www.africasafari.co.za/malaria1.htm
- **Malaria**, health professionals only can obtain advice from the following centres:

London:	020 7927 2437 (09.00–16.30 h on weekdays) PHLS Communicable Disease Surveillance Centre. Tel.: 020 8200 6868 ext. 3412 (09.00–12.30 h on weekdays).
Glasgow:	0141 946 7120.
Liverpool:	0151 708 9393.
Birmingham:	0121 766 6611.
Oxford:	01865 225570 (Ward). 01865 225217 (Outpatients 14.00–17.00 h).

- **Malaria Foundation**: http://www.malaria.org/
- **Malaria Guidelines, UK**, the 1997 British Malaria Prophylaxis Guidelines: http://www.phls.co.uk/advice/cdrr1097.pdf
- **Malaria—Multilateral Initiative**: http://www.malaria.org/MIM.html
- **Malaria Reference Laboratory**. For the Public—Tel.: 0891 600 350—24-h Helpline (payline). For advice to doctors and nurses, Tel.: 020 7927 2437.
- **Manchester—Department of Infectious Diseases**, North Manchester Healthcare Trust, Monsell Wing, Central Drive, Delaunays Road, Crumpsall, Manchester M8 5RB. Tel.: 0161 795 4567 ext. 3320.
- **Medeva Pharma Ltd**, Medeva House, Regent Park, Kingston Road, Leatherhead, Surrey KT22 7PQ. Tel.: 01372 364 000. Fax: 01372 364 018. Tel.: 01372 364 100 (medical information).
- **Medical Advisory Service for Travellers Abroad (MASTA)**, Room 28, Denton House, 40–44 Wicklow Street, London WC1 9HL. Tel.: 020 7837 5540; Travel Health Line Tel.: 0906 8224 100 (24 h advice, payline, 60p per minute); Visa & passport information line Tel.: 0906 5501 100 (calls charged at £1.00 per minute). MASTA Marketing and sales: Moorfield Road, Yeadon, Leeds LS19 7BN. Tel.: 0113 238 7500. Fax: 0113 238 7501. Website: http://www.masta.org/index.html
- **Medical Defence Organizations**:
  - Medical Defence Union 020 7486 6181; http://www.the-mdu.com
  - Medical Protection Society 01132 436436; http://www.mps.org.uk
  - St Paul Healthcare 0808 100 5599; http://www.protection.stpaul.co.uk
- **Medic-Alert Foundation International**, 1 Bridge Wharf, 156 Caledonian Road, London N1 9UU. Tel.: 020 7833 3034. Freephone: 0800 220 386.
- **Medical Expeditions**: Website: http://ourworld.compuserve.com/homepages/medical_expeditions
- **Medicine Planet**, a website full of information on travel, with special pages for women, children and adventure traveller. Connections with many other websites: http://www.medicineplanet.com.
- **Medinfo UK**. Information for parents on immunizations such as MMR: http://www.medinfo.co.uk/immunizations/mmr.html

- **Medisense**, 17 The Courtyard, Gorsey Lane, Coleshill, Birmingham B46 1JA. Tel.: 01675 467 006.
- **Meningococcal vaccine advice.** Tel.: 0141 946 7120 (Scotland); 020 8200 6868 (London).
- **Merck Pharmaceuticals**, Harrier House, High Street, West Drayton, Middlesex UB7 7QG. Tel.: 01895 452 200. Fax: 01895 420 605.
- **Mobility International**, advice for the disabled: http://www.miusa.org
- **Multilateral Initiative on Malaria** website: http://mim.nih.gov/partnerships/index.html
- **National AIDS Helpline.** Tel.: 0800 567 123 (24 h, free).
- **National Association for Maternal and Child Welfare**, 40–42 Osnaburgh Street, London NW1 3ND. Tel.: 020 7383 4117.
- **National Foundation for Infectious Diseases.** Raises awareness about infectious diseases and their management, provides news, factsheets, a library of diseases and information on forthcoming conferences: http://www.nfid.org/
- **Netdoctor**: http://www.netdoctor.co.uk and go to the travel medicine section.
- **New Zealand site** providing comprehensive information on travel health: http://www.travelhealth.co.n2
- **Nomad Medical Ltd**, 3–4 Wellington Terrace, Turnpike Lane, London N8 0PX. Tel.: 020 8365 8698. Fax: 020 8889 9529. E-mail: nomad.travstore@virgin.net A wide range of travel products.
- **Northern Ireland—Infectious Diseases Unit**, Belvoir Park Hospital, Hospital Road, Belfast BT8 8JR. Tel.: 01232 491 942 ext. 236/237.
- **Novartis Pharmaceuticals**, Frimley Business Park, Frimley, Surrey GU16 5SG. Tel.: 01276 698 370; Fax: 01276 692 508.
- **Ohio State University**, College of Biological Sciences: http://www.biosci.ohio-state.educ
- **Pan American Health Organization.** A regional office of the WHO. For advice for travellers to the Western Hemisphere—country-specific information about many health issues, contact their website: http://www.paho.org
- **Parasites and Parasitology, Ohio State University College of Biological Sciences.** A very popular website with an interesting questions and answers section: http://www.biosci.ohio-state.edu/~parasite/home.html
- **Parasitological Research Groups Worldwide** provides links to Parasitology research groups and societies: http://www.biophys.uni-dusseldorf.de/FBBiologie/FB-biologie.html/
- **Passport offices:**
  London: Tel.: 020 7279 3434.
  Glasgow, Belfast, Liverpool, Newport, Peterborough: Tel.: 0990 210 410.
- **Patient Group Directions (Approved Group Protocols)**, is a database of approved protocols for the supply and administration of medicines: http://www.groupprotocols.org.uk
- **Patients' Association**, 8 Guildford Street, London WC1 1DT. Tel.: 020 7242 3460 (09.30–17.30 h).
- **PAX Healthcare Products Ltd**, Stonebridgelands, Woodchurch, Ashford, Kent TN26 3SL. Tel.: 01233 860 832. Fax: 01233 861 373. Provides 'Travel Pax', a selection of nine OTC medicines for common travel illnesses and an advice booklet.
- **Pharmacia and Upjohn Ltd**, Davy Avenue, Knowhill, Milton Keynes MK5 8PH. Tel.: 01908 661 101; Fax: 01908 690 091.
- **Philip Harris Medical Ltd**, Hazelwell Lane, Stirchley, Birmingham B30 2PS. Tel.: 0121 433 3030. Travel aid kit, single, family, large packs with intravenous fluids for expeditions, etc.
- **PHLS (Public Health Laboratory Services)**, Communicable Disease Surveillance Centre, 61 Colindale Avenue, London NW9 5HT. Tel.: 020 8200 6868. Weekdays 9.30 am to 12.30 pm. Fax: 020 8200 7868. http://www.phls.co.uk Influenza activity updates: http://www.phls.co.uk/facts/influenza/fluactivity0001.htm
- **Public Health Laboratory**, Belfast City Hospital, Belfast BT9 7AB, Northern Ireland. Tel.: 028 90 329 241.
- **PHLS Malaria Reference Laboratories:** Tel.: 020 7636 3924 weekdays 9 am to 4.30 pm. UK malaria guidelines: http://www.phls.co.uk/advice/cdrr1097.pdf
  Birmingham: Birmingham Heartlands Hospital, Bordesley Green East, Birmingham B9 5SS. Tel.: 0121 766 6611. Fax: 0121 772 6229.
  Glasgow: Ruchill Hospital, Bilsiand Drive, Glasgow G20 9NB, Scotland. Tel.: 0141 946 7120.

Liverpool: Liverpool School of Tropical Medicine, Pembroke Place, Liverpool L3 5QA. Tel.: 0151 708 9393.

London: London School of Hygiene and Tropical Medicine, Keppel Street, London WC1E 7HT. Tel.: 020 7636 8636; 020 7636 3924; for clinical advice: Tel.: 020 7387 4411; GPs and nurses for advice, Tel.: 020 7927 2437 (09.00–16.30 h); advice to the public on malaria, Tel.: 0891 600 350 (payline).

Oxford: Churchill Hospital, Oxford OX3 7LJ. Tel.: 01865 225 570.

- **PHLS Group Laboratory East**, Public Health & Clinical Microbiology Laboratory, Box 236, Addenbrookes Hospital, Hills Road, Cambridge CB2 2QW. Tel.: 01223 257 036. Fax: 01223 242 775.
- **PHLS Group Laboratory Midlands**, Birmingham Heartlands Hospital, Bordesley Green East, Birmingham B9 5SS. Tel.: 0121 766 6611. Fax: 0121 772 6229.
- **PHLS Group Laboratory North**, Institute of Pathology, Newcastle General Hospital, Westgate Road, Newcastle upon Tyne NE4 6BE. Tel.: 0191 273 8811. Fax: 0191 226 0265. Also, Bridle Path, York Road, Leeds TS15 7TR. Tel.: 0113 264 5011. Fax: 0113 260 3655.
- **PHLS Laboratory North-west**, Fazakerley Hospital, Lower Lane, Liverpool L9 7AL. Tel.: 0151 525 2323. Fax: 0151 530 1647.
- **PHLS Laboratory South-west**, Church Lane, Heavitree, Exeter EX2 5AD. Tel.: 01392 402 977. Fax: 01392 412 835. Also, Salisbury District Hospital, Odstock Road, Salisbury SP2 8BJ. Tel.: 01722 336 020. Fax: 01722 412 636.
- **PHLS Laboratory Wales**, Department of Medical Microbiology, University Hospital of Wales, Heath Park, Cardiff CF4 4XW. Tel.: 029 2074 2047. Fax: 029 2074 4123.
- **PHLS Meningococcal Reference Laboratory**. Tel.: 0161 445 2416.
- **Photographs of people with vaccine-preventable diseases**. Website: http://www.immunize.org/catg.d/pict001.htm/
- **Practice Nurse E-mail Discussion Group**: practicenurse@egroups.com
- **Practice Nurse Website**: http://www.haines.grid9.net/pn

- **Prescription Pricing Authority (PPA)**: *England*: Bridge House, 152 Pilgrim Street, Newcastle upon Tyne NE1 6SN. Tel.: 0191 232 5371. *Wales*: Welsh Health Common Services Authority, Crickhowell House, Pierhead Street, Capital Waterside, Cardiff CF1 5XT. Tel.: 02920 500 500.
- **Primary Care National Electronic Library for Health**: http://www.nelh-pc.nhs.uk/
- **Prodigy net**: Good launch pad to locate relevant material including infectious diseases. Helps locate books on infectious diseases: http://pages.prodigy.net/pdeziel
- **Questions on immunizations**: call CDC's Immunization Information Hotline on 001 800 234 2522. E-mail: nipinfo@cdc.gov
- **Rabies information**: 'Pet Travel Scheme': For up-to-date government information telephone 'The Pet Line' on 0870 2411 710, or e-mail: pets@ahvg.maff.gov.uk Alternatively, use the website: http://www.maff.gov.uk/animalh/guarantine/default.htm
  - The DoH's *Memorandum on rabies: prevention and control* can be found on http://www.doh.gov.uk/memorandumonrabies
  - The WHO report on Rabies: Request by e-mail: on cdsdoc@who-int or on the website: http://www.who.int/emc-documents/rabies/whocdscraph994c.html
  - Pre-exposure: Telephone advice for health professionals on pre-exposure rabies vaccination can be obtained from the Travel Unit, Communicable Disease Surveillance Centre on 020 8200 6868. In Scotland, contact Scottish Centre for Infection and Environmental Health (SCIEH) on 0141 300 1100.
  - Post-exposure: Advice from the PHLS Virus Reference Division in London (Tel.: 020 8200 4400), in Scotland (Tel.: 0141 531 5900 or SCIEH 0141 300 1100), and in Northern Ireland (Tel.: 01232 329 241). Enquiries of foreign health authorities regarding the health of the animal involved in an incident, telephone the Communicable Diseases Branch of the DoH on 020 7972 1522, or out of hours on 020 7210 3000.
  - Country by country rabies risk: The Virus Reference Division, Central Public Health

Laboratory, Colindale, London NW9 5HT, Tel.: 020 8200 4400. In Scotland, SCIEH, Clifton House, Clifton Place, Glasgow G3 7LN, Tel.: 0141 300 1100.

- Rabies vaccine for those at occupational risk: PHLS Virus Division, Tel.: 020 8200 4400. In Scotland details of availability of vaccine from SCIEH, Tel.: 0141 300 1100.

• **Reference vaccination charts:** appear regularly in medical/nursing newspapers and magazines.

• **Regent Labs Ltd,** Cunard Road, London NW10 6PN. Tel.: 020 8965 3637.

• **Regional Pharmacist Procurement Coordinator,** Eastern Health and Social Services Board, 12–21 Linenhall Street, Belfast BT2 8BS, Northern Ireland. Tel.: 028 90 321 313.

• **Regional Virus Laboratory,** Royal Victoria Hospital, Grosvenor Road, Belfast BT12 6BA, Northern Ireland. Tel.: 028 90 240 503.

• **Resuscitation Council (UK) 1999 Guidelines:** http://www.resus.org.uk

• **Roche Diagnostics Ltd,** Bell Lane, Lewes, East Sussex BN7 1LG. Tel.: 01273 480 444.

• **Roche Products Ltd,** PO Box 8, Welwyn Garden City, Hertfordshire AL7 3AY. Tel.: 01707 366 000. Fax: 01707 338 297.

• **Royal Association for Disability and Rehabilitation (RADAR),** Unit 12, City Forum, 250 City Road, London EC1V 8AF. Tel.: 020 7250 3222 for services and leaflets.

• **Royal College of General Practitioners (RCGP),** 14 Princes Gate, Hyde Park, London SW7 1PU. Tel.: 020 7581 3232. Fax: 020 7225 3047. E-mail: info@rcgp.org.uk Website: http://www.rcgp.org.uk

• **Royal College of Nursing,** Travel Health Nurses' Group, 20 Cavendish Square, London W1M 0AB. Tel.: 020 7872 0480. Fax: 020 735 5137. Website: http://www.rcn.org.uk

• **Royal College of Obstetricians and Gynaecologists (RCOG).** Tel.: 020 7772 6224. Website: http://www.rcog.org.uk

• **Royal Free Hospital,** Travel Medicine Unit, London. Diploma in Travel Health and Medicine (1-year course). Tel.: 020 7830 2999. Fax: 020 7830 2268. Advice for the public: 0891 633 433 (payline). Travel Health Clinic: 020 7830 2885 weekdays 9 am to 5 pm.

• **Royal Society for Prevention of Accidents:** http://www.rospa.co.uk

• **Safe Injection Global Network (SIGN):** http://www.injectionsafety.org

• **SAGA,** 0800 300 600.

• **Sanger Centre** has data on nucleotide sequences for many microorganisms: http://www.sanger.ac.uk/Projects/

• **SatelLife** is a non-profit-making humanitarian organization that focuses on the developing countries. A ProMed mail facility provides a rapid, and nonpolitical, infectious disease monitoring service: http://www.healthnet.org

• **Scotland: Common Services Agency,** Trinity Park House, South Trinity Park, Edinburgh EH5 3SH, Scotland. Tel.: 0131 552 6255, ext. 2283

• **Scottish AIDS Monitor,** 26 Anderson Place, Edinburgh EH6 5NP. Tel.: 0131 555 4850.

• **Scottish Centre for Infection and Environmental Health (SCIEH),** Clifton House, Clifton Place, Glasgow G3 7LN. Tel.: 0141 300 1100. Fax: 0141 300 1170. Website: http://www.show.scot.nhs.uk/scieh/ For TRAVAX, see below. *Fit for travel* SCIEH website for the public: http://www.fitfortravel.scot.nhs.uk

• **Scottish Meningococcal and Pneumococcal Reference Laboratory.** Tel.: 0141 201 3836.

• **SmithKline Beecham Pharmaceuticals,** Mundells, Welwyn Garden City, Hertfordshire AL7 1EY. For medical information: Tel.: 0808 100 2228. Orders-Tel.: 0808 100 9997. Orders-Fax: 0808 100 8802. Orders e-mail: ukpharma.customer@sb.com Website: http://www.sb.com

• **SmithKline Beecham Biologicals:** http://www.worldwidevaccines.com

• **Solvay Healthcare Ltd,** Mansbridge Road, West End, Southampton, Hampshire SO18 3JD. Tel.: 023 8046 7000. Fax: 023 8046 5350.

• **Splenectomy Trust,** c/o Swinbrook Post Office, Oxon OX18 4DX.

• **Staffordshire University, School of Health.** Short Course in Travel Health, twice a year. Tel.: 01785 353 696.

• **Swiss Net UK plc,** Hartley House Industrial Estate, Hucknall Road, Sherwood, Nottingham NG5 1FD. Tel.: 0115 969 2500. Fax: 0115 969 3270. A wide range of mosquito nets.

- **Terence Higgins Trust**, 52–54 Gray's Inn Road, London WC1 8JU. Tel.: 020 7242 1010 (daily 10.00–12.00 h).
- **ToxBase: The database of the National Poisons Information Service**. Information on toxins, their effects and how to manage them. Drugs, plants, snake bites and household products. Comprehensive list of antidotes and where to find them. Location of hyperbaric chambers in the UK. Free to NHS professionals but you are required to register (allow a week): http://www.spib.axl.co.uk
- **Trailfinders Travel Clinics** Tel.: 020 7938 3999 (London), 0141 353 00 66 (Scotland).
- **TRAVAX**, a constantly updated travel vaccination and malaria chemoprophylaxis information service for the medical profession, run by SCIEH (Tel.: 0141 300 1100) in Scotland. The system is by subscription and requires a computer and modem. Website: http://www.axl.co.uk/scieh
- **TRAVAX** *Fit for Travel* is a colourful and informative website from SCIEH free for the public. It gives country-specific information on immunizations and other preventive strategies, including information on malaria: http://www.fitfortravel.scot.nhs.uk
- **Travel guides**: http://www.lonelyplanet.com and http://www.wcites.com
- **Travel Health UK**, an independent nurse-led travel health website giving practical advice and useful links for staying healthy while travelling abroad: http://www.TravelHealth.co.uk
- **Travel Health online USA**. Website: http://www.tripprep.com/country/country.html
- **Travel insurance online**: http://www.underthesun.co.uk, http://www.i-travelinsurance.com, http://www.eaglestardirect.co.uk
- **'Traveller'** from **Traveller Direct Ltd**, Aizlewoods Mill, Nursery Street, Sheffield S3 8GG, is a constantly updated system of specific information on vaccinations, health risks, malaria, yellow fever, etc. It is by yearly subscription. Tel.: 0114 282 3488. Fax: 0114 282 3489.
- **Travellers' Medical and Vaccination Centre**, an Australian site providing general and country-specific information on infectious diseases and immunizations: http://www.tmvc.com.au/info.html
- **Traveller's precautions**, from the American University of Beirut: http://www.aub.edu.lb/uhs/chm/travel/

- **Travel Medicine Advisor, American Health Consultants**, online comprehensive resource of travel medicine. To subscribe ring 001 404 262 5476. Fax: 001 404 262 5525.
- **Travel Medicine Bureau, Dublin**. Website: http://www.tmb.i.e.
- **Travel Medicine Matrix**, links to other sites: http://www.medmatrix.org/index.asp
- **Travel News Organization**, a useful site as it gives the telephone number and web address of every airline operating in the UK: http://www.travel-news.org. A similar site is **Travel From Here** but with links to flight specialists, tour operators and hotels, at http://www.infotravel.co.uk
- **Triscope**, Alexandra House, Albany Road, Brentford, Middlesex TW8 0NE. Tel.: 020 8580 7021. Helpline: 08457 585 641. Gives travel advice for people with disabilities. This service is free. E-mail: tripscope@cableinet.co.uk Website: http://www.justmobility.co.uk/tripscope
- **Tropical Medicine in Dublin**: http://www.tmb.i.e.
- **Tropical Screening Service** for returned travellers (private). Tel.: 020 7830 9683. Fax: 0771 2582 023. Website: http://www.tropicalscreening.com.
- **Tulane University School of Public Health and Tropical Medicine, New Orleans, Louisiana**: Website: http://www.tropmed.tulane.edu/tropinfo.htm
- **UK practice.net Ltd** (networks many websites), First Floor, Juniper Court, Boxwell Road, Berkhamsted, Hertfordshire HP4 3ET. Tel.: 01442 873861. Website: http://www.ukpractice.net
- **United Nations Office for the Coordination of Humanitarian Affairs**: http://www.reliefweb.int
- **University of Glasgow, Course in Travel Medicine** for Certificate, Diploma and MSc in Travel Medicine. Enquiries to: The University Secretary, Department of Infectious Diseases, Ruchill Hospital, Bilsiand Drive, Glasgow G20 9NT. Tel.: 0141 946 7120, ext. 1368. The course is open to registered medical practitioners and registered nurses. Website: http://www.dph.gla.ac.uk/TravMed/Index.htm
- **University of Texas**. Information on community-acquired pneumonia. This website has an extensive slide show that covers just about everything: http://www.utexas.edu/pharmacy/courses/

phr385e/community_pneu/index.htm

- **USA information for parents on immunizations** (backed by the USA Department of Health). Website: http://www.ecbt.org/parents.htm#guide
- **USA National Immunization Program**: http:/www.cdc.gov/nip/vacsafe
- **US National Institute of Allergy and Infectious Diseases**, includes the Jordan Report 2000. It gives an overview of 60 infectious diseases: http://www.niaid.nih.gov
- **US National Library of Medicine**. A portal to online health information for the health professionals as well as for the general public. Good information on AIDS: http://www.nlm.nih.gov
- **US State Department Services**, Travel Warnings and Consular Sheets: http://travel.state.gov/travel_warnings.html
- **Vaccine Adverse Event Reporting System** (USA): http://www.vaers.org
- **Virgin**: http://www.fly.virgin.com
- **Web for Women for Women**, information on many aspects of sexuality and contraception: http://www.io.com/~wwwomen?contraception?index.html Additional information from the Durex website: http://www.durex.com
- **Wellcome Foundation**. This trust supports global research in awards and funding initiatives: http://www.wellcome.ac.uk/international/
- **Welsh Health Common Service Authority**, Crickhowell House, Pierhead Street, Capital Waterside, Cardiff CF1 5XT, Wales. Tel.: 029 20 500 500.
- **Wheelchair Travel** 11, Johnston Green, Guildford GU2 6XS. Tel.: 01483 233 640. Fax: 01483 23 7772. E-mail: info@wheelchair-travel.co.uk Website: http://www.wheelchair-travel.co.uk
- **Wilderness Medical Society**: http://http://www.al.com/wms
- **Williams Medical Supplies**, Unit H6, Springhead Enterprise Park, Northfleet, Kent DA11 8HD Tel.: 01474 535 330. Emergency packs.
- **World Health Organization**, Avenue Appia 20, Ch–1211 Geneva 27, Switzerland. Distribution and sales: Tel.: 00 41 22 791 2476. Fax: 00 41 22 7914857.

  Website: http://www.who.int For vaccinations requirements and health advice: http://www.who.int/ith/

Disease outbreak information: http://www.who.ch/outbreak/outbreak_home.html Information on Rabies: http://oms.b3e.jussieu.fr/rabnet/ Immunization schedules: http://www.who.int/gpv-dvacc/service/immschedule.htm Surveillance and epidemic response: http://www.who.ch/emc/surveill/index.html WHO Outbreaks News (regularly updated): http://www.who.int/emc/outbreak_news/index.html Weekly Epidemiological Record from the WHO: http://www.who.ch/wer/wer_home.htm Yellow Book—International Travel and Health: http://www.who.int/ith/english/welcome.html Pan American Health Organization (a regional WHO office) for country-specific information about many health issues for travellers to the Western Hemisphere: http://www.paho.org WHO Division of control of tropical diseases: http://www.who.int/ctd/ WHO special programme for research and training in tropical diseases: http://www.who.int/tdr/ WHO's geographical information system to monitor influenza activity: http://www.who.int/emc/diseases/flu/index.html The WHO report on rabies: request by E-mail: on cdsdoc@who-int or on the website: http://www.who.int/emc-documents/rabies/whocdscraph994c.html Information on vaccines and diseases: http://www.who.int/vaccines/map.htm Latest news: http://www.who.int/vaccines/news/index Vaccine and surveillance: http://www.who.int/vaccines-surveillance/intro.html The Malaria Network: a joint WHO and World Bank project: http://www.malarianetwork.org/ Hepatitis B: http://www.who.int/gpv-fvacc/diseases/hepatitisb Travel information: http://www.who.int/vaccinesdiseases/travel/travel.html Health topics: http://www.health-topics/idindex.htm Emerging and other Communicable Diseases Surveillance and Control (EMC): http://www.who.int/emc/ Information on infectious diseases, safety of vaccines, etc.: http://www.who.int/vaccines-diseases/dislist.htm

Details of the WHO's *Roll-Back Malaria* campaign on: http://www.rbm.who.int/

International Travel and Health—Vaccination requirements and health advice. WHO 2000 edition—ISBN 92 41580240. This (yellow) book can also be viewed and downloaded from the WHO website: http://www.who.int/ith/english/index.htm/.htm

● **Weekender**—an on line directory of weekend breaks in the UK and abroad. Their definition of a weekend is a maximum of 4 nights, at least one of which is Saturday or Sunday, anywhere on earth that can be reached in a weekend: http://www.webweekends.co.uk

● **Wyeth Laboratories**, Huntercombe Lane South, Taplow, Maidenhead, Berkshire SL6 0PH. Tel.: 01628 604 377. Fax: 01628 666 368.

● **Yahoo for travel**: http://dir.yahoo.com/recreation/travel/

● **Yellow Fever Vaccination Centres**, Department of Health, Room 554, Richmond House, 79 Whitehall, London SW1A 2NS. Tel.: 020 7210 5039. Information on yellow fever as well as how to become a Yellow Fever Vaccination Centre contact the Public Health Unit on 020 7972 5047. Fax: 020 7972 5013. Stocks of yellow fever vaccination certificates (mention form Port 37) from 0541 555 455 or Fax: 01623 724 524.

Chapter 65

Embassies and High Commissions in London

	Telephone number
Afghan Embassy, 31 Prince's Gate SW7	020 7589 8891
Albanian Embassy, 6 Wilton Ct, 59–60 Eccleston Sq. SW1	020 7976 5295
Algerian Embassy, 6 Hyde Park Gate SW7	020 7211 7800
American Embassy, 24 Grosvenor Sq. W1	020 7499 9000
Angola Embassy, 98 Park Lane W1	020 7495 1752
Antigua and Bermuda High Commission, 15 Thayer St. W1	020 7486 7073
Argentina Embassy, 53 Hans Place SW1	020 7584 6494
Armenian Embassy, 25 Cheniston Gardens SW7	020 7938 5453
Australian High Commission, Australia House, The Strand WC2	020 7379 4334
Austrian Embassy, 18 Belgrave Mews West SW1	020 7235 3731
Bahamas High Commission, 10 Chesterfield St. W1	020 7408 4488
Bahrain Embassy, 98 Gloucester Rd. SW7	020 7370 5132
Bangladesh High Commission, 28 Queen's Gate SW7	020 7584 0081
Barbados High Commission, 1 Great Russell St. WC1	020 7631 4975
Belarus Embassy, 6 Kensington Court W8	020 7937 3288
Belarus Embassy, 1 St. Stephen's Crescent W2	020 7221 3795
Belgian Embassy, 103 Eaton Sq. SW1	020 7235 0616
Belize High Commission, 10 Harcourt House 19a Cavendish Sq. W1	020 7499 9728
Bolivian Embassy, 106 Eaton Sq. SW1	020 7235 4248
Bosnia-Hercegovina Embassy, 40–41 Conduit St. W1	020 7734 3758
Botswana High Commission, 6 Stratford Place W1	020 7499 0031
Brazilian Embassy, 32 Green St. W1	020 7499 0877
Brunei Darrusalam High Commission, 19–20 Belgrave Sq. SW1	020 7581 0521
Bulgarian Embassy, 186 Queen's Gate SW7	020 7584 9400
Canadian High Commission, 1 Grosvenor Sq. W1	020 7258 6600
Cayman Islands Government Office, 6 Arlington St. SW1	020 7491 7772
Chilean Embassy, Piccadilly House, 33 Regent St. SW1	020 7734 0802
Chinese Embassy, 49 Portland Place W1	020 7636 5726
Columbian Embassy, 76 Chester Sq. SW1	020 7730 1625
Congo Democratic Republic (former Zaire), 22 Chesham Place SW1	020 7235 6137
Congo Republic Consulate, 12 Caxton St. SW1	020 7222 7575
Croatian Embassy, 18–21 Jermyn St. SW1	020 7434 2946
Cuban Embassy, 167 High Holborn WC1	020 7240 2488
Cyprus High Commission, 93 Park St. W1	020 7499 8272
Czech Republic Embassy, 26 Kensington Place Gardens W8	020 7243 1115
Danish Embassy, 55 Sloane St. SW1	020 7333 0200
Dominica High Commission, 1 Collingham Gardens SW5	020 7370 5194
Eastern Caribbean States, High Commission, 10 Kensington Court W8	020 7937 9522

Ecuador Embassy, Flat 3, 3 Hans Crescent SW1	020 7584 2648
Egypt Embassy, 26 South St. W1	020 7499 2401
El Salvador Embassy, 159 Great Portland St. W1	020 7436 8282
Estonia Embassy, 16 Hyde Park Gate SW7	020 7589 3428
Ethiopia Embassy, 17 Prince's Gate SW7	020 7589 7212
European Parliament, 2 Queen Anne's Gate SW1	020 7222 0411
Fiji Embassy, 34 Hyde Park Gate SW7	020 7584 3661
Finland Embassy, 38 Chesham Place SW1	020 7838 6200
France Embassy, 212 Grosvenor Place SW1	020 7235 7080
Gabonese Embassy, 27 Elvaston Place SW7	020 7823 9986
Gambia High Commission, 57 Kensington Court W8	020 7937 6316
Gayana High Commission, 3 Palace Court, Bayswater Rd. W2	020 7229 7684
German Embassy, 23 Belgrave Square SW1	020 7824 1300
Greece Embassy, la Holland Park W11	020 7727 3071
Grenada High Commission, 1 Collingham Gardens SW5	020 7373 7809
Guatemala Embassy, 13 Fawcett St. SW10	020 7351 3042
Guinea Bisau Republic, Consulate General, 8 Palace Gate W8	020 7589 5253
Honduras Consulate, 115 Gloucester Place W1	020 7486 4880
Hungary Embassy, 46 Eaton Place SW1	020 7235 4048
Iceland Embassy, 1 Eaton Terrace SW1	020 7730 5131
India High Commission, India House, Aldwych WC2	020 7836 8484
Indonesia Embassy, 38 Grosvenor Sq. W1	020 7499 7661
Iran Embassy, 16 Prince's Gate SW7	020 7225 3000
Iraqi Interest Section, 21 Queen's Gate SW7	020 7584 7141
Ireland Embassy, 17 Grosvenor Place SW1	020 7235 2171
Israel Embassy, 2 Palace Gate Green W8	020 8957 9500
Italy Embassy, 14 Three Kings Yard W1	020 7312 2200
Ivory Coast Embassy, 2 Upper Belgrave St. SW1	020 7235 6991
Jamaica High Commission, 1–2 Prince Consort Rd. SW7	020 7823 9911
Japan Embassy, 101–104 Piccadilly W1	020 7937 6500
Jordan Embassy, 6 Upper Phillmore Gardens W8	020 7937 3685
Kazakstan Consulate, 3 Warren Mews W1	020 7387 1047
Kenya High Commission, 45 Portland Place W1	020 7636 2371
Korea Embassy, 4 Palace Gate W8	020 7581 0247
Kuwait Embassy, 45 Queen's Gate SW7	020 7589 4533
Latvia Embassy, 45 Nottingham Place W1	020 7312 0040
Lebanon Embassy, 21 Kensington Palace Gardens W8	020 7229 7265
Lesotho High Commission, 7 Chesham Place SW1	020 7235 5686
Liberia Embassy, 2 Penbridge Place W2	020 7221 1036
Libya Interest Section, 119 Harley St. W1	020 7486 8250
Lithuania Embassy, 17 Essex Villas W8	020 7938 2481
Luxembourg Embassy, 27 Wilton Crescent SW1	020 7235 6961
Macedonia Embassy, Suite 10, Harcourt House, Cavendish Sq. W1	020 7499 5152
Malaysia High Commission, 45 Belgrave Sq. SW1	020 7235 8033
Mauritius High Commission, 32–33 Elvaston Place, SW7	020 7581 0294
Mexico Embassy, 42 Hertford St. W1	020 7499 8586
Monaco Consulate General, 4 Cromwell Place SW7	020 7225 2679
Mongolia Embassy, 7 Kensington Close W8	020 7937 5238

Morocco Embassy, 49 Queen's Gate Gardens SW7	020 7581 5001
Mozambique Embassy, Fitzroy Sq. W1	020 7383 3800
Myanmar (Burma) Embassy, 19a Charles St. W1	020 7629 4486
Namibia High Commission, 6 Chandos St. W1	020 7636 6244
Nepal Royal Embassy, 12a Kensington Palace Gardens W8	020 7229 1594
Netherlands Embassy, 38 Hyde Park Gate SW7	020 7584 5040
New Zealand High Commission, 80 Haymarket SW1	020 7930 8422
Nicaragua Consulate, 58–60 Kensington Church St. W8	020 7938 2373
Nigeria High Commission, 9 Northumberland Avenue WC2	020 7839 1244
Norway Embassy, 25 Belgrave Sq. SW1	020 7237 7151
Pakistan High Commission, 36 Lowndes Sq. SW1	020 7235 2044
Panama Embassy, 48 Park St. W1	020 7493 4646
Paraguay Embassy, Braemar Lodge, Cornwall Gardens SW7	020 7937 1253
Peru Embassy, 52 Sloane St. SW1	020 7235 1917
Philippines Embassy, 9a Palace Green W8	020 7937 1600
Poland Embassy, 47 Portland Place W1	020 7580 4324
Portugal Embassy, 11 Belgrave Sq. SW1	020 7235 5331
Qatar Embassy, 115 Queen's Gate SW7	020 7581 8611
Romania Embassy, 4 Palace Green Road W8	020 7937 9666
Russian Embassy, Consular Department, 5 Kensington Palace Gardens W8	020 7229 8027
Saudi Arabia Royal Embassy, 30 Charles St. W1	020 7917 3000
Senegal Embassy, 11 Phillmore Gardens W8	020 7937 0925
Seychelles High Commission, 111 Eros House, Baker St. W1	020 7224 1660
Sierra Leone High Commission, 3 Portland Place W1	020 7636 6483
Singapore High Commission, 9 Wilton Crescent W1	020 7235 8315
Slovak Republic Embassy, 25 Kensington Palace Gardens W8	020 7243 0803
Slovenia Embassy, 11–15 Wigmore St. W1	020 7495 7775
South Africa High Commission, S.A. House, Trafalgar Sq. WC2	020 7930 4488
Spain Embassy, 24 Belgrave Sq. SW1	020 7235 5555
Sri Lanka High Commission, 13 Hyde Park Gardens W2	020 7262 1841
Sudan Embassy, 3 Cleveland Row, St. James SW1	020 7839 8080
Swaziland High Commission, 20 Buckingham Gate SW1	020 7630 6611
Sweden Embassy, 11 Montagu Place W1	020 7917 6400
Syria Embassy, 8 Belgrave Sq. SW1	020 7245 9012
Tanzania High Commission, 43 Hertford St. W1	020 7499 8951
Thailand Royal Embassy, 28 Prince's Gate SW7	020 7584 5421
Tonga High Commission, 36 Molyneux St. W1	020 7724 5828
Trinidad and Tobago High Commission, 42 Belgrave Sq. SW1	020 7245 9351
Tunisia Embassy, 29 Prince's Gate SW7	020 7584 8117
Turkey Embassy, Rudland Lodge, Rudland Garden SW7	020 7584 1078
Uganda High Commission, 58–59 Trafalgar Sq. WC2	020 7839 5783
Ukraine Embassy, 78 Kensington Park Rd. W11	020 7727 6312
United Arab Emirates Embassy, 30 Prince's Gate SW7	020 7581 1281
Uruguay Embassy, 140 Brompton Rd. SW3	020 7584 8192
Venezuela Embassy, 56 Grafton Way W1	020 7387 6727
Vietnam Embassy, 12 Victoria Rd. W8	020 7937 1912
Yemen Embassy, 57 Cromwell Rd. SW7	020 7584 6607
Zimbabwe High Commission, 429 Strand WC2	020 7836 7755

Chapter 66

World travel advice checklist

The travel advice checklist (Table 66.1) is for short-term travellers. This information is constantly updated with some changes being introduced from time to time. For which malaria prophylaxis, please refer to the *British Malaria Guidelines* on p. 383.

All travellers should have their polio and tetanus immunizations up-to-date. Influenza vaccine should be considered when appropriate. All children should have completed their routine immunizations (including the MMR vaccine for those over 1 year of age) before travelling abroad.

SCIEH's *Fit for Travel* is a colourful and informative website from SCIEH free for the public. It gives country-specific information on immunizations and other preventive strategies, including information on malaria: http://www.fitfortravel.scot.nhs.uk

If the practice does not subscribe to a commercial information system, you may wish to connect onto websites already given in Sources of Travel Information in Chapter 64, which include the following websites:

Information on travel problems and requirements by areas (USA): http://www.cdc.gov/travel/

Information from Australia on current requirements for some individual countries: http://www.health-fax.org.au and go to 'Travel Health', or go directly to: http://www.healthfax.org.au/travind. htm

Another good Australian site with general and country-specific information on infectious diseases and immunizations is: http://www.tmvc.com.au/info.html

For a UK site go to: http://www.travelhealth. co.uk

Table 66.1 World travel advice vaccination checklist

Destination	Typhoid	Hepatitis A	Diphtheria	Tuberculosis	Hepatitis B	Rabies	Meningitis	Yellow fever	Japanese B encephalitis	Tick-borne encephalitis	Malaria risk
Abu Dhabi	S	R	S	S	S	S					✓✓
Afghanistan	R	R	S	S	S	S					✓✓
Albania	R	R	S	S	S	S				S	
Algeria	R	R	S	S	S	S					✓✓
Angola	R	R	S	S	S	S	S	R			✓✓
Antigua &Barbuda	S	R	S	S	S						
Argentina	R	R	S	S	S	S					✓✓
Armenia	R	R	S	S	S	S				S	✓✓
Australia										S	
Austria										S	
Azerbaijan	R	R	R	S	S	S				S	✓
Azores											
Bahamas	S	R	S	S	S						
Bahrain	R	R	S	S	S	S					
Bali	R	R	S	S	S	S			S		✓✓
Bangladesh	R	R	S	S	S	S			S		✓✓
Barbados	S	R	S	S	S	S					
Belarus	S	R	R	S	S	S				S	
Belgium											
Belize	R	R	S	S	S	S					✓✓
Benin Republic	R	R	S	S	S	S	S	M			✓✓
Bermuda	S	R	S	S	S	S					
Bhutan	R	R	S	S	S	S	S		S		✓✓
Bolivia	R	R	S	S	S	S	S	R			✓✓
Bosnia	S	R	S	S	S	S				S	
Botswana	R	R	S	S	S	S	S				✓✓
Brazil	R	R	S	S	S	S	S	R			✓✓
Brunei	R	R	S	S	S	S			S		
Bulgaria	S	S	S	S	S	S				S	
Burkina Faso	R	R	S	S	S	S	S	M			✓✓
Burundi	R	R	S	S	S	S	S	R			✓✓
Cambodia	R	R	S	S	S	S			S		✓✓
Cameroon	R	R	S	S	S	S	S	M			✓✓
Canada		S									
Canary Islands		S									
Cape Verde Islands	R	R	S	S	S	S					✓
Cayman Islands	S	R	S	S	S						

416

Country								
Central African Republic	R	R	S		S	S	M	✓
Chad	R	R	S		S	S	M	✓
Chile	S	R	S		S	S		✓
China (Mainland)	R	R	S	S	S			✓
China (Hong Kong)	S	S	S		S			✓
China (Macao)	R	R	S	S	S			
Colombia	R	R	S		S	S	R	✓
Comoros	R	R	S		S	S		✓
Congo	R	R	S		S	S	M	✓
Cook Islands	R	R	S		S			
Corfu	S	S	S					
Corsica								
Costa Rica	R	R	S		S	S		✓
Crete	S	S						
Croatia	S	R	S		S	S		
Cuba	R	R	S		S			
Cyprus Republic	S	S						
Czech Republic	S	S				S		
Democratic Republic of Congo (Zaire)	R	R	S		S	S	M	✓
Denmark								
Djibouti	R	R	S		S	S		✓
Dominica	S	R	S		S			
Dominican Republic	R	R	S		S			✓
East Timor	R	R	S	S	S		R	✓
Ecuador	R	R	S		S			✓
Egypt	R	R	S		S			✓
El Salvador	R	R	S		S			✓
Equatorial Guinea	R	R	S		S	S	R	✓
Eritrea	R	R	S		S	S		✓
Estonia	S	R	S		S			
Ethiopia	R	R	R		S	S	R	✓
Falkland Islands		S	S					
Fiji	R	R	S		S			✓
Finland		S	S			S		
France								
French Guiana	R	R	S		S	S	M	✓
French Polynesia	R	R	S		S			

s, sometimes recommended; r, recommended; m, mandatory

continued p. 418

Table 66.1 *cont.*

Destination	Typhoid	Hepatitis A	Diphtheria	Tuberculosis	Hepatitis B	Rabies	Meningitis	Yellow fever	Japanese B encephalitis	Tick-borne encephalitis	Malaria risk
Gabon	R	R	S	S	S	S	S	M			✓
Gambia	R	R	S	S	S	S	S	R			✓✓
Georgia	S	R	R	S	S	S				S	
Germany										S	
Ghana	R	R	S	S	S	S	S	M			✓
Gibraltar		S									
Greece											
Greenland											
Grenada	S	R	S	S	S	S					
Guadeloupe	S	R	S	S	S						
Guatemala	R	R	S	S	S	S		R			✓✓✓
Guinea Bissau/Africa	R	R	S	S	S	S	S	M			✓✓✓
Guinea Equatorial	R	R	S	S	S	S	S	R			✓✓✓
Guinea Republic/Africa	R	R	S	S	S	S		R			✓✓
Guyana	R	R	S	S	S	S					✓✓
Haiti	R	R	S	S	S	S					✓✓
Hawaii		S	S								
Honduras	R	R	S	S	S	S					✓✓
Hungary		S								S	
Ibiza		S									
Iceland											
India	R	R	S	S	S	S			S		✓✓✓
Indonesia	R	R	S	S	S	S			S		✓✓✓✓
Iran	R	R	S	S	S	S					✓✓✓
Iraq	R	R	S	S	S	S					✓✓✓
Irian Jaya (Indonesia)	R	R	S	S	S	S					✓✓
Ireland											
Israel	S	R	S	S	S						
Italy		S									
Ivory Coast	R	R	S	S	S	S	S	M			✓
Jamaica	S	R	S	S	S						
Japan										S	
Jordan	R	R	S	S	S	S					
Kazakhstan	R	R	S	S	S	S				S	
Kenya	R	R	S	S	S	S	S	R			✓
North Korea	R	R	S	S	S	S			S		
South Korea	S	R	S	S	S	S			S		
Kuwait	S	R	S	S	S	S					

Country	1	2	3	4	5	6	7	8	9	10	11
Kyrgystan	R	R	S	S	S	S			S		
Laos	R	R	S	S	S	S			S		
Latvia	S	R	S	S	S	S				S	✓
Lebanon	R	R	S	S	S	S					
Lesotho	R	R	S	S	S	S					
Liberia	R	R	S	S	S	S	S	M			✓
Libya	R	R	S	S	S	S					✓
Lithuania	S	R	S	S	S	S				S	
Luxembourg		S									
Macedonia	R		S	S	S	S					
Madagascar	R	R	S	S	S	S				S	✓
Madeira	S										
Majorca	S										
Malawi	R	R	S	S	S	S	S				✓
Malaysia	R	R	S	S	S	S					✓
Maldives	R	R	S	S	S	S				S	
Mali	R	R	S	S	S	S	S	M	S		✓
Malta	S		S				S				
Martinique	S	R	S	S	S	S					✓
Mauritania	R	R	S	S	S	S	S	M			✓
Mauritius	R	R	S	S	S	S					✓
Mayotte	R	R	S	S	S	S					✓
Mexico	R	S	S	S	S	S					
Minorca	S	S									
Moldova	S	R	S	S	S	S				S	
Monaco											
Mongolia	R	R	S	S	S	S					
Montenegro	R	S	S	S	S	S				S	
Monteserrat	S	S	S	S	S	S					
Morocco	R	R	S	S	S	S					
Mozambique	R	R	S	S	S	S	S				✓
Myanmar (Burma)	R	R	S	S	S	S			S		✓
Namibia	R	R	S	S	S	S	S		S		✓
Nepal	R	R	S	S	S	S	S		S		✓
Netherlands											
Netherlands Antilles	S	R	S	S	S	S					
New Caledonia	R	R	S	S	S	S					
New Zealand											
Nicaragua	R	R	S	S	S	S	S	M			✓
Niger	R	R	S	S	S	S	S	M			✓

s, sometimes recommended; r, recommended; m, mandatory

continued p.420

Table 66.1 *cont.*

Destination	Typhoid	Hepatitis A	Diphtheria	Tuberculosis	Hepatitis B	Rabies	Meningitis	Yellow fever	Japanese B encephalitis	Tick-borne encephalitis	Malaria risk
Nigeria	R	R	S	S	S	S	S	R			✓
Norway										S	
Oman	R	R	S	S	S	S					✓
Pakistan	R	R	S	S	S	S			S		✓✓
Panama	R	R	S	S	S	S		R			✓✓
Papua New Guinea	R	R	S	S	S	S					✓✓
Paraguay	R	R	S	S	S	S					✓✓
Peru	R	R	S	S	S	S		R			✓✓
Philippines	R	R	S	S	S	S			S		✓✓
Poland		S	S		S				S		
Portugal		S	S								
Puerto Rico	R	R	S	S	S	S					
Qatar	R	R	S	S	S	S					
Reunion Islands	R	R	S	S	S	S					
Romania	R	R	R	S	S	S				S	
Russian Federation	R	R	R	S	S	S				S	
Rwanda	R	R	S	S	S	S	S	M			✓
St. Kitts and Nevis	S	R	S	S	S						
St. Lucia	S	R	S	S	S						
St. Vincent & Grenadines	S	R	S	S	S						
Samoa	R	R	S	S	S						
Sao Tome & Principe	R	R	S	S	S	S	S	M		✓	
Sardinia											
Saudi Arabia	S	R	S	S	S	S	R/M				✓
Senegal	R	R	S	S	S	S	S	R		S	✓✓
Serbia	R	R	S	S	S	S					
Seychelles	R	R	S	S	S	S					
Sierra Leone	R	R	S	S	S	S	S	R			✓
Singapore	S	S	S	S	S						
Slovakia	S	S	S	S	S	S				S	
Slovenia	S	R	S	S	S	S				S	
Solomon Islands	R	R	S	S	S	S	S				✓✓✓
Somalia	R	R	S	S	S	S		R			✓✓✓
South Africa	R	R	S	S	S	S					✓
Spain		R									
Sri Lanka	R	R	S	S	S	S	S		S		✓✓✓
Sudan	R	R	S	S	S	S		M			✓✓✓
Surinam	R	R	S	S	S	S		R			✓✓✓

Swaziland	R	S	S			S			
Sweden	R	S	S		S	S			✓
Switzerland	R	S	S		S	S			✓
Syria	R	S	S		S	S			
Taiwan	R	S	S	S	S	S	S		✓
Tajikistan	S	S	S		S	S			✓
Tanzania	R	S	S	S	S	S	S	R	✓
Thailand	R	S	S		S	S		S	
Tobago	S	S	S	S	S	S		S	
Togo	R	S	S		S	S		M	
Tonga	R	S	S		S	S			✓
Trinidad	S	S	S		S	S		S	
Tunisia	R	S	S		S	S			
Turkey	S	S	S		S	S			✓
Turkmenistan	R	S	S	S	S	S			✓
Uganda	R	S	S		S	S			✓
Ukraine	S	R	R	S	S	S		R	✓
United Arab Emirates	S	S	S		S	S			
United States of America	S								
Uruguay	S	S	S		S	S			✓
Uzbekistan	R	S	S		S	S			✓
Vanuatu	R	S	S		S	S			✓
Venezuela	R	S	S		S	S		R	
Vietnam	R	S	S	S	S	S	S		
Virgin Islands	S								
Windward & Leeward Islands	S	S	S		S	S			
Yemen	R	S	S		S	S			✓
Zambia	R	S	S	S	S	S		S	✓
Zimbabwe	R	S	S		S	S			✓

s, sometimes recommended; r, recommended; m, mandatory

421

Chapter 67 Travel vaccines administration summary

Vaccine	Adult dosage	Child dosage	Primary course	Route	Booster
Diphtheria	Adult low dose, 0.5 mL (consider Td) For all ages over 10 years old	<10 years 0.5 mL Ads diphtheria vaccine (consider DT or DTwP or DtaP depending on age)	3 doses 4 weeks apart	IM/SC	Pre-school (DT) thereafter every 10 years (with Ads low-dose diphtheria vaccine or Td) for the over 10 year olds
Hepatitis A	1 mL Havrix Monodose (16 and over) 0.5 mL Avaxim (16 and over) 1 mL Vaqta (18 and over)	1–15 years 0.5 mL (Havrix Junior monodose) — 2–17 years 0.5 mL Vaqta Paediatric	1 dose	IM	Reinforcing dose: Havrix 6–12 m Avaxim 6–12 m Vaqta Paediatr. 6–18 m Vaqta 6–12 m Thereafter, every 10 years
Hepatitis B	1 mL	0–12 years 0.5 mL (Engerix B paed.) 0–15 years 0.5 mL (HB-Vax II paed.)	3 doses: 0, 1, 6 months. Accelerated course: 0, 1, 2 plus 12 months. For Engerix B adults over 18 years: 0, 7, 21 days plus 12 months	IM	Single booster at 5 years if at increased risk.
Japanese B encephalitis	1 mL	1–3 years 0.5 mL >3 years 1 mL	3 doses 0, 7, 30 days (AP MSD) 0, 7–14, 365 days –three doses (Korea)	SC	2 + years (AM MSD) 2 + years. 3 years but annually if at high risk (Korea)
Meningococcal AC VAX	0.5 mL	≥2 months 0.5 mL	Single dose	SC/IM	<5 years, 1–2 years >5 years, 5 years
Meningivac A + C	0.5 mL	≥18 months 0.5 mL	Single dose	IM/SC	>3 years
MenC conjugate	0.5 mL	2–4 months 5–12 months over 13 months and adults	3 doses 2 doses monthly 1 dose	IM	None
Poliomyelitis OPV	3 drops or monodose	3 drops or monodose	3 doses 4 weeks apart	Orally	Pre-school (fourth) Leaving school (fifth). Every 10+ years if at risk

Vaccine	Dose	Age-specific dose	Schedule	Route	Booster
IPV	0.5 mL		3 doses 4 weeks apart	IM/SC	Every 10+ years if at risk
Rabies	1 mL		3 doses 0, 7, 28 days	IM/SC	2–3 years if at continued risk
Tetanus	0.5 mL		3 doses 4 weeks apart	IM/SC	Pre-school (fourth) (fifth) Leaving school (fifth). No booster after 5 doses unless tetanus-prone injury or travel to high-risk area†
Tick-borne encephalitis	0.5 mL	0.5 mL (under 1 year if at very high risk only)	3 doses: 0, 1–3, 12 months	IM	Every 3 years
Tuberculosis (tuberculin negative, except <3 months) ID BCG	0.1 mL	>3 months 0.1 mL <3 months 0.05 mL	Single dose	Strictly ID	None. If at very high risk: skin test 10-yearly and re-immunize if negative
Typhoid Vi antigen	0.5 mL	0.5 mL ≥18 months (Typhim Vi) ≥24 months (Typherix)	Single dose	IM/SC (Typhim Vi) IM (Typherix)	3 years
Oral typhoid vaccine 1 capsule		≥6 years 1 capsule	3 doses, one capsule on alternate days	Orally	1 year for travel to endemic areas
Yellow fever	0.5 mL	≥9 months 0.5 mL	Single dose	SC	10 years (for travellers)
Combined hepatitis A & B	Twinrix Adult 1 mL	Twinrix Paediatric 0.5 mL	0,1,6 months	IM	With monovalent: Hep. A 10 years Hep. B 5 years if at risk
Combined hepatitis A and Typhoid	Hepatyrix 1 mL	15 years and over Hepatyrix 1 mL	Single dose Reinforcing dose of Hep. A monovalent in 6–12 months	IM	With monovalent: Hep. A 10+ years. Typhoid 3 years.

Index